Cytokine Therapeutics in Infectious Diseases

Cytokine Therapeutics in Infectious Diseases

Editor

Steven M. Holland
Head, Immunopathogenesis Unit
Laboratory of Host Defenses
National Institute of Allergy and Infectious Diseases
National Institutes of Health
Bethesda, Maryland

LIPPINCOTT WILLIAMS & WILKINS
A **Wolters Kluwer** Company
Philadelphia • Baltimore • New York • London
Buenos Aires • Hong Kong • Sydney • Tokyo

Acquisitions Editor: Jonathan Pine
Developmental Editor: Anne Snyder
Production Editor: Rakesh Rampertab
Manufacturing Manager: Tim Reynolds
Cover Designer: Mark Lerner
Compositor: Lippincott Williams & Wilkins Desktop Division
Printer: Edwards Brothers

530 Walnut Street
Philadelphia, PA 19106 USA
LWW.com

Printed in the USA

Library of Congress Cataloging-in-Publication Data

Cytokine therapeutics in infectious disease / [edited by] Steven M. Holland.
p. ; cm.
Includes bibliographical references and index.
ISBN 0-7817-1625-X
1. Cytokines—therapeutic use. 2. Communicable diseases—Chemtherapy. I. Holland, Steven M. (Steven Matthew), 1957–
[DNLM: 1. Cytokines—therapeutic use. 2. Communicable Diseases—drug therapy. QW568 C99449 2001]
RM282.C95 C965 2001

---

10 9 8 7 6 5 4 3 2 1

To
my wife, Maryland, for her understanding, forbearance, and support.

To
my daughters Jennifer, Madeline, and Elizabeth, for their tolerance.
Yes, we can play now.

To
my parents, James and Jimmie, whose shining examples of what
it means to be physicians and parents, burn bright.

Contents

Contributing Authors

Edward Abraham, M.D. *Division of Pulmonary Medicine, University of Colorado Health Sciences Center, Denver, Colorado*

Stephen J. Chanock, M.D. *Senior Investigator, Immunocompromised Host Section, Pediatric Oncology Branch, Advanced Technology Center, National Cancer Institute, National Institutes of Health, Bethesda, Maryland*

Jeffrey I. Cohen, M.D. *Head, Medical Virology Section, Laboratory of Clinical Investigation, National Institutes of Health, Bethesda, Maryland*

Charles A. Dinarello, M.D. *Professor of Medicine, Division of Infectious Diseases, University of Colorado Health Sciences Center, Denver, Colorado*

Samuel Fan, M.D. *Professor of Medicine, Department of Biology, Bradley University, Peoria, Illinois*

David M. Frucht, M.D. *Clinical Associate, Arthritis and Rheumatism Branch, National Institute of Arthritis, Musculoskeletal and Skin Diseases, National Institutes of Health, Bethesda, Maryland*

John I. Gallin, M.D. *Warren Grant Magnuson Clinical Center, National Institutes of Health, Bethesda, Maryland*

Sara M. Garrido, M.D. *Columbia Basin Hermatology and Oncology, Kennewick, Washington*

J. Milton Gaviria, M.D. *Department of Internal Medicine, Infectious Diseases, Mid-Columbia Medical Associates, University of Washington, Seattle, Washington*

Thomas Hartung, M.D. *Department of Biological Pharmacology, University of Konstanz, Konstanz, Germany*

N. Lynn Henry, Ph.D. *Laboratory of Parasitic Diseases, National Institute of Allergy and Infectious Diseases, National Institutes of Health, Bethesda, Maryland*

Steven M. Holland, M.D. *Head, Immunopathogenesis Unit, Laboratory of Host Defenses, National Institute of Allergy and Infectious Diseases, National Institutes of Health, Bethesda, Maryland*

Shin-ichiro Kashiwamura, M.D. *Department of Medical Zoology, Laboratory of Host Defenses, Institute for Advanced Medical Sciences, Hyogo College of Medicine, Nishinomiya, Hyogo, Japan*

Brian L. Kelsall, M.D. *Investigator, Laboratory of Clinical Investigation, National Institute of Allergy and Infectious Diseases, National Institutes of Health, Bethesda, Maryland*

Joseph A. Kovacs, M.D. *Senior Investigator, Critical Care Medicine Department, Warren Grant Magnuson Clinical Center, National Institutes of Health, Bethesda, Maryland*

Janaki C. Kuruppu, M.D. *Critical Care Medicine Department, Warren Grant Magnuson Clinical Center, National Institutes of Health, Bethesda, Maryland*

Thomas L. Lehrnbecher, M.D. *Kinderklinik der Universitat, Wurzburg, Germany*

Darin M. Lerner, M.D. *Weill Medical College, Cornell University, Westchester Division, White Plains, New York*

Daniel R. Lucey, M.D. *Division of Infectious Diseases, Department of Medicine, Washington Hospital Center, Washington, DC*

John F. McDyer, M.D. *Laboratory of Clinical Investigation, National Institute of Allergy and Infectious Diseases, National Institutes of Health, Bethesda, Maryland*

Kirk D. Miller, M.D. *Staff Physician, Warren Grant Magnuson Clinical Center, National Institutes of Health, Bethesda, Maryland*

Kenji Nakanishi, M.D. *Professor, Department of Immunology and Medical Zoology, Hyogo College of Medicine, Nishinomiya, Hyogo, Japan*

Thomas B. Nutman, M.D. *Head, Helminth Immunology Section, Laboratory of Parasitic Diseases, National Institute of Allergy and Infectious Diseases, National Institutes of Health, Bethesda, Maryland*

John J. O'Shea, M.D. *Lymphocyte Cell Biology Section, Arthritis and Rheumatism Branch, National Institute of Arthritis, Musculoskeletal and Skin Diseases, National Institutes of Health, Bethesda, Maryland*

Haruki Okamura, M.D. *Professor, Laboratory of Host Defenses, Institute for Advanced Medical Sciences, Hyogo College of Medicine, Nishinomiya, Hyogo, Japan*

Andriani C. Patera, M.D. *Visiting Fellow, Medical Virology Section, Laboratory of Clinical Investigation, National Institutes of Health, Bethesda, Maryland*

Richard K. Root, M.D. *Chief, Medical Services, Harborview Medical Center, Seattle, Washington*

Donald L. Rosenstein, M.D. *Chief, Psychiatry Consultation-Liaison Service, National Institute of Mental Health, Bethesda, Maryland*

Robert A. Seder, M.D. *Chief, Cellular Immunity Section, Vaccine Research Center, Laboratory of Clinical Investigation, National Institute of Allergy and Infectious Diseases, National Institutes of Health, Bethesda, Maryland*

Richard M. Siegel, M.D. *Research Associate, National Institutes of Allergy and Infectious Diseases, National Institutes of Health, Bethesda, Maryland*

Alan Stoudemire, M.D. *Deceased*

Philip E. Tarr, M.D. *Albert Einstein College of Medicine, Bronx, New York*

Hiroko Tsutsui, M.D. *Associate Professor, Department of Immunology and Medical Zoology, Hyogo College of Medicine, Nishinomiya, Hyogo, Japan*

Roberta Visconti, M.D. *Lymphocyte Cell Biology Section, Arthritis and Rheumatism Branch, National Institute of Arthritis, Musculoskeletal and Skin Diseases, National Institutes of Health, Bethesda, Maryland*

Drew Weissman, M.D., Ph.D. *Assistant Professor, Division of Infectious Diseases, University of Pennsylvania, Philadelphia, Pennsylvania*

Chang-You Wu, M.D. *Visiting Associate, Vaccine Research Center, National Institute of Allergy and Infectious Diseases, National Institutes of Health, Bethesda, Maryland*

Tomohiro Yoshimoto, M.D. *Department of Immunology and Medical Zoology, Laboratory of Host Defenses, Institute for Advanced Medical Sciences, Hyogo College of Medicine, Nishinomiya, Hyogo, Japan*

Foreword

The recent explosion of scientific information resulting from advances in molecular biology and the human genome project has provided unprecedented opportunities for drug development. A great example of how molecular discovery has resulted in new therapeutic targets is exemplified in the fields of inflammation and immunology. *Cytokine Therapeutics in Infectious Diseases* is structured to highlight a vital component of these opportunities. Cytokines are key regulators of inflammation and immunity that together comprise two critical systems of host defense.

The word *cytokine* is relatively new, created in the last quarter of the twentieth century. Cytokines refers to a myriad of cellular proteins with pro-inflammatory and anti-inflammatory effects. They are cellular products released from the cell *cyto*plasm to the extracellular space. The biologic responses they elicit result from ligation of specific receptors on target cells, making them the hormones of the immune system and more. They are pleiotropic and act on many cell types. Cytokines are great communicators, linking the nervous, endocrine, and immune systems.

The terminology describing cytokines can be confusing, since an individual cytokine often has multiple names, based on its cell of origin, biologic effect or molecular size. *Mono*kines and *lympho*kines refer to cytokines originally described as of a monocyte or lymphocyte origin. However, we now know that many cell types can produce monkines and lymphokines. The term *interleukin* was first used to describe cytokines produced by leukocytes that act on leukocytes, but it is now recognized that interleukins may be produced by, and act on, many different cells with diverse functional outcomes. For example, interleukin-1 causes fever, induces sleep, and modulates many aspects of inflammation and immunity. The interleukins are numbered according to their chronology of discovery. *Chemo*kines are cytokines that cause directed migration, *chemo*taxis, of target cells. Today we know that different chemokines share structural similarities, but they may have broad biologic functions beyond initiating chemotaxis, including the facilitation of cell invasion by certain microbial pathogens, such as HIV.

The application of cytokines to the therapy of infectious diseases is a centerpiece of the cytokine story. Not since the introduction of antimicrobials has there been such promise for new therapies for the management of infectious diseases. Cytokines provide an opportunity to amplify the natural host defenses to fight and, in the compromised host, prevent infection. The application of granulocyte colony stimulating factor (G-CSF) to the treatment of neutropenias, especially those induced by chemotherapy, has been spectacular, and has helped spawn the biotechnology industry. Prophylactic use of interferon γ to reduce infections in children with chronic granulomatous disease of childhood and the use of interferon α in the management of hepatitis C illustrate the broad potential of these approaches. Combination of cytokine immune adjuvants with antimicrobials to treat infectious diseases, such as tuberculosis, is an exciting approach currently undergoing clinical trials.

The successful use of competitive molecules for tumor necrosis factor α to treat rheumatoid arthritis has demonstrated the clinical potential of natural or designed anti-cytokines. The identification of specific molecular targets for cytokines and their receptors holds promise for specific regulation of inflammation in infectious diseases and other clinical settings, without the nonspecific and often devastating consequences of steroids.

Cytokine Therapeutics in Infectious Diseases is a timely and ambitious book that pulls together the key components of this rapidly emerging area. Its chapters illustrate the therapeutic opportunities of fine regulation of the components of inflammation and immunity. The use of cytokines to enhance natural host defense to eradicate infections, on the one hand, and the introduction of anti-cytokines to dampen the devastation of uncontrolled responses of the innate and adaptive immune systems, on the other, is now rich with clinical potential. This well-presented and concise book summarizes nicely where the field is at, and where it is likely to go.

John I. Gallin, M.D.
The Laboratory of Host Defenses
National Institute of Allergy and Infectious Diseases
National Institutes of Health
Bethesda, Maryland

Preface

The great Roman philosopher Lucretius (98-55 BCE) went to great pains in his surviving work, *De Rerum Natura*, to give mechanistic explanations for all natural phenomena. At the heart of his system was the idea of indissoluble parts, or atoms, that carried information, allowing us to have knowledge of remote events. Almost 200 years later, the preeminent Greek physician and anatomist, Galen of Pergamum, presented a unified system in which all things were composed of specific elements (earth, air, fire, and water), giving rise to the four humors (blood, yellow bile, black bile, and phlegm) and affected by the primary qualities (hot, cold, wet, and dry). By various combinations of these elements and humors, one might account for all human variations and phenotypes, and these determinations, in turn, helped guide specific therapies. Although these conceptions may seem quaint to our more complicated modern understandings, they were surprisingly prescient. In infection and immunity we now believe that the critical mediators of inflammation, cytokines and chemokines, are central to infection susceptibility, outcome, and, in the last few years, therapy.

Cytokines and chemokines are becoming parts of everyday conversation in infectious diseases. These range from key susceptibility factors (e.g., CCR5 for HIV; interferon γ receptors for mycobacterial infection) to standard therapeutics (e.g., G-CSF for neutropenia; interferon α for hepatitis C). However, despite their progressive importance in daily practice, they have not been dealt with as a whole. Subsequently, finding consolidated information on cytokines and chemokines has been difficult. In addition, since these mediators often act on each other, sometimes in very profound ways, the proper understanding of one cytokine and its action and toxicity is intrinsically bound to those of others as well. Therefore, with the movement of these factors from immunologic mediators to actual therapeutic drugs, it seemed timely and appropriate to bring together expert authors to describe the past, current, and future applications of specific cytokines and chemokines. With the increases in drug resistant organisms, the paucity of newer antimicrobials, and the inexorable progression of therapeutic immune suppression, a working knowledge of those cytokines and chemokines that are near or in clinical use should be useful to practitioners, fellows, and students alike.

Steven M. Holland, M.D.

Acknowledgments

I would like to thank Ruth Weinberg for her helpful discussions and encouragement in the development of this idea, and my developmental editor, Anne Snyder, for her perseverance and professionalism.

Cytokine Therapeutics in Infectious Diseases

1

The Role of Interleukin-1 in Sepsis

Charles A. Dinarello and Edward Abraham

Department of Medicine, Divisions of Infectious Diseases and Pulmonary Medicine, University of Colorado Health Sciences Center, Denver, Colorado

INTRODUCTION

Interleukin-1 (IL-1α and IL-1β) is the prototypic "multifunctional" cytokine. Unlike the lymphocyte and colony stimulating growth factors, IL-1 affects nearly every cell type, and often in concert with other cytokines or small mediator molecules. Although some lymphocyte and colony stimulating growth factors may be therapeutically useful, IL-1 is a highly inflammatory cytokine, and the margin between clinical benefit and unacceptable toxicity in humans is exceedingly narrow. In contrast, agents that reduce or suppress the production and/or activity of IL-1 are likely to have an impact on clinical medicine, particularly infectious diseases. In support of this concept, there is growing evidence that the production and activity of IL-1, particularly IL-1β, are tightly regulated events as if nature has placed specific "road blocks" to reduce the response to IL-1 during disease. In addition to controlling gene expression, synthesis, and secretion, this regulation extends to surface receptors, soluble receptors, and a receptor antagonist.

There are three members of the IL-l gene family: IL-1α, IL-β, and IL-1 receptor antagonist (IL-1Ra). IL-1α and IL-1β are agonists, and IL-1Ra is a specific receptor antagonist. The naturally occurring IL-1Ra appears to be a unique situation in cytokine biology. The intron–exon organization of the three IL-1 genes suggests duplication of a common gene some 350 million years ago. Before this common IL-1 gene, there may have been an ancestral gene from which fibroblast growth factor evolved since IL-1 and fibroblast growth factor share significant amino acid homologies, lack a signal peptide, and form an all β-pleated sheet tertiary structure. IL-1α and β are synthesized as precursors without leader sequences. The molecular weight of each precursor is 31 kDa. Processing of IL-1α or IL-1β to "mature" forms of 17 kd requires specific cellular proteases. In contrast, IL-1Ra evolved with a signal peptide and is readily transported out of the cells and is the most common member of the IL-1 family to measure in the circulation. In most clinical disease states, IL-1Ra levels are markedly elevated and serve as an indicator of the acute phase reaction (1).

Another member of the IL-1 family that participates in infectious disease is IL-18. IL-18 was formerly called IFNγ-inducing factor (2). IL-18 is a proinflammatory cytokine that plays a major role in the so-called T-helper type 1 and type 2 paradigm. The biology of IL-18 has been reviewed (3) (see Chapter 7).

As with other cytokines, the importance of IL-1 in health and disease have been revealed using gene deletion in mice. The IL-1α–deficient mouse and the IL-1β–deficient mouse are normal and show no indication of susceptibility to common pathogens encountered in nonpathogen free facilities, On the other hand, the IL-1Ra–deficient mouse is unusually sensitive to spontaneous development of diseases such as a rheumatoid arthritis-like illness (4).

IL-1 PRODUCTION IN VARIOUS INFECTIOUS DISEASE STATES

The production of IL-1 in various diseases has been examined in many studies. In general, there is increased gene expression and synthesis of IL-1α, IL-1β, or IL-1Ra whether determined by *in situ* hybridization, steady state mRNA levels, antibody staining of tissues, circulating levels, or *ex vivo* production from cultured cells. Increased IL-1 production has been reported in patients with various viral, bacterial, fungal, and parasitic infections but also in high-dose IL-2 therapy, solid tumors, some leukemias, HIV-1 infection, autoimmune disorders, trauma (surgery), hemodialysis, ischemic diseases (myocardial infarction), noninfectious hepatitis, asthma, ultraviolet radiation, closed head injury, pancreatitis, periodontitis, graft versus host disease, and transplant rejection, and in healthy subjects following strenuous exercise. However, in most conditions, IL-1 is not the only cytokine exhibiting increased production. Hence, the specificity of the IL-1 findings as related to the pathogenesis of any particular disease is lacking.

CIRCULATING IL-1 IN HUMANS

In various disease states, IL-1β, but not IL-1α, is detected in the circulation. Detection of IL-1α is rare because this cytokine is primarily cytosolic and is released only under unusual *in vitro* or *in vivo* conditions and probably due to cell death. Significant elevations in plasma IL-1β have been detected in healthy humans injected with LPS (5,6) and in patients with septic shock and burns (7). Circulating IL-1β levels are relatively low compared to levels of IL-6, IL-8, and tumor necrosis factor–alpha (TNFα). Correlations have been shown for plasma IL-1β levels and severity of acute attacks of rheumatoid arthritis (8), thermal burns (9), and mortality in septic shock (10). Circulating levels of IL-6 or IL-1Ra are frequently correlated with severity of sepsis, inflammation, trauma, graft rejection, and autoimmune diseases. Measurement of IL-6 is a surrogate marker for IL-1β.

Why are IL-1β levels low and difficult to detect? Unlike TNF-α, IL-6, or IL-1Ra, a significant amount of precursor IL-1β remains inside the cell. IL-1β also binds to large proteins, such as α-2-macroglobulin, complement (11), and the soluble type II IL-1 receptor. The presence of IL-1sRII at 100 pM reduces the detection of IL-1β in clinical samples by 50% (12).

PRODUCTION OF IL-1 FROM CELLS *IN VITRO* AND *EX VIVO*

In general, IL-1 is not present in PBMC when taken from healthy subjects; however, when incubated for several hours, PBMC from patients with rheumatoid arthritis (13), osteomalacia, sepsis, hemodialysis, myocardial infarction, and some vasculitides produced elevated amounts of IL-1 compared to control subjects. Extreme caution needs to be exercised so that contaminating endotoxins in the tissue culture medium do not artifactually stimulate "spontaneous" IL-1 production during the culture period. IL-1 and other cytokines are also produced in whole blood cultures, eliminating the need to separate the mononuclear population.

GENETIC LINKAGE OF DISEASE AND IL-1

In humans, IL-1α, IL-1β, and IL-1Ra are found on the long arm of chromosome 2 distributed over 430 kilobases. Some autoimmune diseases appear to be linked, in part, to IL-1 gene polymorphisms. For example, there is a *TaqI* polymorphism in the 5th exon of the human IL-1β gene which is a T to C transition. This mutation at amino acid 105 of precursor IL-1β is associated with a significantly greater portion of IL-1β secreted from the monocytes of homozygous diabetic individuals compared to monocytes from control subjects (14).

Fang et al. (15) examined two well-described genetic polymorphisms in the IL-1 family: the A1–5 allele in intron 2 of the IL-1Ra gene and the *Taq1* site in exon 5 of the IL-1β gene. The frequency of these alleles in 93 consecutive patients admitted to the surgical intensive care unit was compared to those in a cohort of 261 local blood donors in apparent health. The results were surprising in that there was a high frequency of the IL-1RaA2 allele in the cohort with severe sepsis compared to the healthy cohort ($p < 0.01$). Although there was no association with outcome (survival or organ failure), the study suggests that persons homozygous for this allele were more likely to find themselves in a surgical intensive care unit with severe sepsis than those without the allele. The internal control for this study was the lack of clinical outcome associated with the *Taq1* allele in this cohort of 93 patients.

Can we believe that this IL-1Ra allele makes one more likely to develop severe sepsis? What is known about this allele and IL-1Ra production? In one study, the amount of IL-1Ra produced from patients with insulin dependent diabetes mellitus was reduced (16). In another study, granulocyte-macrophage colony stimulating factor was used to stimulate IL-1Ra production. Persons with the IL-1RaA2 allele exhibited increased production compared to those without this allele (17). In addition, in that study, there was reduced production of IL-1α in these subjects. Clearly, these results need to be confirmed prospectively, but the concept that a gene polymorphism is associated with a measurable difference in the amount of the gene product and a disease outcome may help resolve some of the problems encountered in new therapeutic clinical trials in septic shock patients. As it now stands, it seems that persons with the IL-1RaA2 allele make more IL-1Ra, which is a risk factor for developing severe sepsis following a surgical procedure.

Linkage of a particular cytokine gene polymorphism to disease is not always found in each population studied. For example, a predisposition to develop severe systemic lupus erythematosus was linked to the IL-1RaA2 allele in a cohort of persons in the United Kingdom (18). In a cohort living in Australia, this association was not found (19). Similarly, the association of the IL-1Ra allele and ulcerative colitis in England (20) was not observed in a cohort of patients living in Southern Germany (21).

The literature on IL-1 contains well over several hundred citations on the production of IL-1 in animals and humans in association with different diseases, particularly infectious diseases. Even if IL-1 production from cells or IL-1 levels in a body fluid were perfectly correlated with a particular disease, the relevance of IL-1 to that disease would be still unproved. Only specific IL-1 neutralization or receptor blockade can establish causation or contribution. This restriction is not limited to IL-1 but exists for each cytokine.

Nevertheless, studying IL-1 production in disease states can be useful as a marker of disease progression or therapeutic efficacy. Increasing evidence demonstrates that the circulating level of IL-6 rather than IL-1 is the best assessment for an association of elevated production of biologically active IL-1 with the severity of disease. IL-6 levels appear to reflect synergistic induction by IL-1 and TNF during most disease states. However, IL-6 itself is not an agonist in the pathogenesis of the sepsis syndrome. Unlike IL-1 or TNF, IL-6 does not cause hypotension in humans or stimulate genes for inflammatory molecules. Most of the importance of IL-1 and infections relates to the patient faced with a life-threatening sepsis syndrome. Clinical studies of blocking IL-1 in patients with sepsis have been carried out and are discussed below.

THE PHYSIOLOGICAL CATASTROPHE OF SEPTIC SHOCK

The diagnosis of sepsis syndrome or septic shock is based on a constellation of physiologic, metabolic and hematologic abnormalities most commonly occurring in patients with a known infection. In most cases, the patient is already hospitalized with an antecedent illness or has experienced recent surgery. Many patients, but not all, are being treated with appropriate antibiotics for a suspected infection. Approximately 25% of patients with sepsis syndrome are in hemodynamic shock at the time of presentation (22). Characteristic of septic shock, the hypotension is unresponsive to rapid fluid replacement. In most circumstances, when blood pressure falls relative to the patient's normotensive level (a 25% to 35% reduction), 500 mL of saline infusion is rapidly administered. If there is no response (increase in mean arterial pressure), a diagnosis of hemodynamic shock is made. In the context of an ongoing infection or suspected new infection, the patient is thought to be in septic shock. There is another disease which will mimic the rapid evolution of septic shock, that is, acute pancreatitis in which there is no associated infection but rather systemic inflammation. Clinically, it is often difficult to distinguish between these two. However, the vast majority of patients with hemodynamic shock have an infection as the cause.

If the hypotension is not corrected, progressive reduction in organ perfusion and increasing acidosis leads to tissue hypoxia and results in organ failure. Although the hypotension is initially treated with pressor drugs and antibiotics are either changed or new ones added, a downhill course can rapidly take place, resulting in death. In some patients, this rapid downhill course can be very dramatic. This physiologic cascade is illustrated in Fig. 1.1. Renal failure is an early sign that the hypotension and acidosis have been of significant magnitude and duration. Liver failure can also be rapid. However, increasing loss of cardiac function is of major concern, since there is no "holdover" therapy such as there is hemodialysis for renal failure.

In the past 5 years, the 28-day mortality in patients with sepsis syndrome has decreased somewhat but still ranges from 20% to 50%; mortality in those with septic shock and multiple organ failure is higher despite aggressive intensive care. Intensive care units deliver hemodynamic, metabolic, ventilatory and renal support and critical care has become a recognized medical subspecialty. Clearly, some patients survive the ordeal, but it remains frustrating for the intensivist who cannot halt and reverse the downhill course leading to multiple organ failure and death. New therapies have been sought and tested in these patients. Ideally, the therapy should be able to "rescue" the patient who continues to deteriorate in the face of considerable support efforts. Unfortunately, there is still no therapeutic agent or combination of treatments which have significantly reduced the mortality of this disease over that achieved with up-to-date intensive care strategies (23).

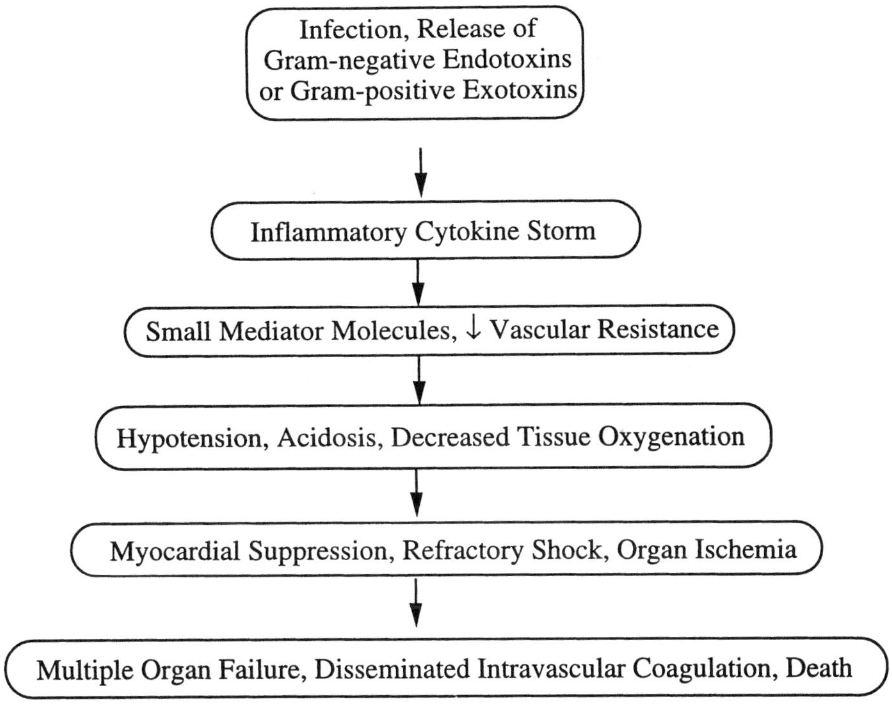

FIG. 1-1. Physiologic events associated with the development of septic shock.

There is little question that the major advance in treating patients with septic shock was the availability of broad spectrum antibiotics. In fact, the sooner broad spectrum antibiotics are administered, the more mortality decreases (24,25). The testing of non–antibiotic-based, novel therapies is based on 50 years of research on how microorganisms trigger the cascade of events in septic shock. Although microbial products such as endotoxins are still targets for therapy, a fundamental concept is that the constellation of abnormalities in these patients is not due to the direct effect of the infectious agent or its products but rather results from the patient's own response to the infection (or in some cases, response to massive trauma and blood loss). Initially, activation of complement was considered causal, particularly the fifth component of complement (c5a), which is a potent neutrophil activator and produces a capillary leak syndrome. The release of platelet activating factor (PAF) was also thought to be responsible, particularly since PAF is a potent hypotensive agent. Using specific inhibitors of PAF, animals given lethal bacterial toxins survive. Similar results were obtained when cyclooxygenase inhibitors were administered to animals lethally challenged with endotoxin or bacteria implicating cyclooxygenase products as contributing causes in septic shock. Numerous animal studies also demonstrated the protective effects of corticosteroids, and several large clinical trials using these potent antiinflammatory agents were undertaken. Clinical trials of PAF antagonists, cyclooxygenase inhibitors, bradykinin antagonists, and corticosteroids have each failed to significantly reduce the 28-day mortality in septic shock patients (Table 1.1).

TABLE 1-1. *Double-blind and placebo-controlled trials for treating patients with sepsis syndrome or septic shock*

Agent	Number of patients enrolled in each trial of the agent
Corticosteroids	75, 223, 59, 382, 60, 48, 172, 85, 194
Anti-endotoxin antibodies	
HA-1A	543, 2,199
E5	448, 847
Bradykinin antagonist	251, 504
PAF antagonists	262, 668
Ibuprofen (cyclooxygenase inhibitor)	29, 30, 455
Anti-TNFα	
Murine anti-TNFα	971, 564, 1,879
Murine anti-TNFα Fab_2' fragment	122, 39, 446
p75 TNF receptor fusion protein	141
p55 TNF receptor fusion protein	498
IL-1 receptor antagonist	99, 893, 696

IL-1 AND TNF IN THE PATHOGENESIS OF SEPSIS AND SEPTIC SHOCK

The field entered a new era when it was shown that neutralizing antibodies to the inflammatory cytokine TNF prevented death in mice (26), rabbits (27), or baboons (28) given a lethal injection of *E. coli* or endotoxin. In the absence of any infection, high doses of TNF in animals induced circulatory collapse and organ necrosis which were very similar to those observed in humans with septic shock. Similar results were observed with high doses of IL-1 in animals. Injecting a combination of low doses of IL-1 plus TNF revealed that these two cytokines acted synergistically in inducing a shock-like state (29). Similar to neutralizing TNF activity, blocking IL-1 receptors was also effective in preventing death in animal models of lethal bacteremia or endotoxemia (30,31). Since TNF induces IL-1 and IL-1 induces TNF, these animal studies showing synergism between the two cytokines made sense. Although a few studies revealed that for some intracellular infections blocking IL-1 or TNF would worsen disease, blocking these cytokines was considered of primary importance compared to loss of host defense function. For the patient without overt infection, for example multiple trauma, the preclinical experimental animal data demonstrated that the systemic injection of either IL-1 or TNF induced physiologic, hematologic, and pathological changes that were nearly identical to those observed during bacteremia or multiple trauma.

Animal studies were confirmed when humans were injected with either IL-1 or TNF. The most impressive physiologic event following the intravenous injection of either cytokine in humans is the fall in blood pressure. Frank hypotension has been reported with doses of IL-1 or TNF as low as 50 ng/kg (32,33). The hypotension is dose-dependent, and despite a short plasma half-life of less than 10 minutes, the biological consequences can be observed for days. In studies in which IL-1 was administered as adjunct therapy for bone marrow transplant recovery, nearly all patients required pressor therapy (33,34). In the few patients in whom the dose of IL-1 was increased to 1 μg/kg, a shock-like state developed. In the case of TNF, an increase in coagulation parameters and an early leukopenia occurred (35,36). The logical clinical conclusion from a vast amount data is that reducing the biological effects of systemic TNF or IL-1 could reduce the risk of dying from septic shock, in that these cytokines are essential for the manifestation of the disease.

THE RATIONALE FOR BLOCKING- IL-1 AND/OR TNF

The biological basis for the development of a shock-like state following systemic IL-1 or TNF has been established at the molecular level. Both cytokines activate the transcription of genes which increase the production of small, potent mediator molecules. For example, IL-1 and TNF increase gene expression and synthesis for phospholipase A2 type II leading to increased PAF synthesis. Similarly, an increase in cyclooxygenase type II (COX-2) by IL-1 and TNF results in elevated levels of PGE_2, reviewed in Dinarello (37). On a molar basis, nitric oxide (NO) is a potent vasodilator and is thought to be primarily responsible for the hypotension and myocardial suppression in septic shock (38). Whereas constitutive NO production is part of hemodynamic homeostasis, increased production of NO in inflammation takes place when NO is produced by inducible nitric oxide synthase (iNOS) (15). IL-1, TNF, and IFNγ, particularly the combination of the three, activate gene expression and synthesis of iNOS.

Trials have been carried out in which TNF was neutralized, either with monoclonal anti-TNF or soluble TNF receptors, and IL-1 activity was blocked with the IL-1 receptor antagonist (23,39–42). Although we discuss below some of the reasons why we believe these trials failed to significantly improve 28-day mortality, nevertheless, the results of trials based on reducing IL-1 or TNF activity have been disappointing. The most recent and largest trial, treating 1,879 patients with septic shock with murine monoclonal antibodies to TNF, improved 28-day mortality by only 2.5% (40.3% for anti-TNF versus 42.8% for the placebo).

METAANALYSIS OF SEPTIC SHOCK INTERVENTION TRIALS

In order to examine the outcomes in terms of safety and efficacy of the many trials in septic shock patients, a metaanalysis was performed (43). The analysis included 39 trials conducted over the past 30 years. There were 20 trials of nonglucocorticoids such as IL-1 receptor antagonist, antibodies to TNF and bradykinin, and PAF antagonists and 10 trials testing antiendotoxin antibodies. There were several conclusions from this analysis: (a) the mortality of the control arm (placebo) for the entire group of 39 trials was consistently 35% to 40%; (b) high-dose glucocorticoids showed a harmful effect on survival; (c) antimediator trials resulted in a small but significant survival benefit; (d) antiendotoxin trials showed no effect. It is important to note that the anticytokine therapy trials did not increase mortality, but rather 28-day mortality was decreased. This latter result is in contrast to predictions that blocking the biological effects of IL-1 or TNF would harmfully reduce host defense systems. In these highly vulnerable patients with severe infection, blocking IL-1 activity or neutralizing TNF had no harmful effect.

Compared to IL-1 and TNF, there is no other cytokine to date that reproduces the dramatic hypotension and physiologic parameters of septic shock in animals or in humans. That does not mean other cytokines do not participate in pathogenesis. For example, animals treated with neutralizing antibodies to IFNγ are protected against the lethal endotoxemia (44). Similar data have been reported for mice lacking the receptor for IFNγ (45). IFNγ is a potent macrophage activator and increases the production of and response to TNF. In contrast to the proinflammatory properties of IFNγ, the administration of IFNγ to certain patients with septic shock appears to be beneficial (46), although those data need confirmation in placebo controlled, blinded trials. Nevertheless, the data in animals for blocking IFNγ, and the ability of IFNγ, to increase gene expression for iNOS is a compelling argument to test anti-IFNγ therapy in humans. The issue of blocking IFNγ is clouded since this cytokine has been injected into several thousand humans (some with infections) without producing hypotension or similar sepsis-like effects.

Other therapeutic approaches in septic patients target the chemokines and adhesion molecules. Although administration of large doses of IL-8 to primates does not result in hypotension, neutralizing antibodies to IL-8 in models of inflammation reduce neutrophil infiltration in the lung, joint, kidney, skin, and myocardium (47). Blocking IL-8 reduces the entrance of neutrophils into inflammatory sites (47). In particular, anti–IL-8 reduces neutrophil accumulation in the lung and myocardium following ischemia-reperfusion injury. If tested in humans, anti–IL-8 therapy would most likely be used in patients with ARDS. IL-8 is increased in bronchoalveolar lavage specimens from patients with ARDS and, in most patients at risk for ARDS, elevated bronchoalveolar lavage IL-8 levels have been predictive of the subsequent development of ARDS (48). Although IL-8 is a sensible target in septic shock patients, particularly for halting the progress of ARDS, the production of IL-8 (and other chemokines) is markedly reduced by the combination of anti-IL-1 and anti-TNF agents. As shown in Fig. 1.2, blocking the biological activities of IL-1 and TNF is an upstream strategy for reducing the cascade of secondary mediators of systemic inflammation. Although the recent metaanalysis of antiinflammatory agents and anti–IL-1–based and anti-TNF–based therapies in septic patients concluded that a consistent, although marginal survival benefit was observed in nonglucocorticoid trials, the

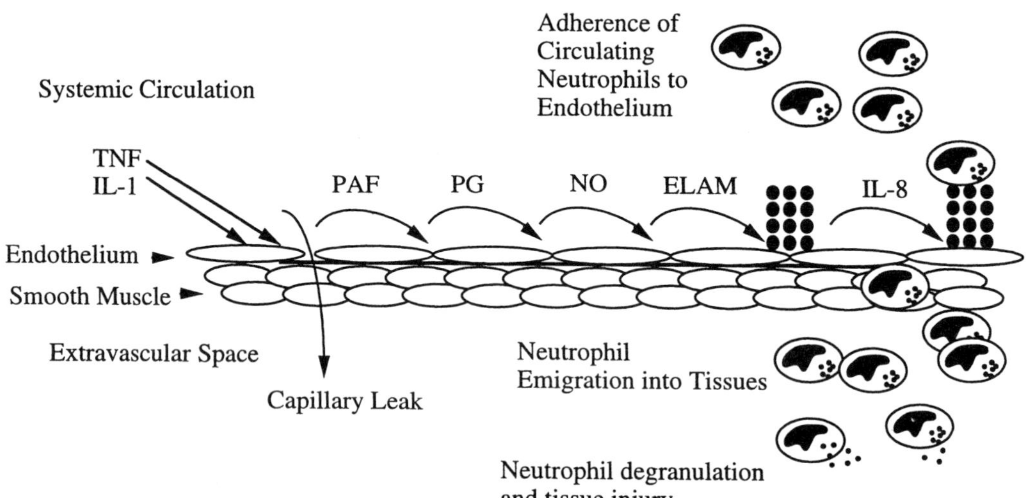

FIG. 1-2. Effect of interleukin-1 (IL-1) and tumor necrosis factor (TNF) on endothelium. TNF and IL-1 activate endothelial cells and trigger the cascade of proinflammatory small molecule mediators. Increased gene expression of phospholipase A2 type II and cyclooxygenase type 2 (COX-2) result in increased prostaglandin synthesis and inducible nitric oxide synthase (iNOS) resulting in elevated production of their products, platelet activating factor (PAF), prostaglandin E_2 (PGE_2), and nitric oxide (NO). Alone or in combination, these mediators decrease the tone of vascular smooth muscle and a decrease in systemic vascular resistance takes place. IL-1 and TNF also cause increased capillary leak. The upregulation of endothelial leukocyte adhesion molecule (ELAM) results in adherence of circulating neutrophils to the endothelium. Increased production of chemokines, such as IL-8, facilitates the emigration of neutrophils into the tissues. Chemokines also activate degranulation of neutrophils. Activated neutrophils lead to tissue destruction, particularly in the lung.

survival benefit for monotherapy using any of these agents never reached a level of significance which would allow approval by regulatory agencies (43).

Is there anything wrong with the concept of anticytokine-based therapies for disease? Anti–TNF-based and anti–IL-1–based therapies have been used in patients with rheumatoid arthritis with clear and often dramatic clinical benefits demonstrating that blocking either cytokine in humans is doable and effective (49–52). Anti-TNF is also very effective when used to pretreat patients with a high risk of the Jarisch-Herxheimer reaction (53) and on a chronic basis in Crohn's (54); IL-1Ra has reduced the severity of graft versus host disease in steroid-resistant bone marrow transplantation patients (55). Moreover, long-term (over 1 year) use of these anticytokine strategies has not been associated with any obvious impairment of host defense, even in patient population with a well-established risk of increased infections. In fact, the metaanalysis of anticytokine therapy trials in septic patients concluded that anticytokine treatment in sepsis is not apparently harmful (43). If there is no harm, then why are the results using these very same agents in patients with septic shock without significant reduction in mortality in the "total" sepsis population?

A CLOSER LOOK AT THE PATIENT POPULATION ENTERING SEPSIS TRIALS

Almost all of the clinical trials investigating new therapies for sepsis have determined patient entry using a broad definition of the "sepsis syndrome," based on clinical criteria including the presence of tachycardia, hyper- or hypothermia, and elevated or decreased peripheral white blood cell counts. These are coupled with the presence of organ system dysfunction, such as lactic acidosis, disseminated intravascular coagulation, hypoxemia, hypotension or decreased urine output. These entry criteria have permitted patients with a wide range of underlying illnesses and sources of infection to be treated. For example, patients with clinical evidence of urinary tract, respiratory or intraabdominal infection, with underlying illnesses as diverse as cancer, autoimmune disorders, chronic renal failure, and diabetes were included in the clinical studies with IL-1Ra or anti-TNF therapies. American and European studies also reflect the dilemma of patient heterogeneity despite identical entry criteria and drug therapy (39,56). The heterogeneity of patients enrolled in sepsis studies can be contrasted to the better defined groups used in studies (39) of IL-1Ra or anti-TNF therapies in rheumatoid arthritis or inflammatory bowel disease.

In animal models of infection, cytokine release is dependent on the source and type of infection. For example, anti-TNF therapies in murine models appear to work best for bacteremia and have poor or no efficacy in intraperitoneal infections. Yet, only a minority of patients in the trials examining anti-TNF therapies were bacteremic. Additionally, in most studies approximately one-third of the patients, despite clinical evidence or suspicion of infection, never have any positive culture results, leaving some question as to the actual nature of the infectious process in these patients.

With the exception of one study, none of the clinical trials has used a measure of enhanced cytokine release as an entry criterion. In that trial employing murine anti-TNF Fab2′ fragments, a single circulating IL-6 level greater than 1,000 pg/mL was utilized to identify a target patient group for therapy (57). Although IL-6 levels consistently correlate with disease severity in most patients with sepsis, patients with infectious and non-infectious diseases show remarkably variable circulating and tissue cytokine levels and a single measurement can be misleading. Since circulating levels of endogenously produced IL-1Ra and soluble TNF receptors are elevated in sepsis, the net biologically active

IL-1 or TNF remains unclear. It would appear more useful to identify for enrollment those patients with increased generation of the biologically active cytokine that is the target of blocking therapy. Unfortunately, such identification is difficult because TNF and IL-1 are released at their greatest concentrations at tissue sites, and rarely do the circulating levels correlate with the levels of local production. Therefore, clinical criteria will probably be required to identify patients with increased tissue IL-1 and TNF production. These patients appear to be those with a rapidly occurring onset of organ system dysfunction secondary to infection, without major underlying and preexistent medical problems. An example would be the young patient with acute onset of meningococcemia, in whom circulating and tissue levels of TNFα are dramatically elevated. In this setting, the greatest survival benefit from anticytokine therapy would be expected when the agent is given very soon after diagnosis and would be observed in the period immediately following therapy, as a direct result of reversal of proinflammatory cytokine driven organ dysfunction.

Humans injected intravenously with either IL-1α or IL-1β also develop hypotension at doses above 50 ng/kg and frank hemodynamic shock at doses above 300 ng/kg (33,34). These studies formed the rational basis for treating patients with sepsis and septic shock with IL-1Ra. Although the overall results of the clinical trials with IL-1Ra were not sufficient to warrant further development in all patients with severe sepsis, some patients during subgroup analyses did show a survival benefit from receiving IL-1Ra (41,58,59). In recently published studies, targeted deletion of the IL-1Ra gene in mice (IL-1Ra knockout mice) has resulted in a phenotype highly vulnerable to endotoxin-induced lethality, whereas mice over expressing IL-1Ra, appear to be protected against lethal endotoxemia (60). These latter experiments suggest that endogenous levels of IL-1Ra may contribute to disease outcome, at least in the case of septic shock.

The working hypothesis is that those individuals with the genetic make-up to produce large amounts of IL-1Ra when septic are afforded a greater level of protection than subjects producing lower levels. The parallel working hypothesis is that those individuals with the genetic make-up to produce less bioactive IL-1β when septic are less likely to die during septic shock compared to those subjects producing larger amounts of IL-1β. Although the ultimate proof of these two hypotheses is to measure the concentrations of IL-1Ra and IL-1β in patients surviving and compare those levels with those patients dying of septic shock, such measurements in the context of the acute setting are affected by nutritional and nongenetic mechanisms present at the time of infection. Hence, an investigation into the genetic determinants which may result in high or low IL-1Ra or IL-1β production should shed light in answering these questions.

mRNA does not cause disease. Even if the promoters for IL-1Ra and the cleavage site for IL-1β are genetically different, unless these differences results in different levels of the gene product, any polymorphisms are of questionable importance to the outcome of disease. Nevertheless, there are lessons to be learned from examination of polymorphisms in cytokine genes. For example, homozygosity for the TNFB2 allele at the TNF locus is associated with nonsurvival in patients with severe sepsis (61). These patients also have elevated TNFα levels in the circulation and higher organ failure scores. Although there is increased mortality with the homozygous TNFB2 allele, there is no difference between the frequency of this polymorphism in the general population and the group of patients in the intensive care unit with a diagnosis of severe sepsis. It appears that if one develops severe sepsis, inheriting the TNFB2 allele makes one particularly at risk for death compared to heterozygotes or patients homozygous for the TNFB1 allele (61).

NEW APPROACHES TO THERAPY

Although specific and successful monotherapy for a particular disease is a desirable goal in therapeutics, there are increasing examples in which treatment is most effective when two or more agents are used. The obvious examples are cancer, autoimmune diseases and HIV-1, where treatment with a single antitumor drug or immunosuppressive regimen or antiviral agent has been replaced with the use of several agents, each targeting a somewhat different mechanism. If more than one agent would benefit the patient with septic shock, there are several possible combinations. In sepsis involving a Gram-negative organism, endotoxin itself acts like a cytokine in that it activates nearly the same genes as do IL-1 and TNFα. A combination of neutralizing antibodies to endotoxin as well as blocking TNF and/or IL-1 may offer the patient with Gram-negative septic shock the greatest chance of survival. Administration of anti–IL-8 with either anti-TNF or anti–IL-1 may be effective for patients with a high risk of developing ARDS. The concept of combining more than one anticytokine agent has sound experimental basis. For example, in animals, a combination of anti-TNF plus anti–IL-1 treatment has increased survival over that using either agent as monotherapy.

Is the failure to rescue patients with anti-TNF or IL-1 blockade due to a delay in intervention? In many patients (75%) with sepsis syndrome, blood pressure and organ perfusion are unimpaired; however, when septic shock develops, circulatory collapse within a few hours is thought to coincide with the onset of a new bacteremia or endotoxemia. In addition, a “cytokine storm” is thought to be responsible for triggering shock. It has been thought that these patients also stand the greatest chance of “rescue” by blocking further cytokine receptor triggering. In patients with similarly serious infections, if fall in blood pressure or the development of organ failure is slower (over days) cytokine receptors are likely to have been engaged before circulatory collapse reaches the level of entry criteria into a trial. In those patients, the administration of anticytokine therapy may be too late to provide a successful rescue. Animal studies have provided a compelling argument for blocking TNF or IL-1 as a therapeutic maneuver in treating septic shock, but in animals the window of time for reversing the events of lethal sepsis is rather small. Does that mean that by the time the patient has overt signs of septic shock it is too late for rescue with anticytokine therapy? In most of the anticytokine trials, the time that passes before a patient actually receives therapy can be 12 to 24 hours after the early indications of altered mental status or blood pressure instability. What can be done to shorten the time between overt evidence of a life threatening process and initiation of anticytokine therapy?

As noted above, the heterogeneity of the acute infectious and underlying disease processes in the patients who were enrolled into sepsis studies may have prevented demonstration of efficacy for anticytokine therapies. Additionally, large numbers of patients with low risk of mortality were enrolled in these clinical trials. Such patients often do not have markedly accelerated proinflammatory responses amenable to anticytokine therapy, and their inclusion in the clinical studies may have diluted out any survival benefit associated with the use of anticytokine therapy for sepsis. Therefore, for future trials it would be important to reduce patient heterogeneity. It has been the common wisdom that larger patient cohorts, similar to the 20,000 patients used to evaluate thrombolytic therapy in acute myocardial infarction, would compensate for the “background noise” of patient heterogeneity in sepsis trials. However, increasing the number of patients and the number of participating hospitals has yielded the same patient heterogeneity.

Nearly every sepsis trial has uncovered a subgroup defined retrospectively with survival benefit using the new therapy. When specific subgroups have been retested prospectively in larger follow-up trials, treating the same subgroup has eluded us, in that patient heterogeneity in the expanded trials dilutes out the efficacy beyond statistical significance. Hence, anticytokine therapy for sepsis still awaits identification of the patient who can be rescued in a timely fashion from the downhill cascade caused by inflammatory cytokines.

ACKNOWLEDGMENTS

This work was supported by NIH grant AI 15614.

REFERENCES

1. Gabay C, Smith MF, Eidlen D, et al. Interleukin 1 receptor antagonist (IL-1Ra) is an acute-phase protein. *J Clin Invest* 1997;99:2930.
2. Nakamura K, Okamura H, Wada M, et al. Endotoxin-induced serum factor that stimulates gamma interferon production. *Infect Immunol* 1989;57:590.
3. Dinarello CA. IL-18: A Th1-inducing, proinflammatory cytokine and new member of the IL-1 family. *J Allergy Clin Immunol* 1999;103:11.
4. Horai R, Asano M, Sudo K, et al. Production of mice deficient in genes for interleukin (IL)-1α, IL-1β, IL-1α/β, and IL-1 receptor antagonist shows that IL-1β is crucial in turpentine-induced fever development and glucocorticoid secretion. *J Exp Med* 1998;187:1463.
5. Cannon JG, Tompkins RG, Gelfand JA, et al. Circulating interleukin-1 and tumor necrosis factor in septic shock and experimental endotoxin fever. *J Infect Dis* 1990;161:79.
6. Granowitz EV, Santos A, Poutsiaka DD, et al. Circulating interleukin-1 receptor antagonist levels during experimental endotoxemia in humans. *Lancet* 1991;338:1423.
7. Cannon JG, Friedberg JS, Gelfand JA, et al. Circulating interleukin-1β and tumor necrosis factor-a after burn injury in humans. *Crit Care Med* 1992;20:1414.
8. Eastgate JA, Symons JA, Wood NC, et al. Correlation of plasma interleukin 1 levels with disease activity in rheumatoid arthritis. *Lancet* 1988;2:706.
9. Wogensen L, Jensen M, Svensson P, et al. Pancreatic beta-cell function and interleukn-1b in plasma during the acute phase response in patients with major burn injuries. *Eur J Immunol* 1993;23:311.
10. Casey LC, Balk RA, Bone RC. Plasma cytokines and endotoxin levels correlate with survival in patients with the sepsis syndrome. *Ann Intern Med* 1993;119:771.
11. Borth W, Urbanski A, Prohaska R, et al. Binding of recombinant interleukin-1 beta to the third complement component and alpha 2-macroglobulin after activation of serum by immune complexes. *Blood* 1990;75:2388.
12. Arend WP, Malyak M, Smith MF, et al. Binding of IL-1α, IL-1β, and IL-1 receptor antagonist by soluble IL-1 receptors and levels of soluble IL-1 receptors in synovial fluids. *J Immunol* 1994;153:4766.
13. Roubenoff R, Roubenoff RA, Cannon JG, et al. Rheumatoid cachexia: cytokine-driven hypermetabolism accompanying reduced body cell mass in chronic inflammation. *J Clin Invest* 1994;93:2379.
14. Pociot F, Molvig J, Wogensen L, et al. A TaqI polymorphism in the human interleukin-1 beta (IL-1 beta) gene correlates with IL-1 beta secretion in vitro. *Eur J Clin Invest* 1992;22:396.
15. Fang FC. Mechanisms of nitric oxide-related antimicrobial activity. *J Clin Invest* 1997;99:2818.
16. Mandrup-Poulsen T, Pociot F, Molvig J, et al. Monokine antagonism is reduced in patients with insulin-dependent diabetes melitus. *Diabetes* 1994;43:1242.
17. Danis VA, Millington M, Hyland V, et al. Cytokine production by normal human monocytes: inter-subject variation and relationship to an IL-1 receptor antagonist (IL-1Ra) gene polymorphism. *Clin Exp Immunol* 1995;99:303.
18. Blakemore AI, Tarlow JK, Cork MJ, et al. Interleukin-1 receptor antagonist gene polymorphism as a disease severity factor in systemic lupus erythematosus. *Arthritis Rheum* 1994;37:1380.
19. Danis VA, Millington M, Huang Q, et al. Lack of association between an interleukin-1 receptor antagonist gene polymorphism and systemic lupus erythematosus. *Dis Markers* 1995;12:135.
20. Mansfield JC, Holden H, Tarlow JK, et al. Novel genetic association between ulcerative colitis and the anti-inflammatory cytokine interleukin-1 receptor antagonist. *Gastroenterology* 1994;106:637.
21. Hacker UT, Gomolka M, Keller E, et al. Lack of association between an interleukin-1 receptor antagonist gene polymorphism and ulcerative colitis. *GUT* 1997;40:623.
22. Sands KE, Bates DW, Lanken PN, et al. Epidemiology of sepsis syndrome in 8 academic centers. *JAMA* 1997;278:234.
23. Abraham E. Therapies for sepsis. Emerging therapies for sepsis and septic shock. *West J Med* 1997;166:195.
24. Kreger BE, Craven DE, McCabe WR. Gram-negative bacteremia. IV. Reevaluation of clinical features and treatment in 612 patients. *Am J Med*1980;68:344.
25. Dunn DL. Gram-negative bacterial sepsis and sepsis syndrome. *Surg Clin North Am* 1994;74:621.

26. Beutler B, Milsark IW, Cerami A. Passive immunization against cachectin/tumor necrosis factor protects mice from lethal effect of endotoxin. *Science* 1985;229:869.
27. Mathison JC, Wolfson E, Ulevitch RJ. Participation of tumor necrosis factor in the mediation of gram negative bacterial lipopolysaccharide-induced injury in rabbits. *J Clin Invest* 1988;81:1925.
28. Tracey K, Fong Y, Hesse DG, et al. Anti-cachectin/TNF monoclonal antibodies prevent septic shock during lethal bacteremia. *Nature* 1987;330:662.
29. Okusawa S, Gelfand JA, Ikejima T, et al. Interleukin 1 induces a shock-like state in rabbits. Synergism with tumor necrosis factor and the effect of cyclooxygenase inhibition. *J Clin Invest* 1-988;81:1162.
30. Wakabayashi G, Gelfand JA, Burke JF, et al. A specific receptor antagonist for interleukin-1 prevents *Escherichia coli*-induced shock. *FASEB J* 1991;5:338.
31. Ohlsson K, Bjork P, Bergenfeldt M, et al. Interleukin-1 receptor antagonist reduces mortality from endotoxin shock. *Nature* 1990;348:550.
32. Chapman PB, Lester TJ, Casper ES, et al. Clinical pharmacology of recombinant human tumor necrosis factor in patients with advanced cancer. *J Clin Oncol* 1987;5:1942.
33. Smith JW, Longo D, Alford WG, et al. The effects of treatment with interleukin-1α on platelet recovery after high-dose carboplatin. *N Engl J Med* 1993;328:756.
34. Smith JW, Urba WJ, Curti BD, et al. The toxic and hematologic effects of interleukin-1 alpha administered in a phase I trial to patients with advanced malignancies. *J Clin Oncol* 1992;10:1141.
35. van der Poll T, Bueller HR, ten Cate H, et al. Activation of coagulation after administration of tumor necrosis factor to normal subjects. *N Engl J Med* 1990;322:1622.
36. van der Poll T, van Deventer SJH, Hack CE, et al. Effects of leukocytes following injection of tumor necrosis factor into healthy humans. *Blood* 1991;79:693.
37. Dinarello CA. Biological basis for interleukin-1 in disease. *Blood* 1996;87:2095.
38. Moncada S, Palmer RMJ, Higgs EA. Nitric oxide: physiology, pathophysiology, and pharmacology. *Pharmacol Rev* 1991;43:109.
39. Abraham E, Wunderink R, Silverman H, et al. Efficacy and safety of monoclonal antibody to human tumor necrosis factor-a in patients with sepsis syndrome. *JAMA* 1995;273:934.
40. Abraham E, Glauser MP, Butler T, et al. p55 tumor necrosis factor receptor fusion protein in the treatment of patients with severe sepsis and septic shock. A randomized controlled multicenter trial. Ro 45-2081 Study Group. *JAMA* 1997;277:1531.
41. Fisher CJJ, Slotman GJ, Opal SM, et al. Initial evaluation of human recombinant interleukin-1 receptor antagonist in the treatment of sepsis syndrome: a randomized, open-label, placebo-controlled multicenter trial. *Crit Care Med* 1994;22:12.
42. Fisher C Jr, Agosti JM, Opal SM, et al. Treatment of septic shock with the tumor necrosis factor receptor:Fc fusion protein. *N Engl J Med* 1996;334:1697.
43. Zeni F, Freeman B, Natanson C. Anti-inflammatory therapies to treat sepsis and septic shock: a reassessment. *Crit Care Med* 1997;25:1095.
44. Heremans H, van Damme J, Dillen C, et al. Interferon-γ, a mediator of lethal lipopolysaccharide-induced Shwartzman-like shock in mice. *J Exp Med* 1990;171:1853.
45. Huang S, Hendriks W, Althage A, et al. Immune response in mice that lack the interferon-gamma receptor. *Science* 1993;259:1742.
46. Doecke WD, Randow F, Syrbe U, et al. Monocyte deactivation in septic patients: restoration by IFN-gamma treatment. *Nat Med* 1997;3:678.
47. Harada A, Mukaida N, Matsushima K. Interleukin-8 as a novel target for intervention therapy in acute inflammatory diseases. *Mol Med Today* 1996;2:482. .
48. Donnelly SC, Strieter RM, Kunkel SL, et al. Interleukin-8 and development of adult respiratory distress syndrome in at-risk patient groups. *Lancet* 1993;341:643.
49. Elliott MJ, Maini RN, Feldmann M, et al. Randomised double-blind comparison of chimeric monoclonal antibody to tumour necrosis factor alpha (cA2) versus placebo in rheumatoid arthritis. *Lancet* 1994;344:1105.
50. Elliott MJ, Maini RN. Anti-cytokine therapy in rheumatoid arthritis. *Baillieres Clin Rheumatol* 1995;9:633.
51. Bresnihan B, Alvaro-Gracia JM, Cobby M, et al. Treatment of rheumatoid arthritis with recombinant human interleukin-1 receptor antagonist. *Arthritis Rheum* 1998;41:2196.
52. Watt I, Cobby M. Recombinant human interleukin-1 receptor antagonist reduces the rate of joint erosion in rheumatoid arthritis. *Arthrit Rheumat* 1996;39:S 123.
53. Fekade D, Knox K, Hussein K, et al. Prevention of Jarisch-Herxheimer reactions by treatment with antibodies against tumor necrosis factor alpha. *N Engl J Med* 1996;335:311.
54. van Dullemen HM, van Deventer SJH, Hommes DW, et al. Treatment of Crohn's disease with anti-tumor necrosis factor chimeric monoclonal antibody (cA2). *Gastroenterology* 1995;109:129.
55. Antin JH, Weinstein HJ, Guinan EC, et al. Recombinant human interleukin-1 receptor antagonist in the treatment of steroid-resistant graft-versus-host disease. *Blood* 1994;84:1342.
56. Cohen J, Carlet J. Intersept: an international, multicenter, placebo-controlled trial of monoclonal antibody to human tumor necrosis factor-alpha in patients with sepsis. *Crit Care Med* 1996;24:1431.
57. Reinhart K, Wiegand-Lohnert C, Grimminger F, et al. Assessment of the safety and efficacy of the . monoclonal anti-tumor necrosis factor antibody-fragment, MAK 195F, in patients with sepsis and septic shock: a multicenter, randomized, placebo-controlled, dose-ranging study. *Crit Care Med* 1996;24:733.

58. Fisher CJJ, Dhainaut JF, Opal SM, et al. Recombinant human interleukin-1 receptor antagonist in the treatment of patients with sepsis syndrome. Results from a randomized, double blind, placebo-controlled trial. *JAMA* 1994;271:1836.
59. Opal SM, Fisher CJJ, Dhainaut JF, et al. Confirmatory interleukin-1 receptor antagonist trial in severe sepsis: A phase III, randomized, double-blind, placebo-controlled, multicenter trial. *Crit Care Med* 1997;25:1115.
60. Hirsch E, Irikura VM, Paul SM, et al. Functions of interleukin-1 receptor antagonist in gene knockout and overproducing mice. *Proc Natl Acad Sci (USA)* 1996;93:11008.
61. Stüber F, Petersen M, Bokelmann F, et al. A genomic polymorphism within the tumor necrosis factor locus influences plasma tumor necrosis factor alpha concentrations and outcome of patients with severe sepsis. *Crit Care Med* 1996;24:381.

2

Interleukin-2

Kirk D. Miller, Janaki C. Kuruppu, and Joseph A. Kovacs

Critical Care Medicine Department, Warren Grant Magnuson Clinical Center, National Institutes of Health, Bethesda, Maryland

HISTORICAL PERSPECTIVE

Discovery and Characterization of Interleukin-2

Investigation of the cytokine that would later be identified as interleukin-2 (IL-2) has origins that have been traced to studies of "lymphocyte stimulating factor" in the mid-1960s (1,2). These early studies ushered in a decade of increasing interest in a number of purported "mitogenic factors" capable of augmenting antigen-mediated lymphoproliferation, or indeed capable of perpetuating lymphoproliferation in the absence of antigen (3). The first compelling evidence for a substance capable of specifically promoting T-cell growth came in the mid-1970s, when Morgan, Ruscetti, and Gallo described an *in vitro* method for maintaining T-lymphocytes derived from bone marrow in exponential growth (4,5). This method required repeated supplementation of the culture medium with supernatants containing a "T-cell growth factor" derived from cultures that had contained lectin-stimulated peripheral lymphocytes. Shortly thereafter, using a similar method, Gillis and Smith reported successful long-term culture of tumor-specific murine cytotoxic T-lymphocytes (CTLs) (6). This led to the generation of antigen-specific CTL clones, which in turn led to the development of a sensitive and quantitative bioassay (7,8).

The stage was now set for an extraordinarily productive second decade of investigation into this newly discovered cytokine (9). By the early 1980s, development of monoclonal antibodies had greatly facilitated purification and amino acid sequencing of the protein; cloning of the cDNA and recombinant expression in both eucaryotic and procaryotic systems followed shortly thereafter (10–13). By the late-1980s, much of its function and structure, including the structure of the IL-2 receptor, had been elucidated (14–16).

Once it became clear that "T-cell growth factor" had biological effects other than promoting T-cell replication (Table 2.1), it was designated as the second in what has become a seemingly ever-expanding family of cytokines classified as interleukins (i.e., cytokines that signal between various types of leukocytes) (17).

IL-2 and the Treatment of Malignancies

The availability of virtually unlimited quantities of recombinant material allowed detailed study of *in vivo* immune responses elicited by IL-2. Among these were studies in mice, which confirmed earlier *in vitro* evidence that IL-2 was capable of inducing cytolytic activity against tumor cells but not against corresponding nonmalignant cells (18). This phenomenon was dependent predominantly upon the ability of IL-2 to transform

TABLE 2-1. *Major biological activities of interleukin-2*

Cell type	Effect of interleukin-2
T cells	
CD4	Proliferation in absence of mitogen or antigen Expansion of antigen-stimulated helper clones
$CD8^+$	Expansion of CTL clones Differentiation into tumor infiltrating lymphocytes
NK cells	Proliferation and augmentation of NK cell activity Production of gamma-interferon
B cells	Proliferation and differentiation Enhancement of antibody production
Monocytes/macrophages	Enhancement of phagocytosis and cytotoxicity Production of IL-1

Data from Smith KA, (*Science* 1988), and Kuziel WA and Greene WC. (*J Invest Dermatol* 1990.)

phenotypic natural killer (NK) cells (and to a lesser extent T-lymphocytes) into "lymphokine-activated killer" (LAK) cells capable of lysing tumor cells that were resistant to killing by untransformed "parent" NK cells (19,20).

Induction of LAK activity in mice was found to be highly dose-dependent; appreciation of the rapid clearance of IL-2 by renal mechanisms led to administration of higher doses by various routes that enhanced anti-tumor responses in mice (21–23).

In an attempt to further enhance LAK activity and mitigate at least some of the toxicities that had been associated with the administration of high-dose IL-2, LAK cells were prepared *ex vivo* by incubation of syngeneic lymphocytes in the presence of IL-2 (24,25). These transformed and expanded cells were in turn reinfused into the tumor-bearing mice along with concomitant administration of IL-2. Tumor responses in animals treated with this "adoptive immunotherapy" were found to be superior to those when high-dose IL-2 was used alone (26–29). An analogous type of therapy utilizing "tumor infiltrating lymphocytes" (TILs) has also been investigated in murine models. Rather than LAK cells, syngeneic lymphocytes are harvested from malignant tissue, expanded *ex vivo* with IL-2, and reinfused in animals receiving systemic IL-2. Regression of certain tumors in mice treated in this fashion was found to be superior to that seen in mice treated with LAK cells and IL-2 (30).

These studies of IL-2 in murine models of malignancy had the overall effect of promoting clinical trials and influencing their design (31). Studies in the mid- to late-1980s using IL-2 alone and IL-2 in combination with LAK cells demonstrated efficacy for both forms of therapy: the highest overall response rates (generally in the 20% to 50% range) were reported in patients with renal cell carcinoma and melanoma who had failed prior antineoplastic regimens (21,32–35). However, substantially lower overall response rates (generally less than 15%) were subsequently reported from a number of studies including large multicenter trials (36–38). Nonetheless, a relatively small subset of patients with renal cell carcinoma and melanoma did achieve prolonged, complete remission (39,40).

Human trials utilizing IL-2 in combination with TILs have been disappointing, owing in part to the technical difficulties involved with this technique (41,42). Also disappointing have been attempts to combine IL-2 and adoptive immunotherapy into regimens that include surgery, radiation, and the use of other cytokines and biological response modifiers, as have attempts to identify predictors of response to IL-2–based therapies. Nor has a survival advantage been shown for any IL-2 containing regimen (43). Moreover, in prospective randomized trials, adoptive immunotherapy in conjunction with IL-2 has not been shown to be superior to high-dose IL-2 administered alone (44,45).

Significant dose-dependent toxicity has been seen in all trials involving the use of IL-2 and IL-2 in combination with LAK cells in the treatment of malignancy (46,47). Constitutional symptoms such a fever, myalgias, and fatigue are seen in essentially all patients. Nausea, vomiting, diarrhea, rash, and fluid retention are common as are laboratory abnormalities including anemia, eosinophilia, thrombocytopenia, and elevated bilirubin, transaminase, and creatinine levels. Severe complications such as the well-described "capillary leak syndrome," hypotension, congestive heart failure, arrhythmias, and myocardial infarction, while less common may be life-threatening and often require care in an intensive care setting (48–51).

Modest response rates—often of limited duration—coupled with considerable toxicity and cost have limited use of IL-2 except in the treatment of renal cell carcinoma and melanoma which at present are the only FDA-approved indications (52). However, the prospect for wider use of IL-2 in the treatment of malignancy will brighten if more efficacious and less toxic regimens can be devised (53–56).

IL-2 and the Treatment of Infectious Diseases

Appreciation of the critical role of IL-2 in maintaining normal cell-mediated immune function was nearly coincident with the appreciation of the profound disturbance in cell-mediated immune function in patients with AIDS (57,58). This fortuitous convergence led to early speculation that IL-2 might have a role in the pathogenesis, and indeed, in the treatment of this syndrome (59,60). Seventeen years later, HIV-1 infection continues, by far, to be the most thoroughly investigated use of IL-2 in the treatment of infectious disease. This chapter will review the use of IL-2 in the treatment of HIV-1 infection, and will also review the small number of studies that have investigated the use of IL-2 in the treatment of other infections.

STRUCTURE AND MECHANISM OF ACTION

Structure of IL-2

IL-2 belongs to a large family of extracellular regulatory molecules that share a four-α helical structure (61). This family includes cytokines, hematopoietic growth factors, interferons, and hormones, all of which are involved in production and regulation of hematopoietic cells, and in innate or acquired immunity. Within this large family of 4-α-helical cytokines, IL-2 belongs to a subgroup, along with IL-4, IL-7, IL-9, IL-13, and IL-15, whose receptors share the common γ (γc) receptor subunit that signals through JAK3.

IL-2 is a 133–amino acid polypeptide with molecular weight of 15.5 kd. X-ray crystallography in conjunction with mutational and functional analyses yielded the 4-α-helical structure analogous to GM-CSF and IL-4 (Fig. 2.1) (62,63). Posttranslational modification includes variable O-linked glycosylation at the threonine residue at position 3, which accounts for variability of reported molecular weights, but does not affect activity of the peptide (64). A single disulfide bond between the cysteine at position 58 and the cysteine at position 105 is essential for interaction of IL-2 with its receptor complex (65). Mutational analysis has demonstrated multiple key amino acids residues involved in binding of IL-2 to its receptor, and therefore required for signal transduction and for targeting T-cell effects (66–72).

The gene for human IL-2 is located on chromosome 4, and is encoded on four exons (73–76). Gene expression is tightly regulated by a 300–base pair (bp) minimal enhancer

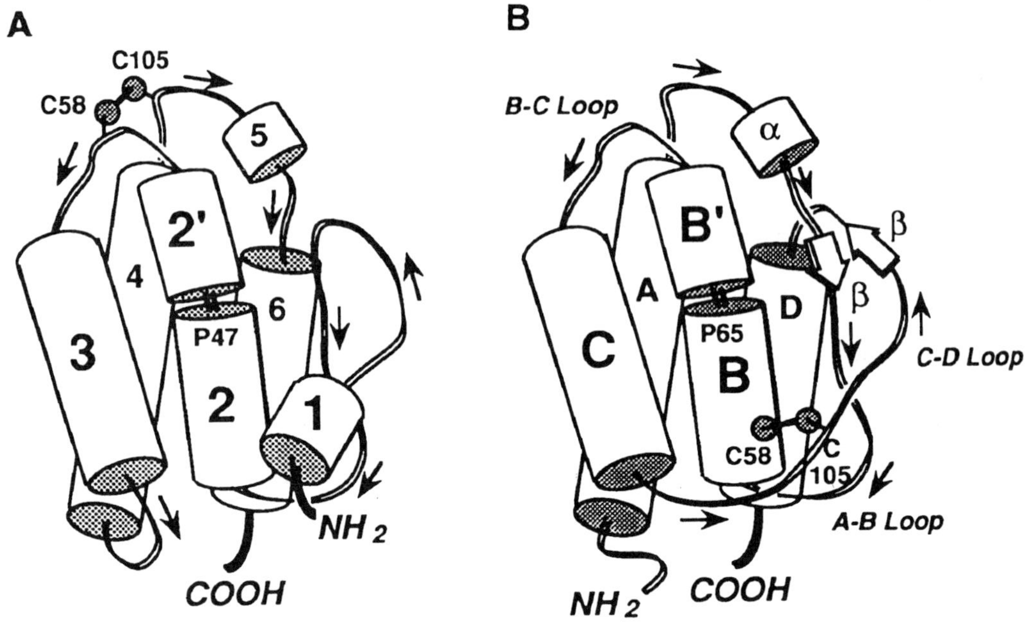

FIG. 2.1. Schematic three-dimensional structure of interleukin-2 (IL-2). **A:** Structure derived from x-ray crystallography. **B:** Model revised based on mutational analysis and comparison with GM-CSF and IL-4. (From Bazan JF. Unraveling the structure of IL-2. *Science* 1992;257:410–413, with permission.)

region located immediately upstream of the transcription start site (77). This domain has NF-KB, and AP-1 sites in addition to sites for binding of Oct-1, Sp-1–like factor, and TGGC factor, which are constitutively expressed in T-cells. Rather than a single regulatory factor being responsible for triggering expression of IL-2, gene expression is stimulated by the simultaneous binding of multiple factors, each enhancing the affinity of its neighbors to bind to the respective sites. Balanced equilibrium of multiple regulatory factors in concert allows for tight gene regulation. An additional upstream sequence, from −300 to −600 bp, appears to promote IL-2 transcription in an, as yet, undetermined manner (78). Lastly, stabilization of the IL-2 mRNA by binding proteins maintains production of peptide (79).

The IL-2 Receptor

The IL-2 receptor (IL-2R) is composed of three separate membrane-bound peptides, IL-2Rα, IL-2Rβ, and the γc-subunit (80). The IL-2Rα subunit, a 55-kd transmembrane protein with a single transmembrane spanning region and small cytoplasmic domain, does not participate in signal transduction (81,82). Its main function is the formation of a high-affinity binding complex with the β and γ subunits of the IL-2R complex (83). IL-2Rα shares homology with the IL-15 receptor α-subunit (84,85). The gene encoding IL-2Rα is located on human chromosome 10, and its expression is regulated by cellular activation, TCR stimulation, IL-1, IL-2, and TNF-α. IL-2Rβ is expressed on early precursor T-cells and B-cells, and on activated T-cells and B-cells (86,87). Resting, mature T-cells and B-cells do not express this subunit.

IL-2Rβ, also a component of the IL-15 receptor complex, is a 75-kd transmembrane protein with a large cytoplasmic domain. IL-2Rβ belongs to the hematopoietin receptor superfamily (88). IL-2Rβ has low affinity for IL-2 by itself (K_d ~ 100 nM), but in association with IL-2Rα demonstrates high affinity binding (K_d ~ 30 pM) (89–91). The IL-2Rβ gene is located on chromosome 22 and consists of 10 exons (92). Three regulatory elements are located upstream from the major transcription start site and include binding sites for Ets-1 and GA-binding protein, Sp1, and Spa and Egr-1 (93,94). IL-2Rβ is constitutively expressed on resting T-cells, B-cells, NK cells, monocytes, macrophages, and neutrophils, and is upregulated in activated T-cells and B-cells (80).

IL-2Rγ (γc) subunit also belongs to the hematopoeitin receptor superfamily, and is shared by receptors for IL-2, IL-4, IL-7, IL-9, IL-13, and IL-15. The γc subunit is a 64-kd transmembrane subunit encoded by a single gene on the X chromosome (95). Mutations of γc are responsible for most cases of X-linked severe combined immunodeficiency (96–98). The γc subunit is expressed on $CD4^+$ and $CD8^+$ T-cells, B-cells, NK cells, monocytes, macrophages, granulocytes, and neutrophils (80).

Signal Transduction

Interaction of IL-2 with its receptor complex begins with binding of IL-2 to IL-2Rα/IL-2Rβ heterodimer (99,100). Subsequently, the γc subunit is recruited by the complex, which results in activation of intracytoplasmic downstream signaling (101,102). The IL-2R has no intrinsic kinase activity, however IL-2/IL-2R activates numerous intracellular kinases leading to phosphorylation of cytoplasmic moieties (103). Six tyrosine residues located on IL-2Rβ are themselves targets of phosphorylation and are required for signaling (104). Two tyrosine residues located on the γc subunit are functionally inactive (105,106).

Three major signal transduction pathways are activated by IL-2: Jak-STAT, Ras-MAPK, and phosphatidylinositol-3 kinase (PI3K) (Fig. 2.2). Jak1 and Jak3, two of the Janus kinase family of tyrosine kinases, bind to the membrane proximal regions of IL-2Rβ and IL-2Rγ, respectively. Jak3 plays a critical role in signaling, and loss-of-function mutations of Jak3 demonstrate a phenotype identical to XSCID (107). Jak activation leads to phosphorylation of tyrosine residues on proteins called STAT (signal transducers and activators of transcription) (108–113). These activated STAT proteins dimerize and translocate to the nucleus, binding to DNA regulatory sites and stimulating gene transcription, including that of IL-2Rα, c-fos, c-myc, and cis (114–117). The end result of the IL-2–stimulated Jak-STAT pathway is cell proliferation.

The Ras-MAP kinase pathway also utilizes Jak3, which phosphorylates the tyrosine residue Y338 on IL-2Rβ, allowing Shc to bind to IL-2Rβ. Shc is then phosphorylated, which then activates Grb2, which in turn activates Ras. Ras activates MAP kinase, which induces c-fos and c-jun (80). Ras signaling has been associated with both proliferative and apoptotic responses (118–120).

The third major signaling pathway involves phosphatidylinositol-3 kinase (PI3K) (121,122). PI3K activates p70 56-kinase and the Akt serine kinase (also called protein kinase B), leading to expression of bcl-2, bcl-x, and c-myc, which are involved in preventing apoptosis (123–126). IL-2 stimulation also leads to association of PI3K with PKCξ, which is involved in cytoskeletal integrity (127,128).

Additional signaling factors include insulin receptor substrates 1 and 2 (IRS-1, IRS-2) (129), Src family kinases, including Lck, Lyn, and Fyn (130–132), SH2 domain-containing tyrosine phosphatases, SHP l and SHP2 (133), and the protooncogenes Cb1 and CrkL (134).

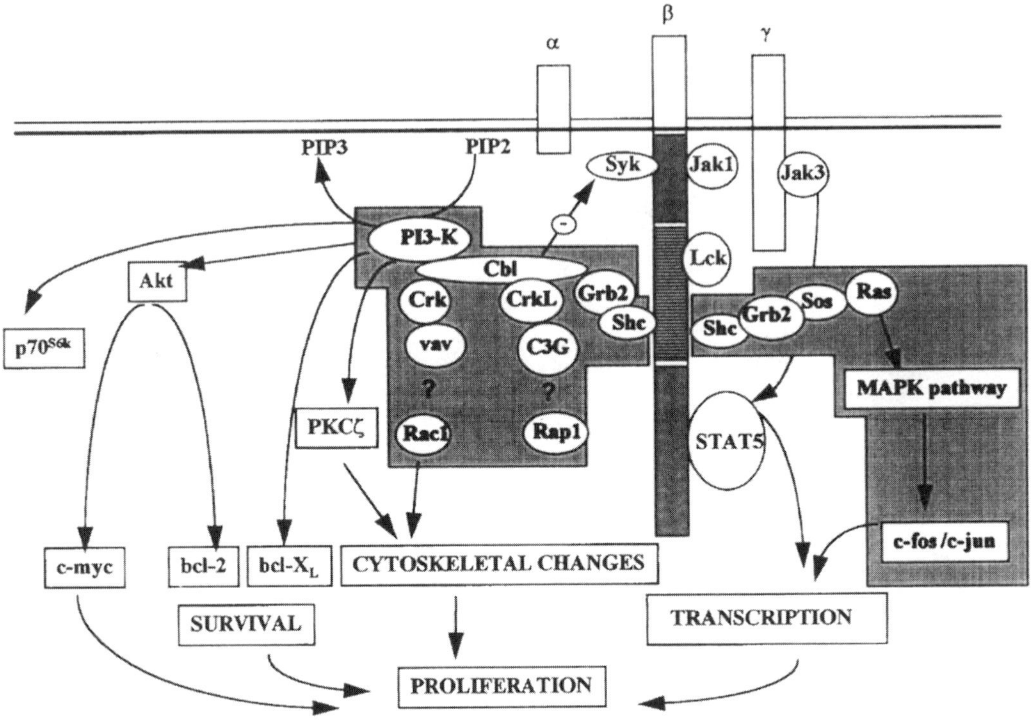

FIG. 2.2. Multiple signaling pathways triggered by interleukin-2 (IL-2). The three major pathways shown are jak-STAT, Ras-MAPK, and PI3K, all of which lead ultimately to production of nuclear factors involved in cell survival and proliferation. (From Gesbert F, Delespine-Carmagnat M, Bertoglio J. Recent advances in the understanding of interleukin-2 signal transduction. *J Clin Immunol* 1998;18:307–320, with permission.)

The signaling pathways and components mentioned above, along with a growing list of factors, interact in a complex fashion in response to IL-2 binding, and also interact with signaling factors generated from activation by other cytokines. Complete understanding of the downstream signaling of IL-2 requires further study. Recent reviews of current understanding of the complex intracellular pathways triggered by IL-2 are available (80,135–137).

ANIMAL MODELS

Transgenic Mice

Introduction of transgenes expressing human IL-2 or IL-2Rα in mice allowed the study of overexpression of these gene products and resulting effects on immune function. It was expected that transgenic expression of high levels of IL-2 would lead to expansion of T-lymphocytes and autoimmunity, however in several mouse models, lymphocyte development and number were normal and no autoimmunity was seen (138–140). In these models, overexpression of IL-2 led to inflammatory processes, such as lymphocytic infiltration of the lungs or macrophage-predominant pancreatitis, without global effects on immune function.

Transgenic expression of both human IL-2 and human IL-2Rα in mice resulted in expansion of large granular lymphocytes with elevated NK activity, and severe interstitial pneumonia and lymphocyte depletion with death of animals by 4 weeks of age (141). These mice had in increased number of intermediate-affinity IL-2 receptors, possibly due to overexpression of IL-2Rβ. Mice overexpressing IL-2RB showed absence of NK cells and dendritic epithelial cells, with no affect on T-cells or B-cells (142). Since IL-15 shares the β and γc subunits with IL-2 (143), and IL-15 is known to be a potent factor for NK differentiation (144), these studies may reflect phenotypic effects of IL-15 rather than IL-2 (145).

IL-2 Knockout Mice

Studies of IL-2 deficiency were possible with the development of an IL-2 knockout mouse (145). A knockout model lacking IL-2Rα was also developed, showing a similar phenotype (146). Surprisingly, these mice had normal T-cell development, and actually had an increased number of T-cells after 3 to 4 weeks of age. Cytotoxic T-cell (CTL) function and humoral immunity were normal in these mice, and NK function was reduced but inducible (147). These mice develop a lethal autoimmune syndrome characterized by hemolytic anemia, splenomegaly, lymphadenopathy, and severe colitis (148,149). Phenotypic expression varies with the genetic background onto which the IL-2 deficiency is introduced. For example, mice with a mixed (129/O1a × C57BL6) genetic background predominantly develop an ulcerative colitis-like disease, whereas the Balb/c strain develops hemolytic anemia without colitis (150). Development of anemia has been shown to depend on the presence of B-cells, while colitis depends on T-cells (151). Development of disease is dependent on thymus-derived IL-2–deficient lymphocytes, as demonstrated by crossing the IL-2–/– gene onto the athymic mouse background, which had normal development (148). Colitis can be prevented in IL-2–/– mice by maintenance in a germ-free environment (152). Colitis can then be induced in these animals by selective exposure to antigens (153,154).

Uncontrolled lymphocyte expansion and autoimmune phenomena seen in IL-2–deficient mice were clarified by the demonstration that IL-2 potentiates Fas-mediated activation-induced cell death (AICD). Subsequently, studies of knockout mice lacking either IL-2 or IL-2Rα showed that IL-2–deficient T-cells were resistant to AICD (155–157). In recent years, investigators have examined different aspects of signaling interactions between IL-2 and Fas/FasL pathways, as well as contributions from other cytokines such as IL-6 and IL-15, to clarify the mechanism by which IL-2 can have opposite effects on cell survival (158–171). One possibility is that T-cells that are activated in the presence of low levels of IL-2 undergo expansion to promote immune responses, but in the presence of high levels of IL-2, as may occur in the thymus, T-cell death occurs (172,173). Another possible mechanism involves modulation of the Fas-inhibitor protein FLIP, which is suppressed by IL-2 (164,174).

Animal Models of Infection

Administration of exogenous IL-2 in animal models of infection has demonstrated efficacy in prevention and treatment of bacterial, parasitic and viral infections. Bacterial infections studied include gram-negative sepsis (175), *Klebsiella* pneumonia (176), mycobacterial infections (177–179), and staphylococcal infections (180,181). IL-2 enhances the murine host response to *Trypanosoma cruzi* (182) and improves survival in mice challenged with a lethal dose of *Toxoplasma gondii* (183). IL-2 has been shown to be important in protection from herpes simplex virus–type 1 (HSV-1) (184–186) and cytomegalovirus

(CMV) (187). Vaccine responses to HIV-1 DNA and tuberculosis are augmented by IL-2 (188,189). Thus, animal models lend support for the concept that IL-2 has the potential for use in the treatment of a variety of infectious diseases.

TREATMENT OF HIV-1 INFECTION

Early Clinical Experience

The ability of IL-2 to induce sustained increases in both the absolute number and percentage of $CD4^+$ T-lymphocytes has made it the cytokine most studied in the treatment of HIV-1 infection (190,191). Interest in this agent was aroused by early *in vitro* studies that demonstrated defective T-cell proliferative responses to antigen and mitogen, as well as defective NK-cell activity, defective antigen-specific cytotoxic lymphocyte activity, and defective production of γ-interferon in patients with AIDS. These defects were at least partially reversed by incubation of peripheral blood mononuclear cells (PBMCs) with IL-2 (192–196).

Such findings provided a rationale for *in vivo* study of IL-2 (60). Early studies were focused on severely immunocompromised patients with clinically defined AIDS and were conducted prior to the availability of specific antiretroviral agents. IL-2 dosing regimens varied widely, and results were largely disappointing due to lack of evidence of long-term immunological or clinical benefit and considerable toxicity (197–205). However, some patients in these studies did experience encouraging, if transient, increases in peripheral $CD4^+$ lymphocytes and improvements in proliferative responses to mitogens.

Intermittent Intravenous Administration

When nucleoside analog antiretroviral drugs became available, these agents were given in conjunction with intermittent cycles of IL-2. Increases in $CD4^+$ lymphocytes were sustained in many patients treated with this combination. The addition of antiretrovirals also addressed the concern that enhanced HIV replication might result from IL-2–induced activation of lymphocytes (206,207).

The maximum tolerated dose of IL-2 by continuous intravenous infusion has been shown to be 12 million international units (mIU) per day when administered for 21 consecutive days and 18 mIU when the period of administration is shortened to 5 days (208). When a regimen based on the latter dosage—18 mIU for 5 days (with dose reductions as needed to alleviate toxicity)—was repeated approximately every 8 weeks, six of 10 patients with baseline $CD4^+$ lymphocyte counts above 200 cells per mm^3 experienced sustained increases in $CD4^+$ lymphocyte counts without a concomitant effect on $CD8^+$ lymphocytes. These patients were also receiving standard doses of zidovudine, didanosine, or zalcitabine alone or in combination. Based on an analysis of the beta chain ($V\beta$) of the T-cell receptor, the $CD4^+$ lymphocyte increases observed in these patients were polyclonal and were associated with increased expression of the high-affinity IL-2 receptor (IL-2Rα) as measured by an increase in the proportion of $CD4^+/CD25^+$ lymphocytes. While $CD8^+$ lymphocyte numbers did not increase, decreases in the number of these lymphocytes expressing activation markers such as HLA-DR were noted. HIV-1 viral loads increased transiently during the infusion of IL-2 but usually returned to baseline levels by the follow-up visit. Sustained increases in $CD4^+$ lymphocyte counts and NK-cell activity were similarly noted in another study of intravenous IL-2 administered with zidovudine (209). In this latter study, escalating doses of IL-2 were administered in 5-day cycles repeated every 7 days to 10 patients with CD4$^+$ lymphocyte counts greater than 400 cells per mm^3. Six of these 10 patients had CD4$^+$ lymphocyte counts above baseline levels six months after the last infusion of IL-2 (210). Increases in CD4$^+$ lymphocyte counts as well as in NK-cell and LAK-cell activity have also been reported in HIV-infected patients with CD4$^+$ lymphocyte counts greater than 100 cells per mm^3 who were treated with four 5-day cycles of intravenous IL-2 and zidovudine for lymphoma (211).

Randomized trials have corroborated the earlier observations outlined above, namely that intermittent intravenous IL-2 therapy can effect statistically significant sustained increases in CD4$^+$ lymphocyte counts without inducing sustained increases in plasma viral load. In the first of these studies, 60 patients with CD4$^+$ lymphocyte counts above 200 cells per mm^3 were randomized to receive only nucleoside analog antiretrovirals (zidovudine, didanosine, or zalcitabine alone or in combination) or these same nucleoside analogs in combination with intermittent 5-day intravenous infusions of IL-2 (212,213). These cycles were repeated every 8 weeks. The starting dose of 18 mIU per day was reduced during the study as needed to treat toxicities. The group receiving IL-2 experienced a mean increase of 37 CD4$^+$ lymphocytes/mm^3/month while the group receiving nucleoside analogs-alone experienced a mean decrease of −5 CD4$^+$ lymphocytes/mm^3/month ($p<0.001$) (Fig. 2.3A). After 12 months of study, the mean CD4$^+$ lymphocyte count of the IL-2 group was more than dou-

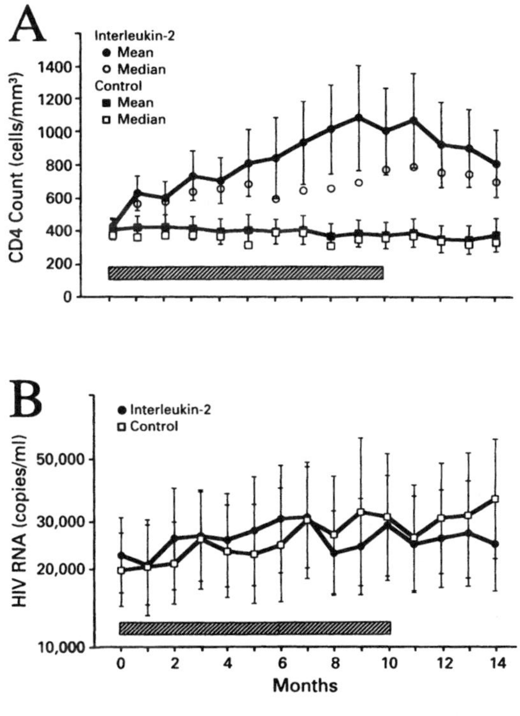

FIG. 2-3. Change in CD4$^+$ lymphocyte counts **(A)** and HIV-1 viral load **(B)** during a randomized trial of intravenously administered interleukin-2 (IL-2) and antiretrovirals or antiretrovirals alone. The *shaded bars* represent the time during which 5-day cycles of IL-2 (repeated every 8 weeks) were administered. (Adapted from Kovacs JA, Vogel S, Albert JM, et al. Controlled trial of interleukin-2 infusions in patients infected with the human immunodeficiency virus. *N Engl J Med* 1996;335:1350–1356, with permission.)

ble the CD4 count of the control group (916 versus 349 cells per mm^3). A concomitant increase in the proportion of $CD4^+$ lymphocytes (CD4%) was also noted in the group that received IL-2. This randomized trial confirmed the earlier observation that $CD8^+$ lymphocyte numbers did not increase while the proportion of $CD8^+$ lymphocytes expressing surface activation markers (HLA-DR^+ and $CD38^+$ lymphocytes) actually decreased. Increased expression of the high-affinity IL-2 receptor as measured by an increase in the proportion of $CD4^+/CD25^+$ lymphocytes was again demonstrated. Also noted was a preferential expansion of naive $CD4^+$ lymphocytes. Importantly, HIV-1 viral loads were not increased in the IL-2 group during the study (Fig. 2.3B), and there was a suggestion of a beneficial effect associated with IL-2 therapy.

Intermittent Subcutaneous Administration

An alternative method of administering IL-2 is by subcutaneous injection. This inviting approach obviates the need for an indwelling infusion catheter, thereby lessening the inconvenience, cost, and complications inherent in continuous IV therapy. Two different formulations of IL-2 have been evaluated: the standard preparation used in the studies of intravenous administration described above, and a polyethylene glycol (PEG)–modified preparation. It should be noted that PEG IL-2 has also been administered intravenously in the setting of HIV infection. PEG IL-2 has a 10- to 20-fold slower clearance than the standard preparation of IL-2 and a resultant pharmacokinetic profile approximating that seen with continuous IV infusion. However, concerns have been raised about the safety of PEG IL-2 and this formulation is no longer being manufactured (214,216).

One controlled trial directly compared the relative efficacy of subcutaneously administered PEG IL-2 (two doses per cycle two days apart, with cycles repeated every two months) with a standard 5-day intravenous regimen (cycles repeated every two months) and also with a control group that was treated with antiretroviral therapy alone. The starting dose of PEG IL-2 was 1.0 mIU per cycle which, if tolerated, was escalated to a final dose 6.5 mIU per cycle. The starting dose of intravenous IL-2 was 12 mIU per day. Patients had baseline $CD4^+$ lymphocyte counts between 200 and 500 cells per mm^3. At the start of the study patients were on a regimen of nucleoside analog antiretrovirals (zidovudine, didanosine, or zalcitabine alone or in combination); after 34 weeks of study, use of lamivudine was permitted. At study week 48, both IL-2 groups experienced an increase in median $CD4^+$ lymphocyte count: 44 cells per mm^3 for the subcutaneous group and 359 cells per mm^3 for the intravenous group. The increases for both of these groups were statistically significant when compared to the control group, which experienced a decline in $CD4^+$ lymphocyte count of 46 cells per mm^3 ($p<.0001$). Nonetheless, the $CD4^+$ lymphocyte response in the PEG-IL-2 group represented a disappointment given the pharmacokinetic-based prediction that this group would respond similarly to the intravenous infusion group (217).

More promising results were obtained when the standard IL-2 preparation was administered subcutaneously at a maximum dose of 15 mIU per day in 5-day cycles repeated every eight weeks. This nonrandomized dose escalation study involved 18 patients with baseline $CD4^+$ lymphocyte counts above 200 cells per mm^3 who were on nucleoside analog antiretroviral therapy (zidovudine, didanosine, or zalcitabine alone or in combination). Patients who failed to respond to the initial once daily subcutaneous dose were eligible to switch to two divided daily doses or intravenous therapy. Twice daily dosing was offered after studies suggested that IL-2 administered on this schedule more closely mimicked the pharmacokinetic profile seen with continuous infusion therapy. Eight of the patients experienced rises in CD4$^+$ lymphocyte counts of at least 200 cells per mm^3 while six others had rises of less than 200 cell per mm^3, and four patients experienced a decline at the end of one year of study. No long-term increases in plasma viral load were seen.

These encouraging results led to a randomized trial of subcutaneously administered IL-2 among patients with CD4$^+$ lymphocyte counts greater than 500 cell per mm^3 at baseline. Forty-nine patients were randomized to either monthly or every other month cycles, and were also randomized to low-dose IL-2 (1.5 mIU twice daily) or high-dose IL-2 (7.5 mIU twice daily). Patients were required to use any combination of FDA-approved antiretroviral agents which, at the time this study was conducted, did include HIV-1 protease inhibitors. Over six months of study, participants in the high-dose groups experienced a mean CD4$^+$ lymphocyte increase of 116 cells per mm^3 per month, while participants in the low-dose group experienced a mean increase of 27 cells per mm^3 per month (Fig. 2.4A). At the end of six months, the high-dose group experienced a mean increase in CD4$^+$ lymphocytes of 95% compared to a 19% increase in the low-dose group. No increases in plasma viral load were seen in either group (Fig. 2.4B).

Another study directly compared subcutaneous and intravenous administration. Ninety-four antiretroviral naive patients with baseline CD4$^+$ lymphocyte counts of 250 to

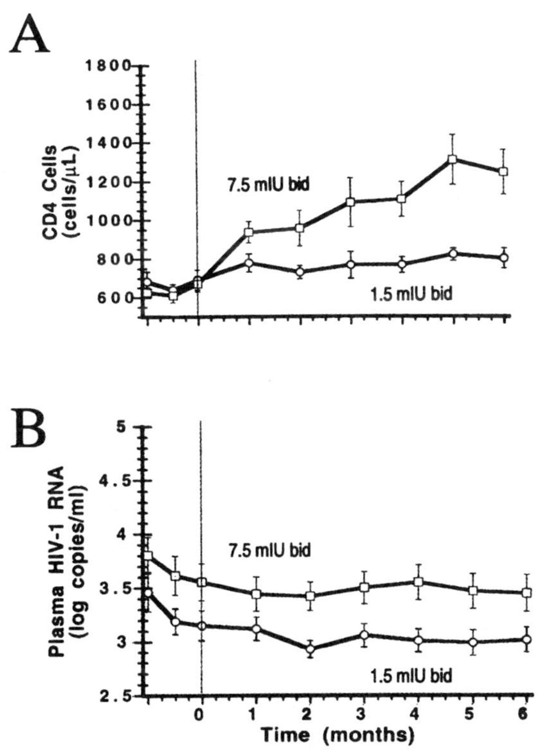

FIG. 2-4. Change in CD4$^+$ lymphocyte counts **(A)** and HIV-1 viral load **(B)** during a trial of subcutanously administered interleukin-2 (IL-2) at two different dosages. (Adapted from Davey R, Chaitt D, Piscitelli S, et al. A randomized trial of high- versus low-dose subcutancous interleukin-2 outpatient therpy for early human immunodeficiency virus type 1 infection. *J Infect Dis* 1999;179:849–858, with permission.)

550 cells/mm^3 were randomized to receive one of four regimens. One group received antiretroviral therapy (zidovudine plus didanosine) alone, while the other three groups were randomized to receive the same antiretrovirals plus IL-2 cycles that were repeated every two months. Participants in these latter three groups received subcutaneously administered IL-2 (3 mIU twice daily for 5 days), or intravenously administered standard IL-2 (12 mIU per day for 5 days), or intravenously administered PEG-IL-2 (2 mIU IV per meter^2 in a single bolus injection). At the end of 50 weeks of study, participants in the three IL-2 groups experienced mean increases in CD4$^+$ lymphocyte counts of 564 cells per mm^3, 676 cells per mm^3 and 105 cells per mm^3 respectively. The increases in the subcutaneous and continuous infusion IL-2 groups were significantly greater than the rise of 55 cells per mm^3 seen in the control group who received antiretrovirals alone (p = .0001 and p = .0002, respectively). The mean increase in CD4$^+$ lymphocyte count experienced by participants in the PEG IL-2 group was not statistically significant when compared to the control group (p = 0.58). Based on this finding, these investigators recommend against further study of PEG IL-2. HIV-1 viral loads were similar in all four groups throughout the study.

Additional studies using a variety of subcutaneous regimens have generally confirmed the findings outlined above: subcutaneously administered IL-2 in combination with antiretrovirals can effect significant increases in CD4$^+$ lymphocyte counts without increasing HIV-1 viral load levels, and at least in select populations immunological changes are similar to those treated with continuous intravenous infusion (213–229).

IL-2 Plus Highly Active Antiretroviral Therapy

The development of highly active antiretroviral therapies (HAART) has lead to a remarkable decrease in morbidity and mortality in conjunction with substantial immune reconstitution in HIV-infected patients. What is the potential role of IL-2 in the HAART era? Prior to the availability of HAART, patients with CD4$^+$ lymphocyte counts less than 200 cells per mm^3 responded poorly to IL-2. In a previously described trial of intravenously administered IL-2, only two of six patients with baseline CD4$^+$ lymphocyte counts between 100 and 200 experienced a 50% or greater increase over baseline, and among those with baseline counts less than 100 none had an increase of this magnitude. HAART has provided the opportunity to reexamine the activity of IL-2 in patients with low baseline CD4$^+$ lymphocyte counts who had previously been treated with IL-2, but were unresponsive (230,231). One trial involved three groups of patients with median CD4$^+$ lymphocyte counts that ranged from 144 to 205 cells per mm^3 who were randomized to either indinavir (using two different dosing regimens) alone or in combination with intravenous IL-2 (maximum dose of 12 mIU IV per day). After 14 weeks of therapy, there was a trend toward better response in the patients who received combined indinavir and IL-2 therapy.

A controlled trial of IL-2 in 72 patients receiving HAART, with CD4$^+$ lymphocyte counts below 200 cells per mm^3 and plasma HIV viral load less than 1,000 copies per mm^3 demonstrated a CD4$^+$ lymphocyte increase of 65 cells per mm^3 after 24 weeks for the IL-2 group (4.5 million IU bid × 5 days q 2 months), compared to an 18 cells per mm^3 increase for the control group (p< 0.0001) (231). Thus, IL-2 can provide potential immunologic benefit to patients responding inadequately to HAART. Other randomized trials of IL-2 in combination with HAART, including trials with patients who have higher baseline CD4$^+$ lymphocyte counts, are also underway to help clarify the potential role of IL-2 in the era of HAART.

Continuous Daily Subcutaneous Administration

Another approach that has been studied in the setting of HIV disease is the daily administration of lower doses of IL-2 than are used in intermittent therapy. Early studies of subcutaneously (and intradermally) administered IL-2 demonstrated increases in eosinophils, NK-cell number and activity, LAK-cell activity, and (γ-interferon levels, but they did not demonstrate increases in $CD4^+$ lymphocyte numbers. Patients in these nonrandomized trials had a wide range of baseline $CD4^+$ lymphocyte counts and the doses of IL-2 utilized were relatively low (232–236). A more recent study of 16 patients with $CD4^+$ lymphocyte counts of 200 to 500 cells per mm^3 evaluated subcutaneous doses that ranged from 62,500 to 250,000 IU/m^2/day (237). All patients were taking nucleoside analog antiretroviral agents (zidovudine, didanosine, zalcitabine, stavudine, or lamivudine alone or in combination). Daily IL-2 therapy was well tolerated and was continued for six months. When changes in cell subtypes in patients who received a lower dose (62,500 to 125,000 IU/m^2/d) were compared to those in patients receiving a higher dose (187,500 to 250,000 IU/m^2d), an increase in NK cells, monocytes, and eosinophils, as well as $CD4^+$ lymphocytes was noted in the latter group. While the mean change in $CD4^+$ lymphocyte count of the higher dose group was significantly different from that of the lower dose group (+28 versus –28 cells/mm^3/month), the difference was primarily due to the rapid decline in $CD4^+$ lymphocyte counts in the lower dose group. The mean monthly increase in $CD4^+$ lymphocyte count from baseline in the higher dose group was not significant (95% CI, –2 to 58 cells per mm^3 per month). Proponents of daily administration argue that this is the preferable approach to IL-2 therapy due to a more favorable side-effect profile. However, while NK cell increases have been consistently demonstrated using daily therapy, to date no controlled trial using such an approach has demonstrated a significant effect on CD4 cell number (238).

Immunological Versus Clinical Benefit of Intermittent IL-2 Therapy

While substantial $CD4^+$ lymphocyte count increases can be induced by intermittently administered IL-2, the clinical benefit of these immunological changes has yet to be demonstrated. Studies examining $CD4^+$ lymphocytes in patients receiving IL-2 suggest that their functionality is similar before and after its administration (239,240). Furthermore, a metaanalysis of three of the already described randomized trials has demonstrated a trend toward reduced risk of disease progression (241). Nonetheless, the clinical efficacy of IL-2 therapy (i.e., its ability to decrease the frequency of opportunistic infections and malignancies and mortality) needs to be addressed in phase 3 trials with clinical endpoints. Such studies are underway (242). Results from these trials are needed before broad recommendations regarding the use of IL-2 in the management of HIV-infected patients can be made.

Frequency And Duration Of Intermittent IL-2 Cycles

Whether intravenously or subcutaneously administered, the intermittent IL-2 regimen most widely studied has been 5-day cycles administered every 8 weeks (208,212,217,218,221,226). This schedule was initially chosen to maximize patient tolerability and minimize patient inconvenience. Also considered was the observation that during prolonged administration of IL-2, the peak in spontaneous lymphocyte blast transformation, which reflects the maximal IL-2–induced proliferative effects, occurs within the first week of therapy, and then diminishes despite continued therapy (203,243).

Three randomized trials have directly compared alternative regimens with the standard IL-2 regimen comprising 5-day cycles repeated every 8 weeks. One study of 22 participants compared $CD4^+$ lymphocyte responses in patients who received cycles of variable duration and variable frequency with those that received the standard 5-day cycles every 8 weeks (244). Participants in this study had baseline $CD4^+$ lymphocyte counts between 200 and 500 cells per mm^3 and were on antiretroviral combinations that included any FDA-approved agents, including protease inhibitors. In one group, the duration of IL-2 administration (at a starting dose of 9 mIU/day) was determined by the pattern of spontaneous lymphocyte blast transformation during individual cycles. In another group, the frequency of administration of IL-2 was determined by the magnitude of individual $CD4^+$ lymphocyte response to previous cycles of IL-2. Another group of participants who received standard 5-day IL-2 cycles served as controls. Dose reductions were more frequent in the group that received longer cycles of IL-2. All three groups experienced significant increases in $CD4^+$ lymphocytes at the end of 32 weeks of study. However, the mean increase of 242 cells per mm^3 in the group that received longer cycles (mean 7.7 days), and the mean increase of 471 cells/mm^3 in the group that received more 5-day cycles (mean 7.1 cycles) were not significantly different from the mean increase of 354 cells/mm^3 observed in the control group ($p > 0.40$).

Another randomized trial of 81 patients examined the relative efficacy of 3- and 4-day intravenous infusions compared to standard 5-day intravenous infusions (at a starting dose of 12 mIU/day) as well as to a control group receiving nucleoside analog antiretroviral therapy alone (245). Participants had baseline $CD4^+$ lymphocyte counts of 100 to 300 cells/mm^3. A higher proportion of patients randomized to 5-day cycles required dose reduction compared to the two groups that received shorter cycles. The median percent change in $CD4^+$ lymphocyte number from baseline for the control, 3-, 4-, and 5-day groups was −25%, −7%, +10%, and +39%, respectively ($p = 0.02$).

An already described randomized trial of subcutaneous IL-2 compared every 4 week and every 8 week cycles. As previously noted, two dosage groups (1.5 mIU and 7.5 mIU SC twice daily for five days) were studied. While $CD4^+$ lymphocyte increases were highly dose dependent, they were only marginally dependent on cycle frequency ($p = 0.096$). Although patients who cycled more frequently experienced more rapid increases in $CD4^+$ lymphocyte counts, this was felt not to outweigh the inconvenience of the more frequent cycles.

Thus, the available experimental evidence lends support to the use of 5-day IL-2 cycles repeated every 8 weeks. Any benefit to cycles of greater frequency than every 8 weeks is marginal and is offset by decreased patient tolerance and increased inconvenience.

Predictors of Response to IL-2

Data from several clinical trials have been used to evaluate predictors of response to IL-2. Two of these trials found a significant correlation between the $CD4^+$ lymphocyte response and the baseline $CD4^+$ lymphocyte count (212,218). While these same studies failed to show a correlation between $CD4^+$ lymphocyte response and baseline viral load, results from two other trials suggest that patients with lower viral loads respond better than patients with higher viral loads (217,226). The data on predictors of response for the most part reflect the experience in trials conducted prior to the advent of HAART.

Side Effects of IL-2 in Treating HIV Infection

The side effects most frequently observed during larger clinical trials of intermittent IL-2 therapy include constitutional symptoms of a "flu-like" illness such as fever, chills, fatigue, myalgias and arthralgias (212,217,221,222,226). Others include nausea, vomiting, diarrhea, stomatitis, sinus congestion, drug rash, pruritus, anxiety, depression, and insomnia. A capillary leak syndrome comprised of fluid retention with edema and weight gain ("third spacing"), decreased urine output, and hypotension may also be seen (208). Elevated serum creatinine and blood urea nitrogen (BUN) levels may result from the capillary leak syndrome or may be associated with use of nonsteroidal antiinflammatory agents during cycles. An odd IL-2–associated side effect is right upper quadrant abdominal pain due to transient edematous thickening of the gallbladder wall as demonstrated by ultrasound (246). Another less common side effect is reactivation of oral or genital herpes (such patients benefit from prophylactic acyclovir during and for several days after cycles). Enhanced growth of anal or genital condylomata has also been seen.

The spectrum of side effects seen with intravenous and subcutaneous administration is generally similar. Local reactions at sites of subcutaneous injection are common: erythema usually clears within several days of completion of the cycle but subcutaneous nodules may take several weeks to resolve (218,226). There has been concern that subcutaneous administration is associated with development of antibodies to recombinant IL-2 that might decrease efficacy (247). This, however, has not been the experience in clinical trials to date (217,218).

Laboratory toxicities seen in clinical trials include low serum levels of calcium, magnesium, albumin and sodium; elevated hepatic aminotransferases and bilirubin; and anemia and thrombocytopenia. Hypothyroidism (elevated TSH levels) as a long-term consequence of IL-2 therapy appears to be immune mediated: hypothyroidism requiring replacement therapy has been noted in 10% of patients treated in clinical trials at the NIH Clinical Center (248). It is usually asymptomatic; rarely, its onset may be preceded by period of transient symptomatic hyperthyroidism.

TABLE 2-2. *Dose-limiting (grade III and grade IV) toxicities of IL-2*[a]

Starting IL-2 dose	18 mIU per day (IV)	7.5 mIU twice daily (SC)	1.5 mIU twice daily (SC)
Side effect			
Fatigue/malaise	44%	20%	5%
Headache	7%	4%	0%
Diarrhea	4%	1%	1%
Stomatitis	4%	0%	1%
Sinus congestion	3%	2%	2%
Myalgia	3%	13%	3%
Laboratory abnormality			
Elevated alanine aminotransferase	1%	2%	1%
Elevated creatinine kinase	1%	2%	1%
Elevated bilirubin	8%	2%	8%
Thrombocytopenia	1%	0%	1%

[a]Percentages represent the proportion of total cycles in which a given side effect was noted. IV, intravenously administered IL-2; SC, subcutaneously administered IL-2. Adapted from Kovacs JA, Vogel S, Albert JM, et al. Controlled trial of interleukin-2 infusions in patients infected with the human immunodeficiency virus. *N Engl J Med* 1996;335:1350–1356, and Davey R, Chaitt D, Piscitelli S, et al. A randomized trial of high- versus low-dose subcutaneous interleukin-2 outpatient therapy for early human immunodeficiency virus type 1 infection. *J Infect Dis* 1999;179:849–858, with permission.

In general, the severity of side effects appears to be dose related (Table 2.2). Although direct comparisons are not easily made because of the various dosing regimens used, subcutaneously administered IL-2 appears to be better tolerated than intravenously administered IL-2.

Infectious Complications of IL-2 Therapy

An increased incidence of bacterial infection among patients treated with intensive regimens for both malignancy and HIV-1 infection has been reported (46,249,250). Gram-positive organisms, such as *Staphylococcus aureus*, have been isolated most frequently, which may reflect an IL-2–induced defect in neutrophil chemotaxis (251). In one study, risk factors for development of bacterial infection in patients with malignancy included indwelling intravenous catheters, open wounds, biliary obstruction, and incomplete treatment of previous infections (252). This study also found that over a period of several years, the incidence of bacterial infection dropped dramatically as monitoring for infection became more vigilant. Recent studies of IL-2 in the setting of HIV-1 infection indicate that bacterial infections are rare with currently used intravenous and subcutaneous regimens (212,217,221,222,226).

Severe Cardiovascular and Pulmonary Toxicity

Life-threatening cardiovascular and pulmonary toxicities associated with high-dose IL-2 therapy in the treatment of malignancy are rarely seen in the treatment of HIV-infected patients. Such severe side effects have not been reported during clinical trials of IL-2 administered subcutaneously (at doses up to 15 mIU/day), which has allowed IL-2 to be safely administered in the outpatient setting (218,221,222,226).

Managing the Side Effects of IL-2 Therapy

Most side effects can be diminished by administration of adjunctive medications. Guidelines for the management of IL-2 associated side effects are presented in Table 2.3. For the most part, these recommendations are tailored to meet the needs of patients treated in an outpatient setting. Side effects that develop during IL-2 therapy will generally improve within a few days of discontinuing IL-2; because immunological responses to IL-2 are not dependent on a single cycle of IL-2, there should be no hesitation in discontinuing a cycle if side effects are of concern. A study that specifically evaluated patients' quality of life during a study of intravenously administered IL-2 found no declines during the 14 months of study (253). Thus, the short-term discomforts associated with IL-2 therapy do not appear to translate into long-term adverse effects on patients' quality of life.

Tumor necrosis factor-alpha (TNF-α) levels increase during IL-2 administration. TNF-alpha may be responsible for many IL-2 side effects including fever and the capillary leak syndrome. Unfortunately, trials of agents that inhibit production of TNF-α, such as thalidomide and monoclonal antibody to TNF, have been disappointing (256). Concern regarding the potential for side effects of corticosteroids, including osteonecrosis of the hip, has dampened enthusiasm for use of these agents in combination with IL-2 (257).

TABLE 2-3. *Outpatient management of IL-2 toxicities in adults*[a]

Side effect	Recommendations for management
Constitutional (fever, chills, aches)	An alternating regimen of acetominophen (650 mg orally every 6 h) alternating with ibuprofen (400–600 mg orally every 6 h) is recommended. It should be started just prior to the start of the IL-2 cycle and continued throughout. Once individual patient tolerances for IL-2 can be assessed, this regimen may be modified. Patients experiencing severe generalized discomfort from IL-2 may be relieved by occasional use of oxycodone (if combined with acetominophen, the total daily dose of acetominophen must be considered).
Rigors	Rigors are extremely uncomfortable. In the inpatient setting, low doses of IV meperidine (25 mg) are very effective. As this is not practicable in the outpatient setting, oral meperidine (50 mg) may be given although the effect is much less dramatic.
Nausea/vomiting	Prochlorperazine (10 mg orally or 25 mg suppositories every 4–6 h) may provide relief (patients should be warned about the possibility of dystonic reactions to prochlorperazine). More severe nausea and vomiting may be treated with ondansetron (8 mg orally) every 8 h. For maximal effect, ondansetron is best used prophylactically by giving it prior to the start of the IL-2 cycle and continuing throughout the cycle.
Diarrhea	Loperamide (1 mg orally every 4–6 h) is usually effective.
Insomnia/anxiety	Temazepam (15–30 mg orally at bedtime) or zolpidem (5–10 mg orally at bedtime) are the agents of choice. Diphenhydramine (50 mg orally at bedtime) may also useful. Lorazepam (0.5–1 mg orally every 6–8 h) is useful in patients who note increased anxiety during IL-2 cycles; it may also be used at bedtime in lieu of temazepam or zolpidem. Triazolam should be avoided. Whenever anxiolytics, hypnotics, and sedative are prescribed, the potential for drug–drug interaction (especially with protease inhibitor antiretroviral agents) should be carefully reviewed.
Sinus congestion	Any of the available combination preparations containing decongestant and guaifenesin are recommended.
Stomatitis	A 2% solution of kaoline pectate, xylocaine, and benadryl as well as other appropriate preparations used in a "swish and spit" fashion will provide temporary relief. IL-2 may precipitate peri-oral herpes outbreaks. Suspicious lesions should be cultured or treated empirically.
Rash/itching	Diphenhydramine (25 to 50 mg orally every 6 h) or hydroxyzine (25 mg orally every 8 h) may provide relief.
Dyspepsia	Esophageal reflux may be exacerbated during IL-2 cycles and may be treated with ranitidine (150 mg orally every 12 h).
Hypomagnesemia	Magnesium oxide (400 mg orally every 8 h). Certain magnesium preparations may exacerbate diarrhea.
Hypocalcemia	Oral calcium supplementation may be used; however, low calcium is usually coincident with low serum albumin and therefore does not need treatment.
Fluid imbalances/low output/hyponatremia	During IL-2 cycles, patients need encouragement to maintain hydration, preferably with "sports beverages" such as Gatorade (or with commercially prepared pediatric oral hydration solutions). Modest weight gains are to be expected. Urine output and specific gravity should be maintained at normal levels. Excessive weight again and low urinary output may respond to discontinuation of ibuprofen or other nonsteroidal antiinflammatory agents. Fluid deficits will usually respond to increased oral intake, but in the setting of hypotension an intravenous fluid bolus (e.g., 250–500 mL of normal saline may be necessary. Hyponatremia (serum sodium of <130 mmol/L) requires close monitoring; if serum sodium levels drop to 125 mmol/L or less, the IL-2 cycle should be interrupted or discontinued.

[a]Side effects other than mild to moderate ones and those that are not responsive to standard measures require dose reduction or cycle interruption (i.e., withholding one or more doses of IL-2), or discontinuation of the cycle. Cycles are not to be extended beyond the usual 5 days to compensate for missed doses during the cycle. Patients should be appropriately warned that a number of the agents mentioned in these guidelines may cause drowsiness and that the effect may be addictive when several such agents are combined.

Practical Considerations

Treatment of HIV-1 infection is not an FDA-approved indication for use of IL-2. Until the clinical benefit of IL-2 is demonstrated, it should primarily be administered as part of clinical trials designed to help elucidate the role of IL-2-in the management of HIV infections. In the interim, physicians and patients who elect to administer IL-2 on an "off label" basis outside of clinical trial settings must be aware of the spectrum of potential toxicities and be prepared to manage them appropriately. Patients with underlying autoimmune of inflammatory processes should probably not receive IL-2 because of a concern that it will exacerbate the process. Although the FDA-approved IL-2 labeling ("package insert") describes experience with the use of IL-2 in the treatment of malignancy which uses daily doses that are several-fold higher than those used in the treatment of HIV infection, the prescribing physician should be familiar with the information presented therein.

Prior to the first cycle, potential side effects should be reviewed in detail with the patient as should guidelines for their treatment (258). Patients should be aware that fevers and generalized aches and pains are to be expected and that routine activities of daily living will likely be disrupted. Around-the-clock availability of medical advice is essential for patients during IL-2 cycles, and they should be given guidelines as to when such advice should be sought.

Patients should be carefully evaluated prior to the start of each cycle. Any indication of an active inflammatory or infectious process, including any but the mildest upper respiratory infections, should delay the start of the cycle. Laboratory studies, including complete blood count and hepatic, renal, and electrolyte panels, should be checked and any new or significant abnormality investigated prior to the start of the cycle. Patients who do start cycles with clinical or laboratory abnormalities and those who develop them during cycles should be closely monitored. Women with childbearing potential should have a pregnancy test prior to each cycle. Thyroid function should be assessed periodically between cycles.

Many HIV-infected patients are co-infected with hepatitis B or hepatitis C. IL-2 has safely been administered to patients with both. Patients included in clinical trials have had only minimal elevations of hepatic aminotransferases and no stigmata of chronic liver disease at the time of enrollment in studies. Although more data would be reassuring, no long-term effects on liver disease have been noted in these patients. Indeed, IL-2 has been investigated in the treatment of chronic hepatitis B and no untoward effects were seen over the short term (259). A small study has provided evidence that hepatitis C viral loads actually tend to drop in HIV-infected patients after 6 months of therapy with IL-2 (260). Larger studies are needed to confirm this finding.

Subcutaneous injection (at a maximum dose of 7.5 mIU twice daily for 5 consecutive days) is the most practical method of IL-2 administration. The starting dose should be decreased in increments of 1.5 to 3.0 mIU to treat toxicities not responsive to standard measures. Cycles can be interrupted by withholding one or more doses of IL-2 for side effects when necessary. Cycles should be discontinued prematurely for severe toxicities or those unresponsive to more conservative measures. If during a cycle, the dose is reduced or doses are withheld, or if the cycle is prematurely discontinued due to toxicity, the subsequent cycle should generally be started at a lower dose. Because transient HIV activation is seen, concomitant antiviral therapy should be part of any IL-2 regimen.

Administration of IL-2 results in transient trafficking effects on lymphocytes, with marked shifts in the numbers of circulating $CD4^+$ cells during and after cycles. It is therefore not helpful to check $CD4^+$ lymphocyte counts during or immediately after IL-2 therapy since the results do not reflect long-term trends. Sustained effects are best assessed by evaluating $CD4^+$ lymphocyte trends at time points one to two months after cycles of IL-2 are completed.

Among patients who have demonstrated a significant increase in $CD4^+$ lymphocyte counts during an initial period when IL-2 cycles are repeated every eight weeks, individualized regimens can be used. Both the IL-2 dose and frequency of administration can usually be decreased while maintaining $CD4^+$ lymphocyte increases achieved during the initial, more intensive period of therapy. Patients initially treated with intravenous IL-2 can be switched to subcutaneous administration. These modified maintenance regimens can be based on a strategy designed to maintain the $CD4^+$ lymphocyte count above a predetermined level (e.g., at a level double the baseline value, or at a level above a threshold level such as 800 or 1,000 cells per mm^3). Such strategies often effect a decrease in the frequency of IL-2 cycles to one every 6 to 12 months, or even less often, thereby greatly improving tolerability of IL-2 therapy and convenience.

Some patients, even those with favorable predictors of response, fail to respond to IL-2. The reasons for this are not understood. An indication that this may be the case is usually evident after the first three to four cycles of IL-2 — at such time the risks and benefits of administering IL-2 should be reassessed.

OTHER USES OF IL-2

Viral, Bacterial, and Protozoal Infections

Even though the potential utility of IL-2 therapy in the treatment of a variety of infections has long been appreciated, remarkably few studies outside of HIV infection have been reported (59,261–263).

While two small preliminary reports suggested some efficacy in treating hepatitis B, subsequent trials of 37 patients found no significant differences in serum hepatitis B-DNA level among patients treated with either IL-2 (at relatively low daily doses) plus α-interferon or α-interferon alone for 5 months (259,264,265). In another small trial of 10 patients in which IL-2 was given at relatively low doses twice weekly, no patients cleared hepatitis B e antigen after three months of study (266). A preliminary dose-escalation study (maximum dose of 5.4 mIU administered by subcutaneous injection for 5 days each week) of IL-2 in 33 patients with chronic hepatitis C has been reported. After 24 weeks of study, aspartate aminotransferase levels and hepatitis C viral load levels were lower. However, all of the participants continued to have measurable hepatitis C viral loads. As mentioned previously, hepatitis C viral loads have also been noted to decrease in patients co-infected with HIV-1 who are treated with IL-2 (260).

Among bacterial infections, only multidrug-resistant tuberculosis (MDRTB) and lepromatous leprosy have been studied in any detail. Several intradermal regimens of low-dose IL-2 have been tried in small numbers of patients with MDRTB in conjunction with conventional antituberculous therapy (270–272). Some patients in these small, uncontrolled studies appeared to demonstrate improved bacillary clearance from sputum as well as improvement in radiographs along with *in vitro* evidence of enhanced immunity to *Mycobacterium tuberculosis.*Two small studies have shown that intradermal injections of low-dose IL-2 over relatively short periods of time cause a reduction in numbers of *Mycobacterium leprae* both in the area of injection and at remote skin sites (268,269). Other effects noted in these studies include cutaneous infiltration of $CD4^+$ lymphocytes, monocytes, and Langerhans' cells as well as increased levels of circulating antibody to *M. leprae* antigens. Inflammation at injection sites and regional lymphadenopathy were noted. A single study of three patients with disseminated cutaneous leishmaniasis demonstrated findings analogous to those reported in leprosy-namely, reduction in numbers of organisms in nodular lesions that were injected with IL-2 along with infiltration by $CD4^+$ lymphocytes and plasma cells (273).

Common Variable Immunodeficiency

IL-2 has been reported to be of benefit in common variable immunodeficiency (274,275). Results of a randomized, crossover trial of 10 patients who were also receiving intravenous gamma globulin (IVIG) have been reported (276). Although requirements for IVIG were not different between the groups receiving PEG IL-2 and placebo, fewer episodes of infection were noted during six months of follow-up in the group that initially received PEG IL-2.

IL-2 as Vaccine Adjuvant

Several cytokines, including IL-2, have been proposed as vaccine adjuvants (277). Results of small human trials of IL-2 as an adjuvant for hepatitis B virus vaccine have been reported. While a preliminary nonrandomized trial suggested that IL-2 promotes antibody responses in patients previously unresponsive to hepatitis B vaccine, a larger randomized trial of 52 hemodialysis patients showed no difference between groups that received IL-2 (74% seroconversion) and placebo (80% seroconversion) (278,279).

FUTURE DIRECTIONS

As discussed above, widespread use of IL-2 in the treatment of HIV infection awaits demonstration of clinical benefit. Large-scale, multicenter, international trials comparing the incidence of opportunistic events and mortality between groups treated with antiretroviral therapy plus intermittent cycles of IL-2 and antiretroviral therapy alone are underway.

A new potential use of IL-2 in the treatment of HIV infection has also emerged: activation of virus in long-lived, dormant T-cells. This theory holds that IL-2 used for this purpose would make latent pools of virus more amenable to eradication with conventional antiretroviral drugs that are only effective against actively replicating virus (280). However, a study in which HAART therapy was discontinued found that all patients had a rebound in viral load, including those who had been receiving IL-2, indicating latent, viable reservoirs from which virus could not be cultured (281,282).

Results from small studies reported to date do not provide sufficient information to predict the future of IL-2 in the treatment of other infections. Future trials will surely continue to focus on infections that are less than effectively treated by more conventional therapies and those that respond very slowly, or only partially, to existing therapies.

ACKNOWLEDGMENTS

The United States Government has been granted a patent for immunological enhancement with intermittent IL-2, listing Dr. Kovacs as an inventor.

REFERENCES

1. Gordon J. ML. A lymphocyte-stimulating factor produced in vitro. *Nature* 1965;208:795.
2. Kasakura L. A factor stimulating DNA synthesis derived from the medium of leucocyte cultures. *Nature* 1965; 208:794.
3. Smith KA. T-cell growth. factor. *Immunol Rev* 1980;51:337–357.
4. Ruscetti FW, Morgan DA, Gallo RC. Functional and morphologic characterization of human T cells continuously grown in vitro. *J Immunol* 1977;119:131–138.
5. Morgan DA, Ruscetti FW, Gallo R. Selective in vitro growth of T lymphocytes from normal human bone marrows. *Science* 1976;193:1007–1008.
6. Gillis S, Smith KA. Long term culture of tumour-specific cytotoxic T cells. *Nature* 1977;268:154–156.
7. Gillis S, Baker PE, Ruscetti FW, et al. Long-term culture of human antigen-specific cytotoxic T-cell lines. *J Exp Med* 1978;148:1093–1098.
8. Gillis S, Ferm MM, Ou W, et al. T cell growth factor: parameters of production and a quantitative microassay for activity. *J Immunol* 1978;120:2027–2032.
9. Gillis S. Interleukin 2: biology and biochemistry. *J Clin Immunol* 1983;3:1–13.
10. Smith KA, Favata MF, Oroszlan S. Production and characterization of monoclonal antibodies to human interleukin 2: strategy and tactics. *J Immunol* 1983;131:1808–1815.
11. Taniguchi T, Matsui H, Fujita T, et al. Structure and expression of a cloned cDNA for human interleukin-2. *Nature* 1983;302:305–310.
12. Devos R, Plaetinck G, Cheroutre H, et al. Molecular cloning of human interleukin 2 cDNA and its expression in E. coli. *Nucleic Acids Res* 1983;11:4307–4323.
13. Rosenberg SA, Grimm EA, McGrogan M, et al. Biological activity of recombinant human interleukin-2 produced in *Escherichia coli. Science* 1984;223:1412–1414.
14. Smith KA. Interleukin-2: inception, impact, and implications. *Science* 1988;240:1169–1176.
15. Kuziel WA, Greene WC. Interleukin-2 and the IL-2 receptor: new insights into structure and function. *J Invest Dermatol* 1990;94:27S–32S.
16. Cosman D, Cerretti DP, Larsen A, et al. Cloning, sequence and expression of human interleukin-2 receptor. *Nature* 1984;312:768–771.
17. Aarden LA. Revised nomenclature for antigen-nonspecific T cell proliferation helper factors. *J Immunol* 1979; 123:2928.
18. Lotze MT, Grimm EA, Mazumder A, et al. Lysis of fresh and cultured autologous tumor by human lymphocytes cultured in T-cell growth factor. *Cancer Res* 1981;41:4420–4425.
19. Burns GF, Triglia T, Werkmeister JA. In vitro generation of human activated lymphocyte killer cells: separate precursors and modes of generation of NK-like cells and "anomalous" killer cells. *J Immunol* 1984;133: 1656–1663.
20. Burns GF, Good MF, Riglar C, et al. Activated lymphocyte killer cells derived from melanoma tissue or peripheral blood. *Clin Exp Immunol* 1984;57:487–494.
21. Rosenberg SA, Lotze MT, Muul LM, et al. Observations on the systemic administration of autologous lymphokine-activated killer cells and recombinant interleukin-2 to patients with metastatic cancer. *N Engl J Med* 1985;313:1485–1492.
22. Donohue JH, Rosenberg SA. The fate of interleukin-2 after in vivo administration. *J Immunol* 1983;130: 2203–2208.
23. Donohue JH, Lotze MT, Robb RJ, et al. In vivo administration of purified Jurkat-derived interleukin 2 in mice. *Cancer Res* 1984;44:1380–1386.
24. Ettinghausen SE, Lipford EH, Mule JJ, et al. Recombinant interleukin 2 stimulates in vivo proliferation of adoptively transferred lymphokine-activated killer (LAK) cells. *J Immunol* 1985;135:3623–3635.
25. Ortaldo JR, Reynolds CW. Natural killer activity: definition of a function rather than a cell type. *J Immunol* 1987;138:4545–4546.
26. Mule JJ, Yang J, Shu S, et al. The anti-tumor efficacy of lymphokine-activated killer cells and recombinant interleukin 2 in vivo: direct correlation between reduction of established metastases and cytolytic activity of lymphokine-activated killer cells. *J Immunol* 1986;136:3899–3909.
27. Mule JJ, Shu S, Rosenberg SA. The anti-tumor efficacy of lymphokine-activated killer cells and recombinant interleukin 2 in vivo. *J Immunol* 1985;135:646–652.
28. Rosenberg SA, Mule JJ. Immunotherapy of cancer with lymphokine-activated killer cells and recombinant interleukin-2. *Surgery* 1985;98:437–444.
29. Thompson JA, Peace DJ, Klarnet JP, et al. Eradication of disseminated murine leukemia by treatment with high-dose interleukin 2. J *Immunol* 1986;137:3675–3680.
30. Rosenberg SA, Spiess P, Lafreniere R. A new approach to the adoptive immunotherapy of cancer with tumor-infiltrating lymphocytes. *Science* 1986;233:1318–1321.
31. Cheever MA, Greenberg PD, Fefer A. Potential for specific cancer therapy with immune T lymphocytes. *J Biol Response Mod* 1984;3:113–127.
32. Rosenberg SA, Lotze MT, Muul LM, et al. A progress report on the treatment of 157 patients with advanced cancer using lymphokine-activated killer cells and interleukin-2 or high-dose interleukin-2 alone. *N Engl J Med* 1987;316:889–897.

33. Rosenberg SA, Lotze MT, Yang JC, et al. Experience with the use of high-dose interleukin-2 in the treatment of 652 cancer patients. *Ann Surg* 1989;210:474–485.
34. Lotze MT, Chang AE, Seipp CA, et al. High-dose recombinant interleukin 2 in the treatment of patients with disseminated cancer: responses, treatment-related morbidity, and histologic findings. *JAMA* 1986;256:3117–3124.
35. West WH, Tauer KW, Yannelli JR, et al. Constant-infusion recombinant interleukin-2 in adoptive immunotherapy of advanced cancer. *N Engl J Med* 1987;316:898–905.
36. Fisher RI, Coltman CA Jr, Doroshow JH, et al. Metastatic renal cancer treated with interleukin-2 and lymphokine- activated killer cells. A phase II clinical trial. *Ann Intern Med* 1988;108:518–523.
37. Dillman RO, Church C, Oldham RK, et al. Inpatient continuous-infusion interleukin-2 in 788 patients with cancer. The National Biotherapy Study Group experience. *Cancer* 1993;71:2358–2370.
38. Voss SD, Sondel PM. The clinical biology and mechanisms of action of systemically administered IL-2. In: Mitchell MS, ed. *Biological approaches to cancer treatment.* New York: McGraw-Hill, 1993:411–439.
39. Fisher RI, Rosenberg SA, Sznol M, et al. High-dose aldesleukin in renal cell carcinoma: long-term survival update. *Cancer J Sci Am* 1997;3:570.
40. Parkinson DR, Abrams JS, Wiernik PH, et al. Interleukin-2 therapy in patients with metastatic malignant melanoma: a phase II study. *J Clin Oncol* 1990;8:1650–1656.
41. Rosenberg SA, Packard BS, Aebersold PM, et al. Use of tumor-infiltrating lymphocytes and interleukin-2 in the immunotherapy of patients with metastatic melanoma. A preliminary report. *N Engl J Med* 1988;319:1676–1680.
42. Parmiani G. An explanation of the variable clinical response to interleukin 2 and LAK cells. *Immunol Today* 1990;11:113–115.
43. Rubin JT, Lotze MT. Adoptive cellular immunotherapy of cancer. In: Mitchell MS, ed. *Biological approaches to cancer treatment.* 1st ed. New York: McGraw-Hill, 1993:379–410.
44. McCabe MS, Stablein D, Hawkins MJ. Phase III randomized trials of IL-2 vs. IL-2/LAK in advanced renal cell carcinoma and advanced melanoma. *Procedings of the American Society of Clinical Oncology* 1991; 10:231.
45. Rosenberg SA, Lotze MT, Yang JC, et al. Prospective randomized trial of high-dose interleukin-2 alone or in conjunction with lymphokine-activated killer cells for the treatment of patients with advanced cancer. *J Natl Cancer Inst* 1993;85:622–632.
46. Siegel JP, Puri RK. Interleukin-2 toxicity. *J Clin Oncol* 1991;9:694–704.
47. Lotze MT, Matory YL, Rayner AA, et al. Clinical effects and toxicity of interleukin-2 in patients with cancer. *Cancer* 1986;58:2764–2772.
48. Ettinghausen SE, Puri RK, Rosenberg SA. Increased vascular permeability in organs mediated by the systemic administration of lymphokine-activated killer cells and recombinant interleukin-2 in mice. *J Natl Cancer Inst* 1988;80:177–188.
49. Ognibene FP, Rosenberg SA, Lotze M, et al. Interleukin-2 administration causes reversible hemodynamic changes and left ventricular dysfunction similar to those seen in septic shock. *Chest* 1988;94:750–754.
50. Gaynor ER, Vitek L, Sticklin L, et al. The hemodynamic effects of treatment with interleukin-2 and lymphokine- activated killer cells. *Ann Intern Med* 1988;109:953–958.
51. White RL Jr, Schwartzentruber DJ, Guleria A, et al. Cardiopulmonary toxicity of treatment with high dose interleukin-2 in 199 consecutive patients with metastatic melanoma or renal cell carcinoma. *Cancer* 1994;74: 3212–3222.
52. Anonymous. Package Insert for Proleukin (human recominbnant interleukin-2). Emeryville, CA: Chiron Corporation, 1998.
53. Sznol M, Parkinson DR. Clinical applications of IL-2. *Oncology (Huntingt)* 1994;8:61–75.
54. Lotze MT, Agarwala SS, Kirkwood JM. Clinical applications of IL-2: the Sznol/Parkinson article reviewed. *Oncology* 1994;8:67–71.
55. Fefer A. Clinical applications of IL-2: the Sznol/Parkinson article reviewed. *Oncology* 1994;8:74–75.
56. Dillman RO. The clinical experience with interleukin-2 in cancer therapy. *Cancer Biother* 1994;9:183–209.
57. Smith KA. Interleukin 2. *Annu Rev Immunol* 1984;2:319–333.
58. Fauci AS, Macher AM, Longo DL, et al. NIH conference. Acquired immunodeficiency syndrome: epidemiologic, clinical, immunologic, and therapeutic considerations. *Ann Intern Med* 1984;100:92–106.
59. Siegel JP, Rook AH, Djeu JY, et al. Interleukin 2 therapy in infectious diseases: rationale and prospects. *Infection* 1984;12:298–302.
60. Lane HC, Siegel JP, Rook AH, et al. Use of interleukin-2 in patients with acquired immunodeficiency syndrome. *J Biol Response Mod* 1984;3:512–516.
61. Nicola NA, Hilton DJ. General classes and functions of four-helix bundle cytokines. In: Cytokines. 1999:1–65.
62. Brandhuber BJ, Boone T, Kenney WC, et al. Three-dimensional structure of interleukin-2. *Science* 1987;238: 1707–1709.
63. Bazan JF. Unraveling the structure of IL-2. *Science* 1992;257:410–413.
64. Robb RJ, Kutny RM, Panico M, et al. Posttranslational modification of human T-cell growth factor. *Biochem Biophys Res Commun* 1983;116:1049–1055.
65. Robb RJ, Kutny RM, Panico M, et al. Amino acid sequence and post-translational modification of human interleukin 2. *Proc Natl Acad Sci U S A* 1984;81:6486–6490.

66. Weir MP, Chaplin MA, Wallace DM, et al. Structure-activity relationships of recombinant human interleukin 2. *Biochemistry* 1988;27:6883–6892.
67. Zurawski SM, Zurawski G. Mouse interleukin-2 structure-function studies: substitutions in the first alpha-helix can specifically inactivate p70 receptor binding and mutations in the fifth alpha-helix can specifically inactivate p55 receptor binding. *Embo J* 1989;8:2583–2590.
68. Landgraf BE, Williams DP, Murphy JR, et al. Conformational perturbation of interleukin-2: a strategy for the design of cytokine analogs. *Proteins* 1991;9:207–216.
69. Kuo LM, Rusk CM, Robb RJ. Structure-function relationships for the IL 2-receptor system. II. Localization of an IL 2 binding site on high and low affinity receptors. *J Immunol* 1986;137:1544–1551.
70. Kuo LM, Robb RJ. Structure-function relationships for the IL 2-receptor system. I. Localization of a receptor binding site on IL 2. *J Immunol* 1986;137:1538–1543.
71. Ju G, Collins L, Kaffka KL, et al. Structure function analysis of human interleukin-2. Identification of amino acid residues required for biological activity. *J Biol Chem* 1987;262:5723–5731.
72. Collins L, Tsien WH, Seals C, et al. Identification of specific residues of human interleukin 2 that affect binding to the 70-kDa subunit (p70) of the interleukin 2 receptor. *Proc Natl Acad Sci USA* 1988;85: 7709–7713.
73. Taniguchi T, Matsui H, Fujita T, et al. Molecular analysis of the interleukin-2 system. *Immunol Rev* 1986;92: 121–133.
74. Fujita T, Takaoka C, Matsui H, et al. Structure of the human interleukin 2 gene. *Proc Natl Acad Sci USA* 1983; 80:7437–7441.
75. Holbrook NJ, Smith KA, Fornace AJ Jr, et al. T-cell growth factor: complete nucleotide sequence and organization of the gene in normal and malignant cells. *Proc Natl Acad Sci USA* 1984;81:1634–1638.
76. Seigel LJ, Harper ME, Wong-Staal F, et al. Gene for T-cell growth factor: location on human chromosome 4q and feline chromosome Bl. *Science* 1984;223:175–178.
77. Rothenberg EV, Ward SB. A dynamic assembly of diverse transcription factors integrates activation and cell-type information for interleukin 2 gene regulation. *Proc Natl Acad Sci USA* 1996;93:9358–9365.
78. Agarwal S, Rao A. Long-range transcriptional regulation of cytokine gene expression. *Curr Opin Immunol* 1998;10:345–352.
79. Hua J, Paetkau V. A binding factor for interleukin 2 mRNA. *Nucleic Acids Res* 1996;24:970–976.
80. Nelson BH, Willerford DM. Biology of the interleukin-2 receptor. *Adv Immunol* 1998;70:1–81.
81. Greene WC, Robb RJ, Svetlik PB, et al. Stable expression of cDNA encoding the human interleukin 2 receptor in eukaryotic cells. *J Exp Med* 1985;162:363–368.
82. Hatakeyama M, Minamoto S, Uchiyama T, et al. Reconstitution of functional receptor for human interleukin-2 in mouse cells. *Nature* 1985;318:467–470.
83. Matsuoka M, Takeshita T, Ishii N, et al. Kinetic study of interleukin-2 binding on the reconstituted interleukin-2 receptor complexes including the human gamma chain. *Eur J Immunol* 1993;23:2472–2476.
84. Anderson DM, Kumaki S, Ahdieh M, et al. Functional characterization of the human interleukin-15 receptor alpha chain and close linkage of IL15RA and IL2RA genes. *J Biol Chem* 1995;270:29862–29869.
85. Giri JG, Kumaki S, Ahdieh M, et al. Identification and cloning of a novel IL-15 binding protein that is structurally related to the alpha chain of the IL-2 receptor. *Embo J* 1995;14:3654–3663.
86. Rothenberg EV. The development of functionally responsive T cells. *Adv Immunol* 1992;51:85–214.
87. Godfrey DI, Zlotnik A. Control points in early T-cell development. *Immunol Today* 1993;14:547–553.
88. Hatakeyama M, Tsudo M, Minamoto S, et al. Interleukin-2 receptor beta chain gene: generation of three receptor forms by cloned human alpha and beta chain cDNA's. *Science* 1989;244:551–556.
89. Wang HM, Smith KA. The interleukin 2 receptor. Functional consequences of its bimolecular structure. *J Exp Med* 1987;166:1055–1069.
90. Lowenthal JW, Greene WC. Contrasting interleukin 2 binding properties of the alpha (p55) and beta (p70) protein subunits of the human high-affinity interleukin 2 receptor. *J Exp Med* 1987;166:1156–1161.
91. Ringheim GE, Freimark BD, Robb RJ. Quantitative characterization of the intrinsic ligand-binding affinity of the interleukin 2 receptor beta chain and its modulation by the alpha chain and a second affinity-modulating element. *Lymphokine Cytokine Res* 1991;10:219–224.
92. Shibuya H, Yoneyama M, Nakamura Y, et al. The human interleukin-2 receptor beta-chain gene: genomic organization, promoter analysis and chromosomal assignment. *Nucleic Acids Res* 1990;18:3697–3703.
93. Lin JX, Bhat NK, John S, et al. Characterization of the human interleukin-2 receptor beta-chain gene promoter: regulation of promoter activity by ets gene products. *Mol Cell Biol* 1993;13:6201–6210.
94. Lin JX, Leonard WJ. The immediate-early gene product Egr-1 regulates the human interleukin- 2 receptor beta-chain promoter through noncanonical Egr and Spl binding sites. *Mol Cell Biol* 1997;17:3714–3722.
95. Noguchi M, Adelstein S, Cao X, et al. Characterization of the human interleukin-2 receptor gamma chain gene. *J Biol Chem* 1993;268:13601–13608.
96. Buckley RH, Schiff RI, Schiff SE, et al. Human severe combined immunodeficiency: genetic, phenotypic, and functional diversity in one hundred eight infants. *J Pediatr* 1997;130:378–387.
97. Fischer A, Cavazzana-Calvo M, De Saint Basile G, et al. Naturally occurring primary deficiencies of the immune system. *Annu Rev Immunol* 1997;15:93–124.
98. Leonard WJ, Noguchi M, Russell SM, et al. The molecular basis of X-linked severe combined immunodefi-

ciency: the role of the interleukin-2 receptor gamma chain as a common gamma chain, gamma c. *Immunol Rev* 1994;138:61–86.
99. Grant AJ, Roessler E, Ju G, et al. The interleukin 2 receptor (IL-2R): the IL-2R alpha subunit alters the function of the IL-2R beta subunit to enhance IL-2 binding and signaling by mechanisms that do not require binding of IL-2 to IL-2R alpha subunit. *Proc Natl Acad Sci USA* 1992;89:2165–2169.
100. Roessler E, Grant A, Ju G, et al. Cooperative interactions between the interleukin 2 receptor alpha and beta chains alter the interleukin 2-binding affinity of the receptor subunits. *Proc Natl Acad Sci USA* 1994;91: 3344–3347.
101. Nakamura Y, Russell SM, Mess SA, et al. Heterodimerization of the IL-2 receptor beta- and gamma-chain cytoplasmic domains is required for signalling. *Nature* 1994;369:330–333.
102. Nelson BH, Lord JD, Greenberg PD. Cytoplasmic domains of the interleukin-2 receptor beta and gamma chains mediate the signal for T-cell proliferation. *Nature* 1994;369:333–336.
103. Saltzman EM, Thom RR, Casnellie JE. Activation of a tyrosine protein kinase is an early event in the stimulation of T lymphocytes by interleukin-2. *J Biol Chem* 1988;263:6956–6959.
104. Friedmann MC, Migone TS, Russell SM, et al. Different interleukin 2 receptor beta-chain tyrosines couple to at least two signaling pathways and synergistically mediate interleukin 2- induced proliferation. *Proc Natl Acad Sci USA* 1996;93:2077–2082.
105. Gaffen SL, Lai SY, Ha M, et al. Distinct tyrosine residues within the interleukin-2 receptor beta chain drive signal transduction specificity, redundancy, and diversity. *J Biol Chem* 1996;271:21381–21390.
106. Nelson BH, Lord JD, Greenberg PD. A membrane-proximal region of the interleukin-2 receptor gamma c chain sufficient for Jak kinase activation and induction of proliferation in T cells. *Mol Cell Biol* 1996;16:309–317.
107. Russell SM, Tayebi N, Nakajima H, et al. Mutation of Jak3 in a patient with SCID: essential role of Jak3 in lymphoid development. *Science* 1995;270:797–800.
108. Gilmour KC, Pine R, Reich NC. Interleukin 2 activates STAT5 transcription factor (mammary gland factor) and specific gene expression in T lymphocytes. *Proc Natl Acad Sci USA* 1995;92:10772–10776.
109. Frank DA, Robertson MJ, Bonni A, et al. Interleukin 2 signaling involves the phosphorylation of Stat proteins. *Proc Natl Acad Sci USA* 1995;92:7779–7783.
110. Nielsen M, Svejgaard A, Skov S, et al. Interleukin-2 induces tyrosine phosphorylation and nuclear translocation of stat3 in human T lymphocytes. *Eur J Immunol* 1994;24:3082–3086.
111. Beadling C, Ng J, Babbage JW, et al. Interleukin-2 activation of STAT5 requires the convergent action of tyrosine kinases and a serine/threonine kinase pathway distinct from the Rafl/ERK2 MAP kinase pathway. *Embo J* 1996;15:1902–1913.
112. Wen Z, Zhong Z, Darnell JE Jr. Maximal activation of transcription by Statl and Stat3 requires both tyrosine and serine phosphorylation. *Cell* 1995;82:241–250.
113. Kirken RA, Malabarba MG, Xu J, et al. Two discrete regions of interleukin-2 (IL2) receptor beta independently mediate IL2 activation of a PD98059/rapamycin/wortmannin-insensitive Stat5a/b serine kinase. *J Biol Chem* 1997;272:15459–15465.
114. Lecine P, Algarte M, Rameil P, et al. Elf-1 and Stat5 bind to a critical element in a new enhancer of the human interleukin-2 receptor alpha gene. *Mol Cell Biol* 1996;16:6829–6840.
115. John S, Robbins CM, Leonard WJ. An IL-2 response element in the human IL-2 receptor alpha chain promoter is a composite element that binds Stat5, Elf-1, HMG-I(Y) and a GATA family protein. *Embo J* 1996;15: 5627–5635.
116. Nakajima H, Liu XW, Wynshaw-Boris A, et al. An indirect effect of Stat5a in IL-2-induced proliferation: a critical role for Stat5a in IL-2-mediated IL-2 receptor alpha chain induction. *Immunity* 1997;7:691–701.
117. Kawahara A, Minami Y, Miyazaki T, et al. Critical role of the interleukin 2 (IL-2) receptor gamma-chain- associated Jak3 in the IL-2-induced c-fos and c-myc, but not bcl-2, gene induction. *Proc Natl Acad Sci USA* 1995;92:8724–8728.
118. Graves JD, Downward J, Izquierdo-Pastor M, et al. The growth factor IL-2 activates p21ras proteins in normal human T lymphocytes. *J Immunol* 1992;148:2417–2422.
119. Satoh T, Minami Y, Kono T, et al. Interleukin 2–induced activation of Ras requires two domains of interleukin 2 receptor beta subunit, the essential region for growth stimulation and Lck-binding domain. *J Biol Chem* 1992;267:25423—25427.
120. Chen CY, Faller DV. Direction of p21ras-generated signals towards cell growth or apoptosis is determined by protein kinase C and Bcl-2. *Oncogene* 1995;11:1487–1498.
121. Augustine JA, Sutor SL, Abraham RT. Interleukin 2- and polyomavirus middle T antigen-induced modification of phosphatidylinositol 3-kinase activity in activated T lymphocytes. *Mol Cell Biol* 1991;11:4431–4440.
122. Merida I, Diez E, Gaulton GN. IL-2 binding activates a tyrosine-phosphorylated phosphatidylinositol-3- kinase.J *Immunol* 1991;147:2202–2207.
123. Ahmed NN, Grimes HL, Bellacosa A, et al. Transduction of interleukin-2 antiapoptotic and proliferative signals via Akt protein kinase. *Proc Natl Acad Sci USA* 1997;94:3627–3632.
124. Gonzalez-Garcia A, Merida I, Martinez AC, et al. Intermediate affinity interleukin-2 receptor mediates survival via a phosphatidylinositol 3-kinase–dependent pathway. *J Biol Chem* 1997;272:10220–10226.
125. Reif K, Burgering BM, Cantrell DA. Phosphatidylinositol 3-kinase links the interleukin-2 receptor to protein kinase B and p70 S6 kinase. *J Biol Chem* 1997;272:14426–14433.
126. Monfar M, Lemon KP, Grammer TC, et al. Activation of pp70/85 S6 kinases in interleukin-2-responsive lym-

phoid cells is mediated by phosphatidylinositol 3-kinase and inhibited by cyclic AMP. *Mol Cell Biol* 1995;15: 326–337.
127. Gomez J, Martinez C, Garcia A, et al. Association of phosphatidylinositol 3 kinase to protein kinase C zeta during interleukin-2 stimulation. *Eur J Immunol* 1996;26:1781–1787.
128. Gomez J, Garcia A, Borlado R, et al. IL,-2 signaling controls actin organization through Rho-like protein family, phosphatidylinositol 3-kinase, and protein kinase C-zeta. *J Immunol* 1997;158:1516–1522.
129. Johnston JA, Wang LM, Hanson EP, et al. Interleukins 2, 4, 7, and 15 stimulate tyrosine phosphorylation of insulin receptor substrates 1 and 2 in T cells. Potential role of JAK kinases. *J Biol Chem* 1995;270:28527–28530.
130. Hatakeyama M, Kono T, Kobayashi N, et al. Interaction of the IL-2 receptor with the src-family kinase p561ck: identification of novel intermolecular association. *Science* 1991;252:1523–1528.
131. Horak ID, Gress RE, Lucas PJ, et al. T-lymphocyte interleukin 2-dependent tyrosine protein kinase signal transduction involves the activation of p561ck. *Proc Natl Acad Sci USA* 1991;88:1996–2000.
132. Molina TJ, Kishihara K, Siderovski DP, et al. Profound block in thymocyte development in mice lacking p561ck. *Nature* 1992;357:161–164.
133. Adachi M, Ishino M, Torigoe T, et al. Interleukin-2 induces tyrosine phosphorylation of SHP-2 through IL-2 receptor beta chain. *Oncogene* 1997;14:1629–1633.
134. Gesbert F, Garbay C, Bertoglio J. Interleukin-2 stimulation induces tyrosine phosphorylation of pl20-Cbl and CrkL and formation of multimolecular signaling complexes in T lymphocytes and natural killer cells. *J Biol Chem* 1998;273:3986–3993.
135. Gesbert F, Delespine-Carmagnat M, Bertoglio J. Recent advances in the understanding of interleukin-2 signal transduction. *J Clin Immunol* 1998;18:307–320.
136. Karnitz LM, Abraham RT. Interleukin-2 receptor signaling mechanisms. *Adv Immunol* 1996;61:147–199.
137. Gomez J, Gonzalez A, Martinez AC, et al. IL-2–induced cellular events. *Crit Rev Immunol* 1998;18:185–220.
138. Ishida Y, Nishi M, Taguchi O, et al. Effects of the deregulated expression of human interleukin-2 in transgenic mice. *Int Immunol* 1989;1:113–120.
139. Allison J, Malcolm L, Chosich N, et al. Inflammation but not autoimmunity occurs in transgenic mice expressing constitutive levels of interleukin-2 in islet beta cells. *Eur J Immunol* 1992;22:1115–1121.
140. Kroemer G, de Cid R, Moreno de Alboran I, et al. Immunological self-tolerance: an analysis employing cytokines or cytokine receptors encoded by transgenes or a recombinant vaccinia virus. *Immunol Rev* 1991;122: 173–204.
141. Ishida Y, Nishi M, Taguchi O, et al. Expansion of natural killer cells but not T cells in human interleukin 2/interleukin 2 receptor (Tac) transgenic mice. *J Exp Med* 1989;170:1103–1115.
142. Suwa H, Tanaka T, Kitamura F, et al. Dysregulated expression of the IL-2 receptor beta-chain abrogates development of NK cells and Thy-1^+ dendritic epidermal cells in transgenic mice. *Int Immunol* 1995;7:1441–1449.
143. DiSanto JP. Cytokines: shared receptors, distinct functions. *Curr Biol* 1997;7:8424–8426.
144. Carson WE, Fehniger TA, Haldar S, et al. A potential role for interleukin-15 in the regulation of human natural killer cell survival. *J Clin Invest* 1997;99:937–943.
145. Schorle H, Holtschke T, Hunig T, et al. Development and function of T cells in mice rendered interleukin-2 deficient by gene targeting. *Nature* 1991;352:621–624.
146. Willerford DM, Chen J, Ferry JA, et al. Interleukin-2 receptor alpha chain regulates the size and content of the peripheral lymphoid compartment. *Immunity* 1995;3:521–530.
147. Kundig TM, Schorle H, Bachmann MF, et al. Immune responses in interleukin-2-deficient mice. *Science* 1993; 262:1059–1061.
148. Kramer S, Schimpl A, Hunig T. Immunopathology of interleukin (IL)–2–deficient mice: thymus dependence and suppression by thymus-dependent cells with an intact IL-2 gene. *J Exp Med* 1995;182:1769–1776.
149. Sadlack B, Merz H, Schorle H, et al. Ulcerative colitis–like disease in mice with a disrupted interleukin-2 gene. *Cell* 1993;75:253–261.
150. Lohler J, Sadlack B, Schorle H, et al. Generalized autoimmune diseases in BALB/c mice with a genetically dependent interleukin-2 deficiency. *Verh Dtsch Ges Pathol* 1996;80:293–296.
151. Ma A, Datta M, Margosian E, et al. T cells, but not B cells, are required for bowel inflammation in interleukin 2–deficient mice. *J Exp Med* 1995;182:1567–1572.
152. Contractor NV, Bassiri H, Reya T, et al. Lymphoid hyperplasia, autoimmunity, and compromised intestinal intraepithelial lymphocyte development in colitis-free gnotobiotic IL-2– deficient mice. *J Immunol* 1998;160: 385–394.
153. Ludviksson BR, Gray B, Strober W, et al. Dysregulated intrathymic development in the IL-2–deficient mouse leads to colitis-inducing thymocytes. *J Immunol* 1997;158:104–111.
154. Ehrhardt RO, Ludviksson BR, Gray B, et al. Induction and prevention of colonic inflammation in IL-2-deficient mice. *J Immunol* 1997;158:566–573.
155. Lenardo ML. Interleukin-2 programs mouse alpha beta T lymphocytes for apoptosis. *Nature*1991;353:858–861.
156. Kneitz B, Herrmann T, Yonehara S, et al. Normal clonal expansion but impaired Fas-mediated cell death and anergy induction in interleukin-2–deficient mice. *Eur J Immunol* 1995;25:2572–2577.
157. Van Parijs L, Biuckians A, Ibragimov A, et al. Functional responses and apoptosis of CD25 (IL-2R alpha)–deficient T cells expressing a transgenic antigen receptor. *J Immunol* 1997;158:3738–3745.
158. Xiao S, Matsui K, Fine A, et al. FasL promoter activation by IL-2 through SP1 and NFAT but not Egr-2 and Egr-3. *Eur J Immunol* 1999;29:3456–3465.

159. Ayroldi E, Zollo O, Cannarile L, et al. Interleukin-6 (IL-6) prevents activation-induced cell death: IL-2–independent inhibition of Fas/fasL expression and cell death. *Blood* 1998;92:4212–4219.
160. Refaeli Y, Abbas AK. Role of cytokines in autoimmunity. *Eur Cytokine Netw* 1998;9:81–82.
161. Van Parijs L, Perez VL, Abbas AK. Mechanisms of peripheral T cell tolerance. *Novartis Found Symp* 1998; 215:5–14.
162. Rodella L, Rezzani R, Zauli G, et al. Apoptosis induced by NK cells is modulated by the NK-active cytokines IL-2 and IL-12. *Int Immunol* 1998;10:719–725.
163. Kung JT, Beller D, Ju ST. Lymphokine regulation of activation-induced apoptosis in T cells of IL-2 and IL-2R beta knockout mice. *Cell Immunol* 1998;185:158–163.
164. Refaeli Y, Van Parijs L, London CA, et al. Biochemical mechanisms of IL-2–regulated Fas-mediated T cell apoptosis. *Immunity* 1998;8:615–623.
165. Wong B, Arron J, Choi Y. T cell receptor signals enhance susceptibility to Fas-mediated apoptosis. *J Exp Med* 1997;186:1939–1944.
166. Chung CD, Lewis LA, Miceli MC. T cell antigen receptor–induced IL-2 production and apoptosis have different requirements for Lck activities. *J Immunol* 1997;159:1758–1766.
167. Eischen CM, Williams BL, Zhang W, et al. ZAP-70 tyrosine kinase is required for the up-regulation of Fas ligand in activation-induced T cell apoptosis. *J Immunol* 1997;159:1135–1139.
168. Esser MT, Dinglasan RD, Krishnamurthy B, et al. IL-2 induces Fas ligand/Fas (CD95L/CD95) cytotoxicity in $CD8^+$ and $CD4^+$ T lymphocyte clones. *J Immunol* 1997;158:5612–5618.
169. Lorenz HM, Hieronymus T, Grunke M, et al. Differential role for IL-2 and IL-15 in the inhibition of apoptosis in short-term activated human lymphocytes. *Scand J Immunol* 1997;45:660–669.
170. Suda T, Okazaki T, Naito Y, et al. Expression of the Fas ligand in cells of T cell lineage. *J Immunol* 1995; 154:3806–3813.
171. Lowry RP, Goebel J. Down-modulation of IL-2–triggered JAK3-STAT5 signaling following $CD4^-$ ligand binding. *Transplant Proc* 1999;31:820–821.
172. Van Parijs L, Refaeli Y, Lord JD, et al. Uncoupling IL-2 signals that regulate T cell proliferation, survival, and Fas-mediated activation-induced cell death. *Immunity* 1999;11:281–288.
173. Matsui K, Jodo S, Xiao S, et al. Hypothesis: A recurrent, moderate activation fosters systemic autoimmunity—the apoptotic roles of TCR, IL-2 and Fas ligand. *J Biomed Sci* 1999;6:306–313.
174. Irmler M, Thorne M, Hahne M, et al. Inhibition of death receptor signals by cellular FLIP. *Nature* 1997; 388:190–195.
175. Chong KT. Prophylactic administration of interleukin-2 protects mice from lethal challenge with gram-negative bacteria. *Infect Immun* 1987;55:668–673.
176. Iizawa Y, Nishi T, Kondo M, et al. Effect of recombinant human interleukin-2 on the course of experimental chronic respiratory tract infection caused by *Klebsiella pneumoniae* in mice. *Infect Immun* 1988;56:45–50.
177. Colizzi V. In vivo and in vitro administration of interleukin-2–containing preparation reverses T-cell unresponsiveness in *Mycobacterium bovis* BCG-infected mice. *Infect Immun* 1984;45:25–28.
178. Jeevan A, Asherson GL. Recombinant interleukin-2 limits the replication of *Mycobacterium lepraemurium* and *Mycobacterium bovis* BCG in mice. *Infect Immun* 1988;56:660–664.
179. Bermudez LE, Stevens P, Kolonoski P, et al. Treatment of experimental disseminated Mycobacterium avium complex infection in mice with recombinant IL-2 and tumor necrosis factor. *J Immunol* 1989;143:2996–3000.
180. Kuroda K, Yagi J, Imanishi K, et al. Implantation of IL-2–containing osmotic pump prolongs the survival of superantigen-reactive T cells expanded in mice injected with bacterial superantigen. *J Immunol* 1996;157: 1422–1431.
181. Daley M, Williams T, Coyle P, et al. Prevention and treatment of *Staphylococcus aureus* infections with recombinant cytokines. *Cytokine* 1993;5:276–284.
182. Choromanski L, Kuhn RE. Use of parasite antigens and interleukin-2 to enhance suppressed immune responses during *Trypanosoma cruzi* infection in mice. *Infect Immun* 1987;55:403–408.
183. Sharma SD, Hofflin JM, Remington JS. In vivo recombinant interleukin 2 administration enhances survival against a lethal challenge with *Toxoplasma gondii*. *J Immunol* 1985;135:4160–4163.
184. Ghiasi H, Cai S, Slanina SM, et al. The role of interleukin (IL)–2 and IL-4 in herpes simplex virus type 1 ocular replication and eye disease. *J Infect Dis* 1999;179:1086–1093.
185. Wiryana P, Bui T, Faltynek CR, et al. Augmentation of cell-mediated immunotherapy against herpes simplex virus by interleukins: comparison of in vivo effects of IL-2 and IL-7 on adoptively transferred T cells. *Vaccine* 1997;15:561–563.
186. Nakao M, Hazama M, Mayumi-Aono A, et al. Immunotherapy of acute and recurrent herpes simplex virus type 2 infection with an adjuvant-free form of recombinant glycoprotein D–interleukin-2 fusion protein. *J Infect Dis* 1994;169:787–791.
187. Dix RD, Giedlin M, Cousins SW. Systemic cytokine immunotherapy for experimental cytomegalovirus retinitis in mice with retrovirus-induced immunodeficiency. *Invest Ophthalmol Vis Sci* 1997;38:1411–1417.
188. Baldwin SL, D'Souza C, Roberts AD, et al. Evaluation of new vaccines in the mouse and guinea pig model of tuberculosis. *Infect Immun* 1998;66:2951–2959.
189. Barouch DH, Santra S, Steenbeke TD, et al. Augmentation and suppression of immune responses to an HIV-1 DNA vaccine by plasmid cytokine/Ig administration. *J Immunol* 1998;161:1875–1882.

190. Smith KA, Jacobson EL, Emert R, et al. Restoration of immunity with interleukin-2 therapy. *AIDS Reader* 1999;9:563–572.
191. Piscitelli SC, Minor JR, Saville MW, et al. Immune-based therapies for treatment of HIV infection. *Ann Pharmacother* 1996;30:62–76.
192. Quinnan GV Jr, Kirmani N, Rook AH, et al. Cytotoxic T cells in cytomegalovirus infection: HLA-restricted T-lymphocyte and non-T-lymphocyte cytotoxic responses correlate with recovery from cytomegalovirus infection in bone-marrow–transplant recipients. *N Engl J Med* 1982;307:7–13.
193. Rook AH, Masur H, Lane HC, et al. Interleukin-2 enhances the depressed natural killer and cytomegalovirus-specific cytotoxic activities of lymphocytes from patients with the acquired immune deficiency syndrome. *J Clin Invest* 1983;72:398–403.
194. Rook AH, Hooks JJ, Quinnan GV, et al. Interleukin 2 enhances the natural killer cell activity of acquired immunodeficiency syndrome patients through a gamma-interferon– independent mechanism. *J Immunol* 1985; 134:1503–1507.
195. Lifson JD, Benike CJ, Mark DF, et al. Human recombinant interleukin-2 partly reconstitutes deficient in-vitro immune responses of lymphocytes from patients with AIDS. *Lancet* 1984;1:698–702.
196. Murray HW, Welte K, Jacobs JL, et al. Production of and in vitro response to interleukin 2 in the acquired immunodeficiency syndrome. *J Clin Invest* 1985;76:1959–1964.
197. Mertelsmann R, Welte K, Sternberg C, et al. Treatment of immunodeficiency with interleukin-2: initial exploration. *J Biol Response Mod* 1984;3:483–490.
198. Kern P, Toy J, Dietrich M. Preliminary clinical observations with recombinant interleukin-2 in patients with AIDS or LAS. *Blut* 1985;50:1–6.
199. Gramatzki M, Nusslein H, Burmester GR, et al. Intralymphatic interleukin 2 treatment in patients with acquired immunodeficiency syndrome: preliminary experience in three cases. *Immunobiology* 1986;172:438–447.
200. Flad HD, Ernst M, Kern P. A phase I/II trial of recombinant interleukin-2 in AIDS/ARC: alterations of phenotypes of peripheral blood mononuclear cells. *Lymphokine Res* 1986;5:S171–S176.
201. Gramatzki M, Burmester GR, Heyder N, et al. Intralymphatic interleukin-2 treatment of a hemophiliac AIDS patient with defective interleukin-2 production. *Klin Wochenschr* 1987;65:380–386.
202. Volberding P, Moody DJ, Beardslee D, et al. Therapy of acquired immune deficiency syndrome with recombinant interleukin-2. *AIDS Res Hum Retroviruses* 1987;3:115–124.
203. Schnittman SM, Vogel S, Baseler M, et al. A phase I study of interferon-alpha 2b in combination with interleukin-2 in patients with human immunodeficiency virus infection. *J Infect Dis* 1994;169:981–989.
204. Ernst M, Kern P, Flad HD, et al. Effects of systemic in vivo interleukin-2 (IL-2) reconstitution in patients with acquired immune deficiency syndrome (AIDS) and AIDS- related complex (ARC) on phenotypes and functions of peripheral blood mononuclear cells (PBMC). *J Clin Immunol* 1986;6:170–181.
205. Lissoni P, Vigore L, Rescaldani R, et al. Neuroimmunotherapy with low-dose subcutaneous interleukin-2 plus melatonin in AIDS patients with CD4 cell number below 200/mm3: a biological phase-II study. *J Biol Regul Homeost Agents* 1995;9:155–158.
206. Clark AG, Holodniy M, Schwartz DH, et al. Decrease in HIV provirus in peripheral blood mononuclear cells during zidovudine and human rIL-2 administration. *J Acquir Immune Defic Syndr* 1992;5:52–59.
207. Schwartz DH, Merigan TC. Interleukin-2 in the treatment of HIV disease. *Biotherapy* 1990;2:119–136.
208. Kovacs JA, Baseler M, Dewar RJ, et al. Increases in CD4 T lymphocytes with intermittent courses of interleukin-2 in patients with human immunodeficiency virus infection. A preliminary study. *N Engl J Med* 1995; 332:567–575.
209. Schwartz DH, Skowron G, Merigan TC. Safety and effects of interleukin-2 plus zidovudine in asymptomatic individuals infected with human immunodeficiency virus. *J Acquir Immune Defic Syndr* 1991;4:11–23.
210. Ramachandran RV, Katzenstein D, Merigan TC. Long-term effects of interleukin-2 on CD4 cell counts in human immunodeficiency virus–infected patients. *J Infect Dis* 1994;170:1044–1046.
211. Mazza P, Bocchia M, Tumietto F, et al. Recombinant interleukin–2 (rIL-2) in acquired immune deficiency syndrome (AIDS): preliminary report in patients with lymphoma associated with HIV infection. *Eur J Haematol* 1992;49:1–6.
212. Kovacs JA, Vogel S, Albert JM, et al. Controlled trial of interleukin-2 infusions in patients infected with the human immunodeficiency virus. *N Engl J Med* 1996;335:1350–1356.
213. Kovacs JA, Davey RTJ, Lane HC. Interleukin-2 infusions in HIV-infected patients. *N Engl J Med* 1997;336: 1260.
214. Wood R, Montoya JG, Kundu SK, et al. Safety and efficacy of polyethylene glycol-modified interleukin-2 and zidovudine in human immunodeficiency virus type 1 infection: a phase I/II study. *J Infect Dis* 1993;167 :519–525.
215. Ramachandran R, Katzenstein DA, Winters MA, et al. Polyethylene glycol–modified interleukin-2 and thymosin alpha 1 in human immunodeficiency virus type 1 infection. *J Infect Dis* 1996;173:1005–1008.
216. Meyers FJ, Paradise C, Scudder SA, et al. A phase I study including pharmacokinetics of polyethylene glycol conjugated interleukin-2. *Clin Pharmacol Ther* 1991;49:307–313.
217. Carr A, Emery S, Lloyd A, et al. Outpatient continuous intravenous interleukin-2 or subcutnaous polyethylene glycol–modified interleukin-2 in human immunodeficiency virus–infected patients: a randomized, controlled, multicenter study. *J Infect Dis* 1998;178:992–999.

218. Davey RT Jr, Chaitt DG, Piscitelli SC, et al. Subcutaneous administration of interleukin-2 in human immunodeficiency virus type 1–infected persons. *J Infect Dis* 1997;175:781–789.
219. Piscitelli SC, Wells MJ, Metcalf JA, et al. Pharmacokinetics and pharmacodynamics of subcutaneous interleukin-2 in HIV-infected patients. *Pharmacotherapy* 1996;16:754–759.
220. Piscitelli SC, Forrest A, Vogel S, et al. Pharmacokinetic modeling of recombinant interleukin-2 in patients with human immunodeficiency virus infection. *Clin Pharmacol Ther* 1998;64:492–498.
221. Davey R, Chaitt D, Piscitelli S, et al. A randomized trial of high- versus low-dose subcutancous interleukin-2 outpatient therpy for early human immunodeficiency virus type 1 infection. *J Infect Dis* 1999;179:849–858.
222. Levy Y, Capitant C, Houhou S, et al. Comparison of subcutaneous and intravenous interleukin-2 in asymptomatic HIV-1 infection: a randomised controlled trial. ANRS 048 study group. *Lancet* 1999;353:1923–1929.
223. De Paoli P, Zanussi S, Simonelli C, et al. Effects of subcutaneous interleukin-2 therapy on CD4 subsets and in vitro cytokine production in HIV^+ subjects. *J Clin Invest* 1997;100:2737–2743.
224. Arno A, Ruiz L, Juan M, et al. Efficacy of low-dose subcutaneous interleukin-2 to treat advanced human immunodeficiency virus type 1. *J Infect Dis* 1999;180:56–60.
225. Bartlett JA. Coadministration of zidovudine and interlukin-2 increases absolute CD4 cells in subjects with Walter Reed Stage 2 Human Immunodericiency Virus Infection: results of ACTG Protocol 042. *J Infect Dis* 1998;178:1170–1173.
226. Hengge UR, Goos M, Esser S, et al. Randomized, controlled phase II trial of subcutaneous interleukin-2 in combination with highly active antiretroviral therapy (HAART) in HIV patients. *AIDS* 1998;12:F225–F234.
227. Simonelli C, Zanussi S, Sandri S, et al. Concomitant therapy with subcutaneous interleukin-2 and zidovudine plus didanosine in patients with early stage HIV infection. *J Acquir Immune Defic Syndr Hum Retrovirol* 1999;20:20–27.
228. Ruxrungtham K, Suwannagool S, Cheuyam M, et al. Dose escalating and biological response study of subcutaneous (sc) IL-2 in HIV-infected Thai patients: the Vanguard study. Australian Society of HIV Medicine Conference, Perth, Australia, 1999.
229. Losso M, Belloso W, Benetucci J, et al. Twenty-month follow-up of the Argentina Vanguard study: a randomized, controlled, phase II trial of intermittent subcutaneous interleukin-2 (scIL2) plus antiretroviral therapy (ARV) vs. ARV alone (Abstract 380). 7th Conference on Retroviruses and Opportunistic Infection, San Francisco, 2000.
230. Falloon J, Owen C, Metcalf J, et al. Indinavir and interleukin-2 in HIV: one year follow-up (Abstract 1108). 36th Interscience Conference on Antimicrobial Agents and Chemotherapy (ICAAC), Toronto, 1997.
231. Katlama C, Duvivier C, Chouquet C, et al. ILSTIM (ANRS 082) A randomized comparative open-label study of interleukin 2(IL2) in patients with CD4 <2000/mm^3 despite effective HAART (Abstract 543). 7th Conference on Retroviruses and Opportunistic Infections, San Francisco, 2000.
232. Teppler H, Kaplan G, Smith KA, et al. Prolonged immunostimulatory effect of low-dose polyethylene glycol interleukin 2 in patients with human immunodeficiency virus type 1 infection. *J Exp Med* 1993;177:483–492.
233. Teppler H, Kaplan G, Smith K, et al. Efficacy of low doses of the polyethylene glycol derivative of interleukin-2 in modulating the immune response of patients with human immunodeficiency virus type 1 infection. *J Infect Dis* 1993;167:291–298.
234. McMahon DK, Armstrong JA, Huang XL, et al. A phase I study of subcutaneous recombinant interleukin-2 in patients with advanced HIV disease while on zidovudine. *AIDS* 1994;8:59–66.
235. Bernstein ZP, Porter MM, Gould M, et al. Prolonged administration of low-dose interleukin-2 in human immunodeficiency virus–associated malignancy results in selective expansion of innate immune effectors without significant clinical toxicity. *Blood* 1995;86:3287–3294.
236. Khatri VP, Fehniger TA, Baiocchi RA, et al. Ultra low dose interleukin-2 therapy promotes a type 1 cytokine profile in vivo in patients with AIDS and AIDS-associated malignancies. *J Clin Invest* 1998;101:1373–1378.
237. Jacobson EL, Pilaro F, Smith KA. Rational interleukin 2 therapy for HIV positive individuals: daily low doses enhance immune function without toxicity. *Proc Natl Acad Sci USA* 1996;93:10405–10410.
238. Lalazari J, Beal J, Ruane P, et al. Low-dose subcutaneous (SC) IL-2 in combination with HAART therapy induces significant increases in NK cells and naive T-cells in patients with <300 $CD4^+$ T-cells/mm3 results of a randomized controlled trial. 7th Conference on Retroviruses and Opportunistic Infections, San Francisco, 2000.
239. Kelleher AD, Roggensack M, Emery S, et al. Effects of IL-2 therapy in asymptomatic HIV-infected individuals on proliferative responses to mitogens, recall antigens and HIV-related antigens. *Clin Exp Immunol* 1998; 113:85–91.
240. Giedlin M, McGrath M, Gascon R, et al. Immunological characterization of HIV seropositive patients treated with subcutaneous Proleukin (aldesleukin) recombinant interleukin-2 (Abstract Th.B.4183). XI International Conference on AIDS, Vancouver, BC, Canada, 1996.
241. Emery S, Capra WB, Cooper DA, et al. Pooled analysis of 3 randomized, controlled trials of interleukin-2 therapy in adult human immunodeficiency virus type 1 disease. *J Infect Dis* 2000;182:428–434.
242. Cohen J. Ambitious clinical trial stirs debate. *Science* 1999;285:41–42.
243. Kovacs JA, Vogel S, Metcalf JA, et al. Interleukin-2 induced immune effects in human immunodeficiency virus-infected patients receiving intermittent interleukin-2 therapy. *Eur J Immunol* 2001;31:1351–1360.
244. Miller KD, Spooner K, Herpin BR, et al. Immunotherapy of HIV-infected patients with intermittent interleukin-2: effect of cycle frequency and duration on degree of $CD4^+$ T-lymphocyte expansion. *Clinical Immunology* 2001;99:30–42.
245. Saravolatz L, Mitsuyasu R, Sneller M, et al. Duration of Proleukin IL-2 therapy is more important than total

dose in achieving CD4 expansion (Abstract 1149). Interscience Conference on Antimicrobial Agents and Chemotherapy (ICAAC), New Orleans, 1996.
246. Walworth CM, Kovacs JA, Vogel SE, et al. Factors associated with symptomatic interleukin-2 induced cholecystopathy in HIV-infected individuals (Abstract G30). Interscience Conference on Antimicrobial Agents and Chemotherapy (ICAAC), New Orleans, 1996.
247. Prummer O. Treatment-induced antibodies to interleukin-2. *Biotherapy* 1997;10:15–24.
248. Sumida S, Miller K, Vogel S, et al. Hypothyroidism is associated with IL-2 therapy in a randomized controlled trial (RCT) of IL-2 treatment of HIV-infection. 36th Annual Meeting of the Infectious Diseases Society of America (IDSA), Denver, 1998.
249. Snydman DR, Sullivan B, Gill M, et al. Nosocomial sepsis associated with interleukin-2. *Ann Intern Med* 1990; 112:102–107.
250. Murphy PM, Lane HC, Gallin JI, et al. Marked disparity in incidence of bacterial infections in patients with the acquired immunodeficiency syndrome receiving interleukin-2 or interferon-gamma. *Ann Intern Med* 1988;108:36–41.
251. Klempner MS, Noring R, Mier JW, et al. An acquired chemotactic defect in neutrophils from patients receiving interleukin-2 immunotherapy. *N Engl J Med* 1990;322:959–965.
252. Pockaj BA, Topalian SL, Steinberg SM, et al. Infectious complications associated with interleukin-2 administration: a retrospective review of 935 treatment courses. *J Clin Oncol* 1993;11:136–147.
253. Barrick B, Vogel SE, Dugan FA, et al. Quality of life and symptom distress in HIV-infected persons receiving intravenous interleukin-2 (IL-2) (Abstract We.B.3201). XI International Conference on AIDS, Vancouver, BC, Canada, 1996.
254. Dubinett SM, Huang M, Lichtenstein A, et al. Tumor necrosis factor–alpha plays a central role in interleukin-2–induced pulmonary vascular leak and lymphocyte accumulation. *Cell Immunol* 1994;157:170–80.
255. Mier JW, Vachino G, van der Meer JW, et al. Induction of circulating tumor necrosis factor (TNF alpha) as the mechanism for the febrile response to interleukin-2 (IL-2) in cancer patients. *J Clin Immunol* 1988;8:426–436.
256. Walker RE, Hahn B, Kelly GG, et al. Effects of TNF-alpha antagonists thalidomide and monoclonal anti-TNF antibody (cA2) on reducing IL-2–associated toxicities: a randomized, controlled trial (Abstract 242). 4th Conference on Retroviruses and Opportunistic Infections, Washington, DC, 1997.
257. Kovacs JA, Miller KD, Jones EJ, et al. High prevalence of avascular necrosis (AVN) of the hip in HIV infection: magnetic resonance imaging of 339 asymptomatic patients. (Abstract 15). Annual Meeting of the Infectious Disease Society of America (IDSA). New Orleans, 2000.
258. Lloyd M, Young KA. Teaching HIV$^+$ outpatients self-administration of subcutaneous interleukin-2 and strategies for symptom management (submitted)
259. Bruch HR, Kom A, Klein H, et al. Treatment of chronic hepatitis B with interferon alpha-2b and interleukin-2. *J Hepatol* 1993;17:S52–S55.
260. Uberti-Foppa C, De Bona A, Morsica G, et al. Recombinant interleukin-2 for treatment of HIV reduces hepatitis C viral load in coinfected patients. *AIDS* 1999;13:140–141.
261. Kaplan G, Cohn ZA, Smith KA. Rational immunotherapy with interleukin 2. *Biotechnology (NY)*1992;10: 157–162.
262. Giedlin MA, Zimmerman RJ. The use of recombinant human interleukin-2 in treating infectious diseases. *Curr Opin Biotechnol* 1993;4:722–726.
263. Vogels MT, van der Meer JW. Use of immune modulators in nonspecific therapy of bacterial infections. *Antimicrob Agents Chemother* 1992;36:1–5.
264. Nishioka M, Kagawa H, Shirai M, et al. Effects of human recombinant interleukin 2 in patients with chronic hepatitis B: a preliminary report. *Am J Gastroenterol* 1987;82:438–442.
265. Onji M, Kondoh H, Horiike N, et al. Effect of recombinant interleukin 2 on hepatitis B e antigen positive chronic hepatitis. *Gut* 1987;28:1648–1652.
266. Tilg H, Vogel W, Tratkiewicz J, et al. Pilot study of natural human interleukin-2 in patients with chronic hepatitis B. Immunomodulatory and antiviral effects. *J Hepatol* 1993;19:259–267.
267. Pardo M, Castillo I, Oliva H, et al. A pilot study of recombinant interleukin-2 for treatment of chronic hepatitis C. *Hepatology* 1997;26:1318–1321.
268. Villahermosa LG, Abalos RM, Walsh DS, et al. Recombinant interleukin-2 in lepromatous leprosy lesions: immunological and microbiological consequences. *Clin Exp Dermatol* 1997;22:134-40.
269. Kaplan G, Britton WJ, Hancock GE, et al. The systemic influence of recombinant interleukin 2 on the manifestations of lepromatous leprosy. *J Exp Med* 1991;173:993-1006.
270. Johnson BJ, Ress SR, Willcox P, et al. Clinical and immune responses of tuberculosis patients treated with low-dose IL-2 and multidrug therapy. *Cytokines Mol Ther* 1995;1:185–196.
271. Johnson BJ, Bekker LG, Rickman R, et al. rhuIL-2 adjunctive therapy in multidrug resistant tuberculosis: a comparison of two treatment regimens and placebo. *Tuber Lung Dis* 1997;78:195–203.
272. Johnson B, Bekker LG, Ress S, et al. Recombinant interleukin 2 adjunctive therapy in multidrug-resistant tuberculosis. *Novartis Found Symp* 1998;217:99–106.
273. Akuffo H, Kaplan G, Kiessling R, et al. Administration of recombinant interleukin-2 reduces the local parasite load of patients with disseminated cutaneous leishmaniasis. *J Infect Dis* 1990;161:775–780.
274. Cunningham-Rundles C, Mayer L, Sapira E, et al. Restoration of immunoglobulin secretion in vitro in common variable immunodeficiency by in vivo treatment with polyethylene glycol- conjugated human recombinant interleukin-2. *Clin Immunol Immunopathol* 1992;64:46–56.
275. Cunningham-Rundles C, Kazbay K, Hassett J, et al. Brief report: enhanced humoral immunity in common vari-

able immunodeficiency after long-term treatment with polyethylene glycol- conjugated interleukin-2. *N Engl J Med* 1994;331:918–921.

276. Rump JA, Jahreis A, Schlesier M, et al. A double-blind, placebo-controlled, crossover therapy study with natural human IL-2 (nhuIL-2) in combination with regular intravenous gammaglobulin (IVIG) infusions in 10 patients with common variable immunodeficiency (CVID). *Clin Exp Immunol* 1997;110:167–173.
277. Heath AW, Playfair JH. The potential of cytokines as adjuvants. *AIDS Res Hum Retroviruses* 1992;8: 1401–1403.
278. Jungers P, Devillier P, Salomon H, et al. Randomised placebo-controlled trial of recombinant interleukin-2 in chronic uraemic patients who are non-responders to hepatitis B vaccine. *Lancet* 1994;344:856–857.
279. Meuer SC, Dumann H, Meyer zum Buschenfelde KH, et al. Low-dose interleukin-2 induces systemic immune responses against HBsAg in immunodeficient non-responders to hepatitis B vaccination. *Lancet* 1989;1:15–18.
280. Cooper DA, Emery S. Latent reservoirs of HIV infection: flushing with IL-2? *Nat Med* 1999;5:611–612.
281. Davey RT Jr, Bhat N, Yoder C, et al. HIV-1 and T cell dynamics after interruption of highly active antiretroviral therapy (HAART) in patients with a history of sustained viral suppression. *Proc Natl Acad Sci USA* 1999;96:15109–15114.
282. Chun TW, Davey RT Jr, Engel D, et al. Re-emergence of HIV after stopping therapy. *Nature* 1999;401:874–875.

3
Interleukin-5

N. Lynn Henry and Thomas B. Nutman

Helminth Immunology Section and Clinical Parasitology Unit, Laboratory of Parasitic Diseases, National Institute of Allergy and Infectious Diseases, National Institutes of Health, Bethesda, Maryland

INTRODUCTION

Interleukin 5 is a member of the cytokine family of polypeptides and glycoproteins that regulates cellular and humoral immune responses. These molecules mediate the interaction of T cells, B cells, and other effector cells of the immune system. The majority of cytokines have a broad range of activity on a variety of target cells, but some cytokines appear to be relatively restricted in the range of target cells. Interleukin (IL)–5 is one such cytokine that acts on selected lineages of cells (1). Although this cytokine was initially described as a growth factor for a murine B cell lymphoma (2), its association with eosinophil differentiation (3) has made IL-5 of special interest in the study of parasitic infections and allergic disorders.

An interesting feature of the biologic activity of IL-5 is its overlap of function with that of IL-3 and granulocyte-macrophage colony-stimulating factor (GM-CSF); however, even though the action and biologic activity of these cytokines overlap substantially, there are cytokine-specific actions that suggest that separate intracellular signaling mechanisms are also activated in addition to common pathways of cell activation (4). Experiments done by several groups have successfully elucidated the molecular basis for this functional overlap; for a review, see Takatsu et al. (5).

In this chapter, we have attempted to summarize current knowledge of the structure and function of IL-5, regulation of the gene encoding this cytokine, the interaction of the molecule with its receptor [the IL-5 receptor (IL-5R)], and its biologic role in selected infectious disease states. Finally, therapeutic strategies that could involve the use of IL-5 or IL-5 blockade either by specific anti–IL-5 antibodies, soluble receptors, or antisense oligonucleotides will be discussed.

HISTORICAL BACKGROUND

IL-5 was initially described as a factor that induces terminal differentiation of murine B cells to immunoglobulin (Ig)-secreting cells (6). The observation that eosinophilia could occur in the absence of changes in populations of other leukocytes suggested not only that there was a control mechanism that was specific for eosinophils but also that there was a T cell dependence of this control. Consequently, other studies examining the role of T cells in the growth and functional activation of B cells revealed that T cell supernatants had the capacity to induce B cell proliferation and antibody secretion (6). This capacity was attributed to a differentiation factor designated T cell Replacing Factor

[TRF] (2,7). B cell growth stimulating activity in T cell supernatants was attributed to another factor designated B cell growth factor (BCGFII), a molecule that was subsequently found to be identical to TRF (8). An eosinophil differentiation factor (EDF) was concurrently reported in supernatants of murine spleen cells (1). The discovery that EDF and TRF activity copurified (9), followed by the demonstration that the factors responsible for these two activities were identical by cDNA cloning and sequence analysis (10,11) established IL-5 to be primarily a T cell-derived cytokine with multiple biologic actions on murine B cells and murine and human eosinophil progenitors (12,13).

ORGANIZATION OF THE IL-5 GENE

The human IL-5 gene is located on chromosome 5 (5q23.3-31) (14–17) in a cluster with the genes for IL-4, IL-3, and GM-CSF. Deletion of the IL-5 gene has been reported with the $5q^-$ syndrome (16), some myeloid leukemias (17), eosinophilic leukemias (18), and certain immunodeficiency states (e.g., severe combined immunodeficiency, SCID) (19).

The organization of the IL-5 gene in the numerous species studied to date show that there are four exons and three introns in IL-5 genes. Conserved TATA-like and cytokine consensus sequences are found 26 and 73 base pairs (bp), respectively, upstream of the transcription initiation sites (20,21). The exon-intron organization and location of cysteine codons in IL-5 genes resemble those of GM-CSF, IL-2, and IL-4 (and are quite distinct from the G-CSF gene), suggesting an overall structural similarity between the IL-5 gene and these others (12,22). There also appear to be regulatory elements 5′ to the coding region of the IL-5 and GM-CSF genes in humans and the mouse that are identical. Furthermore, clustering of the IL-5 gene close to the genes for GM-CSF, IL-4, and IL-3 on chromosome 5 in humans and chromosome 11 in the mouse has been interpreted to indicate that these genes may have derived by duplications from a common ancestral gene. Despite the similarities in localization and gene structure among IL-5, IL-3, IL-4, and GM-CSF, there is no significant nucleotide or amino acid sequence similarity among the cytokines.

REGULATION OF GENE EXPRESSION

The regulation of IL-5 gene expression occurs primarily at the level of transcription (23). Numerous cis-regulatory elements are present in the 5′ flanking region of the IL-5 promoter, which both positively and negatively influence gene expression (Fig. 3.1). CLE0 is located between −56 and −42 and is essential for promoter activity. This site is highly conserved in IL-5 promoters from other species as well as in regulatory regions of other cytokines including IL-3, IL-4, and GM-CSF (24). Transcription factors, including AP-1, Oct 1, Oct 2, ETS1, and ETS2, have been identified that bind this region (24,25). Other sites involved in positive regulation include a constitutive GATA motif at −70 (26), an inducible NF-AT site at −110 with a flanking constitutive GATA site (27–29), and an octamer element at −244 to −237 (30). Mutation of these positive elements has been demonstrated to reduce promoter activity. Negative regulatory elements identified to date include the region from −90 to −79, which binds Oct 1 and YY1 (31), as well as two less well-characterized regions from −127 to −172 (28) and from −312 to −404 (30). A YY1 and NF-AT binding site has also been identified in the distal promoter region from −448 to −460 that appears to be involved in downregulation of IL-5 gene expression (32).

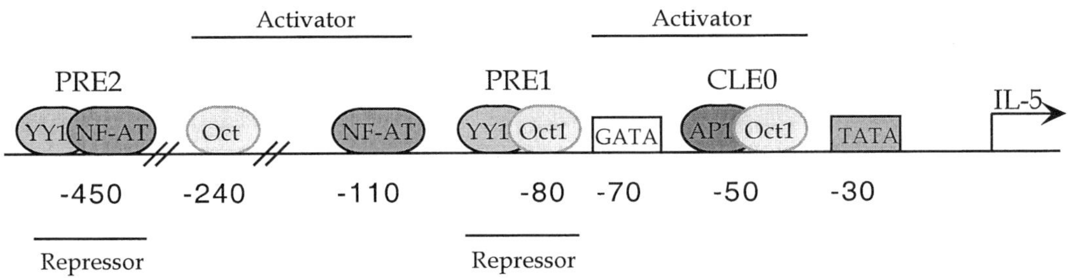

FIG. 3.1. Diagram of IL-5 promoter showing transcription factors active in gene transcription regulation. Regions involved in activation of transcription are indicated above the diagram, and regions involved in repression of transcription are indicated below. Details of the individual transcription factors are given in the text.

PROTEIN STRUCTURE OF IL-5

The human IL-5 gene contains four exons that encode a protein of 134 amino acids (10). The molecular mass of hIL-5 is 45 to 60 kDa, which drops to 25 to 30 kDa under reducing conditions. The active form of the protein exists as an antiparallel homodimeric glycoprotein containing two interchain disulfide bonds between residues 42 and 84. The crystal structure of IL-5 revealed two left-handed bundles of 4 α-helices in an up-up, down-down array and two short antiparallel β-strands packed on opposite sides of the dimer (33). Each bundle comprises three helices from one monomer and one helix from the second monomer. The four-helix structure is similar to that of the monomers GM-CSF and IL-3 (34,35), although only IL-5 exists in dimeric form. IL-5 is glycosylated at two sites *in vivo* (36), and although glycosylation is not required for activity (37), it apparently is important for thermostability (38). Table 3.1 summarizes the biochemical, molecular, and functional properties of human IL-5 and its receptor.

TABLE 3-1. *Molecular and biochemical characteristics of human IL-5 and IL-5 receptor*

Structure	IL-5	IL-5Rα	IL-5Rβ
Molecular			
M_r (Da)	30,000–40,000	60,000	120,000–130,000
No. of amino acids			
Total	134	420	897
Mature product	115		850
Predicted size of peptide	13,149 Da	47,670 Da	92,010 Da
Active form	Homodimer	Bound to β	Bound to IL-5Rα
N-glycosylation sites	2		
Genomic	4 exons, 3 introns	1 exon	1 exon
Chromosomal location	5q23-31	3p24-26	22q12.2-13.1
Copy number	1		
Cell sources	T cells; eosinophils; basophils; epithelial cells; EBV-transformed B cells; Reed-Sternberg cells	B cells; eosinophils; basophils; mast cells; CD34$^+$ stem cells	B cells; eosinophils; basophils; airway neutrophils; monocytes; dendritic cells; endothelial cells; mast cells; macrophages

Human IL-5 is 70% homologous to murine IL-5. It should be noted that, while cross-reactivity in terms of bioassays and immunoassays has been observed between murine and human IL-5, the human cytokine is approximately 100-fold less active on mouse target cells than on human bone marrow cells, while mouse IL-5 is 20-fold less active on human than on homologous bone marrow (39).

IL-5 RECEPTORS

IL-5 has multiple biologic activities that appear to be exerted by interactions with cell surface receptors. These receptors have been shown to be heterogeneous in terms of their affinity and specificity and are low in numbers per cell (typically 100 to 1,000 per cell), features that have hindered their purification (4). The availability of highly purified rIL-5 and anti–IL-5 monoclonal antibodies (mAbs), however, made it possible to examine binding sites for IL-5. The high-affinity IL-5R for both humans and the mouse have been cloned (40,41) using expression strategies, making it possible to define their affinities and specificities (4,42).

Binding kinetics with ^{35}S-labeled or radioiodinated murine rIL-5 have revealed two classes of IL-5 binding sites. Approximately 10% to 15% of these receptors have high-affinity binding (dissociation constant, K_d of ~150 pM), while the remainder have much lower affinity [K_d ~20 nM (43,44)]. Lipopolysaccharide has been shown to upregulate the number of high-affinity IL-5R on murine B cells, and both IL-2 and IL-5 downregulate the same receptor (43). As would be expected, the number of high-affinity IL-5R correlates with responsiveness to IL-5. The concentration of IL-5 that is required for interaction with the two receptors (high and low affinity) indicates that the biologic activity of IL-5 occurs only on engagement of the high-affinity receptor; for a review, see Tominaga et al. (42).

Receptors for IL-5 consist of an α subunit (IL5Rα), specific for IL-5, and a β subunit, common to the receptors for GM-CSF and IL-3. On eosinophils, the receptor has been found to have higher affinity for IL-5 on activated hypodense eosinophils (45) than on normodense, "resting" eosinophils. IL-3 and GM-CSF, whose receptors share the common β subunit with the IL-5 receptor, can cross-compete with IL-5 for binding and biologic activity (46), consistent with the finding that the two IL-5 receptor subunits are not associated in the absence of IL-5 (47).

The gene for the α chain is located on chromosome 3 (3p24-3p26) (48) and is expressed only in eosinophils and basophils (49), and this restricted expression of IL5Rα is probably responsible for the lineage specificity of IL-5. Multiple forms of IL5Rα are produced by alternative splicing, including a membrane-associated form and two soluble forms (50). Soluble IL5Rα is unable to associate with membrane-bound β receptor. The soluble form is able to bind IL-5 with only two to three times lower affinity than the IL-5 receptor complex and inhibits IL-5-dependent proliferation of cells *in vitro* , but its biologic function is unknown. The IL5Rα promoter has been partially characterized. It contains an enhancer-like cis-element (EOS1) between –430 and –422 that binds an unknown myeloid-specific factor and is necessary for full promoter activity and for lineage-specific activity in myeloid and eosinophilic cell lines (51). Other transcription factor binding sites have been identified including an AP-1 site between –440 and –432, which may act synergistically with the EOS1 site (52).

IL5Rα binds IL-5 with low affinity, and the binding affinity is increased two to three times in the presence of the β chain (53). The β chain does not independently bind IL5. The α subunit confers IL-5 specificity but is unable to transmit a signal into the cell. The β chain, in association with IL5Rα, is responsible for signal transduction (54,55). Mutation analysis has demonstrated a number of regions important for the interaction between IL-5 and its receptor, specifically the CD loop and the N-terminus of helix D. Important residues include Glu89 and Arg91 (53,56), which cluster around the interface between the two helix bundles, and Glu110 and Trp 111 (57). Glu13, located at the distal ends of the dimer, is involved in β chain interactions (56). The stoichiometry of the IL5-IL5R interaction is 1:1, and monomeric isomers of IL-5 have been used to demonstrate that the four-helix bundle is sufficient for activity (58).

The IL-5 Signaling Cascade

Receptors belonging to the cytokine receptor superfamily generally fall into two categories—those with and those without intrinsic protein tyrosine kinase activity. Receptors that lack tyrosine kinase activity appear to use intracellular kinases in common pathways of activation and transcription of a variety of genes. The IL-5 receptor does not contain intrinsic tyrosine kinase activity and, therefore, signal transduction via the receptor occurs through multiple cytoplasmic kinases, including the JAK-STAT and Ras-MAP kinase pathways.

According to the model of JAK-STAT-dependent IL-5 signal transduction, binding of IL-5 to IL-5R induces dimerization of receptor components and activation of the closely associated JAKs (59). In the absence of IL-5, JAK-2 has been shown to associate with IL-5Rα, and the proline-rich region of the cytoplasmic domain is necessary for JAK-2 binding (47). IL-5–induced dimerization of IL-5R subunits causes JAK-2 activation and phosphorylation of the β subunit (47). IL-5 has also been shown to activate JAK-1, which associates with the β subunit. The activated JAKs can then phosphorylate the receptors as well as cytoplasmic proteins belonging to a family of transcription factors called signal transduction and activators of transcription (STATs) (60–62). Multiple STATs have been identified that are activated by JAKs, including STAT1α, STAT3, and STAT5 (63–65). Activated STATs then translocate to the nucleus and bind gamma interferon activating sequences (GAS) (62,66,67) in the upstream regulatory regions of the genes encoding IL-5-inducible proteins (Fig. 3.1).

Apart from the JAK-STAT pathway, IL-5 has also been found to induce tyrosine phosphorylation and activation of a number of other kinases belonging to the Ras-Raf-MAP kinase pathway (68). This pathway involves interactions between multiple enzymes and adapter proteins. Two species of *lyn* kinases are phosphorylated and activated rapidly (within 1 minute) in human eosinophils exposed to IL-5 (68,69). These proteins are closely associated with the IL-5β chain. Involvement of the Ras pathway in these cells was demonstrated by increased binding of ^{32}P-GTP to Ras and enzyme activation of a MAP kinase after stimulation with IL-5 (68). A number of adapter proteins involved in signaling in IL-5–induced eosinophils have been identified, including a Shc isomer and Grb2 (70). Shc interacts with the cytoplasmic region of the β subunit and is tyrosine phosphorylated upon stimulation by IL-5. Compelling evidence for the involvement of this pathway in murine B cells also comes from the *xid* mouse, B cells of which are unresponsive to IL-5 and have been demonstrated to have defects in the activation of *btk* following IL-5 stimulation (69,71,72).

A third mechanism of signal transduction stimulated by IL-5 involves the activation of phosphatidylinositol 3-kinase (PI3K) (73). PI3K does not interact directly with IL5R but rather presumably requires additional molecules to mediate the association. Factors identified that interact between the β subunit and PI3K in IL-3- or GM-CSF-activated signaling include SHP-2, *Tec*, and an *src*-associated protein (74–76). PI3K transduces signals to a number of serine/threonine kinases, but its role in IL-5 signaling is not yet known.

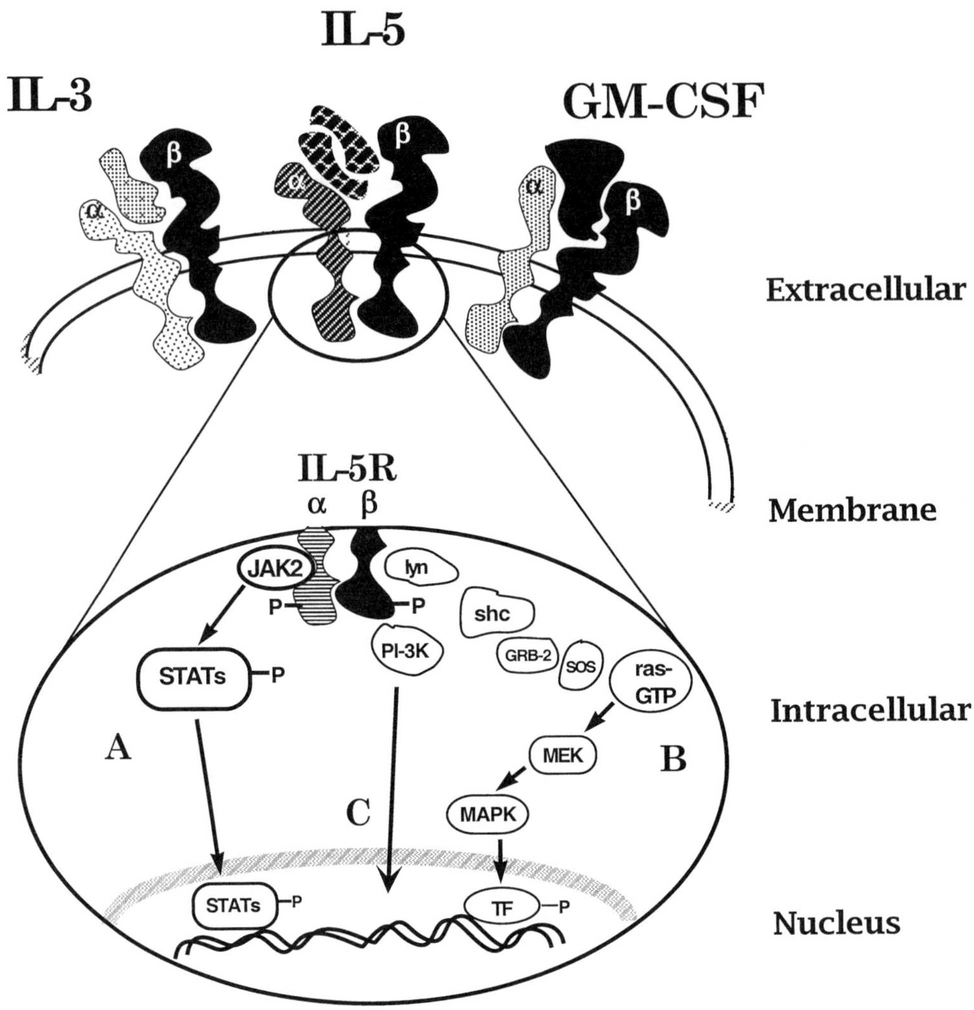

FIG. 3.2. Schematic representation of signal transduction pathways activated by IL-5 receptor binding. The initial event is ligand-dependent aggregation of receptors, bringing jaks in close proximity to each other and to other receptors. Two major pathways activated by cytokine binding depicted in this schematic diagram are the JAK-STAT pathway **(A)** and the *ras* pathway **(B)**. Activation of PI3K **(C)** may also have a role in IL-5 signaling, but the mechanism has not yet been elucidated. The membrane-proximal region of the β chain is required for activation of the JAK-STAT pathway, via JAK2 (for IL-5), and jaks do not necessarily interact with the a subunit, as shown in this illustration. Activation of the *ras* pathway through SHC binding and phosphorylation requires the membrane-distal region, whereas *lyn* phosphorylation requires the membrane-proximal region of the b chain. The b chains of IL-5, IL-3, and GM-CSF are identical. It is likely that similar or identical signal transduction pathways are activated by the cytokines. JAK, Janus kinase; STAT, signal transducer and activator of transcription; PI3K, phosphoinositol-3 kinase; *lyn,* tyrosine kinase of the *src* family of proto-oncogenes; MAPK, mitogen-activated protein kinase; MEK, MAP or Erk kinase;TF, transcription factor (unidentified). *Arrows* indicate phosphorylation of tyrosine residues.

Figure 3.2 depicts a proposed scheme for signal transduction after ligand binding of the IL-5R complex based on current knowledge of intracellular phosphorylation events immediately following IL-5 stimulation of responsive cells.

SOURCES OF IL-5

Activated T cell populations (particularly $CD4^+$ $CD45R0^+$ cells) are the main source of IL-5, but secretion of IL-5 from other cell types has been reported. These include $CD8^+$ T cells (77), natural killer cells (78), mast cells (79), eosinophils (80,81), and airway epithelial cells (82). Epstein-Barr virus (EBV)–transformed B cells from humans can produce large amounts of IL-5 (83). Reed Sternberg cells in individuals with Hodgkin's disease accompanied by eosinophilia have also been found to produce IL-5 and may be involved in generation of eosinophilia associated with this disorder (84).

IL-5 mRNA has also been demonstrated in sites of allergic reactions, such as the airway mucosa in individuals with asthma and seasonal allergic rhinitis. Although most (>70%) of the IL-5 $mRNA^+$ cells in nasal and tracheal mucosa and bronchoalveolar lavage fluid in allergic individuals are T cells (85,86), mast cells and eosinophils have also been shown to express mRNA for IL-5 (87–89). IL-5 mRNA expression in mast cells appears to be restricted to the $tryptase^+$ $chymase^+$ subpopulation (90) and is upregulated by cross-linkage of high-affinity Fc receptors (79). IL-5 has been demonstrated by in situ hybridization in eosinophils found in human intestinal mucosa (91) and in human airway epithelial cells (82).

MAJOR BIOLOGIC ACTIVITIES OF IL-5

The eosinophilopoietic action of IL-5 was first demonstrated in mouse bone marrow cultures and was found to be cell-lineage specific (1). The production of eosinophils in this system is markedly enhanced in parasite-infected mice, and anti–IL-5 administration *in vivo* to parasitized mice completely abolishes the eosinophilia, suggesting that IL-5 is the main factor responsible for eosinophilia in this model (92). The effect of IL-5 on human eosinophils is very similar to that seen in mice; IL-5 prolongs eosinophil survival *in vitro* (93,94), and eosinophilic colonies are preferentially expanded by IL-5 from human bone marrow in culture (95). Studies of the kinetics of IL-5–mediated generation of eosinophils from bone marrow have concluded that IL-5 is only active at a late stage of eosinophil differentiation (96,97). Indeed, preincubation of murine marrow cells with IL-3, GM-CSF, or M-CSF induced a marked increase in eosinophil precursor cells that are IL-5 responsive (5,98,99).

Not only does IL-5 mediate the generation of eosinophils, it also promotes eosinophil survival, most commonly by preventing eosinophil apoptosis (100). IL-5 has also been shown to enhance adhesion of human eosinophils to plasma-coated glass, a phenomenon probably mediated by augmented expression of integrin molecules of the CD11/18 family [(101); for a review, see Weller (102)]. IL-5 has been shown to enhance eosinophil-related cytotoxicity and the respiratory burst in eosinophils (103). In states of hypereosinophilia, such as the idiopathic hypereosinophilic syndrome and the eosinophilia-myalgia syndrome, circulating eosinophils have a higher proportion of hypodense ("activated" versus normodense, inactivated) eosinophils, which have been shown to correlate with IL-5 in serum (104,105). Similar rises in serum IL-5 levels are observed in helminth-infected individuals who develop post treatment eosinophilia (106), in individuals receiving IL-2/lymphokine-activated killer cells (107), and in episodic angioedema with eosinophilia syndrome (108).

Apart from its effect on eosinophil generation and activation, a variety of other effects, mainly related to allergic phenomena, have been attributed to IL-5. rIL-5 induces release of histamine and generation of leukotriene C4 from human basophils *in vitro* (46,109,110), and IL-5 appears to be a basophilopoietic cytokine in humans (111).

The effect of IL-5 on human B cells remains controversial. Although it has been shown to induce IgA and IgM production by peripheral blood B cells *in vitro* (112) and to augment Ig production by *Staphylococcus aureus* Cowan I–stimulated or pokeweed mitogen-stimulated human B cell blasts in the presence of IL-2, hIL-5 has been shown to have no detectable effect on B cell function as determined by a variety of standard B cell functional assays (113).

PATHOPHYSIOLOGY OF THE IL-5 TRANSGENIC MOUSE

Transgenic mice carrying the murine IL-5 gene with promoters for constitutive expression of the cytokine have been used to investigate the role of IL-5 in eosinophil development and B cell function. Two such models of transgenic IL-5 production have been studied (114,115); both sets of transgenic mice exhibited elevated serum IL-5 levels and eosinophilia. A prominent feature of IL-5 transgenic mice is a marked increase in the numbers of circulating lymphocytes and eosinophils. The increase in eosinophil populations is 75-fold compared with age-matched normal mice (115), but cell-cycle analysis of these eosinophils suggests that there is no increase in the proliferative capacity of eosinophils in these animals (116). Tissue infiltration with eosinophils is apparent, and the spleen is typically enlarged approximately five times (in the number of cells). Of interest, the expanded population of eosinophils in these animals appears to be a resting population that requires activation for release of granule contents.

Other abnormalities noted in these mice include expansion of a distinctive population of B cells with a high density of surface IgM and the IL-5 receptor (IL-5R) in the bone marrow and peritoneum. The significance and function of this population is not clearly understood, but this cell population has been postulated to be involved in the generation of autoantibodies (5,117).

The IL-5 transgenic mouse may serve as a model for diseases characterized by eosinophilia such as idiopathic hypereosinophilic syndrome, myositis, and fasciitis, although the fact that the eosinophils are in the resting state in these animals, as opposed to increased proportions of activated eosinophils that are commonly seen in these disease states, must be kept in mind.

IL-5 AND ITS ROLE IN INFECTIOUS DISEASES

Among those infectious agents that cause disease, only the helminth parasites (as opposed to protozoa, bacteria, fungi, and viruses) appear to have IL-5–mediated processes (e.g., eosinophilia) and an expansion of IL-5-producing cells as an almost universal consequence of infection of humans (118–128). Data from animal models, however, have more clearly demonstrated the role of IL-5 in mediating both protection and pathology following infection with helminth parasites. These effects are summarized in Table 3.2 and below.

Although increased IL-5 levels in serum and tissues have been associated with resistance in some experimental models of intestinal helminth infection (129), the absence of

TABLE 3-2. *The role of IL-5 in mediating protection in selected helminth infections*

Organism	IL-5$^{-/-a}$	IL-5 mAb[b]	IL-5R$^{-/-c}$	IL-5 transgenic[d]	References
Angyostrongylus catonensis		Increase	Increase	Decrease	141, 182–184
Heligosomoides polygyrus	Increase	No change			185, 186
Hymenolepis diminuta	No change				186
Litomosomoides sigmodontis	Decrease				
Mesocestoides corti	No change			No change	186, 187
Nipostrongylus brasiliensis		No change		Decrease	129, 131, 188
Onchocerca spp.		Increase			136, 189
Schistosoma spp.		No change		Increase	156, 187
Strongyloides spp.	Increase	Increase			139, 142, 186, 190
Toxocara canis	No change	No change		No change	186, 191–193
Trichinella spp.	No change	No change		Increase	187, 194, 195

[a]IL-5$^{-/-}$; mice with targeted deletion of the IL-5 gene.
[b]IL-5 mAb; mice treated with neutralizing IL-5 mAb.
[c]IL-5R$^{-/-}$; mice with targeted deletion of the IL-5Rα gene.
[d]IL-5 transgenic; mice overexpressing the IL-5 gene.
Results are expressed as an increase, decrease, or no change in the infection of the various murine models.

IL-5 (mice treated with anti–IL-5 antibodies or genetically IL-5–deficient strains of mice) appears to have little or no effect on intestinal parasite survival (130,131) despite a marked effect on helminth-induced eosinophilia (131,132). In contrast, immunity to tissue-invasive helminths appears to be at least partially dependent on IL-5. Immunity to both schistosomal and filarial infection in humans has been correlated with parasite antigen-induced production of IL-5 in some (but not all) studies (118,133). Similarly, animals multiply vaccinated with radiation-attenuated filarial larvae (134) or schistosome cercariae (135) develop partial protective immunity to challenge infection that is accompanied by increased IL-5 production to parasite antigens. This immunity is impaired in the absence of IL-5 in mice immunized with microfilariae or attenuated filarial infective larvae (136,137), but not in murine models of schistosomiasis (138).

Further support for the hypothesis that IL-5 is important in protective immunity to helminths in the tissues but not in the intestine comes from studies with intestinal helminths that have a tissue-migrating phase, such as the murine nematodes *Strongyloides venezuelensis* (139) and *Angiostrongylus cantonensis* (140). Whereas depletion of IL-5 has no effect on intestinal worm burden or egg output following primary infection with *S. venezuelensis*, the characteristic decrease in worm recovery seen following secondary infection is abolished, consistent with an effect of IL-5 on the immune response to tissue-migrating larvae in the lung (139). In *A. cantonensis* infection in mice, immature worms develop in the brain before migrating to the lungs. Prolonged survival of intracranial worms resulting in a larger parasite burden in the lungs has been demonstrated in normal mice treated with anti–IL-5 antibody (140) as well as in IL-5Rα–deficient mice (141), again consistent with a role for eosinophils in tissue-based larval killing.

The dependence of larval killing on IL-5 has also been demonstrated by the implantation of infective Strongyloides larvae in diffusion chambers under the skin of control mice and mice treated with anti–IL-5 antibody (142). Not only were eosinophils the only cells that accumulated in the chamber concomitant with larval killing (143), but such killing could be prevented by inhibition of eosinophil migration into the chamber or treatment of the mice with anti–IL-5 antibody (142,143).

Animal models of protective immunity to the exclusively tissue-dwelling nematode Onchocerca further support the role of IL-5 in mediating resistance to infection. In diffusion chamber studies of infective larvae survival in immune mice, eosinophils were the only cells that accumulated in the chambers concomitant with larval killing (136). In a different murine model system, mice infected with *Onchocerca lienalis* depleted of eosinophils (but not macrophages or neutrophils) with anti–IL-5 mAb showed delayed clearance of primary infection and abrogation of resistance to secondary infection (144).

In humans with onchocerciasis, the picture is somewhat more complex. Some studies of *in vitro* cytokine production in response to parasite antigens have demonstrated increased levels of IL-5 production by peripheral blood mononuclear cells from putatively immune individuals living in areas endemic for onchocerciasis in comparison with those from infected individuals (133), whereas others have detected no difference in parasite antigen-induced IL-5 production between these groups (145).

IL-5–mediated eosinophil production and recruitment have also been implicated in the pathology associated with helminth infection. Clinical similarities between the sequelae of hypereosinophilic syndrome, a syndrome characterized by extremely high levels of eosinophilia and eosinophil-mediated end organ damage (146), and the pathologic consequences of infection with filaria (147) and toxocara (148) are suggestive of a role for eosinophils in the pathologic sequelae of these infections. Increased eosinophil activation as measured by increased responsiveness to the inflammatory mediator, platelet activating factor, has been described in patients with sowda (localized onchodermatitis, a chronic hyperreactive form of onchocerciasis associated with severe skin pathology, compared with normal individuals or onchocerciasis-infected patients with milder symptomatology, providing additional indirect support for this hypothesis (149).

Post-treatment reactions in onchocerciasis (the Mazzotti reaction) can be severe and are believed to reflect an acute exacerbation of the host immune response to microfilariae in the skin and other organs. One of the characteristics of this response is an increase in blood and tissue levels of eosinophils and eosinophil granule proteins that is temporally related to the onset of symptomatology (150) and preceded by an increase in serum levels of IL-5 (106). Although localization of eosinophils and their products in the skin is most pronounced at sites of microfilarial degeneration (150), consistent with the hypothesis that eosinophil-mediated parasite killing plays a major role in pathogenesis, the possibility that recruitment of eosinophils occurs secondarily in response to parasite death cannot be excluded.

More direct evidence that eosinophils mediate the pathology seen in onchocerciasis comes from animal models of corneal keratitis (151,152). Eosinophil infiltration is a characteristic component of the keratitis seen in the corneas of sensitized mice injected intrastromally with onchocercal antigens (153).

Although it seems clear that eosinophils play a role in some types of helminth-induced pathology, they do not appear to be essential to the development of pathologic sequelae in all cases. Liver granulomas in schistosomiasis typically contain a high percentage of eosinophils; however, anti–IL-5-treated mice infected with schistosomiasis produce normal-sized granulomas despite the absence of eosinophils (138,154). Similarly, lung infiltrates in *Nippostrongylus brasiliensis*-infected mice treated with anti–IL-5 differed from *N. brasiliensis*-infected control mice in the absence of eosinophils but not in size or number (131).

POTENTIAL THERAPEUTIC ROLES FOR IL-5 AND IL-5 INHIBITION

In general, increased IL-5 production is observed in situations where there is an expansion of Th2 cell populations or basophilia. In experimental helminth infections of the mouse, IL-5 does not appear to have an important role in the induction of protective immunity, as evidenced by the lack of protection afforded to mice treated with anti–IL-5 at doses that abolish eosinophilia (92,155,156); however, eosinophils have been demonstrated to have helminthotoxic activity against *Schistosoma mansoni* and *S. hematobium* both *in vitro* and in reinfection surveys of children; for a review, see Sanderson (12).

The association of eosinophilia and neoplasia has been noted for many years (157), and its presence has been associated with a favorable prognosis in some cancers, notably carcinomas of the urinary bladder (158), uterine cervix (159), and head and neck (160). Although local production of eosinophilopoietic cytokines (GM-CSF, IL-3, and IL-5) by tumor cells has not been investigated extensively, a study of bone marrow and blood eosinophilia in two patients with solid malignancies found that tumor cells secreted IL-3 and GM-CSF *in vitro*, measured by a sensitive bioassay and neutralizable by antibodies to GM-CSF and IL-3; however, in these experiments, no IL-5 was measured in the supernatants (161). Eosinophilia has also been reported to accompany Hodgkin's lymphoma (162) and some cases of nonlymphocytic leukemias. In some leukemia-associated eosinophilia, chromosomal translocations involving chromosome 5, the location of the IL-5 gene (163,164), have been observed, although there has been no demonstration of elevated IL-5 in these cases.

The role of eosinophil-derived toxic products in necrosis of tumor tissue (165) and correlation of eosinophilia with clinical response in patients treated with IL-2 (166) raises interesting possibilities for the use IL-5 as a therapeutic modality in treatment for certain tumors. Thus, in neoplasms where eosinophilia appears to be associated with better prognosis or where it can be demonstrated that the eosinophilia is primarily mediated by IL-5, treatment with exogenous IL-5 may be an adjunct to the chemotherapeutic regimens available.

Alternatively, there is compelling evidence that an excess of eosinophils and their products can be involved in the pathogenesis of several diseases. There is increasing evidence that eosinophils may be a major factor in the development of respiratory malfunction in asthma, as seen both by the ability of eosinophil products such as major basic protein, eosinophilic cationic protein, and eosinophil peroxidase to cause direct cytotoxicity to lung epithelium *in vitro* and by deposition of these products in damaged lung tissue from asthmatic patients (97,102). In the idiopathic hypereosinophilic syndrome and allergic granulomatosis (Churg-Strauss syndrome), deposits of eosinophil products have been demonstrated in the heart, kidney, and neural tissue. Prolonged peripheral eosinophilia with extremely elevated eosinophil counts from any cause can potentially result in end organ damage to the heart (endomyocardial fibrosis) or nerves (peripheral neuropathy).

IL-5 is considered the most important cytokine involved in the regulation of eosinophilia because of its specificity for the development of eosinophils and, therefore, inhibition of the action of IL-5 is likely to be therapeutic for diseases associated with hypereosinophilia. Numerous methods of blocking IL-5 have been proposed, including antibodies directed against IL-5, soluble IL-5 receptors to block the cytokine-receptor interaction, and antisense oligonucleotides to block the production of IL-5.

Multiple mAbs that neutralize IL-5 have been developed. Initially, two rat antibodies were generated, TRFK-5 (anti-mouse IL-5) and 39D10 (anti-human IL-5), which inhibited airway eosinophilia and bronchial hyperreactivity in multiple animal models. These antibodies inhibited 75% to 95% of challenge-induced eosinophilia in an allergic mouse model when administered intraperitoneally (167,168), and a similar reduction was seen when the antibody was administered intranasally (169). Inhibition was also demonstrated both in allergic guinea pigs (170,171) and in cynomolgus monkeys, in whom the effect lasted for 3 months following a single dose of antibody (172).

To develop a therapeutic neutralizing antibody, the rat mAb, 39D10, was humanized using complementarity determining region grafting technology into a human IgG_4 framework (173). A similar humanized anti–IL-5 antibody has been developed using an IgG_1 framework (174). Using epitope mapping, the antibody was shown to bind the region of IL-5 that is essential for interacting with the α subunit of the IL-5 receptor (175). Similar to the original 39D10 mAb, the humanized antibody displays high-affinity binding to hIL-5, inhibits the binding of IL-5 to cells *in vitro*, and blocks IL-5–mediated proliferation of human erythroleukemic cells *in vitro* (173). Pharmacologic studies in monkeys demonstrate that the antibody is completely absorbed into the systemic circulation following subcutaneous drug administration and that the half-life of the antibody after either intravenous or subcutaneous drug administration is about 2 weeks (174). The maximal decline in eosinophil counts occurred 3 weeks after administration of a single dose (174). The antibody blocks pulmonary eosinophilia and airway hyperreactivity in allergic mice, guinea pigs, and cynomolgus monkeys, and blocks cutaneous eosinophilia in rabbits (173,176). In monkeys, the effect was present up to 6 months following a single dose of antibody (173). Studies are under way to determine the safety and efficacy of these antibodies in humans.

Another proposed IL-5 antagonist is the soluble form of the IL-5 receptor (shIL-5Rα). The soluble isoform is generated *in vivo* by alternative splicing of the mRNA and consists of the extracellular portion of the α receptor chain. IL-5 binds shIL-5Rα with comparable affinity to membrane-bound hIL-5Rα, but the complex containing the soluble isoform is unable to associate with the common β chain, thereby acting as an IL-5 antagonist (177). *In vitro*, shIL-5Rα blocks IL-5–mediated receptor activation, inflammatory mediator production, and cell proliferation and inhibits IL-5–induced eosinophil differentiation from human cord blood cultures (177,178). To increase the half-life of the soluble form in the circulation, a fusion of the soluble human IL-5Rα and the constant domain of the human Ig κ chain has been developed (177).

A third method of blocking the action of IL-5 is interfering with the production of the cytokine using antisense oligonucleotides. Oligonucleotides have been synthesized that block IL-5 expression and secretion *in vitro* (179,180). In murine models, intravenous administration of the antisense oligonucleotide reduced IL-5 protein levels, and challenge-induced eosinophilia, airway hyperreactivity, and late-phase airway hyperresponsiveness (179). This inhibition of eosinophilia was observed for up to 17 days postadministration. In sensitized rats injected with IL-5 antisense-treated T cells, however, an inhibition of the late allergic response was not demonstrated (181).

CONCLUSION

IL-5 is a cytokine that has multiple regulatory functions on eosinophils and (in the mouse) on antibody secreting B cells. Many of these functions overlap with those of IL-3 and GM-CSF. A complex network of cytokines appears to regulate the transcription and translation of the gene for IL-5. Molecular events that follow engagement of the IL-5 receptor have been elucidated in IL-5-responsive cells. The functional overlap of IL-5 with

IL-3 and GM-CSF can be explained on the basis of a common receptor molecule and intracellular portions of the receptors resulting in the activation of similar, if not identical, intracellular events after receptor-ligand binding. Abnormally high levels of this cytokine are associated with infections with tissue-dwelling parasites and a diverse group of hypereosinophilic conditions of unknown etiology. Our understanding of the biologic role of IL-5 in the regulation of eosinophilia and the development of immunity to parasites is far from complete, but basic knowledge of its action at the cellular level has been accumulated and will be critical for the intelligent application of immunotherapy with IL-5 or inhibition of its activity in infectious, neoplastic, and other diseases.

REFERENCES

1. Sanderson CJ, Warren DJ, Strath M. Identification of a cytokine that stimulates eosinophil differentiation in vitro. Its relationship to IL-3, and functional properties of eosinophils produced in cultures. *J Exp Med* 1985; 162:60–74.
2. Swain S, Dutton RW. Production of a B cell growth-promoting activity, DL(BCGF), from a cloned T cell line and its assay on the BCL_1, B cell tumor. *J Exp Med* 1982;156:1821–1834.
3. Sanderson CJ. Control of eosinophilia. *Int Arch Allergy Appl Immunol* 1991;94:122–126.
4. Goodall GJ, Bagley CJ, Vadas MA, et al. A model for the interaction of GM-CSF, IL-3 and IL-5 receptors with their ligands. *Growth Factors* 1993;8:87–97.
5. Takatsu K, Takaki S, Hitoshi Y. Interleukin-5 and its receptor system: implications in the immune system and inflammation. *Adv Immunol* 1994;57:145–190.
6. Schimpl A, Wecker E. Replacement of T-cell function by a T cell product. *Nature* 1972;237:15–17.
7. Takatsu K, Tominaga A, Hamaoka T. Antigen-induced T cell–replacing factor (TRF). I. Functional characterization of a TRF-producing helper T cell subset and genetic studies of TR production. *J Immunol* 1980;124: 2414–2422.
8. Harada N, Kikuchi Y, Tominaga A, et al. BCGFII activity on activated B cells of purified murine T cell replacing factor (TRF) from a T cell hybridoma (B151K12). *J Immunol* 1985;134:3944–3951.
9. Sanderson CJ, Campbell HD, Young IG. Molecular and cellular biology of eosinophil differentiating factor (interleukin-5) and its effect on human and mouse B cells. *Immunol Rev* 1988;102:29–50.
10. Azuma C, Tanabe T, Konishi M, et al. Cloning of the cDNA for human T-cell replacing factor (interleukin-5) and comparison with the murine homologue. *Nucl Acids Res* 1986;14:9149–9158.
11. Kinashi TN, Harada E, Severinson E, et al. Cloning of a complementary DNA encoding T cell replacing factor and identity with B cell growth factor II. *Nature* 1986;324:70–73.
12. Sanderson CJ. The biological role of interleukin 5. *Int J Cell Cloning* 1990;1:147–153.
13. Sanderson CJ. Eosinophil differentiation factor (interleukin-5). *Immunol Ser* 1990;49:231–256.
14. Campbell HD, Sanderson CJ, Wang Y, et al. Isolation, structure and expression of cDNA and genomic clones for murine eosinophil differentiation factor. Comparison with other eosinophilopoietic lymphokines and identity with interleukin-5. *Eur J Biochem* 1988;174:345–352.
15. Campbell HD, Tucker WQJ, Hort Y, et al. Molecular cloning, nucleotide sequence, and expression of the gene encoding human eosinophil differentiation factor. *Proc Natl Acad Sci USA* 1987;84:6629–6633.
16. Sutherland GR, Baker E, Callen DF, et al. Interleukin-5 is at 5q31 and is deleted in the $5q^-$- syndrome. *Blood* 1988;71:1150–1152.
17. Le Beau MM, Lemons RS, Espinosa R, et al. Interleukin-4 and interleukin-5 map to human chromosome 5 in a region encoding growth factors and receptors and are deleted in myeloid leukemias with a del(5q). *Blood* 1989;73:647–650.
18. Yates P, Potter MN. Eosinophilic leukaemia with an abnormality of 5q31, the site of the IL-5 gene. *Clin Lab Haematol* 1991;13:211–215.
19. Geha RS, Castigli E, Chatila T. Novel immune deficiencies: defective transcription of lymphokine genes. *Clin Immunol Immunopathol* 1991;61:S16–S20.
20. Taga T, Kishimoto T. Role of a two-chain IL-6 receptor system in immune and hematopoietic cell regulation. *Crit Rev Immunol* 1992;11:265–280.
21. Tanabe T, Konishi M, Mizuta T, et al. Molecular cloning and structure of the human interleukin-5 gene. *J Biol Chem* 1987;262:16580–16584.
22. Takatsu K. Interleukin 5 (IL-5) and its receptor. *Microbiol Immunol* 1991;35:593–606.
23. Naora H, Young IG. Mechanisms regulating the mRNA levels of interleukin-5 and two other coordinately expressed lymphokines in the murine T lymphoma EL4.23. *Blood* 1994;83:3620–3628.
24. Mori A, Kaminuma O, Mikami T, et al. Dissection of human IL-5 promoter—essential role of CLE0 element in human IL-5 gene transcription. *Int Arch Allergy Immunol* 1997;113:272–274.
25. Blumenthal SG, Aichele G, Wirth T, et al. Regulation of the human interleukin-5 promoter by Ets transcription factors: ETS1 and ETS2, but not ELF-1, cooperate with GATA3 and HTLV-I TAX1. *J Biol Chem* 1999;274:12910–12916.

26. Siegel MD, Zhang D-H, Ray P, et al. Activation of the interleukin-5 promoter by cAMP in murine EL-4 cells requires the GATA-3 and CLE0 elements. *J Biol Chem* 1995;270:24548–24555.
27. Prieschl EE, Gouilleux-Gruart V, Walker C, et al. A nuclear factor of activated T cell–like transcription factor in mast cells is involved in IL-5 gene regulation after IgE plus antigen stimulation. *J Immunol* 1995;154: 6112–6119.
28. Stranick KS, Zambas DN, Uss AS, et al. Identification of transcription factor binding sites important in the regulation of the human interleukin-5 gene. *J Biol Chem* 1997;272:16453–16465.
29. De Boer ML, Mordvinov VA, Thomas MA, et al. Role of nuclear factor of activated T cells (NFAT) in the expression of interleukin-5 and other cytokines involved in the regulation of hemopoietic cells. *Int J Biochem Cell Biol* 1999;31:1221–1236.
30. Gruart-Gouilleux V, Engels P, Sullivan M. Characterization of the human interleukin-5 gene promoter: involvement of octamer binding sites in the gene promoter activity. *Eur J Immunol* 1995;25:1431–1435.
31. Mordvinov VA, Peroni SE, De Boer ML, et al. A human T-cell line with inducible production of interleukins 5 and 4. A model for studies of gene expression. *J Immunol Methods* 1999;228:163–168.
32. Schwenger GTF, Fournier R, Hall LM, et al. Nuclear factor of activated T cells and YY1 combine to repress IL-5 expression in a human T-cell line. *J Allergy Clin Immunol* 1999;104:820–827.
33. Milburn MV, Hassell AM, Lambert MH, et al. A novel dimer configuration revealed by the crystal structure at 2.4. A resolution of human interleukin-5. *Nature* 1993;363:172–176.
34. Feng Y, Klein BK, Vu L, et al. ^{1}H, ^{13}C, and ^{15}N NMR resonance assignments, secondary structure, and backbone topology of a variant of human interleukin-3. *Biochemistry* 1995;34:6540–6551.
35. Diederichs K, Boone T, Karplus PA. Novel fold and putative receptor binding site of granulocyte-macrophage colony-stimulating factor. *Science* 1991;254:1779–1782.
36. Minamitake Y, Kodama S, Katayama T, et al. Structure of recombinant human interleukin 5 produced by Chinese hamster ovary cells. *J Biochem (Tokyo)* 1990;107:292–297.
37. Tominaga A, Takahashi T, Kikuchi Y, et al. Role of carbohydrate moiety of IL-5. Effect of tunicamycin on the glycosylation of IL-5 and the biologic activity of deglycosylated IL-5. *J Immunol* 1990;144:1345–1352.
38. Kodama S, Tsujimoto M, Tsuruoka N, et al. Role of sugar chains in the in-vitro activity of recombinant human interleukin 5. *Eur J Biochem* 1993;211:903–908.
39. Takatsu K, Yamaguchi N, Hitoshi Y, et al. Signal transduction through interleukin-5 receptors. *Cold Spring Harb Symp Quant Biol* 1989;2:745–751.
40. Takaki S, Tominaga A, Hitoshi Y, et al. Molecular cloning and expression of the murine interleukin-5 receptor. *EMBO J* 1990;9:4367–4374.
41. Takaki S, Mita S, Kitamura T, et al. Identification of the second subunit of the murine interleukin-5 receptor: interleukin-3 receptor-like protein, AIC2B, is a component of the high affinity interleukin-5 receptor. *EMBO J* 1991;10:2833–2838.
42. Tominaga A, Takaki A, Hitoshi Y, et al. Role of the interleukin 5 receptor system in hematopoiesis: molecular basis for overlapping function of cytokines. *Bioessays* 1992;14:527–533.
43. Mita S, Tominaga A, Hitoshi Y, et al. Characterization of high affinity receptors for interleukin 5 on interleukin 5–dependent cell lines. *Proc Natl Acad Sci USA* 1989;86:2311–2315.
44. Mita S, Harada N, Naomi S, et al. Receptors for T cell–replacing factor/interleukin 5: specificity, quantitation and its implication. *J Exp Med* 1988;168:863–878.
45. Chihara J, Plumas J, Gruart V, et al. Characterization of a receptor for interleukin 5 on human eosinophils: variable expression and induction by granulocyte/macrophage colony–stimulating factor. *J Exp Med* 1990;172:1347–1351.
46. Lopez AF, Vadas MA, Woodcock JM, et al. Interleukin-5, interleukin-3, and granulocyte-macrophage colony–stimulating factor cross-compete for binding to cell surface receptors on human eosinophils. *J Biol Chem* 1991;266:24741–24747.
47. Ogata N, Kouro T, Yamada A, et al. JAK2 and JAK1 constitutively associate with an interleukin-5 (IL-5) receptor α and β subunit, respectively, and are activated upon IL-5 stimulation. *Blood* 1998;91:2264–2271.
48. Tuypens T, Plaetinck G, Baker E, et al. Organization and chromosomal localization of the human interleukin 5 receptor α-chain gene. *Eur Cytokine Netw* 1992;3:451–459.
49. Lopez AF, Elliott MJ, Woodcock J, et al. GM-CSF, IL-3 and IL-5: cross-competition on human haemopoietic cells. *Immunol Today* 1992;13:495–500.
50. Tavernier J, Tuypens T, Plaetinck G, et al. Molecular basis of the membrane-anchored and two soluble isoforms of the human interleukin 5 receptor α subunit. *Proc Natl Acad Sci USA* 1992;89:7041–7045.
51. Sun Z, Yergeau DA, Wong IC, et al. Interleukin-5 receptor α subunit gene regulation in human eosinophil development: identification of a unique cis-element that acts like an enhancer in regulating activity of the IL-5Rα promoter. *Curr Top Microbiol Immunol* 1996;211:173–187.
52. Baltus B, van Dijk TB, Caldenhoven E, et al. An AP-1 site in the promoter of the human IL-5Rα gene is necessary for promoter activity in eosinophilic HL60 cells. *FEBS Letts* 1998;434:251–254.
53. Tavernier J, Tuypens T, Verhee A, et al. Identification of receptor-binding domains on human interleukin 5 and design of an interleukin 5–derived receptor antagonist. *Proc Natl Acad Sci USA* 1995;92:5194–5198.
54. Murata Y, Takaki S, Migita M, et al. Molecular cloning and expression of the human interleukin 5 receptor. *J Exp Med* 1992;175:341–351.
55. Takaki S, Murata Y, Kitamura T, et al. Reconstitution of the functional receptors for murine and human interleukin 5. *J Exp Med* 1993;177:1523–1529.

56. Graber P, Proudfoot AEI, Talabot F, et al. Identification of key charged residues of human interleukin-5 in receptor binding and cellular activation. *J Biol Chem* 1995;270:15762–15769.
57. Morton T, Li J, Cook R, et al. Mutagenesis in the C-terminal region of human interleukin 5 reveals a central patch for receptor α chain recognition. *Proc Natl Acad Sci USA* 1995;92:10879–10883.
58. Li J, Cook R, Doyle ML, et al. Monomeric isomers of human interleukin 5 show that 1:1 receptor recruitment is sufficient for function. *Proc Natl Acad Sci USA* 1997;94:6694–6699.
59. Taga T, Kishimoto T. Signaling mechanisms through receptors that share signal transducing receptor components. *Curr Opin Immunol* 1995;7:17–23.
60. Silvennoinen O, Witthuhn B, Quelle FW, et al. Structure of the JAK2 protein kinase and its role in IL-3 signal transduction. *Proc Natl Acad Sci USA* 1993;90:8429–8433.
61. Rothman P, Kreider B, Azam M, et al. Cytokines and growth factor signal through tyrosine phosphorylation of a family of related transcription factors. *Immunity* 1994;1:457–468.
62. Darnell JE, Kerr IM, Stark GR, Jak-STAT pathways and transcriptional activation in response to IFNs and other extracellular signaling proteins. *Science* 1994;264:1415–1421.
63. van der Bruggen T, Caldenhoven E, Kanters D, et al. Interleukin-5 signaling in human eosinophils involves JAK2 tyrosine kinase and STAT1 α. *Blood* 1995;85:1442–1448.
64. Caldenhoven E, van Dijk T, Raaijmakers JAM, et al. Activation of the STAT3/acute phase response factor transcription factor by interleukin-5. *J Biol Chem* 1995;270:25778–25784.
65. Mui AL, Wakao H, O'Farrell AM, et al. Interleukin-3, granulocyte-macrophage colony stimulating factor and interleukin-5 transduce signals through two STAT5 homologs. *EMBO J* 1995;14:1166–1175.
66. Pazdrak K, Stafford S, Alam R. The activation of the Jak-STAT 1 signaling pathway by IL-5 in eosinophils. *J Immunol* 1995;155:397–402.
67. Ihle JN, Kerr IM. Jaks and Stats in signaling by the cytokine receptor superfamily. *Trends Genet* 1995;11:69–74.
68. Pazdrak K, Schreiber D, Forsythe P, et al. The intracellular signal transduction mechanism of interleukin 5 in eosinophils: the involvement of lyn tyrosine kinase and the Ras-Raf-1-MEK-microtubule-associated protein kinase pathway. *J Exp Med* 1995;181:1827–1834.
69. Koike M, Kikuchi Y, Tominaga A, et al. Defective IL-5-receptor–mediated signaling in B cells of X-linked immunodeficient mice. *Int Immunol* 1995;7:21–30.
70. Bates ME, Busse WW, Bertics PJ. Interleukin 5 signals through Shc and Grb2 in human eosinophils. *Am J Respir Cell Mol Biol* 1998;18:75–83.
71. Appleby MW, Kerner JD, Chien S, et al. Involvement of p59fynT in interleukin-5 receptor signaling. *J Exp Med* 1995;182:811–820.
72. Li T, Tsukada S, Satterthwaite A, et al. Activation of Bruton's tyrosine kinase (BTK) by a point mutation in its pleckstrin homology (PH) domain. *Immunity* 1995;2:451–460.
73. Coffer PJ, Schweizer RC, Dubois GR, et al. Analysis of signal transduction pathways in human eosinophils activated by chemoattractants and the T-helper 2–derived cytokines interleukin-4 and interleukin-5. *Blood* 1998; 91:2547–2557.
74. Jucker M, Feldman RA. Identification of a new adapter protein that may link the common β subunit of the receptor for granulocyte/macrophage colony–stimulating factor, interleukin (IL)–3, and IL-5 to phosphatidylinositol 3-kinase. *J Biol Chem* 1995;270:27817–27822.
75. Welham MJ, Dechert U, Leslie KB, et al. Interleukin (IL)–3 and granulocyte/macrophage colony–stimulating factor, but not IL-4, induce tyrosine phosphorylation, activation, and association of SHPTP2 with Grb2 and phosphatidylinositol 3-kinase. *J Biol Chem* 1994;269:23764–23768.
76. Takahashi-Tezuka M, Hibi M, Fujitani Y, et al. Tec tyrosine kinase links the cytokine receptors to PI-3 kinase probably through JAK. *Oncogene* 1997;14:2273–2282.
77. Erb KJ, Le Gros G. The role of Th2 type $CD4^+$ T cells and Th2 type $CD8^+$ T cells in asthma. *Immunol Cell Biol* 1996;74:206–208.
78. Warren HS, Kinnear BF, Phillips JH, et al. Production of IL-5 by human NK cells and regulation of IL-5 secretion by IL-4, IL-10, and IL-12. *J Immunol* 1995;154:5144–5152.
79. Okayama Y, Petit-Frere C, Kassel O, et al. IgE-dependent expression of mRNA for IL-4 and IL-5 in human lung mast cells. *J Immunol* 1995;155:1796–1808.
80. Tanaka Y, Delaporte E, Dubucquoi S, et al. Interleukin-5 messenger RNA and immunoreactive protein expression by activated eosinophils in lesional atopic dermatitis skin. *J Invest Dermatol* 1994;103:589–592.
81. Dubucquoi S, Desreumaux P, Janin A, et al. Interleukin 5 synthesis by eosinophils: association with granules and immunoglobulin-dependent secretion. *J Exp Med* 1994;179:703–708.
82. Salvi S, Semper A, Blomberg A, et al. Interleukin-5 production by human airway epithelial cells. *Am J Respir Cell Mol Biol* 1999;20:984–991.
83. Paul CC, Keller JR, Armpriester JM, et al. Epstein-Barr virus transformed B lymphocytes produce interleukin-5. *Blood* 1990;75:1400–1403.
84. Samoszuk M, Nansen L. Detection of interleukin-5 messenger RNA in Reed-Sternberg cells of Hodgkin's disease with eosinophilia. *Blood* 1990;75:13–16.
85. Ying S, Durham SR, Barkans J, et al. T cells are the principal source of interleukin-5 mRNA in allergen-induced rhinitis. *Am J Respir Cell Mol Biol* 1993;9:356–360.
86. Krishnaswamy G, Liu MC, Su SN, et al. Analysis of cytokine transcripts in the bronchoalveolar lavage cells of patients with asthma. *Am J Respir Cell Mol Biol* 1993;9:279–286.

87. Kay AB, Ying S, Durham SR. Phenotype of cells positive for interleukin-4 and interleukin-5 mRNA in allergic tissue reactions. *Int Arch Allergy Immunol* 1995;107:208–210.
88. Bradding P, Roberts JA, Britten KM, et al. Interleukin-4, -5, and -6 and tumor necrosis factor–α in normal and asthmatic airways: evidence for the human mast cell as a source of these cytokines. *Am J Respir Cell Mol Biol* 1994;10:471–480.
89. Bradding P, Feather IH, Wilson S, et al. Immunolocalization of cytokines in the nasal mucosa of normal and perennial rhinitic subjects. The mast cell as a source of IL-4, IL-5, and IL-6 in human allergic mucosal inflammation. *J Immunol* 1993;151:3853–3865.
90. Bradding P, Okayama Y, Howarth PH, et al. Heterogeneity of human mast cells based on cytokine content. *J Immunol* 1995;155:297–307.
91. Desreumaux P, Janin A, Colombel JF, et al. Interleukin 5 messenger RNA expression by eosinophils in the intestinal mucosa of patients with coeliac disease. *J Exp Med* 1992;175:293–296.
92. Rennick DM, Thompson SL, Coffman RL, et al. In vivo administration of antibody to interleukin-5 inhibits increased generation of eosinophils and their progenitors in bone marrow of parasitized mice. *Blood* 1990;76: 312–316.
93. Her E, Frazer J, Austen KF, et al. Eosinophil hematopoietins antagonize the programmed cell death of eosinophils. Cytokine and glucocorticoid effects on eosinophils maintained by endothelial cell–conditioned medium. *J Clin Invest* 1991;88:1982–1987.
94. Tai PC, Sun L, Spry CJ. Effects of IL-5, granulocyte/macrophage colony–stimulating factor (GM-CSF) and IL-3 on the survival of human blood eosinophils in vitro. *Clin Exp Immunol* 1991;85:312–316.
95. Lu L, Lin ZH, Shen RN, et al. Influence of interleukins 3, 5 and 6 on the growth of eosinophil progenitors in highly enriched human bone marrow in the absence of serum. *Exp Hematol* 1990;18:1180–1186.
96. Yamaguchi Y, Suda T, Suda J, et al. Purified IL-5 supports the terminal differentiation and proliferation of murine eosinophil precursors. *J Exp Med* 1988;167:43–56.
97. Gleich GJ, Adolphson CR, Leiferman KM. The biology of the eosinophilic leukocyte. *Annu Rev Med* 1993; 44:85–101.
98. Lu P, Zhou X, Chen SJ, et al. CTLA-4 ligands are required to induce an in vivo interleukin 4 response to a gastrointestinal nematode parasite. *J Exp Med* 1994;180:693–698.
99. Warren DJ, Sanderson CJ. Production of a T cell hybrid producing a lymphokine stimulating eosinophil differentiation. *Immunology* 1985;54:615–623.
100. Yamaguchi Y, Suda T, Ohta S, et al. Analysis of the survival of mature human eosinophils: interleukin-5 prevents apoptosis in mature human eosinophils. *Blood* 1991;78:2542–2547.
101. Walsh GM, Wardlaw AJ, Hartnell A, et al. Interleukin-5 enhances the in vitro adhesion of human eosinophils, but not neutrophils, in a leucocyte integrin (CD11/18)–dependent manner. *Int Arch Allergy Appl Immunol* 1991; 94:174–178.
102. Weller PF. Cytokine regulation of eosinophil function. *Clin Immunol Immunopathol* 1992;62:S55–S59.
103. Lopez AF, Sanderson CJ, Gamble JR, et al. Recombinant human interleukin-5 is a selective activator of human eosinophil function. *J Exp Med* 1988;167:219–224.
104. Owen WF, Rothenberg ME, Petersen J, et al. Interleukin 5 and phenotypically altered eosinophils in the blood of patients with the idiopathic hypereosinophilic syndrome. *J Exp Med* 1989;170:343–348.
105. Owen WF, Petersen J, Sheff DM, et al. Hypodense eosinophils and interleukin 5 activity in the blood of patients with the eosinophilia-myalgia syndrome. *Proc Natl Acad Sci USA* 1990;87:8647–8651.
106. Limaye AP, Abrams JS, Silver JE, et al. Interleukin-5 and the posttreatment eosinophilia in patients with onchocerciasis. *J Clin Invest* 1991;88:1418–1421.
107. van Haelst Pisani C, Kovach JS, Kita H, et al. Administration of interleukin-2 (IL-2) results in increased plasma concentrations of IL-5 and eosinophilia in patients with cancer. *Blood* 1991;78:1538–1544.
108. Butterfield JH, Leiferman KM, Abrams J, et al. Elevated serum levels of interleukin-5 in patients with the syndrome of episodic angioedema and eosinophilia. *Blood* 1992;79:688–692.
109. Bischoff SC, Brunner T, Deweck AL, et al. Interleukin 5 modifies histamine release and leukotriene generation by human basophils in response to diverse agonists. *J Exp Med* 1990;172:1577–1582.
110. Hirai K, Yamaguchi M, Misaki Y, et al. Enhancement of human basophil histamine release by interleukin 5. *J Exp Med* 1990;172:1525–1528.
111. Denburg JA, Silver JE, Abrams JS. Interleukin-5 is a human basophilopoietin: induction of histamine content and basophilic differentiation of HL-60 cells and of peripheral blood basophil-eosinophil progenitors. *Blood* 1991;77:1462–1468.
112. Yokota T, Coffman RL, Hagiawara H, et al. Isolation and characterization of lymphokine cDNA clones encoding mouse and human IgA-enhancing factor and eosinophil colony–stimulating factor activities: relationship to interleukin 5. *Proc Natl Acad Sci USA* 1987;84:7388–7392.
113. Clutterbuck EJ, Shields J, Gordon J, et al. Recombinant human interleukin-5 is an eosinophil differentiation factor but has no activity in standard human B cell growth factor assays. *Eur J Immunol* 1987;17:1743–1750.
114. Dent LA, Strath M, Mellor AL, et al. Eosinophilia in transgenic mice expressing interleukin 5. *J Exp Med* 1990; 172:1425–1431.
115. Tominaga A, Takaki S, Koyama N, et al. Transgenic mice expressing a B cell growth and differentiation factor gene (interleukin 5) develop eosinophilia and autoantibody production. *J Exp Med* 1991;173:429–437.
116. Hitoshi Y, Yamaguchi N, Korenaga M, et al. In vivo administration of antibody to murine IL-5 receptor inhibits eosinophilia of IL-5 transgenic mice. *Int Immunol* 1991;3:135–139.

117. Takatsu K. Interleukin-5. *Curr Opin Immunol* 1992;4:299–306.
118. Medhat A, Shehata M, Bucci K, et al. Increased interleukin-4 and interleukin-5 production in response to *Schistosoma haematobium* adult worm antigens correlates with lack of reinfection after treatment. *J Infect Dis* 1998;178:512–519.
119. Mahanty S, Abrams JS, King CL, et al. Parallel regulation of IL-4 and IL-5 in human helminth infections. *J Immunol* 1992;148:3567–3571.
120. Mahanty S, Abrams JS, Limaye AP, et al. Linkage of IL-4 and IL-5 production in human helminth infections. *Trans Am Assoc Phys* 1991;104:296–303.
121. Mahanty S, King CL, Kumaraswami V, et al. IL-4- and IL-5-secreting lymphocyte populations are preferentially stimulated by parasite-derived antigens in human tissue invasive nematode infections. *J Immunol* 1993; 151:3704–3711.
122. Montenegro SM, Miranda P, Mahanty S, et al. Cytokine production in acute versus chronic human Schistosomiasis mansoni: the cross-regulatory role of interferon-γ and interleukin-10 in the responses of peripheral blood mononuclear cells and splenocytes to parasite antigens. *J Infect Dis* 1999;179:1502–1514.
123. Limaye AP, Abrams JS, Silver JE, et al. Regulation of parasite-induced eosinophilia: selectively increased interleukin 5 production in helminth-infected patients. *J Exp Med* 1990;172:399–402.
124. Kan H, Ogata T, Taniyama A, et al. Extraordinarily high eosinophilia and elevated serum interleukin-5 level observed in a patient infected with *Paragonimus westermani*. *Pediatrics* 1995;96:351–354.
125. Matsumoto R, Ando M, Kohrogi H, et al. Interleukin-5 levels of pleural fluid and serum samples in a patient with PIE syndrome. *Chest* 1992;102:1296–1297.
126. Rigano R, Profumo E, Teggi A, et al. Production of IL-5 and IL-6 by peripheral blood mononuclear cells (PBMC) from patients with *Echinococcus granulosus* infection. *Clin Exp Immunol* 1996;105:456–459.
127. Evans CA, Garcia HH, Hartnell A, et al. Elevated concentrations of eotaxin and interleukin-5 in human neurocysticercosis. *Infect Immun* 1998;66:4522–4525.
128. Matsumoto T, Kimura S, Yamauchi M, et al. Soluble CD23 and IL-5 levels in the serum and culture supernatants of peripheral blood mononuclear cells in a girl with cutaneous paragonimiasis: case report. *Ann Trop Paediatr* 1998;18:49–53.
129. Zhou Y, Bao S, Rothwell TL, et al. Differential expression of interleukin-5 $mRNA^+$ cells and eosinophils in *Nippostrongylus brasiliensis* infection in resistant and susceptible strains of mice. *Eur J Immunol* 1996;26: 2133–2139.
130. Urban JF Jr, Katona IM, Paul WE, et al. Interleukin 4 is important in protective immunity to a gastrointestinal nematode infection in mice. *Proc Natl Acad Sci USA* 1991;88:5513–5517.
131. Coffman RL, Seymour BW, Hudak S, et al. Antibody to interleukin-5 inhibits helminth-induced eosinophilia in mice. *Science* 1989;245:308–310.
132. Kopf M, Brombacher F, Hodgkin PD, et al. IL-5–deficient mice have a developmental defect in $CD5^+$ B-1 cells and lack eosinophilia but have normal antibody and cytotoxic T cell responses. *Immunity* 1996;4:15–24.
133. Steel C, Nutman TB. Regulation of IL-5 in onchocerciasis. A critical role for IL-2. *J Immunol* 1993;150: 5511–5518.
134. Bancroft AJ, Grencis RK, Else KJ, et al. Cytokine production in BALB/c mice immunized with radiation attenuated third stage larvae of the filarial nematode, *Brugia pahangi*. *J Immunol* 1993;150:1395–1402.
135. Wynn TA, Jankovic D, Hieny S, et al. IL-12 enhances vaccine-induced immunity to *Schistosoma mansoni* in mice and decreases T helper 2 cytokine expression, IgE production, and tissue eosinophilia. *J Immunol* 1995; 154:4701–4709.
136. Lange AM, Yutanawiboonchai W, Scott P, et al. IL-4– and IL-5–dependent protective immunity to *Onchocerca volvulus* infective larvae in BALB/cBYJ mice. *J Immunol* 1994;153:205–211.
137. Hogarth PJ, Taylor MJ, Bianco AE. IL-5–dependent immunity to microfilariae is independent of IL-4 in a mouse model of onchocerciasis. *J Immunol* 1998;160:5436–5440.
138. Sher A, Coffman RF, Hieny S, et al. Ablation of eosinophil and IgE responses with anti–IL-5 or anti–IL-4 antibodies fails to affect immunity against *Schistosoma mansoni* in the mouse. *J Immunol* 1990;145:3911–3916.
139. Korenaga M, Hitoshi Y, Yamaguchi N, et al. The role of interleukin-5 in protective immunity to *Strongyloides venezuelensis* infection in mice. *Immunology* 1991;72:502–507.
140. Sasaki O, Sugaya H, Ishida K, et al. Ablation of eosinophils with anti–IL-5 antibody enhances the survival of intracranial worms of *Angiostrongylus cantonensis* in the mouse. *Parasite Immunol* 1993;15:349–354.
141. Yoshida T, Ikuta K, Sugaya H, et al. Defective B-1 cell development and impaired immunity against *Angiostrongylus cantonensis* in IL-5Rα–deficient mice. *Immunity* 1996;4:483–494.
142. Rotman HL, Yutanawiboonchai W, Brigandi RA, et al. *Strongyloides stercoralis*: eosinophil-dependent immune-mediated killing of third stage larvae in BALB/cByJ mice. *Exp Parasitol* 1996;82:267–278.
143. Abraham D, Rotman HL, Haberstroh HF, et al. *Strongyloides stercoralis*: protective immunity to third-stage larvae in BALB/cByJ mice. *Exp Parasitol* 1995;80:297–307.
144. Folkard SG, Hogarth PJ, Taylor MJ, et al. Eosinophils are the major effector cells of immunity to microfilariae in a mouse model of onchocerciasis. *Parasitology* 1996;112:323–329.
145. Elson LH, Calvopina M, Paredes W, et al. Immunity to onchocerciasis: putative immune persons produce a Th1-like response to *Onchcocerca volvulus*. *J Infect Dis* 1995;171:652–658.
146. Weller PF, Bubley GJ, The idiopathic hypereosinophilic syndrome. *Blood* 1994;83:2759–2779.
147. Nutman TB, Miller KD, Mulligan M, et al. *Loa loa* infection in temporary residents of endemic regions: recognition of a hyperresponsive syndrome with characteristic clinical manifestations. *J Infect Dis* 1986;154:10–18.

148. Kayes SG. Human toxocariasis and the visceral larva migrans syndrome: correlative immunopathology. *Chem Immunol* 1997;66:99–124.
149. de Krömer MT, Medina-de-la-Garza CE, Brattig NW. Differences in eosinophil and neutrophil chemotactic responses in sowda and generalized form of onchocerciasis. *Acta Tropica* 1995;60:21–33.
150. Ackerman SJ, Kephart GM, Francis H, et al. Eosinophil degranulation: an immunologic determinant in the pathogenesis of the Mazzotti reaction in human onchocerciasis. *J Immunol* 1990;144:3961–3969.
151. Pearlman E. Immunopathology of onchocerciasis: a role for eosinophils in onchocercal dermatitis and keratitis. *Chem Immunol* 1997;66:26–40.
152. Pearlman E, Lass JH, Bardenstein DS, et al. IL-12 exacerbates helminth-mediated corneal pathology by augmenting inflammatory cell recruitment and chemokine expression. *J Immunol* 1997;158:827–833.
153. Pearlman E, Lass JH, Bardenstein DS, et al. Interleukin 4 and T helper type 2 cells are required for the development of onchocercal keratitis (river blindness). *J Exp Med* 1995;182:931–940.
154. Sher A, Coffman RL, Hieny S, et al. Interleukin 5 is required for the blood and tissue eosinophilia but not granuloma formation induced by infection with *Schistosoma mansoni*. *Proc Natl Acad Sci USA* 1990;87:61–65.
155. Pearce EJ, Sher A. Immunity to helminths. *Curr Opin Immunol* 1989;2:375–379.
156. Sher A, Coffman RL, Hieny S, et al. Ablation of eosinophil and IgE responses with anti–IL-5 or anti–IL-4 antibodies fails to affect immunity against *Schistosoma mansoni* in the mouse. *J Immunol* 1990;145:3911–3916.
157. Lowe D, Jorizzo J, Hutt MSR. Tumour-associated eosinophilia: a review. *J Clin Pathol* 1981;34:1343–1348.
158. Lowe W, Fletcher CDM, Gower RL. Tumour-associated eosinophils in the bladder. *J Clin Pathol* 1984;37:500–502.
159. Kapp DS, Livolsi VA. Intense eosinophilic stromal infiltrate in carcinoma of the uterine cervix. *Gynecol Oncol* 1983;16:19–30.
160. Goldsmith MM, Gresson DH, Askin FB. The prognostic significance of stromal eosinophilia in head and neck cancer. *Otolaryngol Head Neck Surg* 1987;96:319–324.
161. Stefanini M, Claustro JC, Motos RA, et al. Blood and bone marrow eosinophilia in malignant tumors. Role and nature of blood and tissue eosinophil colony–stimulating factor(s) in two patients. *Cancer* 1991;68:543–548.
162. Desenne JJ, Acquatella G, Stern R, et al. Blood eosinophilia in Hodgkin's disease. A follow-up of 25 cases in Venezuela. *Cancer* 1992;69:1248–1253.
163. Srivastava A, Boswell HS, Heerema NA, et al. KRAS2 oncogene overexpression in myelodysplastic syndrome with translocation 5;12. *Cancer Genet Cytogenet* 1988;35:61–71.
164. Berkowicz M, Rosner E, Rechavi G, et al. Atypical chronic myelomonocytic leukemia with eosinophilia and translocation (5;12). A new association? *Cancer Genet Cytogenet* 1991;51:277–278.
165. Huland E, Huland H. Tumor-associated eosinophilia in interleukin-2–treated patients: evidence of toxic eosinophil degranulation on bladder cancer cells. *Cancer Res Clin Oncol* 1992;118:463–467.
166. Arinaga S, Karimine N, Takamuku K, et al. Correlation of eosinophilia with clinical response in patients with advanced carcinoma treated with low-dose recombinant interleukin-2 and mitomycin C. *J Immunol* 1990;144:4898–4905.
167. Kung TT, Jones H, Adams GKI, et al. Characterization of a murine model of allergic pulmonary inflammation. *Int Arch Allergy Immunol* 1994;105:83–90.
168. Kung TT, Stelts DM, Zurcher JA, et al. Involvement of IL-5 in a murine model of allergic inflammation: prophylactic and therapeutic effect of an anti–IL-5 antibody. *Am J Respir Cell Mol Biol* 1995;13:360–365.
169. Shardonofsky FR, Venzor J, Barrios R, et al. Therapeutic efficacy of an anti–IL-5 monoclonal antibody delivered into the respiratory tract in a murine model of asthma. *J Allergy Clin Immunol* 1999;104:215–221.
170. van Oosterhout AJ, van Ark I, Folkerts G, et al. Antibody to interleukin-5 inhibits virus-induced airway hyperresponsiveness to histamine in guinea pigs. *Am J Respir Crit Care Med* 1995;151:177–183.
171. Mauser PJ, Pitman A, Fernandez X, et al. Inhibitory effect of the TRFK-5 anti–IL-5 antibody in a guinea pig model of asthma. *Am Rev Respir Dis* 1993;148:1623–1627.
172. Mauser PJ, Pitman AM, Fernandez X, et al. Effects of an antibody to interleukin-5 in a monkey model of asthma. *Am J Respir Crit Care Med* 1995;152:467–472.
173. Egan RW, Athwal D, Bodmer MW, et al. Effect of Sch 55700, a humanized monoclonal antibody to human interleukin-5, on eosinophilic responses and bronchial hyperreactivity. *Arzneim-Forsch/Drug Res* 1999;49:779–790.
174. Zia-Amirhosseini P, Minthorn E, Benincosa LJ, et al. Pharmacokinetics and pharmacodynamics of SB-240563, a humanized monoclonal antibody directed to human interleukin-5, in monkeys. *J Pharmacol Exp Ther* 1999;291:1060–1067.
175. Zhang J, Kuvelkar R, Murgolo NJ, et al. Mapping and characterization of the epitope(s) of Sch 55700, a humanized mAb, that inhibits human IL-5. *Int Immunol* 1999;11:1935–1943.
176. Egan RW, Athwahl D, Chou CC, et al. Pulmonary biology of anti-interleukin 5 antibodies. *Mem Inst Oswaldo Cruz* 1997;92:S69–S73.
177. Devos R, Plaetinck G, Cornelis S, et al. Interleukin-5 and its receptor: a drug target for eosinophilia associated with chronic allergic disease. *J Leukoc Biol* 1995;57:813–819.
178. Monahan J, Siegel N, Keith R, et al. Attenuation of IL-5–mediated signal transduction, eosinophil survival, and inflammatory mediator release by a soluble human IL-5 receptor. *J Immunol* 1997;159:4024–4034.
179. Karras J, McGraw K, McKay R, et al. Inhibition of antigen-induced eosinophilia and late-phase ariway hyperresponsiveness by an interleukin-5 antisense oligonucleotide in mouse models of asthma. *J Immunol* 2000:164;5409–5415.

180. Weltman JK, Karim AS. Interleukin-5: a proeosinophil cytokine mediator of inflammation in asthma and a target for antisense therapy. *Allergy Asthma Proc* 1998;19:257–261.
181. Molet S, Ramos-Barbon D, Martin JG, et al. Adoptively transferred late allergic response is inhibited by IL-4, but not IL-5, antisense oligonucleotide. *J Allergy Clin Immunol* 1999;104:205–214.
182. Aoki M, Sugaya H, Ishida K, et al. The role of $CD4^+$ and $CD8^+$ T-cells in host morbidity and innate resistance to angiostrongylus cantonensis in the mouse. *Parasitol Res* 1998;84:91–99.
183. Sugaya H, Aoki M, Abe T, et al. Cytokine responses in mice infected with *Angiostrongylus cantonensis*. *Parasitol Res* 1997;83:10–15.
184. Sugaya H, Aoki M, Yoshida T, et al. Eosinophilia and intracranial worm recovery in interleukin-5 transgenic and interleukin-5 receptor α chain-knockout mice infected with *Angiostrongylus cantonensis*. *Parasitol Res* 1997;83:583–590.
185. Urban JJ, Katona IM, Paul WE, et al. Interleukin 4 is important in protective immunity to a gastrointestinal nematode infection in mice. *Proc Natl Acad Sci USA* 1991;88:5513–5517.
186. Ovington KS, Behm CA. The enigmatic eosinophil: investigation of the biological role of eosinophils in parasitic helminth infection. *Mem Inst Oswaldo Cruz* 1997;92:S93–S104.
187. Dent LA, Daly C, Geddes A, et al. Immune responses of IL-5 transgenic mice to parasites and aeroallergens. *Mem Inst Oswaldo Cruz* 1997;92:S45–S54.
188. Shin EH, Osada Y, Chai JY, et al. Protective roles of eosinophils in *Nippostrongylus brasiliensis* infection. *Int Arch Allergy Immunol* 1997;114:S45–S50.
189. Folkard SG, Taylor MJ, Butcher GA, et al. Protective responses against skin-dwelling microfilariae of *Onchocerca lienalis* in severe combined immunodeficient mice. *Infect Immun* 1997;65:2846–2851.
190. Korenaga M, Hitoshi Y, Takatsu K, et al. Cross-resistance between *Strongyloides venezuelensis* and *S. ratti* in mice. *J Helminthol* 1995;69:119–123.
191. Dent LA, Daly CM, Mayrhofer G, et al. Interleukin-5 transgenic mice show enhanced resistance to primary infections with *Nippostrongylus brasiliensis* but not primary infections with *Toxocara canis*. *Infect Immun* 1999; 67:989–993.
192. Sugane K, Kusama Y, Takamoto M, et al. Eosinophilia, IL-5 level and recovery of larvae in IL-5 transgenic mice infected with *Toxocara canis*. *J Helminthol* 1996;70:153–158.
193. Parsons JC, Coffman RL, Grieve RB. Antibody to interleukin 5 prevents blood and tissue eosinophilia but not liver trapping in murine larval toxocariasis. *Parasite Immunol* 1993;15:501–508.
194. Herndon FJ, Kayes SG. Depletion of eosinophils by anti–IL-5 monoclonal antibody treatment of mice infected with *Trichinella spiralis* does not alter parasite burden or immunologic resistance to infection. *J Immunol* 1992; 149:3642–3647.
195. Hokibara S, Takamoto M, Tominaga A, et al. Marked eosinophilia in interleukin-5 transgenic mice fails to prevent *Trichinella spiralis* infection. *J Parasitol* 1997;83:1186–1189.

4

Interleukin-10

Drew Weissman

Division of Infectious Diseases, University of Pennsylvania Medical Center, Philadelphia, Pennsylvania

BRIEF HISTORY

Activities attributed to interleukin (IL)-10 were initially identified in 1989 (1). The cloning of the gene for mouse and human (h) IL-10 followed in 1990 and 1991. Broad immunologic activities have been described, including both enhancing and deactivating actions. Even within a single cell type, IL-10 can have both activating and inhibitory activities, as observed in macrophages. IL-10 potently deactivates macrophages as measured by cytokine production, antigen presentation, and reactive oxygen and nitrogen production, but it also enhances Fc receptor–mediated endocytosis and killing. The roles of IL-10 in modulating murine models and human diseases, including parasitic infection, rheumatoid arthritis, systemic lupus erythematosus, and inflammatory bowel disease (IBD), to name a few, have been investigated. This chapter discusses the history of IL-10, the mechanisms of action, animal model data, and preliminary data in human trials.

IL-10 was initially identified by three different *in vitro* biologic activities. Cytokine synthesis inhibitory factor (CSIF), later named IL-10, was isolated from murine T helper 2 (Th2) clones in a search for factors that inhibited proliferation and function of Th1 cells, analogous to the interferon (IFN)–γ inhibitory effect on Th2 cells. CSIF inhibited IFN-γ production from Th1 cells (1). In an alternate series of experiments, an activity produced by mouse lymphoma cells was found to increase growth of mast cells in culture in the presence of IL-3 or IL-4 and alone sustained the viability of mast cells (2–5). These supernatants were also found to enhance murine thymocyte proliferation when grown in IL-2 and IL-4 (6).

IL-10 was found to have high amino acid (84%) and nucleotide sequence (71%) homology to an open reading frame in the Epstein-Barr virus (EBV), BCRF1 (7–9). The viral (v) IL-10 has no introns and does not share 5′ and 3′ regions, suggesting that EBV captured a processed hIL-10 ancestral gene (9). vIL-10 has threefold to 10-fold lower activity than IL-10 depending on the activity being measured (9). Viral IL-10 has been demonstrated to be important in multiple stages of EBV infection, ranging from lytic infection to tumorigenesis (7,8,10–17).

OVERVIEW OF ACTIVITY

IL-10 (Fig. 4.1) has activity on most cells of the immune system and includes both direct activity through its receptor expressed on the surface of the cell, and indirect activ-

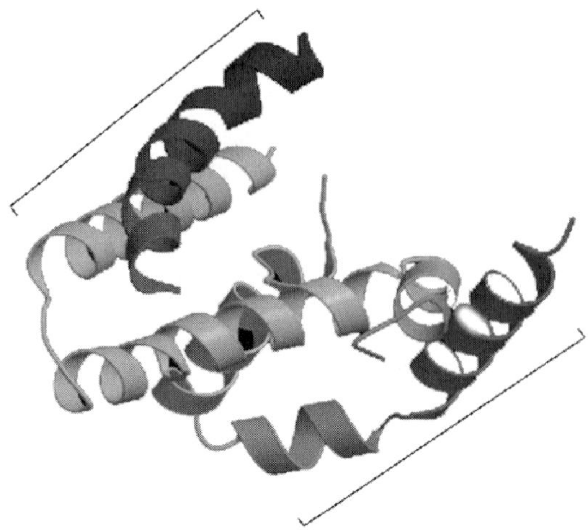

FIG. 4.1. Diagram of interleukin-10 (IL-10) structure based on x-ray crystallography. *Brackets* indicate regions that interact with the alpha chain of the IL-10 receptor.

ity, in which the cell affected is not directly acted on by IL-10, but, rather, another cell important in inducing the activity is affected (Table 4.1). IL-10 activity in mice does not always correlate with human action. Herein is an attempt to limit the discussion to hIL-10 unless the activity being described is similar in both systems. The action on individual cells will be described first followed by the effect of IL-10 on immune functions.

Many immune and certain nonimmune cells produce hIL-10. Human $CD4^+$ T cells, including Th0, Th1, and Th2 clones, secrete IL-10 (18). Monocytes, macrophages (19,20), B cells, including EBV-infected cell lines (21,22), keratinocytes (23–26), and melanoma and certain carcinomas (27–30) produce IL-10. Depending on the cell type, the produced IL-10 may act as a growth factor or as a modulator of immune function on the cells producing it (autocrine activity) or surrounding cells (paracrine activity).

T Cells/Thymocytes

hIL-10 has been demonstrated to act directly on T cells and $CD4^+$ T cell clones and inhibit proliferation. The inhibition of proliferation is independent of activation, coactiva-

TABLE 4-1. *Effect of human IL-10 on immune functions*

Positive
Enhances ADCC activity of monocytes
B cell growth and differentiation factor
Increases CTL activity in certain systems
Increases NK cell activity in certain systems
Chemotactic for $CD8^+$ T cells
Negative
Blocks monocyte/macrophage reactive oxidant production
Inhibits pro-inflammatory cytokine secretion
Decreases antigen presentation
Down regulates IL-12
Blocks T-cell activation
Inhibits chemotaxis of $CD4^+$ T cells

tion, or adhesion molecules but is overcome by the addition of IL-2, suggesting that IL-10's direct effect on T cells is to inhibit IL-2 production (31). The inhibition of IL-2 also is observed at the level of mRNA, but IL-10 does not affect IL-4, IL-5, IFN-γ, or granulocyte-macrophage-colony stimulating factor (GM-CSF) production. IL-10 is chemotactic for hCD8$^+$ T cells but not hCD4$^+$ T cells, and it inhibits chemotaxis of CD4$^+$ T cells towards IL-8 (32). hIL-10 does not appear to have any action on thymocytes. Thus, unlike murine IL-10, which has multiple direct effects in promoting T cell differentiation, CTL generation, and CTL activity, hIL-10 only has an inhibitory activity directly on CD4$^+$ T cell clones and T cells with the exception of its chemoattraction for CD8$^+$ T cells.

B Lymphocytes

hIL-10 enhances multiple aspects of B cell growth, differentiation, and function. hIL-10 enhances *Staphylococcus aureus* Cowan (SAC) strain and surface Ig cross-linking induced B lymphocyte proliferation (33–35). A greater effect on proliferation was observed when CD40 was used as a stimulator and when IL-4 was added (33,36). The action of IL-10 on B cells depends in part on the stage of activation of the cells. IL-10 blocked apoptosis of germinal center B cells (37) but induced apoptosis of chronic lymphocytic leukemia cells (38). This dichotomy of action has been explained by the observation that IL-10 added early during SAC activation resulted in apoptosis while delaying addition for 72 hours blocked apoptosis and increased the differentiation of B cells (33). IL-10 also acts as a differentiation factor for B cells. It increases the total amount of IgG, IgM, and IgA produced by SAC or CD40 stimulated B cells (33). IL-10 also directly induces IgG isotype class switching (39,40). Interesting reports have investigated the role of IL-10 in IgA secretion. It was demonstrated that IL-10 with TGF-β induced IgA subclass switching in anti-CD40 stimulated B cells (41). In two studies of IgA-deficient individuals, B cells from a subset of individuals in each study produced IgA when IL-10 was added to their *in vitro*–stimulated cells. No IgA was produced with stimulation alone in the absence of IL-10 (42,43). These observations suggest that a subset of IgA-deficient individuals may have a defect in IL-10–induced IgA production. Thus, hIL-10 increases the activation and differentiation of human B cells, which is in part dependent on the stage of differentiation of the cell. In addition, it induces IgG and IgA class switching. An inhibitory effect on B cell development by IL-10 has been described, but this occurs indirectly through accessory cells.

Natural Killer Cells

Natural killer (NK) cells represent a small population of cells that lyse tumor and virally infected cells without prior sensitization. IL-2–activated NK cells produce IFN-γ, tumor necrosis factor (TNF)–α, and GM-CSF in response to IL-10 stimulation. IL-10 in combination with low concentrations of IL-2 increases NK cytotoxicity, while IL-10 alone, when added to NK cells, enhances their killing ability on NK-resistant target cells. IL-10 led to an increase in proliferation when added to certain populations of NK cells in the presence of IL-2 (44). Not all studies are in agreement with the ability of IL-10 to upregulate IFN-γ secretion by NK cells (45). An additional study has demonstrated that IL-10 increases NK activity by downregulating major histocompatibility complex (MHC) class I expression on tumor cells (46). Thus, although not all studies are in agreement with regard to mechanism, most agree that IL-10 increases NK cytotoxic activity.

Monocyte/Macrophages

One of the most prominent functions of IL-10 is its macrophage-deactivating property. It alters the function, cytokines produced, morphology, and phenotype of monocytes and macrophages, but not all of IL-10 effects on monocyte/macrophages are inhibitory. Surface antigen expression of human monocytes treated with exogenous IL-10 demonstrates a downregulation of MHC class II molecules and an inhibition of IL-4 or IFN-γ induced upregulation of MHC class II (7). In addition, when monocytes are stimulated with lipopolysaccharide (LPS), the endogenously produced IL-10 also downregulates MHC class II expression (7,20). IL-10 has no effect on the baseline or induced expression of CD14, CD54 (ICAM-1), CD58 (LFA-3), or CD11a,b,c in monocyte/macrophages. The effect of IL-10 downregulation of MHC class II on antigen presenting cell function will be discussed below.

IL-10 strongly inhibits cytokine synthesis at both protein and mRNA levels. IL-1α, IL-1β, IL-6, IL-8, TNF-α, GM-CSF, MIP-1α, prostaglandin E_2, migration inhibitory factor (MIF), and granulocyte colony-stimulating factor (G-CSF) induced by LPS or LPS plus IFNγ and other activation events are potently inhibited by IL-10 (20,47–51). IL-10 inhibits proinflammatory cytokines (52,53) and chemokines (D. Weissman and Anthony S. Fauci, unpublished observations) when administered *in vivo* to normal volunteers as a single infusion. In a mouse model of endotoxin shock, the administration of IL-10 with a lethal amount of LPS resulted in protection from death and an inhibition of the proinflammatory cytokine TNF-α (54). IL-10 acts in an autoregulatory role in monocytes. It is produced following activation and acts to inhibit further proinflammatory cytokine release as well as its own release (20,55,56). In addition to inhibiting cytokines, it also inhibits the production of reactive oxygen (O_2^-) and nitrogen species used by macrophages to kill ingested organisms (57).

IL-10, unlike its overall inhibition of most cytokines, induces IL-1 receptor antagonist (RA), which also has antiinflammatory properties (58–60). In addition, IL-10 enhances certain monocyte functions. Monocytes treated with IL-10 increase their expression of CD64 (FcγRI) and enhance their ability to lyse anti-D–coated RBC, a measure of antibody-dependent cell cytotoxicity (ADCC) (61,62). Thus, IL-10 potently inhibits the activation of, cytokine release by, and most effector functions of human monocyte/macrophages by direct and indirect mechanisms with the exception that it enhances ADCC activity.

Cytokine Network Interactions

As detailed in almost every chapter of this book, cytokines act in a network. In addition to the IL-10 ability to modulate immune functions, it is extremely potent at modifying cytokine secretion from multiple cell types. As described above, its action on monocyte/macrophages results in the inhibition of proinflammatory cytokine secretion. Another main cytokine involved in cell-mediated immunity is IL-12 (see Chapter 5). IL-10 is a major regulator of IL-12 production and inhibits its production from dendritic cells and other antigen presenting cells (63–68). As IL-12 is important in Th1 cellular immunity, IL-10 inhibition of IL-12 blocks the induction of potent cell mediated immunity and IFN-γ production. IL-12 both directly and synergistically with other cytokines and signaling events induces IL-10, suggesting a regulatory role for IL-12 on its own production (66,67,69–75). Thus, in addition to IL-10's other effects on antigen presenting cell function described below, one of its most potent effects is mediated by its inhibition of IL-12.

Antigen-Presenting Cell Function

The presentation of antigen to and activation of T cells occurs through both antigen-specific and antigen independent interactions between an antigen-presenting cell (APC) and a T cell. Antigens obtained by an APC are processed into peptides and associated with MHC class I (for $CD8^+$ T cells) and II (for $CD4^+$ T cells) molecules and expressed on the surface. A T cell that can recognize the antigenic peptide in association with the MHC molecule forms an interaction between its T cell receptor (TCR) and the MHC–peptide complex on the APC. Other interactions between adhesion molecules and costimulatory molecules are also required. Adhesion molecule interactions including LFA-1 and CD2 on the T cell and ICAM-1 and LFA-3 on the APC, respectively, stabilize cellular interaction and may also deliver activation signals to the cells. Costimulation between CD28 on the T cell and CD80 and CD86 on the APC and CD40 and CD40L allow for efficient T cell activation and enhance APC activity. T cell activation leads to the release of IL-2 and the expression of the high-affinity IL-2 receptor (IL-2R) leading to an autocrine loop and T cell proliferation. IL-10 acts on many pathways to inhibit antigen presentation, including direct effects on T cells, inhibition of cytokines and cytokine receptors, and downregulation of surface molecules important in T cell activation.

Costimulation has been demonstrated to be essential for efficient T cell activation *in vivo* (76,77). Stimulation of CD28 in concert with TCR signaling switches the signaling program of the T cell from death to activation and proliferation. One mechanism of IL-10 inhibition of T cell activation occurs through its ability to downregulate CD80 and CD86 expression on APC, including macrophages and dendritic lineage cells (78–80). In addition, ICAM-1 expression on monocytes (78), and CTLA4, a ligand for CD80 and CD86 on T cells (81), is also downregulated by IL-10. This interference with CD80/CD86–CD28/CTLA4 costimulation leads to a reduced ability to activate T cells. IL-10 downregulates MHC class II expression on DC, monocytes, and Langerhans cells (tissue DC), which is necessary for presentation of antigenic peptide to T cells (7,82–85). IL-10 also downregulates the ability of MHC class I and II molecules to present antigenic peptides to T cell hybridomas (86). Thus, IL-10 inhibits T cell activation by APC through multiple mechanisms, including an inhibition of IL-12 secretion by the APC and IL-2 secretion by the T cell, a downregulation of MHC and adhesion molecule expression, and a decrease in costimulatory molecules.

IL-10 Signal Transduction/Gene Regulation

IL-10 maps to human chromosome 1 (87–89) and is flanked by regulatory sequences found in other cytokine genes including a cytokine responsive element 3 to 4 kb upstream from the start site (88,90). The hIL-10 receptor shares structural homology with and is a member of the IFN-γ receptor (R) family, but unlike IFN-γ, it shares signaling pathways with the IL-6R (91). The receptor has a molecular weight of 90 to 110 kDa and is located on chromosome 11. A second receptor also of the IFN-γ family, called CFR2-4 in the mouse, has also been identified and characterized as a component of the IL-10 receptor (92,93). Both receptors are needed for signal transduction (Fig. 4.2). The cytoplasmic tail of the IL-10R contains two box 3 sequences. Upon binding of IL-10, they phosphorylate and activate the Janus kinase/STAT pathway. Janus kinase phosphorylates STAT 3 and likely also 1 and 5 leading to DNA binding complexes that activate specific genes. In macrophages, IL-10 mediates both an inhibition of proliferation and a deactivation. Both of these responses require tyrosine phosphorylation of the receptor, but the inhibition of

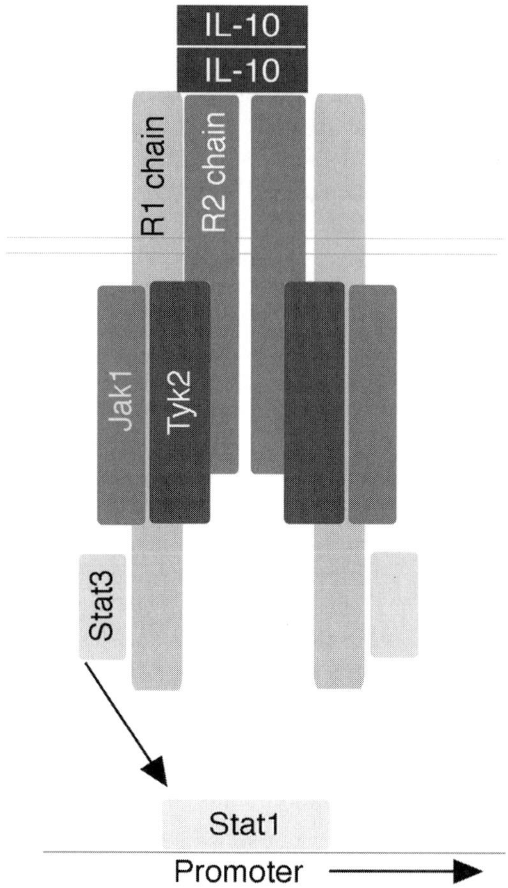

FIG. 4.2. Potential signaling sequences for interleukin-10 (IL-10). IL-10 binds as a dimer to the alpha and beta chains of the IL-10 receptor. Tyrosine phosphorylation leads to activation of a janus kinase and STAT3, STAT1, and STAT5 in certain systems. Activation leads to nuclear binding and gene regulation. STAT3-independent signaling has also been described.

proinflammatory cytokines appears independent of STAT 3 (94), suggesting multiple second messenger pathways. To this end, IL-10 has also been demonstrated to stimulate TYK2, phosphatidyl inositol-3 kinase and p70 S6 kinase (95).

The IL-10 gene is tightly regulated, and a low level of constitutive expression by macrophages is observed. Upon activation of macrophages, high levels of gene transcription occur. EBV-transformed B cells, or EBV-positive Burkitt's lymphoma cells, have high levels of constitutive gene expression (90). The IL-10 promoter contains a TATA box and numerous upstream regulatory sequences. Positive regulatory sequences are found between 900 and 1,100 base pairs upstream while negative regulatory sequences have been identified between 300 and 800 base pairs upstream (90). In a study of transformed T cell lines, nuclear factor kappa B (NFkB), a transcription factor important in the activation of proinflammatory cytokines, was shown to act on the IL-10 gene to increase IL-10 transcription independent of TNF-α, a major inducer of NFkB (96).

The IL-10 promoter contains multiple polymorphisms, some of which have been associated with increased or decreased IL-10 production. In addition, polymorphisms in the

TNF-α promoter that increase TNF-α production lead to a decrease in IL-10 production (97–100). An analysis of the frequency of specific polymorphisms in the IL-10 promoter with SLE demonstrates that certain polymorphisms correlate with certain forms of SLE and may lead to and be part of a genetic background of SLE susceptibility (101,102). A study of IL-10 promoter polymorphisms in rheumatoid arthritis did not find any association with disease, although a polymorphism associated with low IL-10 production and IgA rheumatoid factor and worse disease was observed. Given IL-10's IgA class-switching activity, it is not directly apparent how a decrease in IL-10 would lead to an increase in IgA rheumatoid factor, suggesting an indirect effect (103). A study of TNF-α and IL-10 inducibility in families with a history of fatal meningococcal disease found a 20-fold increased risk of fatal meningococcal disease in subjects with decreased TNF-α and increased IL-10 production (97). These studies suggest that genetic polymorphisms of the IL-10 promoter, and likely of other cytokine promoters that subsequently affect IL-10 production, can affect IL-10 responses to certain pathologic processes and affect disease development or course.

IL-10 Production and Regulation

IL-10 is produced by multiple cell types including T cells, B cells, monocyte/macrophages, mast cells, eosinophils, keratinocytes, and epithelial cells (104) as well as by numerous tumor cells. The production and regulation of IL-10 depends on both the cell being studied and the environment of the cell.

Monocyte/macrophages stimulated with LPS or endotoxin produce high levels of IL-10. This IL-10 production is increased if the cells are treated with substance P (105) or adenosine or adenosine agonists (106–108). IL-10 potently autoregulates its production in monocyte/macrophages (20,55) and is regulated by other cytokines as well. IL-4, IL-13, and IFN-γ all downregulate IL-10 production by activated monocytes (109,110).

Viral IL-10

Homologues of IL-10 have been found in herpes viruses, including EBV (7) and equine herpesvirus 2 (111). The BCRF1 gene of EBV shares high amino acid sequence homology with hIL-10 (85%) and results in a 17-kDa protein that shares many activities with IL-10. vIL-10 inhibits cytokine secretion and induces macrophage deactivation although at a lower efficiency (1,000-fold less for blocking IL-2 secretion from $CD4^+$ T cells) (17). Recent studies demonstrated that vIL-10 is an agonist for the IL-10R with impaired binding (17). vIL-10 is expressed early during EBV-induced transformation of human B cells and is a growth factor for EBV-transformed lymphomas (112–115). EBV-infected B cells also produce hIL-10, usually 20 to 30 hours after vIL-10, which has also been demonstrated to be important as a growth factor as well (21,116,117). Both vIL-10 and host IL-10 enhance the transformation of B cells by at least two mechanisms, first by acting as a growth factor and second by inhibiting IFN-γ, a cytokine that inhibits EBV transformation (11).

In addition to acting as a growth factor for EBV-transformed B cells, viral IL-10, similar to hIL-10, inhibits antigen presentation and T cell activation, and may act to depress immune responses against EBV-induced tumor cells (7). The level and significance of immune suppression by EBV-induced (host) or -produced (viral) IL-10 is not fully understood. vIL-10 is produced during the lytic stage of EBV infection. vIL-10, produced by or added to B cells presenting EBV antigen to form CTL or MHC-unrestricted (NK) cells led to an enhancement of cytotoxic activity (16). Opposite results were observed in EBV-induced nasopharyngeal carcinomas. An inverse correlation between the number of CTL and the presence of IL-10 was observed, suggesting that tumor produced IL-10 inhibited the immune response to the tumor (118). In EBV mononucleosis, both viral and host IL-10 are produced. IL-10 decreased apoptosis in T cells from mononucleosis subjects. This block in programmed cell death should lead to more antigen-specific effector cells, although the effect of IL-10 on effector function was not addressed (119). Overall, it is not clear whether this block in apoptosis occurs *in vivo* and, if so, what is its overall effect on immune function. Thus, EBV uses its own production of vIL-10 and its ability to induce host IL-10 to promote B cell transformation and growth and inhibit immune destruction of transformed cells.

Animal Data

Considerable animal data, mainly in murine systems, on the role of IL-10 in various disease processes, exist. The use of the mouse as a model to study IL-10 has certain limitations. In the mouse, IL-10 is a Th2 cytokine produced by Th2 T cells, while, in humans, IL-10 is produced by both Th1 and Th2 cells. In inbred mice, certain distinct Th cytokine patterns are observed in response to particular organisms: Balb/c mice respond with a Th2 response, while CBA/CaH-T6J mice have a Th1 response to Leishmania (120). In humans, cytokine responses are not so straightforward. In this section, I will discuss studies involving IL-10 knockout mice (mice where the gene for IL-10 has been inactivated). The relevance of murine models of IL-10 activity will be discussed below in the human diseases they are meant to model.

IL-10 knockout mice develop normal numbers of T and B cells and mount normal antibody responses to multiple antigens (121). As expected, they are much more susceptible to endotoxin challenge than wild type controls (122). Mice lacking IL-10 develop a diffuse enterocolitis over time that resembles IBD in humans (121). $CD4^+$ T cells from these mice demonstrate severe polarity towards a Th1 phenotype and transfer of these $CD4^+$ T cells to immunodeficient mice leads to the appearance of enterocolitis in the recipient. A proposed mechanism of immune hyperactivation against normal bowel flora was suggested (123–125) and has been confirmed in IL-10 knockout mice maintained in germ-free conditions (126). Immunization with other antigens or infection with other types of organisms leads to similar immune hyperactivation (127). *Toxoplasma gondii* infection of IL-10–deficient mice leads to early death in the absence of increased parasite growth (128). This suggests that the mice succumb to immune hyperstimulation. IL-10 is also important in the immune privilege of the anterior chamber of the eye. In IL-10 knockout mice immunized with ovalbumin into the anterior chamber, significant delayed type hypersensitivity (DTH) responses were noted, while in wild-type mice no response was observed (129). Together the data suggest that endogenous IL-10 plays an important role *in vivo* in downregulating monokine and IFN-γ responses to antigens and infections, thereby preventing host immunopathology.

HUMAN EXPERIENCE, TOXICITY, EFFICACY, AND CLINICAL TRIALS

IL-10 has been implicated in the disease process of many human diseases. Early human clinical trials have been performed in IBD and HIV and are underway in other diseases. In all trials, thus far, minimal toxicity has been observed. In certain trials, headaches and decreased platelets were observed above placebo-treated subjects at high doses (25 μg/kg). Given IL-10's multiple activities on the immune system, it is often difficult to determine the effect of the various functions modulated by IL-10 on the disease process. In subjects with IBD, characterized by colonic lesions that often develop infectious complications, no increased incidence of infections has been observed, suggesting that IL-10's immunosuppressive activity is not pronounced or is overshadowed by other actions in IBD. Multiple IL-10 promoter polymorphisms have been identified, some of which associate with particular disease syndromes suggesting a correlation between IL-10 gene control and certain diseases.

Autoimmune Disorders

Rheumatoid arthritis is characterized by inflammatory joint disease and the presence of rheumatoid factor. Studies of rheumatoid arthritis joint synovial tissue demonstrate proliferative synovitis with high levels of the proinflammatory cytokines IL-1, IL-6, IL-8, and TNF-α; IL-10 has been demonstrated to be increased (103–133). It has been suggested that the predominance of proinflammatory cytokines is responsible for joint destruction. The addition of IL-10 to synovial cells led to a downregulation of costimulatory molecules and cytokine secretion by the synovial cells and a decrease in T cell activation (134). IL-10 treatment of activated peripheral blood or synovial cells from subjects with rheumatoid arthritis led to a reversal of cartilage degradation in *in vitro* models (135). These studies suggest that the addition of IL-10 may ameliorate the inflammatory process in rheumatoid arthritis. This has been confirmed in murine trials of collagen-induced arthritis, a model of rheumatoid arthritis (136,137). Certain studies implicate a possible role for IL-10 in promoting rheumatoid arthritis, as IL-10 has been observed to be required for terminal differentiation of IgM-RF–producing B cells (138).

A study of IL-10 promoter polymorphisms demonstrated that alleles associated with high or low production of IL-10 were not correlated with increased risk of disease, suggesting that IL-10 production was not directly related to rheumatoid arthritis (103). However, this does not rule out that other unknown IL-10 regulatory mutations, or polymorphisms in other genes that indirectly regulate IL-10, may exist. Therapeutic approaches to reducing proinflammatory cytokines, namely TNF-α are in clinical use with good success. The ability of IL-10 to inhibit a broader range of proinflammatory cytokines will likely lead to future approaches to treatment of rheumatoid arthritis.

Systemic lupus erythematosus (SLE) is an autoimmune disorder characterized by polyclonal B cell activation. Unlike rheumatoid arthritis, where the major pathologic process appears to be joint inflammation which is downregulated by IL-10, in SLE, IL-10 appears to be deleterious. Elevated levels of IL-10 and imbalances between IL-2/IFN-γ and IL-10 are associated with SLE disease activity (139–144). Two polymorphic dinucleotide repeats in the IL-10 promotor region (IL10-G and IL10-R) have been identified. An analysis of patients and matched controls demonstrates that the IL10-G microsatellite, which is associated with increased IL-10 production, is associated with SLE (101). A second study found that the presence of IL-10 promotor polymorphisms associated with increased production was associated with auti-R autoantibodies and renal disease (102). A suggested mechanism is that autoantibody production in SLE is driven by IL-10; for a review, see Emilie et al. (145). Thus, the pathological process of SLE appears to be dependent upon and driven by IL-10.

Inflammatory Bowel Disease

Ulcerative colitis and Crohn's disease have been suggested to represent immune hyperstimulation to bacterial or viral pathogens or a lack of tolerance to enteric organisms in the GI tract. Circulating or intestinal IL-10 protein or mRNA is reduced while proinflammatory cytokines are increased suggesting a dysregulation of cytokines (146–151). Strong evidence for a role of IL-10 in IBD has been observed in a mouse model. IL-10–deficient mice develop an inflammatory bowel disorder that is reduced with the administration of IL-10 (121). IL-10 has entered early clinical trials for the treatment of IBD, usually given as daily subcutaneous injections. At the time of the writing of this chapter, the code had not been broken, but the data suggest that IL-10 decreases the symptoms of moderate to severe IBD.

Infectious Diseases

Sepsis

IL-10 is an important cytokine in the pathogenesis of sepsis, but depending on the system used, a variety of conclusions have been reached. IL-10 is an appealing candidate for the treatment of sepsis given its ability to inhibit TNF, IL-1, and IL-8 and its potentiation of IL-1RA and TNF receptor (p55) release. Initial murine studies suggested that IL-10–protected mice from lethal endotoxin challenge (54). Most murine models of sepsis have demonstrated a protective effect of endogenously produced or exogenously given IL-10 (122,152–157). These models include treating mice with endotoxin, inducing infections with virulent organisms, or cecal ligation. They typically demonstrate that IL-10 reduces the production of most proinflammatory cytokines. Most also find that IL-10 is elevated after endotoxin or bacterial challenge. From a simplistic point of view, sepsis leads to the production of proinflammatory cytokines and proinflammatory cytokine levels correlate with death from sepsis. Thus, blocking proinflammatory cytokines should be beneficial.

Further murine and human studies have identified complications to this reasoning. Other model studies using Candida, Listeria, and Klebsiella infection suggest the opposite result, that IL-10 increases mortality; for a review, see Remick et al. (158). In a comprehensive study of cecal ligation in the rat, purported to be very similar to human sepsis, no increased survival with IL-10 treatment was observed. In both mouse models and studies of septic humans, IL-10 levels have been found to be elevated (159–164). In certain human studies, a correlation between IL-10 and poor outcome has been observed (162,164). Other defects, including immune suppression due to IL-10, have been described (165–169). A potential mechanism for IL-10/endotoxin immune suppression has been suggested in a study in which normal human volunteers were given a low dose challenge with endotoxin. Resulting cytokine levels demonstrated a shift towards Th2 cytokines, which could lead to less cellular immune reactivity (170). As a whole, the study of IL-10 in sepsis is complicated by the specific system used to study sepsis, our lack of knowledge of the role of all of the various mediators, and our lack of understanding of sepsis itself.

Chagas' Disease

Infections with *Trypanasoma cruzi* can develop into a chronic process characterized by cardiomyopathy, Chagas' disease, or remain in an indolent state, which is regulated by the immune system. Murine models of *T. cruzi* infection offer a direct role for IL-10, through its ability to modulate other cytokines and macrophages, in the regulation of disease.

Initial studies of *T. cruzi* infection in mice demonstrated susceptible and resistant strains. It was known that endogenous and exogenous IFN-γ was important in protection. A study designed to identify the source of resistance searched for soluble mediators in spleen cell supernatants and identified IL-10 (171). In addition to IL-10's ability to inhibit IFN-γ release, it also blocked IFN-γ's ability to inhibit organism growth in macrophages (171). This occurs through IL-10's direct ability to block macrophage activation by multiple stimuli including IFN-γ and engulfment of foreign organisms.

Both innate and acquired immunity to *T. cruzi* is determined by IFN-γ and modulated by IL-10. NK cells have been determined to be a major producer of IFN-γ in early infection and the inhibition of IL-10 activity by monoclonal antibodies increases IFN-γ production (172–174). As the immune system is a delicate balance between activating and suppressing factors and mechanisms, it is assumed that the presence of IL-10, which increases parasite growth, is required for an efficient balance between parasite replication and self-destruction. In IL-10 knockout mice, *T. cruzi* infection was better controlled (lower parasitemia), but the animals died faster. The addition of IL-10 or an antibody to IL-12 led to a reversal of early mortality. These data suggest that IL-10 is required to prevent immune hyperactivation and the development of pathologic immune responses (175).

The data on IL-10 in *T. cruzi* infection in humans is more limited. Acutely infected children demonstrated a primarily Th1 cytokine pattern (IFN-γ), while the cytokine pattern of the post-acute, early indeterminate phase was Th0, with both IFN-γ and IL-4 (176). Elevated levels of IL-10, IL-5, and IFN-γ but not IL-2 or IL-4 mRNA were observed in subjects with Chagas' disease compared to controls (177), but a direct correlation between increased IL-10 production and worse disease has not been established. In human *T. cruzi* infection, the cytokine response is usually Th0. Further studies in subjects with limited compared to progressive *T. cruzi* infection may determine whether a correlation with IL-10 promoter polymorphisms exists.

Role of IL-10 Modulation of Immune Functions in Infectious Diseases

IL-10 has been studied for its ability to modulate numerous immune functions, T cell and macrophage deactivation, and B cell activation in many infectious diseases. In murine models, IL-10 has been studied for its ability to turn off Th1 responses and turn on Th2 responses. Diseases that are controlled by Th1 immune responses, such as *T. cruzi*, do worse when IL-10 is added, while diseases that result from overactive Th1 responses, such as Toxoplasmosis, improve when IL-10 is added. In humans, the dichotomy of IL-10 in Th2 versus Th1 responses is less pronounced.

Human lymphatic filariasis is caused by the nematode *Wuchereria bancrofti*. Organisms circulate in the blood as microfilaria or are contained leading to chronic lymphatic obstruction. Individuals with chronic lymphatic obstruction exhibit both Th2 and Th1 parasite antigen-driven responses. In peripheral blood mononuclear cells (PBMCs) from individuals with microfilaria, there was a marked downregulation of cellular response to parasite antigens, with decreased expression of mRNA for the Th1 cytokines, IFN-γ and IL-2. An increase in IL-10 mRNA expression was observed in concert with the decreased Th1 cytokines. Unexposed controls had a Th1 pattern of cytokine secretion with no IL-4 or IL-5 mRNA expression. A significant negative correlation between IL-10 mRNA expression and PBMC proliferation in individuals with circulating microfilaria was observed, suggesting a possible role for IL-10 in antigen-specific hyporesponsiveness (178,179). A possible mechanism for increased IL-10 association with a Th2 response and a loss of T cell activation was suggested in studies using cytokine modulation of antigen-activated PBMC from infected subjects. The addition of IL-10 neutralizing antibodies resulted in an increase in IFN-γ secretion, suggesting that IL-10 downregulated the Th1 response. The addition of IL-12 increased the Th1 response (180). These studies suggest that the antigen-specific hyporesponsiveness of T cells in subjects with microfilaria is due to IL-10 downregulation of Th1 responses through its ability to inhibit IL-12 release.

Infection with the protozoan *Leishmania donovani* can cause subclinical infection, disease limited to the skin and/or mucous membranes, or serious visceral disease in humans. In an early study, IL-10 production correlated with disease severity (181). IL-10 was found to inhibit intracellular killing of Leishmania by macrophages through its inhibition of reactive nitrogen production (182). Infected individuals who developed visceral Leishmaniasis had abundant IL-10 mRNA but no IFN-γ or IL-12. The addition of IL-12 *in vitro* reversed the defect in Th1 responsiveness and increased IFN-γ and cytotoxic responses (183,184). This suggests that similar to filariasis, visceral Leishmania disease occurs in the setting of IL-10 inhibition of IL-12 production and Th1 cellular immune responsiveness. In addition, IL-10 also decreases the ability of macrophages to kill the organism through its deactivating ability.

IL-10 is a potent deactivator of macrophage function, but under certain circumstances, it increases macrophage activity. IL-10–treated macrophages from normal volunteers had decreased ability to kill ingested Aspergillus hyphae, but had increased ability to phagocytose organisms (185). Another function of macrophages affected by IL-10 is antigen presentation leading to T cell activation. Respiratory syncytial virus (RSV) causes repeated infections in childhood thought to be due in part to an ineffective immune response. It has been suggested that the incomplete immunity results from IL-10 production from RSV-infected alveolar macrophages that interferes with the production of immunoregulatory cytokines and efficient T cell activation (186).

HIV

As in all of HIV, IL-10 appears to be multifactorial in its production and activities on the host and virus. IL-10 and TNF-α mirror each other in most disease states and experimental systems. Both are increased in sepsis, autoimmune disorders, and after endotoxin challenge. In HIV infection, a similar pattern is observed. With advancing disease stage, increasing levels of plasma IL-10 are observed (187–192). Some researchers have found IL-10 to be in part responsible for the immune dysfunction of HIV (193,194), while others disagree (195). The addition of IL-10 to monocyte/macrophage lineage cells leads to either enhancement or inhibition of viral infection, depending on the system used. IL-10 has multiple effects on lymphoid development, particularly as a stimulant of activated B-cell proliferation and differentiation. It is thought that IL-10 may play a role in the development of B lymphoid malignancies. This is based on the observations that (a) lymphomatous tissues from HIV-infected patients contain numerous cells expressing IL-10 mRNA and protein; and (b) EBV induces cellular IL-10, requires IL-10 as a growth factor, and has been found in lymphomas in HIV-infected subjects (196). The anti-TNF and antiinflammatory properties of IL-10 have resulted in clinical trials using IL-10.

The amount of IL-10 protein in plasma, mRNA in PBMC, or IL-10 protein induced by polyclonal activators from PBMC increases with advancing HIV disease stage (187,188,192).There are similar results for TNF-α; for a review, see Navikas et al. (192). The source of the elevated IL-10 is likely due to a number of factors. IL-10 increases in response to TNF, and TNF levels increase in advancing HIV disease due to infections and inflammatory stimuli. The direct effect of IL-10 on HIV replication *in vitro* is inhibition of viral growth in $CD4^+$ T cells (197) Results are dichotomous in cells of the monocyte/macrophage lineage. In monocyte derived macrophages, IL-10 inhibits HIV infection by at least two mechanisms, by blocking the autocrine loops of proinflammatory and HIV-inducing cytokines, TNF-α and IL-6 (198), and by inhibition of maturation (47,199). IL-10 also synergizes with multiple cytokines in enhancing HIV replication in chronically infected cell lines of monocyte lineage (200–202).

Based on the *in vitro* results of IL-10, it was used in a phase I clinical trial in HIV infected humans. The results of these trials mirrored that observed when IL-10 was given to uninfected controls (52,53). There was a profound decrease in proinflammatory cytokine secretion induced by endotoxin, and a transient decrease in $CD3^+$ T cells with an increase in monocytes. In HIV-infected subjects, a transient decrease in plasma viral load (50% to 60%) after IL-10 was observed in the lowest dose (1 μg/kg) group (D. Weissman and A.S. Fauci, unpublished observations). In multiple dosing trials, no persistent decrease in plasma viral load was noted, and the trials were terminated. The cause of this transient HIV decrease and its inability to be sustained is unknown.

FUTURE DIRECTIONS

IL-10 has multiple suppressive and enhancing immune activities. Its ability to decrease macrophage and T cell activation appears to be beneficial in the treatment of IBD. Its role in the treatment of other diseases is currently being investigated. The search for inhibitors of IL-10 for use in diseases such as SLE, where IL-10 has a direct role in disease pathogenesis, may yield additional therapies. Given IL-10's broad ability to inhibit proinflammatory cytokines, it has advantages over agents that block a single cytokine, such as anti-TNF antibodies or soluble receptors. However, because of the numerous immune actions of IL-10, its use has to be tempered based on the overall effect of its administration. Further clinical trials in various diseases will expand our knowledge of IL-10's *in vivo* effects and direct its use to diseases where its advantages outweigh its drawbacks.

REFERENCES

1. Fiorentino DF, Bond MW, Mosmann TR. Two types of mouse T helper cell. IV. Th2 clones secrete a factor that inhibits cytokine production by Th1 clones. *J Exp Med* 1989;170:2081–2095.
2. O'Garra A, Howard M. Cytokines and Ly-1 (B1) B cells. *Int Rev Immunol* 1992;8:219–234.
3. Rennick D, Hunte B, Dang W, et al. Interleukin-10 promotes the growth of megakaryocyte, mast cell, and multilineage colonies: analysis with committed progenitors and Thy1loSca1$^+$ stem cells. *Exp Hematol* 1994;22: 136–141.
4. Tsuji K, Koike K, Komiyama A, et al. Synergistic action of interleukin-10 (IL-10) with IL-3, IL-4 and stem cell factor on colony formation from murine mast cells in culture. *Int J Hematol* 1995;61:51–60.
5. Lalani I, Bhol K, Ahmed AR. Interleukin-10: biology, role in inflammation and autoimmunity. *Ann Allergy Asthma Immunol* 1997;79:469–483.
6. Suda T, MacNeil I, Fischer M, et al. Identification of a novel thymocyte growth factor derived from B cell lymphomas. *Adv Exp Med Biol* 1991;292:115–120.
7. de Waal Malefyt R, Haanen J, Spits H, et al. Interleukin 10 (IL-10) and viral IL-10 strongly reduce antigen-specific human T cell proliferation by diminishing the antigen-presenting capacity of monocytes via downregulation of class II major histocompatibility complex expression. *J Exp Med* 1991;174:915–924.
8. Niiro H, Otsuka T, Abe M, et al. Epstein-Barr virus BCRF1 gene product (viral interleukin 10) inhibits superoxide anion production by human monocytes. *Lymphokine Cytokine Res* 1992;11:209–214.
9. Moore KW, Rousset F, Banchereau J. Evolving principles in immunopathology: interleukin 10 and its relationship to Epstein-Barr virus protein BCRF1. *Springer Semin Immunopathol* 1991;13:157–166.
10. Touitou R, Cochet C, Joab I. Transcriptional analysis of the Epstein-Barr virus interleukin-10 homologue during the lytic cycle. *J Gen Virol* 1996;77:1163–1168.

11. Stuart AD, Stewart JP, Arrand JR, et al. The Epstein-Barr virus encoded cytokine viral interleukin-10 enhances transformation of human B lymphocytes. *Oncogene* 1995;11:1711–1719.
12. Taga H, Taga K, Wang F, et al. Human and viral interleukin-10 in acute Epstein-Barr virus–induced infectious mononucleosis. *J Infect Dis* 1995;171:1347–1350.
13. Stewart JP, Behm FG, Arrand JR, et al. Differential expression of viral and human interleukin-10 (IL-10) by primary B cell tumors and B cell lines. *Virology* 1994;200:724–732.
14. Miyazaki I, Cheung RK, Dosch HM. Viral interleukin 10 is critical for the induction of B cell growth transformation by Epstein-Barr virus. *J Exp Med* 1993;178:439–447.
15. Ryon JJ, Hayward SD, MacMahon EM, et al. In situ detection of lytic Epstein-Barr virus infection: expression of the NotI early gene and viral interleukin-10 late gene in clinical specimens. *J Infect Dis* 1993;168:345–351.
16. Stewart JP, Rooney CM. The interleukin-10 homolog encoded by Epstein-Barr virus enhances the reactivation of virus-specific cytotoxic T cell and HLA-unrestricted killer cell responses. *Virology* 1992;191:773–782.
17. Ying L, de Waal Malefyt R, Briere F, et al. The EBV IL-10 homologue is a selective agonist with impaired binding. *J Immunol* 1997;158:604–613.
18. Yssel H, De Waal Malefyt R, Roncarolo MG, et al. IL-10 is produced by subsets of human $CD4^+$ T cell clones and peripheral blood T cells. *J Immunol* 1992;149:2378–2384.
19. Ralph P, Nakoinz I, Sampson-Johannes A, et al. IL-10, T lymphocyte inhibitor of human blood cell production of IL-1 and tumor necrosis factor. *J Immunol* 1992;148:808–814.
20. de Waal Malefyt R, Abrams J, Bennett B, et al. Interleukin 10 (IL-10) inhibits cytokine synthesis by human monocytes: an autoregulatory role of IL-10 produced by monocytes. *J Exp Med* 1991;174:1209–1220.
21. Benjamin D, Knobloch TJ, Dayton MA. Human B-cell interleukin-10: B-cell lines derived from patients with acquired immunodeficiency syndrome and Burkitt's lymphoma constitutively secrete large quantities of interleukin-10. *Blood* 1992;80:1289–1298.
22. Benjamin D, Park CD, Sharma V. Human B cell interleukin 10. *Leuk Lymphoma* 1994;12:205–210.
23. Enk CD, Sredni D, Blauvelt A, et al. Induction of IL-10 gene expression in human keratinocytes by UVB exposure *in vivo* and *in vitro*. *J Immunol* 1995;154:4851–4856.
24. Becherel PA, LeGoff L, Frances C, et al. Induction of IL-10 synthesis by human keratinocytes through CD23 ligation: a cyclic adenosine 3′,5′-monophosphate-dependent mechanism. *J Immunol* 1997;159:5761–5765.
25. Enk AH, Katz SI. Identification and induction of keratinocyte-derived IL-10. *J Immunol* 1992;149:92–95.
26. Nickoloff BJ, Fivenson DP, Kunkel SL, et al. Keratinocyte interleukin-10 expression is upregulated in tape-stripped skin, poison ivy dermatitis, and Sezary syndrome, but not in psoriatic plaques. *Clin Immunol Immunopathol* 1994;73:63–68.
27. Dummer W, Bastian BC, Ernst N, et al. 1996. Interleukin-10 production in malignant melanoma: preferential detection of IL-10-secreting tumor cells in metastatic lesions. *Int J Cancer* 1996;66:607–610.
28. Lattime EC, Mastrangelo MJ, Bagasra O, et al. Expression of cytokine mRNA in human melanoma tissues. *Cancer Immunol Immunother* 1995;41:151–156.
29. Kruger-Krasagakes S, Krasagakis K, Garbe C, et al. Expression of interleukin 10 in human melanoma. *Br J Cancer* 1994;70:1182–1185.
30. Gastl GA, Abrams JS, Nanus DM, et al. Interleukin-10 production by human carcinoma cell lines and its relationship to interleukin-6 expression. *Int J Cancer* 1993;55:96–101.
31. de Waal Malefyt R, Yssel H, de Vries JE. Direct effects of IL-10 on subsets of human $CD4^+$ T cell clones and resting T cells. Specific inhibition of IL-2 production and proliferation. *J Immunol* 1993;150:4754–4765.
32. Jinquan T, Larsen CG, Gesser B, et al. Human IL-10 is a chemoattractant for $CD8^+$ T lymphocytes and an inhibitor of IL-8–induced $CD4^+$ T lymphocyte migration. *J Immunol* 1993;151:4545–4551.
33. Rousset F, Garcia E, Defrance T, et al. Interleukin 10 is a potent growth and differentiation factor for activated human B lymphocytes. *Proc Natl Acad Sci U S A* 1992;89:1890–1893.
34. Itoh K, Hirohata S. The role of IL-10 in human B cell activation, proliferation, and differentiation. *J Immunol* 1995;154:4341–4350.
35. Li L, Krajewski S, Reed JC, et al. The apoptosis and proliferation of SAC-activated B cells by IL-10 are associated with changes in Bcl-2, Bcl-xL, and Mcl-1 expression. *Cell Immunol* 1997;178:33–41.
36. Armitage RJ, Macduff BM, Spriggs MK, et al. Human B cell proliferation and Ig secretion induced by recombinant CD40 ligand are modulated by soluble cytokines. *J Immunol* 1993;150:3671–3680.
37. Pound JD, Gordon J. Maintenance of human germinal center B cells *in vitro*. *Blood* 1997;89:919–928.
38. Fluckiger AC, Durand I, Banchereau J. Interleukin 10 induces apoptotic cell death of B-chronic lymphocytic leukemia cells. *J Exp Med* 1994;179:91–99.
39. Malisan F, Fluckiger AC, Ho S, et al. B-chronic lymphocytic leukemias can undergo isotype switching *in vivo* and can be induced to differentiate and switch *in vitro*. *Blood* 1996;87:717–724.
40. Fujieda S, Saxon A, Zhang K. Direct evidence that gamma 1 and gamma 3 switching in human B cells is interleukin-10 dependent. *Mol Immunol* 1996;33:1335–1343.
41. Defrance T, Vanbervliet B, Briere F, et al. Interleukin 10 and transforming growth factor beta cooperate to induce anti-CD40-activated naive human B cells to secrete immunoglobulin A. *J Exp Med* 1992;175:671–682.
42. Briere F, Bridon JM, Chevet D, et al. Interleukin 10 induces B lymphocytes from IgA-deficient patients to secrete IgA. *J Clin Invest* 1994;94:97–104.
43. Friman V, Hanson LA, Bridon JM, et al. IL-10–driven immunoglobulin production by B lymphocytes from IgA-deficient individuals correlates to infection proneness. *Clin Exp Immunol* 1996;104:432–438.

44. Carson WE, Lindemann MJ, Baiocchi R, et al. The functional characterization of interleukin-10 receptor expression on human natural killer cells. *Blood* 1995;85:3577–3585.
45. Hunter CA, Subauste CS, Van Cleave VH, et al. Production of gamma interferon by natural killer cells from *Toxoplasma gondii*–infected SCID mice: regulation by interleukin-10, interleukin-12, and tumor necrosis factor alpha. *Infect Immun* 1994;62:2818–2824.
46. Kundu N, Fulton AM. Interleukin-10 inhibits tumor metastasis, downregulates MHC class I, and enhances NK lysis. *Cell Immunol* 1997;180:55–61.
47. Naif HM, Chang J, Ho-Shon M, et al. Inhibition of human immunodeficiency virus replication in differentiating monocytes by interleukin 10 occurs in parallel with inhibition of cellular RNA expression. *AIDS Res Hum Retroviruses* 1996;12:1237–1245.
48. Berkman N, John M, Roesems G, et al. Inhibition of macrophage inflammatory protein-1 alpha expression by IL-10. Differential sensitivities in human blood monocytes and alveolar macrophages. *J Immunol* 1995;155: 4412–4418.
49. Geng Y, Gulbins E, Altman A, et al. Monocyte deactivation by interleukin 10 via inhibition of tyrosine kinase activity and the Ras signaling pathway. *Proc Natl Acad Sci USA* 1994;91:8602–8606.
50. Niiro H, Otsuka T, Kuga S, et al. IL-10 inhibits prostaglandin E_2 production by lipopolysaccharide-stimulated monocytes. *Int Immunol* 1994;6:661–664.
51. Wu J, Cunha FQ, Liew FY, et al. IL-10 inhibits the synthesis of migration inhibitory factor and migration inhibitory factor–mediated macrophage activation. *J Immunol* 1993;151:4325–4332.
52. Chernoff AE, Granowitz EV, Shapiro L, et al. A randomized, controlled trial of IL-10 in humans. Inhibition of inflammatory cytokine production and immune responses. *J Immunol* 1995;154:5492–5499.
53. Fuchs AC, Granowitz EV, Shapiro L, et al. Clinical, hematologic, and immunologic effects of interleukin-10 in humans. *J Clin Immunol* 1996;16:291–303.
54. Howard M, Muchamuel T, Andrade S, et al. Interleukin 10 protects mice from lethal endotoxemia. *J Exp Med* 1993;177:1205–1208.
55. Knolle PA, Uhrig A, Protzer U, et al. Interleukin-10 expression is autoregulated at the transcriptional level in human and murine Kupffer cells. *Hepatology* 1998;27:93–99.
56. van der Poll T, Jansen J, Levi M, et al. Regulation of interleukin 10 release by tumor necrosis factor in humans and chimpanzees. *J Exp Med* 1994;180:1985–1988.
57. Bogdan C, Vodovotz Y, Nathan C. Macrophage deactivation by interleukin 10. *J Exp Med* 1991;174:1549–1555.
58. Cassatella MA, Meda L, Gasperini S, et al. Interleukin 10 (IL-10) upregulates IL-1 receptor antagonist production from lipopolysaccharide-stimulated human polymorphonuclear leukocytes by delaying mRNA degradation. *J Exp Med* 1994;179:1695–1699.
59. Jenkins JK, Malyak M, Arend WP. The effects of interleukin-10 on interleukin-1 receptor antagonist and interleukin-1 beta production in human monocytes and neutrophils. *Lymphokine Cytokine Res* 1994;13:47–54.
60. Seitz M, Loetscher P, Dewald B, et al. Interleukin-10 differentially regulates cytokine inhibitor and chemokine release from blood mononuclear cells and fibroblasts. *Eur J Immunol* 1995;25:1129–1132.
61. Capsoni F, Minonzio F, Ongari AM, et al. IL-10 up-regulates human monocyte phagocytosis in the presence of IL-4 and IFN-gamma. *J Leukoc Biol* 1995;58:351–358.
62. te Velde AA, de Waal Malefijt R, Huijbens RJ et al. IL-10 stimulates monocyte Fc gamma R surface expression and cytotoxic activity. Distinct regulation of antibody-dependent cellular cytotoxicity by IFN-gamma, IL-4, and IL-10. *J Immunol* 1992;149:4048–4052.
63. Koch F, Stanzl U, Jennewein P, et al. 1996. High level IL-12 production by murine dendritic cells: upregulation via MHC class II and CD40 molecules and downregulation by IL-4 and IL-10. *J Exp Med* 1996;184:741–746. [For erratum, see *J Exp Med* 1996;184: following 1590.]
64. D'Andrea A, Aste-Amezaga M, Valiante NM, et al. Interleukin 10 (IL-10) inhibits human lymphocyte interferon gamma-production by suppressing natural killer cell stimulatory factor/IL-12 synthesis in accessory cells. *J Exp Med* 1993;178:1041–1048.
65. Gazzinelli RT, Hayashi S, Wysocka M, et al. Role of IL-12 in the initiation of cell mediated immunity by *Toxoplasma gondii* and its regulation by IL-10 and nitric oxide. *J Eukaryot Microbiol* 1994;41:9S.
66. Peng X, Kasran A, Ceuppens JL. Interleukin 12 and B7/CD28 interaction synergistically upregulate interleukin 10 production by human T cells. *Cytokine*1997;9:499–506.
67. Spencer NF, Daynes RA. IL-12 directly stimulates expression of IL-10 by CD5+ B cells and IL-6 by both CD5+ and CD5$^-$ B cells: possible involvement in age-associated cytokine dysregulation. *Int Immunol* 1997;9:745–754.
68. Anitescu M, Chace JH, Tuetken R, et al. Interleukin-10 functions *in vitro* and *in vivo* to inhibit bacterial DNA-induced secretion of interleukin-12. *J Interferon Cytokine Res* 1997;17:781–788.
69. Meyaard L, Hovenkamp E, Otto, SA et al. 1996. IL-12–induced IL-10 production by human T cells as a negative feedback for IL-12–induced immune responses. *J Immunol* 156:2776–2782.
70. Uyemura K, Demer LL, Castle SC, et al. Cross-regulatory roles of interleukin (IL)-12 and IL-10 in atherosclerosis. *J Clin Invest* 1996;97:2130–2138.
71. Daftarian PM, Kumar A, Kryworuchko M, et al. IL-10 production is enhanced in human T cells by IL-12 and IL-6 and in monocytes by tumor necrosis factor–alpha. *J Immunol* 1996;157:12–20.
72. Snijders A, Hilkens CM, van der Pouw Kraan TC, et al. Regulation of bioactive IL-12 production in lipopolysaccharide-stimulated human monocytes is determined by the expression of the p35 subunit. *J Immunol* 1996;156:1207–1212.

73. Windhagen A, Anderson DE, Carrizosa A, et al. IL-12 induces human T cells secreting IL-10 with IFN-gamma. *J Immunol* 1996;157:1127–1131.
74. Jeannin P, Delneste Y, Seveso M, et al. IL-12 synergizes with IL-2 and other stimuli in inducing IL-10 production by human T cells. *J Immunol* 1996;156:3159–3165.
75. Chen YM, Yang WK, Ting CC, et al. Cross regulation by IL-10 and IL-2/IL-12 of the helper T cells and the cytolytic activity of lymphocytes from malignant effusions of lung cancer patients. *Chest* 1997;112:960–966.
76. Green JM, Noel PJ, Sperling AI, et al. Absence of B7-dependent responses in CD28-deficient mice. *Immunity* 1994;1:501–508.
77. Sharpe AH. Analysis of lymphocyte costimulation *in vivo* using transgenic and. *Curr Opin Immunol* 1995; 7:389–395.
78. Willems F, Marchant A, Delville JP et al. Interleukin-10 inhibits B7 and intercellular adhesion molecule–1 expression on human monocytes. *Eur J Immunol* 1994;24:1007–1009.
79. Kubin M, Kamoun M, Trinchieri G. Interleukin 12 synergizes with B7/CD28 interaction in inducing efficient proliferation and cytokine production of human T cells. *J Exp Med* 1994;180:211–222.
80. Chang CH, Furue M, Tamaki K. 1995. B7-1 expression of Langerhans cells is up-regulated by proinflammatory cytokines, and is down-regulated by interferon-gamma or by interleukin-10. *Eur J Immunol* 25:394–398.
81. Gong JH, Zhang M, Modlin RL, et al. Interleukin-10 downregulates *Mycobacterium tuberculosis*–induced Th1 responses and CTLA-4 expression. *Infect Immun* 1996;64:913–918.
82. Bejarano MT, de Waal Malefyt R, Abrams JS, et al. Interleukin 10 inhibits allogeneic proliferative and cytotoxic T cell responses generated in primary mixed lymphocyte cultures. *Int Immunol* 1992;4:1389–1397.
83. Caux C, Massacrier C, Vanbervliet B, et al. Interleukin 10 inhibits T cell alloreaction induced by human dendritic cells. *Int Immunol* 1994;6:1177–1185.
84. Peguet-Navarro J, Moulon C, Caux C, et al. Interleukin-10 inhibits the primary allogeneic T cell response to human epidermal Langerhans cells. *Eur J Immunol* 1994;24:884–891.
85. Peguet-Navarro J, Moulon C, Caux C, et al. Inhibitory effect of IL-10 on human Langerhans cell antigen presenting function. *Adv Exp Med Biol* 1995;378:359–361.
86. Hiltbold EM, Ziegler HK. Interferon-gamma and interleukin-10 have cross-regulatory roles in modulating the class I and class II MHC-mediated presentation of epitopes of *Listeria monocytogenes* by infected macrophages. *J Interferon Cytokine Res* 1996;16:547–554.
87. Eskdale J, Kube D, Gallagher G. A second polymorphic dinucleotide repeat in the 5′ flanking region of the human IL10 gene. *Immunogenetics* 1996;45:82–83.
88. Eskdale J, Kube D, Tesch H, et al. Mapping of the human IL10 gene and further characterization of the 5′ flanking sequence. *Immunogenetics* 1997;46:120–128.
89. Kim JM, Brannan CI, Copeland NG, et al. Structure of the mouse IL-10 gene and chromosomal localization of the mouse and human genes. *J Immunol* 1992;148:3618–3623.
90. Kube D, Platzer C, von Knethen A, et al. Isolation of the human interleukin 10 promoter. Characterization of the promoter activity in Burkitt's lymphoma cell lines. *Cytokine* 1995;7:1–7.
91. Lai CF, J. Ripperger, K. K. Morella, et al. Receptors for interleukin (IL)–10 and IL-6–type cytokines use similar signaling mechanisms for inducing transcription through IL-6 response elements. *J Biol Chem* 1996;271: 13968–13975.
92. Spencer SD, Di Marco F, Hooley J, et al. The orphan receptor CRF2-4 is an essential subunit of the interleukin 10 receptor. *J Exp Med* 1998;187:571–578.
93. Kotenko SV, Krause CD, Izotova LS, et al. Identification and functional characterization of a second chain of the interleukin-10 receptor complex. *EMBO J* 1997;16:5894–5903.
94. O'Farrell AM, Liu Y, Moore KW, et al. IL-10 inhibits macrophage activation and proliferation by distinct signaling mechanisms: evidence for Stat3-dependent and -independent pathways. *EMBO J* 1998;17:1006–1018.
95. Crawley JB, Williams LM, Mander T, et al. Interleukin-10 stimulation of phosphatidylinositol 3-kinase and p70 S6 kinase is required for the proliferative but not the antiinflammatory effects of the cytokine. *J Biol Chem* 1996;271:16357–16362.
96. Mori N, Prager D. Activation of the interleukin-10 gene in the human T lymphoma line HuT 78: identification and characterization of NF-kappa B binding sites in the regulatory region of the interleukin-10 gene. *Eur J Haematol* 1997;59:162–170.
97. Westendorp RG, Langermans JA, Huizinga TW, et al. Genetic influence on cytokine production and fatal meningococcal disease. *Lancet*1997;349:170–173. [For erratum, see *Lancet* 1997;349:656.]
98. Eskdale J, Gallagher G. A polymorphic dinucleotide repeat in the human IL-10 promoter. *Immunogenetics* 1995;42:444–445.
99. Platzer C, Volk HD, Platzer M. 5′ noncoding sequence of human IL-10 gene obtained by oligo-cassette PCR walking. *DNA Seq* 1994;4:399–401.
100. Turner DM, Williams DM, Sankaran D, et al. An investigation of polymorphism in the interleukin-10 gene promoter. *Eur J Immunogenet* 1997;24:1–8.
101. Eskdale J, Wordsworth P, Bowman S, et al. Association between polymorphisms at the human IL-10 locus and systemic lupus erythematosus. *Tissue Antigens* 1997;49:635–639.
102. Lazarus M, Hajeer AH, Turner D et al. Genetic variation in the interleukin 10 gene promoter and systemic lupus erythematosus. *J Rheumatol* 1997;24:2314–2317.

103. Hajeer AH, Lazarus M, Turner D, et al. IL-10 gene promoter polymorphisms in rheumatoid arthritis. *Scand J Rheumatol* 1998;27:142–145.
104. Bonfield TL, Konstan MW, Burfeind P, et al. Normal bronchial epithelial cells constitutively produce the anti-inflammatory cytokine interleukin-10, which is downregulated in cystic fibrosis. *Am J Respir Cell Mol Biol* 1995;13:257–261.
105. Ho WZ, Kaufman D, Uvaydova M, et al. Substance P augments interleukin-10 and tumor necrosis factor-alpha release by human cord blood monocytes and macrophages. *J Neuroimmunol* 1996;71:73–80.
106. Hasko G, Szabo C, Nemeth ZH, et al. Adenosine receptor agonists differentially regulate IL-10, TNF-alpha, and nitric oxide production in RAW 264.7 macrophages and in endotoxemic mice. *J Immunol* 1996;157: 4634–4640.
107. Le Moine O, Stordeur P, Schandene L, et al. Adenosine enhances IL-10 secretion by human monocytes. *J Immunol* 1996;156:4408–4414.
108. Benbernou N, Esnault S, Shin HC, et al. Differential regulation of IFN-gamma, IL-10 and inducible nitric oxide synthase in human T cells by cyclic AMP–dependent signal transduction pathway. *Immunology* 1997;91: 361–368.
109. de Waal Malefyt R, Figdor CG, Huijbens R, et al. Effects of IL-13 on phenotype, cytokine production, and cytotoxic function of human monocytes. Comparison with IL-4 and modulation by IFN-gamma or IL-10. *J Immunol* 1993;151:6370–6381.
110. Chomarat P, Rissoan MC, Banchereau J, et al. 1993. Interferon gamma inhibits interleukin 10 production by monocytes. *J Exp Med* 1993;177:523–527.
111. Rode HJ, Janssen W, Rosen-Wolff A, et al. The genome of equine herpesvirus type 2 harbors an interleukin 10 (IL10)–like gene. *Virus Genes* 1993;7:111–116.
112. Beatty PR, Krams SM, Martinez OM. Involvement of IL-10 in the autonomous growth of EBV-transformed B cell lines. *J Immunol* 1997;158:4045–4051.
113. Burdin N, Peronne C, Banchereau J, et al. Epstein-Barr virus transformation induces B lymphocytes to produce human interleukin 10. *J Exp Med* 1993;177:295–304.
114. Burdin N, Rousset F, Banchereau J. B-cell–derived IL-10: production and function. *Methods* 1997;11:98–111.
115. Kanegane H, Wakiguchi H, Kanegane C, et al. Viral interleukin-10 in chronic active Epstein-Barr virus infection. *J Infect Dis* 1997;176:254–257.
116. Klein SC, Kube D, Abts H, et al. Promotion of IL8, IL10, TNF alpha and TNF beta production by EBV infection. *Leuk Res* 1996;20:633–636.
117. Nakagomi H, Dolcetti R, Bejarano MT, et al. The Epstein-Barr virus latent membrane protein-1 (LMP1) induces interleukin-10 production in Burkitt lymphoma lines. *Int J Cancer* 1994;57:240–244.
118. Yao M, Ohshima K, Suzumiya J, et al. Interleukin-10 expression and cytotoxic-T-cell response in Epstein-Barr-virus–associated nasopharyngeal carcinoma. *Int J Cancer* 1997;72:398–402.
119. Taga K, Chretien J, Cherney B, et al. Interleukin-10 inhibits apoptotic cell death in infectious mononucleosis T cells. *J Clin Invest* 1994;94:251–260.
120. Soares MB, David JR, Titus RG. An *in vitro* model for infection with *Leishmania major* that mimics the. *Infect Immun* 1997;65:2837–2845.
121. Kuhn R, Lohler J, Rennick D, et al. Interleukin-10–deficient mice develop chronic enterocolitis. *Cell* 1993;75: 263–274.
122. Berg DJ, Kuhn R, Rajewsky K, et al. Interleukin-10 is a central regulator of the response to LPS in murine models of endotoxic shock and the Shwartzman reaction but not endotoxin tolerance. *J Clin Invest* 1995;96: 2339–2347.
123. MacDonald TT. Gastrointestinal inflammation. Inflammatory bowel disease in knockout mice. *Curr Biol* 1994; 4:261–263.
124. Davidson NJ, Leach MW, Fort MM, et al. T helper cell 1-type CD4$^+$ T cells, but not B cells, mediate colitis in interleukin 10–deficient mice. *J Exp Med* 1996;184:241–251.
125. Berg DJ, Davidson N, Kuhn R, et al. Enterocolitis and colon cancer in interleukin-10–deficient mice are associated with aberrant cytokine production and CD4($^+$) TH1-like responses. *J Clin Invest* 1996;98:1010–1020.
126. Sellon RK, Tonkonogy S, Schultz M, et al. Resident enteric bacteria are necessary for development of spontaneous colitis and immune system activation in interleukin-10–deficient mice. *Infect Immun* 1998;66: 5224–5231.
127. Rennick DM, Fort MM, Davidson NJ. Studies with IL-10$^{-/-}$ mice: an overview. *J Leukoc Biol* 1997;61: 389–396.
128. Gazzinelli RT, Wysocka M, Hieny S, et al. In the absence of endogenous IL-10, mice acutely infected with *Toxoplasma gondii* succumb to a lethal immune response dependent on CD4$^+$ T cells and accompanied by overproduction of IL-12, IFN-gamma and TNF-alpha. *J Immunol* 1996;157:798–805.
129. D'Orazio TJ, Niederkorn JY. A novel role for TGF-beta and IL-10 in the induction of immune privilege. *J Immunol* 1998;160:2089–2098.
130. Cush JJ, Splawski JB, Thomas R, et al. Elevated interleukin-10 levels in patients with rheumatoid arthritis. *Arthritis Rheum* 1995;38:96–104.
131. Cohen SB, Katsikis PD, Chu CQ, et al. High level of interleukin-10 production by the activated T cell population within the rheumatoid synovial membrane. *Arthritis Rheum* 1995;38:946–952.

132. Isomaki P, Punnonen J. Pro- and anti-inflammatory cytokines in rheumatoid arthritis. *Ann Med* 1997;29: 499–507.
133. Klimiuk PA, Goronzy JJ, J. Bjornsson, et al. Tissue cytokine patterns distinguish variants of rheumatoid synovitis. *Am J Pathol* 1997;151:1311–1319.
134. Kawakami A, Eguchi K, Matsuoka N, et al. Inhibitory effects of interleukin-10 on synovial cells of rheumatoid arthritis. *Immunology* 1997;91:252–259.
135. van Roon JA, van Roy JL, Gmelig-Meyling FH, et al. Prevention and reversal of cartilage degradation in rheumatoid arthritis by interleukin-10 and interleukin-4. *Arthritis Rheum* 1996;39:829–835.
136. Tanaka Y, Otsuka T, Hotokebuchi T, et al. Effect of IL-10 on collagen-induced arthritis in mice. *Inflamm Res* 1996;45:283–288.
137. Walmsley M, Katsikis PD, Abney E, et al. Interleukin-10 inhibition of the progression of established collagen-induced arthritis. *Arthritis Rheum* 1996;39:495–503.
138. Perez L, Orte J, Brieva JA. Terminal differentiation of spontaneous rheumatoid factor–secreting B cells from rheumatoid arthritis patients depends on endogenous interleukin-10. *Arthritis Rheum* 1995;38:1771–1776.
139. Takahashi S, Fossati L, Iwamoto M, et al. Imbalance towards Th1 predominance is associated with acceleration of lupus-like autoimmune syndrome in MRL mice. *J Clin Invest* 1996;97:1597–1604.
140. Houssiau FA, Lefebvre C, Vanden Berghe M, et al. Serum interleukin-10 titers in systemic lupus erythematosus reflect disease activity. *Lupus* 1995;4:393–395.
141. Llorente L, Richaud-Patin Y, Wijdenes J, et al. Spontaneous production of interleukin-10 by B lymphocytes and monocytes in systemic lupus erythematosus. *Eur Cytokine Netw* 1993;4:421–427.
142. Liu TF, Jones BM. Impaired production of IL-12 in systemic lupus erythematosus. I. Excessive production of IL-10 suppresses production of IL-12 by monocytes. *Cytokine* 1998;10:140–147.
143. Mongan AE, Ramdahin, Warrington RJ. Interleukin-10 response abnormalities in systemic lupus erythematosus. *Scand J Immunol* 1997;46:406–412.
144. al-Janadi M, al-Dalaan A, al-Balla S, et al. Interleukin-10 (IL-10) secretion in systemic lupus erythematosus and rheumatoid arthritis: IL-10–dependent $CD4^+CD45RO^+$ T cell-B cell antibody synthesis. *J Clin Immunol* 1996;16:198–207.
145. Emilie D, Zou W, Fior R, et al. Production and roles of IL-6, IL-10, and IL-13 in B-lymphocyte malignancies and in B-lymphocyte hyperactivity of HIV infection and autoimmunity. *Methods* 1997;11:133–142.
146. Nielsen OH, Koppen T, Rudiger N, et al. Involvement of interleukin-4 and -10 in inflammatory bowel disease. *Dig Dis Sci* 1996;41:1786–1793.
147. Niessner M, Volk BA. Altered Th1/Th2 cytokine profiles in the intestinal mucosa of patients with inflammatory bowel disease as assessed by quantitative reversed transcribed polymerase chain reaction (RT-PCR). *Clin Exp Immunol* 1995;101:428–435.
148. Kucharzik T, Stoll R, Lugering N, et al. Circulating antiinflammatory cytokine IL-10 in patients with inflammatory bowel disease (IBD). *Clin Exp Immunol* 1995;100:452–456.
149. Schreiber S, Heinig T, Thiele HG, et al. Immunoregulatory role of interleukin 10 in patients with inflammatory bowel disease. *Gastroenterology* 1995;108:1434–1444.
150. Narula SK, Cutler D, Grint P. Immunomodulation of Crohn's disease by interleukin-10. *Agents Actions Suppl* 1998;49:57–65.
151. van Hogezand RA, Verspaget HW. New therapies for inflammatory bowel disease: an update on chimeric anti-TNF alpha antibodies and IL-10 therapy. *Scand J Gastroenterol Suppl* 1997;223:105–107.
152. Drazan KE, Wu L, Bullington D, et al. Viral IL-10 gene therapy inhibits TNF-alpha and IL-1 beta, not IL-6, in the newborn endotoxemic mouse. *J Pediatr Surg* 1996;31:411–414.
153. Cusumano V, Genovese F, Mancuso G, et al. Interleukin-10 protects neonatal mice from lethal group B streptococcal infection. *Infect Immun* 1996;64:2850–2852.
154. Kato T, Murata A, Ishida H, et al. Interleukin 10 reduces mortality from severe peritonitis in mice. *Antimicrob Agents Chemother* 1995;39:1336–1340.
155. Standiford TJ, Strieter RM, Lukacs NW, et al. Neutralization of IL-10 increases lethality in endotoxemia. Cooperative effects of macrophage inflammatory protein–2 and tumor necrosis factor. *J Immunol* 1995;155: 2222–2229.
156. Rogy MA, Auffenberg T, Espat NJ, et al. Human tumor necrosis factor receptor (p55) and interleukin 10 gene transfer in the mouse reduces mortality to lethal endotoxemia and also attenuates local inflammatory responses. *J Exp Med* 1995;181:2289–2293.
157. Marchant A, Bruyns C, Vandenabeele P, et al. The protective role of interleukin-10 in endotoxin shock. *Prog Clin Biol Res* 1994;388:417–423.
158. Remick DG, Garg SJ, Newcomb DE, et al. Exogenous interleukin-10 fails to decrease the mortality or morbidity of sepsis. *Crit Care Med* 1998;26:895–904.
159. Sherry RM, Cue JI, Goddard JK, et al. Interleukin-10 is associated with the development of sepsis in trauma patients. *J Trauma* 1996;40:613–617.
160. Brandtzaeg P., Osnes L, Ovstebo R, et al. Net inflammatory capacity of human septic shock plasma evaluated by a monocyte-based target cell assay: identification of interleukin-10 as a major functional deactivator of human monocytes. *J Exp Med* 1996;184:51–60. [For erratum, see *J Exp Med* 1996;184:2075.]
161. Derkx B, Marchant A, Goldman M, et al. High levels of interleukin-10 during the initial phase of fulminant meningococcal septic shock. *J Infect Dis* 1995;171:229–232.

162. Parsons PE. Interleukin-10: the ambiguity in sepsis continues [Editorial; Comment]. *Crit Care Med* 1998; 26:818–819.
163. Kasai T, Inada K, Takakuwa T, et al. Anti-inflammatory cytokine levels in patients with septic shock. *Res Commun Mol Pathol Pharmacol* 1997;98:34–42.
164. Neidhardt R, Keel M, Steckholzer U, et al. Relationship of interleukin-10 plasma levels to severity of injury and clinical outcome in injured patients. *J Trauma* 1997;42:863–71.
165. Junger WG, Hoyt DB, Liu FC, et al. Immunosuppression after endotoxin shock: the result of multiple anti-inflammatory factors. *J Trauma* 1996;40:702–709.
166. Ayala A, Lehman DL, Herdon CD, et al. Mechanism of enhanced susceptibility to sepsis following hemorrhage. Interleukin-10 suppression of T-cell response is mediated by eicosanoid-induced interleukin-4 release. *Arch Surg* 1994;129:1172–1178.
167. Lyons A, Kelly JL, Rodrick ML, et al. Major injury induces increased production of interleukin-10 by cells of the immune system with a negative impact on resistance to infection. *Ann Surg* 1997;226:450–460.
168. Burke GW, Ciancio G, Cirocco R, et al. Association of interleukin-10 with rejection-sparing effect in septic kidney transplant recipients. *Transplantation* 1996;61:1114–1116.
169. Platz KP, Mueller AR, Rossaint R, et al. Cytokine pattern during rejection and infection after liver transplantation—improvements in postoperative monitoring? *Transplantation* 1996;62:1441–1450.
170. Zimmer S, Pollard V, Marshall GD, et al. The 1996 Moyer Award. Effects of endotoxin on the Th1/Th2 response in humans. *J Burn Care Rehabil* 1996;17:491–496.
171. Silva JS, Morrissey PJ, Grabstein KH, et al. Interleukin 10 and interferon gamma regulation of experimental *Trypanosoma cruzi* infection. *J Exp Med* 1992;175:169–174.
172. Abrahamsohn IA. Cytokines in innate and acquired immunity to *Trypanosoma cruzi*. *Braz J Med Biol Res* 1998;31:117–121.
173. Abrahamsohn IA, Coffman RL. *Trypanosoma cruzi:* IL-10, TNF, IFN-gamma, and IL-12 regulate innate and acquired immunity to infection. *Exp Parasitol* 1996;84:231–244.
174. Cardillo F, Voltarelli JC, Reed SG, et al. Regulation of *Trypanosoma cruzi* infection in mice by gamma interferon and interleukin 10: role of NK cells. *Infect Immun* 1996;64:128–134.
175. Hunter CA, Ellis-Neyes LA, Slifer T, et al. IL-10 is required to prevent immune hyperactivity during infection with *Trypanosoma cruzi*. *J Immunol* 1997;158:3311–3316.
176. Samudio M, Montenegro-James S, Cabral M, et al. Cytokine responses in *Trypanosoma cruzi* –infected children in Paraguay. *Am J Trop Med Hyg* 1998;58:119–121.
177. Dutra WO, Gollob KJ, Pinto-Dias JC, et al. Cytokine mRNA profile of peripheral blood mononuclear cells isolated from individuals with *Trypanosoma cruzi* chronic infection. *Scand J Immunol* 1997;45:74–80.
178. Ravichandran M, Mahanty S, Kumaraswami V, et al. Elevated IL-10 mRNA expression and downregulation of Th1-type cytokines in microfilaraemic individuals with *Wuchereria bancrofti* infection. *Parasite Immunol* 1997;19:69–77.
179. Mahanty S, Mollis SN, Ravichandran M, et al. High levels of spontaneous and parasite antigen-driven interleukin-10 production are associated with antigen-specific hyporesponsiveness in human lymphatic filariasis. *J Infect Dis* 1996;173:769–773.
180. Mahanty S, Ravichandran M, Raman U, et al. Regulation of parasite antigen-driven immune responses by interleukin-10 (IL-10) and IL-12 in lymphatic filariasis. *Infect Immun* 1997;65:1742–1747.
181. Ghalib HW, Piuvezam MR, Skeiky YA, et al. Interleukin 10 production correlates with pathology in human *Leishmania donovani* infections. *J Clin Invest* 1993;92:324–329.
182. Vouldoukis I, Becherel PA, Riveros-Moreno V, et al. Interleukin-10 and interleukin-4 inhibit intracellular killing of *Leishmania infantum* and *Leishmania major* by human macrophages by decreasing nitric oxide generation. *Eur J Immunol* 1997;27:860–865.
183. Bacellar O, Brodskyn C, Guerreiro J, et al. Interleukin-12 restores interferon-gamma production and cytotoxic responses in visceral leishmaniasis. *J Infect Dis* 1996;173:1515–1518.
184. Ghalib HW, Whittle JA, Kubin M, et al. IL-12 enhances Th1-type responses in human *Leishmania donovani* infections. *J Immunol* 1995;154:4623–4629.
185. Roilides E, Dimitriadou A, Kadiltsoglou I, et al. IL-10 exerts suppressive and enhancing effects on antifungal activity of mononuclear phagocytes against *Aspergillus fumigatus*. *J Immunol* 1997;158:322–329.
186. Panuska JR, Merolla R, Rebert NA, et al. Respiratory syncytial virus induces interleukin-10 by human alveolar macrophages. Suppression of early cytokine production and implications for incomplete immunity. *J Clin Invest* 1995;96:2445–2453.
187. Ameglio F, Cordiali Fei P, Solmone M, et al. Serum IL-10 levels in HIV-positive subjects: correlation with CDC stages. *J Biol Regul Homeost Agents* 1994;8:48–52.
188. Chehimi J, Ma X, Chouaib S, et al. Differential production of interleukin 10 during human immunodeficiency virus infection. *AIDS Res Hum Retroviruses* 1996;12:1141–1149.
189. De Luca A, Antinori A, Cingolani A, et al. Evaluation of cerebrospinal fluid EBV-DNA and IL-10 as markers for *in vivo* diagnosis of AIDS-related primary central nervous system lymphoma. *Br J Haematol* 1995;90: 844–849. [For erratum, see *Br J Haematol* 1995;91:1035.]
190. Khatissian E, Chakrabarti L, Hurtrel B. Cytokine patterns and viral load in lymph nodes during the early stages of SIV infection. *Res Virol* 1996;147:181–189.
191. Klein SA, Dobmeyer JM, Dobmeyer TS, et al. Demonstration of the Th1 to Th2 cytokine shift during the course

of HIV-1 infection using cytoplasmic cytokine detection on single cell level by flow cytometry. *AIDS* 1997; 11:1111–1118.
192. Navikas V, Link J, Persson C, et al. Increased mRNA expression of IL-6, IL-10, TNF-alpha, and perforin in blood mononuclear cells in human HIV infection. *J Acquir Immune DeficSyndr Hum Retrovirol* 1995;9: 484–489.
193. Clerici M, Wynn TA, Berzofsky JA, et al. Role of interleukin-10 in T helper cell dysfunction in asymptomatic individuals infected with the human immunodeficiency virus. *J Clin Invest* 1994;93:768–775.
194. Clerici M, Balotta C, Salvaggio A, et al. Human immunodeficiency virus (HIV) phenotype and interleukin-2/interleukin-10 ratio are associated markers of protection and progression in HIV infection. *Blood* 1996; 88:574–579.
195. Graziosi C, Pantaleo G, Gantt KR, et al. Lack of evidence for the dichotomy of TH1 and TH2 predominance in HIV-infected individuals. *Science* 1994;265:248–252.
196. Marsh, JW, Herndier B, Tsuzuki A, et al. Cytokine expression in large cell lymphoma associated with acquired immunodeficiency syndrome. *J Interferon Cytokine Res* 1995;15:261–268.
197. Weissman D, Daucher J, Barker T, et al. Cytokine regulation of HIV replication induced by dendritic cell-CD4-positive T cell interactions. *AIDS Res Hum Retroviruses* 1996;12:759–767.
198. Weissman D, Poli G, Fauci AS. Interleukin 10 blocks HIV replication in macrophages by inhibiting the autocrine loop of tumor necrosis factor alpha and interleukin 6 induction of virus. *AIDS Res Hum Retroviruses* 1994;10:1199–1206.
199. Chang J, Naif HM, Li S, et al. The inhibition of HIV replication in monocytes by interleukin 10 is linked to inhibition of cell differentiation. *AIDS Res Hum Retroviruses* 1996;12:1227–1235.
200. Finnegan A, Roebuck KA, Nakai BE, et al. IL-10 cooperates with TNF-alpha to activate HIV-1 from latently and acutely infected cells of monocyte/macrophage lineage. *J Immunol* 1996;156:841–851.
201. Weissman D, Poli G, Fauci AS. IL-10 synergizes with multiple cytokines in enhancing HIV production in cells of monocytic lineage. *J Acquir Immune Defic Syndr Hum Retrovirol* 1995;9:442–449.
202. Angel JB, Saget BM, Wang MZ, et al. Interleukin-10 enhances human immunodeficiency virus type 1 expression in a chronically infected promonocytic cell line (U1) by a tumor necrosis factor alpha-independent mechanism. *J Interferon Cytokine Res* 1995;15:575–584.

5

Interleukin-12

John F. McDyer, *Chang-You Wu, Brian L. Kelsall, and *Robert A. Seder

*Laboratory of Clinical Investigation; and *Vaccine Research Center, National Institute of Allergy and Infectious Diseases, National Institutes of Health, Bethesda, Maryland*

INTRODUCTION

Interleukin 12 (IL-12) is a heterodimeric molecule (IL-12 p70) composed of the p35 and p40 subunits (1). Its physiologic source *in vivo* has primarily been from antigen-presenting cells (APC), including monocytes/macrophages and dendritic cells (DC); however, neutrophils, keratinocytes, and B cells have also been shown to be involved in its production (2). The biologic activities of IL-12 are mediated through a specific high-affinity receptor that is expressed primarily on activated T and freshly isolated NK cells (3–9). Functionally, the most remarkable biologic property of IL-12 as it relates to infectious disease is its potent ability to induce IFN-γ from a variety of immune regulatory cells. In this regard, the presence of IL-12 strongly influences differentiation of naive $CD4^+$ T cells toward a Th1 phenotype (10,11). Moreover, IL-12 enhances cytotoxic T cell (CTL)–mediated lysis and NK cell activity (12). Taken together, these effector functions place IL-12 at a critical juncture in regulating cellular immune responses and mediating protection against a variety of intracellular infections. This chapter will review the basic biology of IL-12 and its role in several experimental animal models of infectious disease. This will provide a framework for understanding the therapeutic potential of IL-12 both as a vaccine adjuvant and as a treatment for infections requiring enhanced cellular immunity.

REGULATION OF IL-12 PRODUCTION

Role of IFN-γ in Regulation of IL-12 Production

The most important functional role of IL-12 as it relates to infectious disease is its capacity to induce IFN-γ (13). Remarkably, as in other biologic systems in which there are regulatory feedback loops, IFN-γ also has an important role in IL-12 regulation. In this regard, one of the early questions addressed by many investigators was whether IFN-γ precedes production of IL-12 or vice versa. It was initially reported that human monocytes stimulated with IFN-γ alone did not induce IL-12 p40 mRNA or protein production; however, IFN-γ was able to "prime" cells for lipopolysaccharide (LPS)–induced transcription of the IL-12 p40 gene (14,15). Furthermore, it was reported that induction of IL-12 p40 from macrophages in response to mycobacterial infection was dependent on the presence of both IFN-γ and TNF-α (16). Taken together, these data suggested a requisite role for IFN-γ in "priming" for IL-12 production from human monocytes (14,15) or bone marrow–derived macrophages (16).

With regard to the mechanism by which IFN-γ controls IL-12 transcription, one must have an understanding of the factors involved in IFN-γ transcription. In this regard, the ability of IFN-γ to regulate transcription is controlled in large part by a group of proteins such as IRF-1, IRF-2, and ICSBP, which belong to the interferon regulatory factor (IRF) family of transcription factors (17–21). These proteins function by binding to the interferon-stimulated response element (ISRE) found in promoters of IFN-inducible genes. Recently, several studies have used ISCBP$^{-/-}$ mice to examine its role in regulating the immune response to a variety of infectious pathogens (22–25). In murine models of *Listeria monocytogenes* (23), *Leishmania major* (24), and *Toxoplasma gondii* (25), the fact that ICSBP$^{-/-}$ mice had enhanced susceptibility provided clear evidence for its importance for infections requiring IL-12-dependent production of IFN-γ. In these studies, it was directly shown that IL-12 production was markedly reduced (24,25). Moreover, IL-12 production could not be restored from cells of ICSBP$^{-/-}$ mice in response to microbial stimuli, even in the presence of exogenous IFN-γ (24,25). These results provided clear molecular evidence for the importance of ICSBP in IL-12 induction in response to intracellular pathogens as well as the ability of IFN-γ to enhance IL-12 transcription (14).

Finally, although the previous discussion highlights the importance of IFN-γ in regulating IL-12 transcription, there have been several studies showing that IL-12 can be induced in an IFN-γ–independent manner. First, IFN-γ receptor–deficient mice infected with *Listeria monocytogenes* produced significant amounts of both IL-12 p40 and IFN-γ following restimulation of spleen cells *in vitro* (26). Second, cells from IFN-γ–deficient mice infected with *Toxoplasma gondii* were also able to produce IL-12 p40 and p70 following *in vitro* stimulation. Remarkably, in a separate report, it was shown that IL-12 p40 could be detected following injection of IFN-γ$^{-/-}$ mice with an antigen derived from *T. gondii* (27). Moreover, in this study, IL-12 p40 was detected only from CD8$^+$CD11c$^+$ lymphoid DC (27). These data clearly show that in response to certain infectious pathogens, IL-12 p40 production *in vivo* can be induced in the absence of IFN-γ. In addition, these data raise the issue of whether DC production of IL-12 may be less dependent on IFN-γ than that required for monocyte/macrophage production of IL-12.

Role of CD40L/CD40 Costimulation in Production of IL-12

A central role of CD40L/CD40 costimulation in regulating humoral and cellular immune responses was first appreciated in patients with hyperimmunoglobulin M (hyper-IgM) syndrome (28,29). These patients had, in addition to a defect in T cell–dependent antibody production, increased susceptibility to *Pneumocystis carinii* and cryptosporidium infections. These latter infections strongly suggested that there was a defect in the cellular immune response. The central role that CD40/CD40L costimulation had in mediating cellular immune responses was subsequently shown in studies using mice deficient in either CD40 or CD40L. In these studies, T cell activation and production of cytokines such as IFN-γ were markedly impaired in response to protein antigens (30,31). Furthermore, additional *in vitro* studies showed that CD40L/CD40 regulated T cell activation and production of IL-12 and IFN-γ through at least two mechanisms. First, CD40L directly induces production of IL-12 from APC (macrophages and DC) expressing CD40 (32–35). Second, CD40L/CD40 stimulation enhances expression of costimulatory molecules (e.g., B7-1, B7-2) on APC, leading to increased T cell stimulation (20,36,37). Taken together, these data illustrate the central role that CD40L/CD40 stimulation has in regulating Th1 responses following stimulation with a protein antigen. By contrast, IL-12 production from mononuclear cells stimulated with microbial stimuli such as LPS or heat-killed *Listeria monocytogenes* induced IL-12 production in a CD40L-independent manner (38), suggesting that certain intracellular pathogens can directly induce IL-12 in the absence of CD40/CD40L stimulation and raising the question as to the requirements for CD40L/CD40 stimulation *in vivo* to a variety of infectious stimuli. In the following section, the role of CD40L/CD40 stimulation was evaluated in those experimental infectious disease models in which IL-12-dependent production of IFN-γ is critical for protection.

The first studies to evaluate the role of CD40L in host immunity against an intracellular parasite used the experimental model of murine leishmania infection. *Leishmania major* infection has been shown to require IL-12–dependent production of IFN-γ from $CD4^+$ T cells for effective immunity. In these experiments, $CD40L^{-/-}$ mice were markedly impaired in production of both IL-12 and IFN-γ, which correlated with enhanced susceptibility to infection (39,40). Similar results were seen from $CD40L^{-/-}$ mice infected with *L. amazonensis* (41), suggesting that CD40L/CD40 stimulation was required *in vivo* for effective Th1 response to this infectious stimulus. In marked contrast, CD40L-deficient mice infected *in vivo* with *Histoplasma capsulatum* (42) or *Mycobacterium tuberculosis* (43) were not more susceptible compared with wild-type animals. These data are consistent with the *in vitro* studies alluded to above in which microbial stimuli such as LPS or *L. monocytogenes* readily induce IL-12 in the absence of CD40L/CD40 stimulation. Thus, with the exception of Leishmania, most intracellular pathogens can directly induce IL-12 in a CD40L/CD40-independent manner. These *in vivo* mouse data are consistent with the clinical observation that patients with X-linked hyper-IgM (who have a mutation in CD40L) do not appear to be more vulnerable to infection with *H. capsulatum* or *M. tuberculosis*.

Microbial Stimuli Affecting IL-12 Induction

As noted above, certain microorganisms or bacterial products can directly induce IL-12 in the absence of IFN-γ or CD40L/CD40 stimulation. The list of potent IL-12 inducers includes *L. monocytogenes*, *T. gondii*, *H. capsulatum*, *M. tuberculosis*, and LPS. Furthermore, the recent finding that a protein derived from *T. gondii* (Stag) can elicit IL-12 p40 from lymphoid DC in an IFN-γ–, CD40L–independent manner (27), underscores the importance of DC in priming immune responses following infection.

Inhibitory Regulation of IL-12 Production

In contrast to these positive regulators of IL-12 production, it has become clear that signals that inhibit IL-12 production from APC may be important for regulation of cell-mediated immune responses. Initially described were cytokine inhibitors of IL-12 such as IL-10, TGF-β, IL-4, and IL-13, the latter two having more complex effects than the former in that preincubation with these cytokines can also enhance IL-12 production (13,44). Recently, engagement of noncytokine receptors (45–47), such as IgG in the form of Ig-opsonized bacteria (48) or immune complexes (49), complement components (47,48,50), thalidomide (51), pentoxifylline (52), tetrahydrocannabinol (THC) (53,54), chemokines and chemoattractants (55–58), 1,25,dihydroxyvitamin D3 (59), adrenergic agonists (60), prostaglandin E_2 (PGE_2) (61), and ADP-ribosylating toxins such as cholera toxin (62) have all been shown to inhibit IL-12 p70 production from human monocytes *in vitro*. Of interest, the inhibitory effect of these factors on DC production of IL-12 has been more variable; i.e., it has been shown that the latter three factors above inhibit CD40–induced IL-12 production from human monocyte-derived DC, while signaling via chemokine/chemoattractant receptors and Fc receptors has little effect on DC.

In addition to these *in vitro* studies, there is evidence that many of these factors also suppress IL-12 production *in vivo*. Thus, it has been shown that treatment of mice with antibodies to complement receptor 3 (CR3, CD11b/CD18) or cholera toxin results in suppression of IL-12 and IFN-γ production following systemic injection of LPS (50,62). In addition, mice given THC or the chemokine MCP-1 have a decreased ability to mount Th1 responses to infectious pathogens, consistent with their ability to inhibit IL-12 production (53,56). Finally, treatment of humans with selective β2-adrenergic agonists has been shown to suppress production of IL-12 by whole-blood lymphocytes stimulated *in vitro* (60).

While the mechanisms by which these various inhibitory factors act on IL-12 production remain largely unknown, several features of this inhibition are clear. The first is that all of these inhibitors, despite acting through discrete surface receptors, appear to inhibit IL-12 in a more or less selective fashion, in that production of other proinflammatory cytokines such as TNF-α, IL-1 and IL-6, remain largely unaffected. The one exception to this is cholera toxin, which inhibits production of TNF-α as well as IL-12 (62). The second feature is that most IL-12 inhibitors do not appear to act via the induction of autocrine production of cytokines or prostaglandins that can suppress IL-12, such as IL-10, TGF-β, or PGE_2. The possible exceptions to this rule are the chemokines MCP 1–4 and IgG complexes, which may be partially dependent on IL-10 (55,63). Finally, it is clear that induction of high levels of intracellular cAMP can directly inhibit IL-12 production. This is shown by the fact that treatment of cells with forskolin, which induces production of cAMP, or with dibutyryl-cAMP, which enters the cell directly, suppresses the ability of those cells to produce IL-12 (61). This mechanism is also consistent with the effects of cholera toxin, which acts to activate G_s proteins, which subsequently induce production of intracellular cAMP. The induction of cAMP, however, cannot explain why C5a or fMLF, acting via the C5a receptor and the high-affinity formyl-peptide receptor, respectively, can dramatically and selectively suppress production of IL-12, because these agents act via G_i proteins that inhibit production of cAMP. Clearly, more needs to be done to identify the signaling pathways that are responsible for inhibition of IL-12 production and for the differential effects of many of these inhibitors on monocytes and DC, as well as to determine whether these inhibitory signaling pathways can be therapeutically manipulated for treatment of Th1-mediated autoimmunity or for enhancement of vaccine efficacy.

Summary of the Factors Regulating IL-12 Production

To conclude, IL-12 is a central cytokine in regulating cellular immunity. As it relates to intracellular infections, it has a positive role in enhancing the production of IFN-γ, the effector cytokine that leads to intracellular killing. In contrast, IL-12 can have a deleterious role in mediating proinflammatory responses associated with organ-specific autoimmune disease. Thus, with regard to infection, it is critical that rapid production of IL-12 occur soon after exposure to provide protection. This can occur through a confluence of factors (direct induction, CD40L/CD40 interaction, and IFN-γ), as noted above. Soon thereafter, there are many factors by which IL-12 production and Th1 responses are limited. This careful balance ensures protection against lethal pathogens but prevents untoward reactivity against self antigens. When this regulation becomes unlinked, there are pathologic consequences.

IL-12 RECEPTOR/IL-12 RESPONSIVENESS

The biologic activities of IL-12 are mediated through a specific, high-affinity receptor composed of IL-12Rβ1 and IL-12Rβ2 subunits, which exist primarily on T and NK cells.

The cDNA for two IL-12R subunits have been cloned from human and mouse T cells and designated as IL-12Rβ1 and IL-12Rβ2 (3,9). Both of these subunits are type I transmembrane glycoproteins (gp) with molecular sizes of about 100 kd for IL-12Rβ1 and 130 kd for IL-12Rβ2. These subunits are members of the cytokine receptor superfamily and are related to the β type cytokine receptor gp130, a common receptor subunit for IL-6, IL-11, oncostatin M, granulocyte colony-stimulating factor (G-CSF), leukemia inhibitory factor (LIF), and ciliary neurotrophic factor. The mouse and human IL-12Rβ1 and IL-12Rβ2 are 54% and 68% identical on the amino acid sequence level, respectively. When individually expressed on COS cells, IL-12Rβ1 and IL-12Rβ2 subunits bound labeled IL-12 with only low affinity (5 nM); however, coexpression of IL-12Rβ1 and IL-12Rβ2 displayed high (50 pM)–affinity and low (5 nM)–affinity IL-12 binding sites (3,64). In addition, when the IL-3-dependent mouse pro-B cell line Ba/F3 was stably transfected with the two IL-12R subunits, it also revealed high and low affinity for IL-12 binding sites, and these cells proliferated in response to IL-12 (3). These data indicate that both IL-12Rβ1 and IL-12Rβ2 are required to generate a functional receptor. In comparison to IL-12Rβ1, IL-12Rβ2 appears to function as a signal-transducing component of the high-affinity receptor complex, due to the presence of conserved tyrosine residues in its cytoplasmic domain. Furthermore, analysis of the interactions of IL-12 with IL-12Rβ1 and IL-12Rβ2 subunits indicates that IL-12 appears to interact with IL-12Rβ1 via the p40 subunit, while IL-12Rβ2 interacts with both p35 and p40 subunits (4).

Upon binding of IL-12R on T and NK cells, IL-12 stimulates tyrosine phosphorylation of the Jak2 and Tyk2 protein kinases, which in turn activate multiple STATs, including STAT1, STAT3, STAT4, and STAT5 (65–68). Among these, STAT4 appears to be essential for mediating the response to IL-12, as demonstrated in STAT4-deficient mice, which have defects in IFN-γ induction and proliferation, enhancement of NK cytolytic function, and Th1 differentiation in response to IL-12 (69).

With regard to cellular distribution of the IL-12 receptors, studies using flow cytometry show that the IL-12Rβ1 chain is expressed on several human T, NK, and B cell lines but not on nonlymphohemotopoietic cell lines (5,70–72). IL-12Rβ1 expression is upregulated on activated human T, NK, and B cells. Expression of IL-12Rβ1 and IL-12Rβ2 subunits on human peripheral blood mononuclear cells (PBMC), and specifically on T cells, can be positively or negatively regulated by cytokines (6), steroids (73), and accessory signals (74). Factors that enhance T cell proliferation and activation appear to have a positive influence on IL-12R expression. Thus, IL-2, IL-7, IL-15, and CD28 costimulation upregulates IL-12Rβ1 expression (6,74). Furthermore, cytokines that promote Th1 responses also enhance IL-12R expression; in this regard, IL-12 and IL-18 are perhaps the most potent inducers of IL-12R expression (75–77). Moreover, IFN-γ in the mouse (70) and IFN-α in the human (71) also upregulate IL-12Rβ2 subunit expression. By contrast, factors such as IL-4, IL-10, TGF-β, PGE_2, and dexamethasone, which inhibit Th1 induction, are found to inhibit expression of the IL-12R (6,70,71,73).

Functional evidence for the importance of IL-12 receptor subunits in IFN-γ production and NK activity was provided by several studies. Polyclonal and monoclonal antibodies against the human IL-12Rβ1 subunit inhibit IL-12–induced proliferation, secretion of IFN-γ, and development of LAK activity by human PBMC (5). These observations were confirmed in an animal study showing that splenocytes from IL-12Rβ1–deficient (IL-12Rβ1$^{-/-}$) mice are also deficient in IL-12–induced proliferation, IFN-γ secretion, Th1 development, and enhancement of NK lytic activity (7). These results demonstrate that IL-12Rβ1 not only contributes to the generation of high-affinity IL-12 binding sites but is also essential for formation of functional IL-12R.

ROLE OF IL-12 RECEPTOR IN HUMAN DISEASE

The role of IL-12R expression in humans has been studied both directly and in a correlative manner. Correlative evidence for a role of IL-12Rβ2 in human disease was obtained by analyzing expression of IL-12Rβ1 and IL-12Rβ2 in tuberculosis patients and healthy tuberculin reactors. In this report, the percentages of T cells expressing IL-12Rβ1 and IL-12Rβ2 in tuberculosis patients were significantly decreased compared with those of the healthy tuberculin reactors (78). The best and most demonstrative evidence in humans that functional IL-12 receptors have a role in mediating protection against intracellular infections comes from studies of patients with mutations in the IL-12Rβ1 receptor. PBMC from these patients are markedly impaired in their production of IFN-γ, IL-12–induced enhancement of NK activity, and IL-12R signaling. Furthermore, these patients suffer from severe nontuberculous mycobacterial and salmonella infections (79,80). These unique patients have provided us with a compelling example of the importance of IL-12 responsiveness in maintaining sufficient production of IFN-γ to mediate control of specific intracellular infections.

INFECTIOUS DISEASE MODELS

The previous sections outlined the basic biology of IL-12 and the factors governing its regulation. This section will provide an in-depth analysis of the role that IL-12 has in mediating protective immunity to a variety of infectious pathogens.

Leishmania Major

The murine model of *L. major* infection has provided valuable insight into the role of cellular immunity in mediating protection against intracellular pathogens. Effective primary immunity to *L. major* infection is due to the development of a Th1 response characterized by the IL-12-dependent production of IFN-γ (81,82). In contrast, disease susceptibility is correlated with early production of Th2 cytokines, which appear to inhibit both IL-12 responsiveness and the subsequent development of protective Th1-type cells (83). The ability of IL-12 treatment at the time of infection to induce protective Th1-type responses in susceptible strains of mice was the first *in vivo* evidence that IL-12 could direct T helper differentiation *in vivo* (81,82).

The *L. major* model also provided the first demonstration that IL-12 could be an effective Th1-inducing adjuvant when combined with a protein antigen. In the initial study, effective vaccination against *L. major* in susceptible strains was achieved using IL-12 with soluble leishmanial antigen (SLA) and a recombinant leishmanial protein (LACK) (84,85). In a subsequent study, it was demonstrated that subcutaneous administration of plasmid DNA encoding the LACK antigen was sufficient to confer protection to susceptible BALB/c mice challenged 2 or 12 weeks postvaccination (86). In the same study, although vaccination with leishmanial protein plus IL-12 protein protected mice challenged 2 weeks postvaccination (similar to the previous reports), these mice failed to control infection when challenged 12 weeks postvaccination. These studies demonstrated that vaccination with plasmid DNA encoding a specific leishmanial antigen is more effective than leishmanial protein plus IL-12 protein in eliciting long-term immunity capable of controlling *L. major* infection. Of note, leishmanial protein plus IL-12 DNA was able to confer longer-lasting immunity (87). Taken together, these data suggest that, in this vaccine model, the persistence of adjuvant (IL-12) may be the critical determinant in maintaining durable cell-mediated immune responses capable of protecting mice following infection.

Use of IL-12 as a Vaccine Adjuvant for Cutaneous Leishmaniasis Infection

Based on the original report that IL-12 could be an effective adjuvant in conferring protection to susceptible mice following vaccination with leishmanial protein, an additional study in primates using a single vaccination with clinical-grade leishmanial protein plus human IL-12 and alum conferred protection to monkeys that were challenged 4 weeks postvaccination (88). Of importance, vaccination with this regimen was found to be safe. Thus, this model provides a standard by which to compare other vaccine regimens. In light of the mouse data described above, one important issue will be to challenge monkeys at later time points postvaccination to ensure that a sufficient memory immune response is elicited to control infection.

Listeria monocytogenes

Listeria monocytogenes is a Gram-positive rod existing in animal reservoirs, soil, vegetation, and in normal gastrointestinal flora in healthy individuals. Human disease caused by *L. monocytogenes* (listeriosis) occurs in the setting of immunosuppression, pregnancy, or through food-borne transmission. Thus, patients with underlying solid or hematologic malignancies, HIV infection, diabetes mellitus, renal disease, or on long-term glucocorticoid treatment or chemotherapy are predisposed to infection with *L. monocytogenes*.

The *L. monocytogenes* mouse model has been critical for understanding the importance of how the innate and acquired immune response are linked to provide a protective response (89,90). In these studies, it was shown that IL-12 could have a protective role in severe combined immunodeficient (SCID) mice following infection with *L. monocytogenes* by its ability to enhance production of IFN-γ by NK cells (91). Furthermore, neutralization of endogenous IL-12 resulted in an increase in bacterial burden, providing further evidence for the importance of IL-12 (92,93). Finally, APC that had been exposed to *Listeria* were able to influence differentiation of naive $CD4^+$ T cells into IFN-γ–producing T cells in an IL-12–dependent manner showing a role for IL-12 in Th1 priming *in vitro* (10). Taken together, these data show that IL-12 plays a central role in augmenting production of IFN-γ in both innate (NK cell) and acquired (T cell) immune responses.

Role Of IL-12 In Human Listeria Infection

Because infections with *L. monocytogenes* (predominantly gastroenteritis secondary to food poisoning or meningitis in the immunocompromised host) are readily treatable with antibiotics (i.e., ampicillin), there does not appear to be a clinical role for cytokine therapy with IL-12 in human listeriosis.

Toxoplasma gondii

Toxoplasma gondii, a protozoan parasite belonging to the coccidia family and Apicomplexa phylum, is widespread, with a large number of mammal and bird species known to serve as host. Among humans, it is estimated that more than 500 million people are infected worldwide. The life cycle of *T. gondii* is complex, with the definitive host being the cat. Ingestion of sporulated oocysts by intermediary hosts (e.g., humans) results in infection that can persist for life. In the intermediary host, the tachyzoite (rapidly multiplying form) replicates until the cell bursts and infectious parasites are released to the extracellular environment, repeating the cycle. Tachyzoites are cleared with the development of immunity. If not controlled by the immune system, tachyzoites can reemerge from dormant cysts, resulting in disease, particularly in the setting of cellular immunodeficiency. Such is the case with toxoplasmic encephalitis in patients with advanced HIV infection (94,95).

Similar to *L. monocytogenes* infection, multiple components of the immune system play an important role in resistance to *T. gondii*, including cells from the innate immune response in the initial stages of infection, to the development of the adaptive immune response, in which T cells play a predominant role. The innate immune response is particularly dependent on cytokine release by macrophages and DC following exposure to the parasite. In this regard, production of IL-12 by these cells is central for an effective immune response to *T. gondii*, culminating in IL-12–dependent IFN-γ release, initially from NK cells and subsequently from T cells (96,97).

The mouse experimental data provide clear evidence for both exogenous and endogenous IL-12 having a role in mediating protective immunity. First, with regard to the role of endogenous IL-12, both SCID mice and immunocompetent mice infected with *T. gondii* had accelerated mortality when treated with anti-IL-12 antibodies (98–100). Moreover, treatment with recombinant IL-12 prolonged survival of T cell–deficient mice infected with *T. gondii* (101) and protected immunocompetent animals against a lethal challenge with a virulent strain of *T. gondii* (100). The protective effect of IL-12 was shown to be mediated by production of IFN-γ from NK cells in SCID mice as well as T cell-derived production of IFN-γ in immunocompetent animals. Finally, with regard to human disease, it is worth noting that tachyzoite extracts can trigger synthesis of IFN-γ by NK cells associated with monocytes (but in the absence of T cells) derived from PBMC of healthy or HIV-infected donors (102). These findings indicate that the T cell-independent pathway for IFN-γ synthesis is also operative in humans infected with *T. gondii*.

Of interest, although macrophages have been assumed to be the major source of IL-12 following infection with *T. gondii* as alluded to above, a recent study indicates that DC are perhaps the major source of IL-12 in lymphoid tissue responsible for T cell priming during the very early response to tachyzoite products (27). Although these results may be specific for *T. gondii*, they raise the question of whether lymphoid DC also have an important role in regulating immunity to other intracellular infections.

Role of IL-12 in Human Toxoplasmosis Infection

Over the past 15 years, there has been an increase in *T. gondii* infection, especially in patients infected with HIV. In addition to a progressive decrease in $CD4^+$ T cells, IL-12 production is diminished in HIV infection. Thus, due to the importance of IL-12 in mediating host protection against *T. gondii*, there appears to be a good scientific basis for its use as treatment in HIV-infected patients with toxoplasmosis not responding to conventional therapy. There is reluctance to use a proinflammatory cytokine such as IL-12 as therapy for a closed-space infection in the central nervous system at this time.

Histoplasma capsulatum

Histoplasma capsulatum is a dimorphic fungus that exists in a mycelial form in the soil of various geographic regions of the world. Primary infection occurs through inhalation of conidial or mycelial fragments, which are ingested by macrophages and subsequently converted into the yeast form. In most instances, immunocompetent hosts develop a mild, self-limited upper respiratory infection involving only the lungs. Protective immunity is achieved by the interaction of T cells and macrophages and is usually long-lasting. By contrast, in immunocompromised hosts, disseminated infection can occur either through primary infection or by reactivation of a previous infection (103–105). Clinically, disseminated histoplasmosis is an important clinical complication in HIV-infected individuals as well as in immunocompromised hosts living in certain geographic regions of the United States (104,105). Thus, understanding the factors involved in protective immunity may lead to effective immune-based therapies for immunocompromised patients with disseminated infection.

Similar to murine models of *T. gondii* and *L. monocytogenes*, the innate and acquired immune responses lead to effective intracellular killing of *H. capsulatum*. As with the other intracellular infectious pathogens discussed in this chapter, IL-12 is the central regulator affecting both the induction and magnitude of the IFN-γ response. Thus, in both pulmonary and systemic murine models of *H. capsulatum* infection, neutralization of IL-12 is associated with diminished production of IFN-γ, resulting in overwhelming infection and accelerated mortality (106,107). Several studies have examined which cell types are critical in *H. capsulatum* infection. A role for IL-12–dependent production of IFN-γ independent of T cells was shown in studies using SCID mice. In these studies, treatment of SCID mice with exogenous IL-12 prolonged survival through an IFN-γ–dependent mechanism. T cells also play a critical role in the adaptive immune response to *H. capsulatum* infection. Immunodeficient mice (SCID or Nu/Nu) display increased susceptibility to *H. capsulatum*, as do normal mice depleted of $CD4^+$ or $CD8^+$ T cells (108–110). Finally, IL-12 treatment of normal mice infected with a lethal dose of *H. capsulatum* enhances production of IFN-γ by $CD4^+$ and $CD8^+$ T cells and protects mice from a fatal outcome. Taken together, these data suggest that IL-12 is the central regulator in mediating production of IFN-γ from both NK and T cells.

Role of IL-12 in Disseminated Histoplasmosis in Humans

The current standard treatment for disseminated histoplasmosis in immunocompromised patients is Amphotericin B (AmB). Although treatment with AmB is quite effective, there have been rare therapeutic failures. Moreover, AmB treatment is toxic and cumbersome. The systemic model of *H. capsulatum* infection in SCID mice has been used to evaluate the role of IL-12 as a potential therapy in the presence or absence of conventional chemotherapy with AmB (111). These studies demonstrate what might occur in patients with disseminated histoplasmosis and advanced HIV infection, because these patients often have significant numbers of NK cells and $CD8^+$ T cells but lack $CD4^+$ T cells. Mice treated with IL-12 or AmB alone had an increase in survival and reduction in organism load. Remarkably, *H. capsulatum*-infected mice treated with both IL-12 and AmB developed sterilizing immunity that persisted for several months. In this protocol, IL-12 was given only once a week and AmB three times per week. Based on these data, it is possible that combination therapy with IL-12 and AmB may maximize the clinical outcome but reduce the duration of treatment with AmB, thereby minimizing any side effects associated with this treatment. Thus, HIV-infected patients with disseminated histoplasmosis who are unresponsive or suffer from relapsing disease could be candidates for this therapeutic approach.

Mycobacterial Infections

Currently, one-third of the world population is infected with *M. tuberculosis*; this results in approximately 3 million deaths per year (112). In addition, other mycobacterial infections, including *M. leprae* and *M. avium* complex, contribute to significant morbidity worldwide. A common feature of mycobacterial disease is the requirement for an adequate cell-mediated immune response for both protection and control of infection. As with other intracellular pathogens, IFN-γ plays a central part in mediating resistance to mycobacteria. Therefore, the role of IL-12 has been studied in several murine models of mycobacterial infection (i.e., *M. tuberculosis*, *M. avium,* and *M. bovis*) as well as in human *in vitro* systems.

M. tuberculosis/M. bovis

Because IL-12 is a crucial regulator of Th1 immune responses, its role has been investigated in both *M. tuberculosis* and *M. bovis* BCG mouse models of infection. Infection of IL-12 p40-deficient mice with *M. tuberculosis* resulted in uncontrolled bacterial growth and profoundly impaired production of IFN-γ (113). In addition, these IL-12-mutant mice generated defective granuloma formation. Similarly, neutralization of endogenous IL-12 by treatment with antibodies in susceptible mice infected with *M. bovis* demonstrated markedly impaired production of IFN-γ, and mice failed to control infection (114). Taken together, these data show that IL-12 is essential for control of *M. tuberculosis* and *M. bovis* infections in the mouse model.

A series of studies has examined the role of IL-12 in cells from patients exposed to or infected with *M. tuberculosis*. In several reports examining cytokine production from pleural fluid mononuclear cells, it was shown that IFN-γ and IL-12 were increased preferentially compared with those derived from peripheral blood (115–117). Because patients with pleural disease have an apparently effective immune response, it was inferred that production of these cytokines may have a role in the protective response. In comparing the immune responses from PPD^+ patients to those of patients with pulmonary tuberculosis, it was shown that patients with tuberculosis had reduced production of IL-2 and IFN-γ (118–121). Studies of IL-12 and IFN-γ regulation were extended to HIV-infected individuals with tuberculosis. In these studies, it was found that PBMC from HIV-infected patients had deficient proliferation and IFN-γ production compared with HIV tuberculosis patients in response to stimulation with *M. tuberculosis* (122). These responses could be enhanced by addition of IL-12 *in vitro*. In a subsequent study, PBMC from HIV-negative patients infected with multidrug resistant tuberculosis (MDR-TB) who had variable $CD4^+$ T cell counts were found to have diminished Th1 responses (proliferation and IFN-γ production) when the CD4 count was below 500 (123). Of interest, production of IL-12 p70 by MDR-TB patients was similar when compared with that of healthy PPD^+ or normal controls; however, addition of exogenous IL-12 to *in vitro* cultures of PBMC resulted in a striking increase in production of IFN-γ in both the MDR-TB patients and PPD^+ and PPD-controls. These results suggest a potential benefit of IL-12 therapy for treatment of patients with various mycobacterial infections and functionally impaired immunity.

M. avium

Nontuberculous mycobacterial infections are becoming increasingly recognized as an etiology for both isolated pulmonary infections and disseminated disease in various populations, including patients with advanced HIV infection. *M. avium* is the most common nontuberculous mycobacterial infection (124).

In the mouse model, the roles of both endogenous and exogenous IL-12 have been extensively studied. First, mice treated with antibody to IL-12 throughout the course of infection were unable to control infection (125). Second, mice lacking a functional IL-12 p40 gene are highly susceptible to *M. avium* infection, with markedly increased bacterial loads. In contrast, SCID mice infected with *M. avium* are partially resistant, suggesting a T cell–independent pathway to control *M. avium* infection, likely mediated by NK cells (126); however, neutralizing antibody to IL-12 in these animals impairs resistance. Thus, endogenous IL-12 appears to play a crucial role in the protective immune response to *M. avium* in the murine model of infection. The role of exogenous IL-12 is discussed below.

In addition to the murine models, there is evidence in human mycobacterial disease that IL-12 plays an indispensable role in immunity. In a familial cohort with disseminated *M. avium* complex infection, adherent patient monocytes made abnormally low amounts of IL-12 p70 after stimulation with *Staphylococcus aureus* Cowan I strain (127). Moreover, cocultures of familial patient monocytes with either familial or normal T cells made undetectable IL-12 in response to PHA stimulation. In another report, a child with disseminated BCG infection (*M. bovis*) and *Salmonella enteritidis* infection was found to have a large homozygous deletion within the IL-12 p40 subunit that precluded expression of functional IL-12 p70 protein (128). Notably, these two groups of patients responded to antimycobacterial therapy only after the initiation of subcutaneous IFN-γ treatment. Thus, abnormal regulation of IL-12 production may result in susceptibility to mycobacterial infections. Finally, as noted above, two groups simultaneously reported several patients with severe nontuberculous infections, including *M. bovis* or *M. avium*, as well as Salmonella infections, who lacked the IL-12Rβ1 (79,80). Collectively, this body of evidence suggests that IL-12 is irreplaceable for protective immunity to mycobacteria.

IL-12 Treatment for Mycobacterial Infections

As with other models of intracellular infection, exogenous IL-12 treatment in murine mycobacterial infections has provided valuable insight into its potential use as a therapeutic agent. This was first shown when a susceptible mouse strain was given IL-12 at the initiation of infection with *M. tuberculosis* (129). In these experiments, mean survival time doubled and lung pathology was delayed in the IL-12–treated mice compared with control animals. Moreover, mice with the same genetic background in which the IFN-γ gene was disrupted were not protected by IL-12 treatment, indicating that IL-12 mediates protection against *M. tuberculosis* in an IFN-γ–dependent manner. Finally, when highly susceptible mouse strains lacking T cells were infected with *M. tuberculosis* and treated with IL-12, their survival was extended (130). This T cell–independent resistance was likely due to the production of IFN-γ by NK cells. Taken together, these data show that IL-12 affects IFN-γ production from both NK and T cells.

For *M. avium* infection, a series of studies has examined the role of IL-12 with or without chemotherapy in the mouse model. In these studies, treatment of SCID mice with IL-12 combined with a cocktail of antimycobacterial drugs resulted in a decrease in bacterial load that was significantly greater than that resulting from the administration of IL-12 or drugs alone (126). A similar synergistic effect was seen when immunocompetent mice were treated with IL-12 in combination with antibiotics. The activity of IL-12 in these studies was also shown to be dependent on induction of endogenous IFN-γ. Thus, these data suggest a synergy between IL-12 and antimycobacterial therapy for *M. avium* infection.

Currently, IL-12 adjuvant therapy is being investigated in patients with severe nontuberculous mycobacterial infections. These include several patients with familial *M. avium* infections in whom IL-12 production appears to be abnormally low (127) or HIV-infected individuals poorly responsive to conventional chemotherapy. In addition, patients with MDR-TB are also being treated with IL-12 therapy in addition to chemotherapy. Finally, non-HIV patients with *M. tuberculosis* infection who also have accompanying lymphopenia have been shown to have impaired Th1 responses (123). These patients, too, would be potential candidates for adjuvant IL-12 therapy.

VIRAL INFECTIONS

The ability of IL-12 to enhance production of IFN-γ, CTL, and NK lytic activity and to induce production of opsonizing IgG antibodies makes it potentially important for resistance to viral infections. Consequently, IL-12 has been studied extensively in several animal models of viral infection, including murine cytomegalovirus (MCMV), lymphocytic choriomeningitis virus (LCMV), herpes simplex, influenza, and murine AIDS (MAIDS). In addition, there has been extensive investigation into the role of IL-12 in patients with chronic hepatitis B viral infection and HIV infection. The following section reviews the importance of IL-12 and its potential role as a therapeutic agent in a broad range of viral infections.

Animal Models in Viral Disease

Mouse models of MCMV and LCMV infection have provided great insight into the role of IL-12 in viral immunity. It was first shown that low doses of IL-12 enhanced immunity to LCMV infection (131). Of interest, high doses of IL-12 were detrimental to resistance and actually led to inhibition of virus-specific CTL activity. Moreover, treatment of the mice with anti–TNF-α antibodies abrogated all IL-12–induced effects (132). These studies were the first demonstration that excessive IL-12 may actually be harmful in the setting of acute viral infection. In the MCMV model of infection, IL-12 therapy increased NK cell cytotoxicity and IFN-γ production, and substantially decreased viral burdens in treated animals. These beneficial effects were prevented by depletion of either NK cells or IFN-γ (133).

In studying the role of endogenous IL-12 following infection, IL-12 was detected following MCMV but not LCMV infection. Moreover, as a functional correlate anti–IL-12 treatment blocked NK cell production of IFN-γ in the MCMV model but had no effect on LCMV replication. In the MCMV model, anti–IL-12 treatment failed to alter later T cell responses, including IFN-γ production and viral clearance (134).

In addition to the studies with anti–IL-12, two recent reports examined immune responses in IL-12–deficient mice following viral infection. In response to mouse hepatitis virus (MHV) infection, IL-12–deficient mice effectively controlled liver damage similar to control animals (135). This was in contrast to IFN-γ receptor–deficient mice, who had increased susceptibility to MHV in the same studies. Remarkably, following MHV infection IL-12–deficient mice had high IFN-γ production by $CD4^+$ splenocytes. In response to LCMV or VSV infection, IL-12–deficient mice also had virus-specific Th1 production (136). Taken together, these data suggest that, for certain viral infections, IL-12 is not essential for generation of Th1-type cytokine responses.

HIV Infection

Advanced infection with HIV has long been recognized to substantially impair cellular immune function. This leads to diminished resistance to many opportunistic pathogens characteristic of AIDS (e.g., *Pneumocystis carinii, Mycobacterium tuberculo-*

sis, Mycobacterium avium, Toxoplasma gondii, Candida albicans, and others). As noted before, IL-12 plays a major role in regulating immunity to many of these pathogens. Thus, the study of IL-12 in HIV disease has been of great interest.

PBMC and alveolar macrophages from HIV-infected individuals have an impaired ability to produce IL-12 in response to *Staphylococcus aureus* Cowan strain (SAC) even in patients with relatively normal $CD4^+$ T cell counts (137,138). Moreover, PBMC from HIV-infected individuals have an impaired ability to upregulate the IL-12Rβ2 chain in response to mitogenic stimuli (139). The mechanisms involved in these defects are incompletely understood and may be multifactorial. The IL-12-producing capacity of stimulated monocytes is diminished following *in vitro* infection with HIV, suggesting a direct viral inhibitory effect. Recently, the HIV protein Tat has been shown to decrease IL-12 production from stimulated PBMC, whereas other HIV proteins (Nef and gp120) had no effect (140). Hyperproduction of the antagonistic cytokine IL-10 has also been postulated to account for decreased IL-12 production by HIV-infected patients; however, increased production of IL-10 by HIV patient cells has been demonstrated in some studies but not others, and thus remains controversial (137,141). Although bacterial stimulation of monocytes from HIV patients results in abnormally low IL-12 production, the HIV gp120 envelope induces IL-12 (and IL-10) production in monocytes from healthy donors (142). Therefore, patients with HIV infection may be in a perpetual state of immune activation in vivo, expressing low levels of the proinflammatory cytokines, including IL-12. Consequently, they may be unable to generate a high-level spike of IL-12 in response to acute infectious stimulation (143).

Therapeutic Role for IL-12 in HIV

Despite some of the promising early *in vitro* data using IL-12 to restore immune function in HIV (144), studies in the monkey and Phase I human studies have been rather disappointing. In a study examining administration of IL-12 to chronically SIV-infected rhesus monkeys, IL-12 treatment was well tolerated (145). Although both NK activity and IFN-γ-producing capacity were enhanced in vitro, there were no detectable changes in viral load in the treated animals. Furthermore, in phase I studies of IL-12 treatment in HIV-infected individuals, there did not appear to be any significant increase or decrease in viral load, nor was there a change in $CD4^+$ T cell count (146). Based on these data, there does not appear to be a role for IL-12 therapy for treatment of HIV disease as a single agent. As noted above, IL-12 therapy is being used as adjunctive immunotherapy in HIV-infected patients with disseminated *M. avium* complex infection. Moreover, IL-12 may be considered as a means to enhance the immune response in patients on highly active anti-retroviral therapy (HAART). Alternatively, IL-12 could be used as an adjuvant with a prophylactic or therapeutic vaccine to enhance cellular immunity.

Hepatitis

Chronic hepatitis B and hepatitis C viruses (HBV and HCV) are both associated with the serious clinical consequences of cirrhosis and/or hepatocellular carcinoma. Immunotherapy with IFN-γ is currently being used in patients with chronic HBV and HCV infections, with response rates of 35% to 50%. Those HBV patients who respond to IFN-γ therapy appear to have an increased Th1 response compared with non-responders, with higher detectable serum levels of IL-12 and IFN-γ. *In vitro* studies have shown that IL-12 enhances PBMC proliferation and IFN-γ production following stimulation with HBV surface antigen in patients with chronic HBV infection (147). In patients with chronic HCV infection, IL-12 enhanced *in vitro* PBMC HCV antigen-specific Th1 responses (148). These data suggest that IL-12 may be useful as an immunotherapeutic agent in patients with chronic viral hepatitis, either in the form of monotherapy (e.g., IFN-γ) or as an adjuvant to antiviral chemotherapy (e.g., with lamivudine).

Therapeutic Potential of IL-12 in Human Infectious Disease

Having highlighted the potential therapeutic roles of IL-12 for particular infections, we conclude with the following points. Because the major effect of IL-12 is to augment production of IFN-γ (the effector molecule for a Th1 response, critical for control of the aforementioned infections), it is often asked whether IL-12 is a better therapeutic agent than IFN-γ directly. There are several reasons why IL-12 may be more advantageous as an adjuvant cytokine therapeutic agent. First, IL-12 has a longer biologic half-life than IFN-γ (24 h versus 6 h). Second, IL-12 treatment leads to induction of IFN-γ from host-activated T cells and NK cells, which may be more physiologic in a cognate manner in which the immune cells secreting the IFN-γ are in proximity to the infected target cell. Third, IFN-γ treatment would primarily act as a direct effector cytokine. By contrast, IL-12 could influence the differentiation of antigen-specific T cells, leading to specific IFN-γ–producing memory cells. Finally, IL-12 is a potent regulator of its own receptor. In this regard, it would serve to enhance its own responsiveness. In humans, IFN-γ has substantially less effect on IL-12 responsiveness.

Another important point with regard to IL-12 therapy is that, in most murine models of infection, IL-12 treatment for established infections has been less successful than IL-12 given immediately before or at the time of infection. Thus, its potential as a therapeutic in established human infectious diseases remains to be determined. Nevertheless, IL-12 remains a potentially important therapeutic agent when combined with existing chemotherapy in patients with disseminated or refractory disease.

TOXICITIES

Immunotherapy with IL-12 is currently under investigation in human trials for cancer and several infectious diseases. As with any drug therapy, it is important to be aware of the potential toxicities to assess risks versus benefits of treatment. One general potential concern with IL-12 is its role in mediating proinflammatory responses. In this regard, IL-12—through its induction of a cytokine (e.g., IFN-γ or TNF-α)—could affect underlying conditions such as autoimmune disease. Clinical experience to date derives from over 400 patients treated. The most common adverse effects (greater than 50%) include flu-like symptoms such as fever, chills, sweats, nausea, vomiting, headache, and fatigue. Less common adverse events include insomnia, hypotension, dyspnea, abdominal pain/gastrointestinal bleeding, and injection site reactions. The most common laboratory abnormalities associated with IL-12 therapy include transient elevations of liver enzymes as well as azotemia/proteinuria, neutropenia, anemia, thrombocytopenia, and hyperglycemia. Overall, IL-12 has been well tolerated thus far in early human clinical studies, particularly when given via subcutaneous injection. There were several deaths in an early study using high-dose (500 ng/kg) IL-12 intravenously in patients with advanced renal cell cancer for 5 consecutive days. Two deaths were attributed to IL-12 therapy. This unforeseen and unexpected toxicity was determined to be due to the elimination of a previously used single initial dose of IL-12 at 2 weeks before high-dose therapy. Subsequent studies in mice and primates demonstrated that this initial "priming" dose 2 weeks before high-dose therapy resulted in attenuated IFN-γ production and greatly reduced the severe toxicity associated with high-dose intravenous IL-12 therapy (149). A priming dose is now given within 2 weeks for consecutive-day therapy; however, most regimens are lower dose, subcutaneous, and two to three times per week.

CONCLUSION

IL-12, a potent cytokine produced by multiple cell types, plays a central role in regulation of cellular immunity to many infectious organisms. Its predominant effects include production of IFN-γ and enhancement of cytolytic function of T and NK cells. Multiple animal and human models of infection demonstrate that IL-12 and its receptor are critical, if not indispensable, for induction of a protective Th1 immune response. These studies have led to ongoing clinical investigations to determine whether IL-12 may be used in humans, either as an adjuvant to conventional chemotherapy in resistant intracellular infections (e.g., in mycobacterial disease) or as a potential vaccine adjuvant (e.g., in leishmanial infections). As with any new therapeutic strategy with possible toxicities, the potential clinical benefit must be carefully balanced with safe administration in the target populations.

REFERENCES

1. Wolf SF, Temple PA, Kobayashi M, et al. Cloning of cDNA for natural killer cell stimulatory factor, a heterodimeric cytokine with multiple biologic effects on T and natural killer cells. *J Immunol* 1991;146: 3074–3081.
2. Trinchieri G, Scott P. Interleukin-12: a proinflammatory cytokine with immunoregulatory functions. *Res Immunol* 1995;146:423–431.
3. Presky DH, Yang H, Minetti LJ, et al. A functional interleukin 12 receptor complex is composed of two β-type cytokine receptor subunits. *Proc Natl Acad Sci USA* 1996;93:14002–14007.
4. Presky DH, Minetti LJ, Gillessen S, et al. Analysis of the multiple interactions between IL-12 and the high affinity IL-12 receptor complex. *J Immunol* 1998;160:2174 –2179.
5. Wu CY, Warrier RR, Carvajal DM, et al. Biological function and distribution of human interleukin-12 receptor β chain. *Eur J Immunol* 1996;26:345–350.
6. Wu C, Warrier RR, Wang X, et al. Regulation of interleukin-12 receptor β1 chain expression and interleukin-12 binding by human peripheral blood mononuclear cells. *Eur J Immunol* 1997;27:147–154.
7. Wu C, Ferrante J, Gately MK, et al. Characterization of IL-12 receptor β1 chain (IL-12Rβ1)–deficient mice: IL-12Rβ1 is an essential component of the functional mouse IL- 12 receptor. *J Immunol* 1997;159: 1658–1665.
8. Chua AO, Chizzonite R, Desai BB, et al. Expression cloning of a human IL-12 receptor component. A new member of the cytokine receptor superfamily with strong homology to gp130. *J Immunol* 1994;153:128–136.
9. Chua AO, Wilkinson VL, Presky DH, et al. Cloning and characterization of a mouse IL-12 receptor-β component. *J Immunol* 1995;155:4286–4294.
10. Hsieh CS, Macatonia SE, Tripp CS, et al. Development of Th1 CD4[+] T cells through IL-12 produced by Listeria-induced macrophages. *Science* 1993;260:547–549.
11. Seder RA, Gazzinelli R, Sher A, et al. Interleukin 12 acts directly on CD4[+] T cells to enhance priming for interferon γ production and diminishes interleukin 4 inhibition of such priming. *Proc Natl Acad Sci USA* 1993;90:10188–10192.
12. Chan SH, Perussia B, Gupta JW, et al. Induction of interferon γ production by natural killer cell stimulatory factor: characterization of the responder cells and synergy with other inducers. *J Exp Med* 1991;173:869–879.
13. D'Andrea A, Aste AM, Valiante NM, et al. Interleukin 10 (IL-10) inhibits human lymphocyte interferon γ production by suppressing natural killer cell stimulatory factor/IL-12 synthesis in accessory cells. *J Exp Med* 1993;178:1041–1048.
14. Ma X, Chow JM, Gri G, et al. The interleukin 12 p40 gene promoter is primed by interferon γ in monocytic cells. *J Exp Med* 1996;183:147–157.
15. Hayes MP, Wang J, Norcross MA. Regulation of interleukin-12 expression in human monocytes: selective priming by interferon-γ of lipopolysaccharide-inducible p35 and p40 genes. *Blood* 1995;86:646–650.
16. Flesch IE, Hess JH, Huang S, et al. Early interleukin 12 production by macrophages in response to mycobacterial infection depends on interferon γ and tumor necrosis factor α. *J Exp Med* 1995;181:1615–1621.

17. Driggers PH, Ennist DL, Gleason SL, et al. An interferon γ-regulated protein that binds the interferon-inducible enhancer element of major histocompatibility complex class I genes. *Proc Natl Acad Sci USA* 1990;87: 3743–3747.
18. Miyamoto M, Fujita T, Kimura Y, et al. Regulated expression of a gene encoding a nuclear factor, IRF-1, that specifically binds to IFN-β gene regulatory elements. *Cell* 1988;54:903–913.
19. Harada H, Fujita T, Miyamoto M, et al. Structurally similar but functionally distinct factors, IRF-1 and IRF- 2, bind to the same regulatory elements of IFN and IFN-inducible genes. *Cell* 1989;58:729–739.
20. Veals SA, Schindler C, Leonard D, et al. Subunit of an α-interferon–responsive transcription factor is related to interferon regulatory factor and Myb families of DNA-binding proteins. *Mol Cell Biol* 1992;12:3315–3324.
21. Au WC, Moore PA, Lowther W, et al. Identification of a member of the interferon regulatory factor family that binds to the interferon-stimulated response element and activates expression of interferon-induced genes. *Proc Natl Acad Sci USA* 1995;92:11657–11661.
22. Holtschke T, Lohler J, Kanno Y, et al. Immunodeficiency and chronic myelogenous leukemia-like syndrome in mice with a targeted mutation of the ICSBP gene. *Cell* 1996;87:307–317.
23. Fehr T, Schoedon G, Odermatt B, et al. Crucial role of interferon consensus sequence binding protein, but neither of interferon regulatory factor 1 nor of nitric oxide synthesis for protection against murine listeriosis. *J Exp Med* 1997;185:921–931.
24. Giese NA, Gabriele L, Doherty TM, et al. Interferon (IFN) consensus sequence-binding protein, a transcription factor of the IFN regulatory factor family, regulates immune responses *in vivo* through control of interleukin 12 expression. *J Exp Med* 1997;186:1535–1546.
25. Scharton-Kersten T, Contursi C, Masumi A, et al. Interferon consensus sequence binding protein–deficient mice display impaired resistance to intracellular infection due to a primary defect in interleukin 12 p40 induction. *J Exp Med* 1997;186:1523–1534.
26. Szalay G, Ladel CH, Blum C, et al. IL-4 neutralization or TNF-α treatment ameliorate disease by an intracellular pathogen in IFN-γ receptor–deficient mice. *J Immunol* 1996;157:4746–4750.
27. Sousa CR, Hieny S, Scharton-Kersten T, et al. *In vivo* microbial stimulation induces rapid CD40 ligand-independent production of interleukin 12 by dendritic cells and their redistribution to T cell areas. *J Exp Med* 1997;186:1819–1829.
28. Noelle RJ. CD40 and its ligand in host defense. *Immunity* 1996;4:415–419.
29. Grewal IS, Flavell RA. CD40 and CD154 in cell-mediated immunity. *Annu Rev Immunol* 1998;16:111–135.
30. van Essen D, Kikutani H, Gray D. CD40 ligand-transduced co-stimulation of T cells in the development of helper function. *Nature* 1995;378:620–623.
31. Grewal IS, Xu J, Flavell RA. Impairment of antigen-specific T-cell priming in mice lacking CD40 ligand. *Nature* 1995;378:617–620.
32. Cella M, Scheidegger D, Palmer LK, et al. Ligation of CD40 on dendritic cells triggers production of high levels of interleukin-12 and enhances T cell stimulatory capacity: T-T help via APC activation. *J Exp Med* 1996; 184:747–752.
33. Shu U, Kiniwa M, Wu CY, et al. Activated T cells induce interleukin-12 production by monocytes via CD40-CD40 ligand interaction. *Eur J Immunol* 1995;25:1125–1128.
34. Kennedy MK, Picha KS, Fanslow WC, et al. CD40/CD40 ligand interactions are required for T cell-dependent production of interleukin-12 by mouse macrophages. *Eur J Immunol* 1996;26:370–378.
35. Koch F, Stanzl U, Jennewein P, et al. High level IL-12 production by murine dendritic cells: upregulation via MHC class II and CD40 molecules and downregulation by IL-4 and IL-10. *J Exp Med* 1996;184:741–746. [For erratum, see *J Exp Med* 1996;184: following 1590.]
36. Caux C, Massacrier C, Vanbervliet B, et al. Activation of human dendritic cells through CD40 cross-linking. *J Exp Med* 1994;180:1263–1272.
37. McDyer JF, Goletz TJ, Thomas E, et al. CD40 ligand/CD40 stimulation regulates the production of IFN-γ from human peripheral blood mononuclear cells in an IL-12- and/or CD28-dependent manner. *J Immunol* 1998;160: 1701–1707.
38. DeKruyff RH, Gieni RS, Umetsu DT. Antigen-driven but not lipopolysaccharide-driven IL-12 production in macrophages requires triggering of CD40. *J Immunol* 1997;158:359–366.
39. Campbell KA, Ovendale PJ, Kennedy MK, et al. CD40 ligand is required for protective cell-mediated immunity to *Leishmania major*. *Immunity* 1996;4:283–289.
40. Kamanaka M, Yu P, Yasui T, et al. Protective role of CD40 in *Leishmania major* infection at two distinct phases of cell-mediated immunity. *Immunity* 1996;4:275–281.
41. Soong L, Xu JC, Grewal IS, et al. Disruption of CD40-CD40 ligand interactions results in an enhanced susceptibility to Leishmania amazonensis infection. *Immunity* 1996;4:263–273.
42. Zhou P, Seder RA. CD40 ligand is not essential for induction of type 1 cytokine responses or protective immunity after primary or secondary infection with *Histoplasma capsulatum*. *J Exp Med* 1998;187:1315–1324.
43. Campos-Neto A, Ovendale P, Bement T, et al. CD40 ligand is not essential for the development of cell-mediated immunity and resistance to *Mycobacterium tuberculosis*. *J Immunol* 1998;160:2037–2041.
44. D'Andrea A, Ma X, Aste AM, et al. Stimulatory and inhibitory effects of interleukin (IL)-4 and IL-13 on the production of cytokines by human peripheral blood mononuclear cells: priming for IL-12 and tumor necrosis factor α production. *J Exp Med* 1995;181:537–546.
45. Belkaid Y, Butcher B, Sacks DL. Analysis of cytokine production by inflammatory mouse macrophages at the

single-cell level: selective impairment of IL-12 induction in Leishmania-infected cells. *Eur J Immunol* 1998; 28:1389–1400.
46. Carrera L, Gazzinelli RT, Badolato R, et al. Leishmania promastigotes selectively inhibit interleukin 12 induction in bone marrow-derived macrophages from susceptible and resistant mice. *J Exp Med* 1996;183: 515–526.
47. Karp CL, Wysocka M, Wahl LM, et al. Mechanism of suppression of cell-mediated immunity by measles virus. *Science* 1996;273:228–231. [For erratum, see *Science* 1997;275:1053.]
48. Sutterwala FS, Noel GJ, Clynes R, et al. Selective suppression of interleukin-12 induction after macrophage receptor ligation. *J Exp Med* 1997;185:1977–1985.
49. Berger S, Chandra R, Ballo H, et al. Immune complexes are potent inhibitors of interleukin-12 secretion by human monocytes. *Eur J Immunol* 1997;27:2994–3000.
50. Marth T, Kelsall BL. Regulation of interleukin-12 by complement receptor 3 signaling. *J Exp Med* 1997;185: 1987–1995.
51. Moller DR, Wysocka M, Greenlee BM, et al. Inhibition of IL-12 production by thalidomide. *J Immunol* 1997;159:5157–5161.
52. Moller DR, Wysocka M, Greenlee BM, et al. Inhibition of human interleukin-12 production by pentoxifylline. *Immunology* 1997;91:197–203.
53. Klein TW, Newton C, Zhu W, et al. 9-Tetrahydrocannabinol, cytokines, and immunity to Legionella pneumophila. *Proc Soc Exp Biol Med* 1995;209:205–212.
54. Newton C, Klein T, Friedman H. The role of macrophages in THC-induced alteration of the cytokine network. *Adv Exp Med Biol* 1998;437:207–214.
55. Braun MC, Lahey E, Kelsall BL. Selective suppression of IL-12 production by chemoattractants. *J Immunol* 2000;164:3009–3017.
56. Chensue, Warmington SW, Ruth KS, et al. Role of monocyte chemoattractant protein-1 (MCP-1) in Th1 (mycobacterial) and Th2 (schistosomal) antigen-induced granuloma formation-Relationship to local inflammation, Th cell expression, and IL-12 production. *J Immunol* 1996;157:7.
57. Karpus WJ, Kennedy KJ. MIP-1α and MCP-1 differentially regulate acute and relapsing autoimmune encephalomyelitis as well as Th1/Th2 lymphocyte differentiation. *J Leukoc Biol* 1997;62:681–687.
58. Karpus WJ, Kennedy KJ, Kunkel SL, et al. Monocyte chemotactic protein 1 regulates oral tolerance induction by inhibition of T helper cell 1–related cytokines. *J Exp Med* 1998;187:733–741.
59. D'Ambrosio D, Cippitelli M, Cocciolo MG, et al. Inhibition of IL-12 production by 1,25-dihydroxyvitamin D3. Involvement of NF-κB downregulation in transcriptional repression of the p40 gene. *J Clin Invest* 1998;101: 252–262.
60. Panina BP, Mazzeo D, Lucia PD, et al. β2-agonists prevent Th1 development by selective inhibition of interleukin 12. *J Clin Invest* 1997;100:1513–1519.
61. van der Pouw Kraan TC, Boeije LC, Smeenk RJ, et al. Prostaglandin-E_2 is a potent inhibitor of human interleukin 12 production. *J Exp Med* 1995;181:775–779.
62. Braun MC, He J, Wu CY, et al. Cholera toxin suppresses interleukin (IL)–12 production and IL-12 receptor β1 and β2 chain expression. *J Exp Med* 1999;189:541–552.
63. Sutterwala FS, Noel GJ, Salgame P, et al. Reversal of proinflammatory responses by ligating the macrophage Fcγ receptor type I. *J Exp Med* 1998;188:217–222.
64. Gubler U, Presky DH. Molecular biology of interleukin-12 receptors. *Ann N Y Acad Sci* 1996;795:36–40.
65. Gollob JA, Murphy EA, Mahajan S, et al. Altered interleukin-12 responsiveness in Th1 and Th2 cells is associated with the differential activation of STAT5 and STAT1. *Blood* 1998;91:1341–1354.
66. Bacon CM, McVicar DW, Ortaldo JR, et al. Interleukin 12 (IL-12) induces tyrosine phosphorylation of JAK2 and TYK2: differential use of Janus family tyrosine kinases by IL-2 and IL-12. *J Exp Med* 1995;181: 399–404.
67. Bacon CM, Petricoin EF III, Ortaldo JR, et al. Interleukin 12 induces tyrosine phosphorylation and activation of STAT4 in human lymphocytes. *Proc Natl Acad Sci USA* 1995;92:7307–7311.
68. Jacobson NG, Szabo SJ, Weber-Nordt RM, et al. Interleukin 12 signaling in T helper type 1 (Th1) cells involves tyrosine phosphorylation of signal transducer and activator of transcription (STAT)3 and STAT4. *J Exp Med* 1995;181:1755–1762.
69. Thierfelder WE, van Deursen JM, Yamamoto K, et al. Requirement for STAT4 in interleukin-12-mediated responses of natural killer and T cells. *Nature* 1996;382:171–174.
70. Szabo SJ, Dighe AS, Gubler U, et al. Regulation of the interleukin (IL)-12Rβ2 subunit expression in developing T helper 1 (Th1) and Th2 cells. *J Exp Med* 1997;185:817–824.
71. Rogge L, Barberis-Maino L, Biffi M, et al. Selective expression of an interleukin-12 receptor component by human T helper 1 cells. *J Exp Med* 1997;185:825–831.
72. Rogge L, Papi A, Presky DH, et al. Antibodies to the IL-12 receptor β2 chain mark human Th1 but not Th2 cells *in vitro* and in vivo. *J Immunol* 1999;162:3926–3932.
73. Wu CY, Wang K, McDyer JF, et al. Prostaglandin E_2 and dexamethasone inhibit IL-12 receptor expression and IL-12 responsiveness. *J Immunol* 1998;161:2723–2730.
74. Igarashi O, Yamane H, Imajoh-Ohmi S, et al. IL-12 receptor (IL-12R) expression and accumulation of IL-12Rβ1 and IL-12Rβ2 mRNAs in $CD4^+$ T cells by costimulation with B7-2 molecules. *J Immunol* 1998;160: 1638–1646.

75. Chang JT, Shevach EM, Segal BM. Regulation of interleukin (IL)-12 receptor β2 subunit expression by endogenous IL-12: a critical step in the differentiation of pathogenic autoreactive T cells. *J Exp Med* 1999;189: 969–978.
76. Xu D, Chan WL, Leung BP, et al. Selective expression and functions of interleukin 18 receptor on T helper (Th) type 1 but not Th2 cells. *J Exp Med* 1998;188:1485–1492.
77. Yoshimoto T, Takeda K, Tanaka T, et al. IL-12 up-regulates IL-18 receptor expression on T cells, Th1 cells, and B cells: synergism with IL-18 for IFN-γ production. *J Immunol* 1998;161:3400–3407.
78. Zhang M, Gong J, Presky DH, et al. Expression of the IL-12 receptor β1 and β2 subunits in human tuberculosis. *J Immunol* 1999;162:2441–2447.
79. Altare F, Durandy A, Lammas D, et al. Impairment of mycobacterial immunity in human interleukin-12 receptor deficiency. *Science* 1998;280:1432–1435.
80. de Jong R, Altare F, Haagen IA, et al. Severe mycobacterial and Salmonella infections in interleukin-12 receptor-deficient patients. *Science* 1998;280:1435–1438.
81. Heinzel FP, Schoenhaut DS, Rerko RM, et al. Recombinant interleukin 12 cures mice infected with *Leishmania major*. *J Exp Med* 1993;177:1505–1509.
82. Sypek JP, Chung CL, Mayor SE, et al. Resolution of cutaneous leishmaniasis: interleukin 12 initiates a protective T helper type 1 immune response. *J Exp Med* 1993;177:1797–1802.
83. Launois P, Swihart KG, Milon G, et al. Early production of IL-4 in susceptible mice infected with *Leishmania major* rapidly induces IL-12 unresponsiveness. *J Immunol* 1997;158:3317–3324.
84. Afonso LC, Scharton TM, Vieira LQ, et al. The adjuvant effect of interleukin-12 in a vaccine against *Leishmania major*. *Science* 1994;263:235–237.
85. Mougneau E, Altare F, Wakil AE, et al. Expression cloning of a protective Leishmania antigen. *Science* 1995;268:563–566.
86. Gurunathan S, Sacks DL, Brown DR, et al. Vaccination with DNA encoding the immunodominant LACK parasite antigen confers protective immunity to mice infected with *Leishmania major. J Exp Med* 1997;186: 1137–1147.
87. Gurunathan S, Prussin C, Sacks DL, et al. Vaccine requirements for sustained cellular immunity to an intracellular parasitic infection. *Nat Med* 1998;4:1409–1415.
88. Kenney RT, Sacks DL, Sypek JP, et al. Protective immunity using recombinant human IL-12 and alum as adjuvants in a primate model of cutaneous leishmaniasis. *J Immunol* 1999;163:4481–4488.
89. Kaufmann SH. Immunity to intracellular bacteria. *Annu Rev Immunol* 1993;11:129–163.
90. Unanue ER. Studies in listeriosis show the strong symbiosis between the innate cellular system and the T-cell response. *Immunol Rev* 1997;158:11–25.
91. Tripp CS, Wolf SF, Unanue ER. Interleukin 12 and tumor necrosis factor α are costimulators of interferon γ production by natural killer cells in severe combined immunodeficiency mice with listeriosis, and interleukin 10 is a physiologic antagonist. *Proc Natl Acad Sci USA* 1993;90:3725–3729.
92. Tripp CS, Gately MK, Hakimi J, et al. Neutralization of IL-12 decreases resistance to Listeria in SCID and C.B-17 mice. Reversal by IFN-γ. *J Immunol* 1994;152:1883–1887.
93. Wagner RD, Steinberg H, Brown JF, et al. Recombinant interleukin-12 enhances resistance of mice to *Listeria monocytogenes* infection. *Microb Pathog* 1994;17:175–186.
94. Cesbron MF, Dubremetz JF, Sher A. The immunobiology of toxoplasmosis. *Res Immunol* 1993;144:7–8.
95. Frenkel JK. Toxoplasmosis in human beings. *J Am Vet Med Assoc* 1990;196:240–248.
96. Scharton-Kersten T, Denkers EY, Gazzinelli R, et al. Role of IL-12 in induction of cell-mediated immunity to *Toxoplasma gondii. Res Immunol* 1995;146:539–545. [For erratum, see *Res Immunol* 1996;147:121.]
97. Biron CA, Gazzinelli RT. Effects of IL-12 on immune responses to microbial infections: a key mediator in regulating disease outcome. *Curr Opin Immunol* 1995;7:485–496.
98. Gazzinelli RT, Wysocka M, Hayashi S, et al. Parasite-induced IL-12 stimulates early IFN-γ synthesis and resistance during acute infection with *Toxoplasma gondii. J Immunol* 1994;153:2533–2543.
99. Hunter CA, Subauste CS, Van Cleave VH, et al. Production of γ interferon by natural killer cells from *Toxoplasma gondii*-infected SCID mice: regulation by interleukin-10, interleukin- 12, and tumor necrosis factor α. *Infect Immunol* 1994;62:2818–2824.
100. Khan IA, Matsuura T, Kasper LH. Interleukin-12 enhances murine survival against acute toxoplasmosis. *Infect Immunol* 1994;62:1639–1642.
101. Gazzinelli RT, Hieny S, Wynn TA, et al. Interleukin 12 is required for the T-lymphocyte-independent induction of interferon γ by an intracellular parasite and induces resistance in T-cell–deficient hosts. *Proc Natl Acad Sci U S A* 1993;90:6115–6119.
102. Khatri VP, Fehniger TA, Baiocchi RA, et al. Ultra low dose interleukin-2 therapy promotes a type 1 cytokine profile *in vivo* in patients with AIDS and AIDS-associated malignancies. *J Clin Invest* 1998;101:1373–1378.
103. Goodwin RA Jr, Shapiro JL, Thurman GH, et al. Disseminated histoplasmosis: clinical and pathologic correlations. *Medicine (Baltimore)* 1980;59:1–33.
104. Johnson PC, Khardori N, Najjar AF, et al. Progressive disseminated histoplasmosis in patients with acquired immunodeficiency syndrome. *Am J Med* 1988;85:152–158.
105. Wheat LJ, Connolly-Stringfield PA, Baker RL, et al. Disseminated histoplasmosis in the acquired immune deficiency syndrome: clinical findings, diagnosis and treatment, and review of the literature. *Medicine (Baltimore)* 1990;69:361–374.

106. Allendoerfer R, Biovin GP, Deepe GS Jr. Modulation of immune responses in murine pulmonary histoplasmosis. *J Infect Dis* 1997;175:905–914.
107. Zhou P, Sieve MC, Bennett J, et al. IL-12 prevents mortality in mice infected with *Histoplasma capsulatum* through induction of IFN-γ. *J Immunol* 1995;155:785–795.
108. Williams DM, Graybill JR, Drutz DJ. *Histoplasma capsulatum* infection in nude mice. *Infect Immunol* 1978;21:973–977.
109. Gomez AM, Bullock WE, Taylor CL, et al. Role of L3T4$^+$ T cells in host defense against *Histoplasma capsulatum. Infect Immunol* 1988;56:1685–1691.
110. Deepe GS Jr. Role of CD8$^+$ T cells in host resistance to systemic infection with *Histoplasma capsulatum* in mice. *J Immunol* 1994;152:3491–3500.
111. Zhou P, Sieve MC, Tewari RP, et al. Interleukin-12 modulates the protective immune response in SCID mice infected with *Histoplasma capsulatum. Infect Immunol* 1997;65:936–942.
112. Dolin PJ, Raviglione MC, Kochi A. Global tuberculosis incidence and mortality during 1990–2000. *Bull World Health Organ* 1994;72:213–220.
113. Cooper AM, Magram J, Ferrante J, et al. Interleukin 12 (IL-12) is crucial to the development of protective immunity in mice intravenously infected with *Mycobacterium tuberculosis. J Exp Med* 1997;186:39–45.
114. Thompson-Snipes L, Skamene E, Radzioch D. Acquired resistance but not innate resistance to *Mycobacterium bovis* bacillus Calmette-Guerin is compromised by interleukin-12 ablation. *Infect Immunol* 1998;66: 5268–5274.
115. Barnes PF, Fong SJ, Brennan PJ, et al. Local production of tumor necrosis factor and IFN-γ in tuberculous pleuritis. *J Immunol* 1990;145:149–154.
116. Barnes PF, Lu S, Abrams JS, et al. Cytokine production at the site of disease in human tuberculosis. *Infect Immunol* 1993;61:3482–3489.
117. Zhang M, Gately MK, Wang E, et al. Interleukin 12 at the site of disease in tuberculosis. *J Clin Invest* 1994; 93:1733–1739.
118. Zhang M, Lin Y, Iyer DV, et al. T-cell cytokine responses in human infection with *Mycobacterium tuberculosis. Infect Immunol* 1995;63:3231–3234.
119. Onwubalili JK, Scott GM, Robinson JA. Deficient immune interferon production in tuberculosis. *Clin Exp Immunol* 1985;59:405–413.
120. Vilcek J, Klion A, Henriksen-DeStefano D, et al. Defective γ-interferon production in peripheral blood leukocytes of patients with acute tuberculosis. *J Clin Immunol* 1986;6:146–151.
121. Sanchez FO, Rodriguez JI, Agudelo G, et al. Immune responsiveness and lymphokine production in patients with tuberculosis and healthy controls. *Infect Immunol* 1994;62:5673–5678.
122. Zhang M, Gong J, Iyer DV, et al. T cell cytokine responses in persons with tuberculosis and human immunodeficiency virus infection. *J Clin Invest* 1994;94:2435–2442.
123. McDyer JF, Hackley MN, Walsh TE, et al. Patients with multidrug-resistant tuberculosis with low CD4$^+$ T cell counts have impaired Th1 responses. *J Immunol* 1997;158:492–500.
124. Horsburgh CR Jr. Epidemiology of disease caused by nontuberculous mycobacteria. *Semin Respir Infect* 1996;11:244–251.
125. Castro AG, Silva RA, Appelberg R. Endogenously produced IL-12 is required for the induction of protective T cells during *Mycobacterium avium* infections in mice. *J Immunol* 1995;155:2013–2019.
126. Doherty TM, Sher A. IL-12 promotes drug-induced clearance of *Mycobacterium avium* infection in mice. *J Immunol* 1998;160:5428–5435.
127. Frucht DM, Holland SM. Defective monocyte costimulation for IFN-γ production in familial disseminated *Mycobacterium avium* complex infection: abnormal IL-12 regulation. *J Immunol* 1996;157:411–416.
128. Altare F, Lammas D, Revy P, et al. Inherited interleukin 12 deficiency in a child with bacille Calmette-Guerin and *Salmonella enteritidis* disseminated infection. *J Clin Invest* 1998;102:2035–2040.
129. Flynn JL, Goldstein MM, Triebold KJ, et al. IL-12 increases resistance of BALB/c mice to *Mycobacterium tuberculosis* infection. *J Immunol* 1995;155:2515–2524.
130. Cooper AM, Roberts AD, Rhoades ER, et al. The role of interleukin-12 in acquired immunity to *Mycobacterium tuberculosis* infection. *Immunology* 1995;84:423–432.
131. Orange JS, Wolf SF, Biron CA. Effects of IL-12 on the response and susceptibility to experimental viral infections. *J Immunol* 1994;152:1253–1264.
132. Orange JS, Salazar-Mather TP, Opal SM, et al. Mechanism of interleukin 12–mediated toxicities during experimental viral infections: role of tumor necrosis factor and glucocorticoids. *J Exp Med* 1995;181:901–914.
133. Orange JS, Wang B, Terhorst C, et al. Requirement for natural killer cell-produced interferon γ in defense against murine cytomegalovirus infection and enhancement of this defense pathway by interleukin 12 administration. *J Exp Med* 1995;182:1045–1056.
134. Orange JS, Biron CA. An absolute and restricted requirement for IL-12 in natural killer cell IFN-γ production and antiviral defense. Studies of natural killer and T cell responses in contrasting viral infections. *J Immunol* 1996;156:1138–1142.
135. Schijns VE, Haagmans BL, Wierda CM, et al. Mice lacking IL-12 develop polarized Th1 cells during viral infection. *J Immunol* 1998;160:3958–3964.
136. Oxenius A, Karrer U, Zinkernagel RM, et al. IL-12 is not required for induction of type 1 cytokine responses in viral infections. *J Immunol* 1999;162:965–973.

137. Chehimi J, Starr SE, Frank I, et al. Impaired interleukin 12 production in human immunodeficiency virus-infected patients. *J Exp Med* 1994;179:1361–1366.
138. Denis M, Ghadirian E. Dysregulation of interleukin 8, interleukin 10, and interleukin 12 release by alveolar macrophages from HIV type 1–infected subjects. *AIDS Res Hum Retroviruses* 1994;10:1619–1627.
139. Marshall JD, Chehimi J, Gri G, et al. The interleukin-12-mediated pathway of immune events is dysfunctional in human immunodeficiency virus-infected individuals. *Blood* 1999;94:1003–1011.
140. Ito M, Ishida T, He L, et al. HIV type 1 Tat protein inhibits interleukin 12 production by human peripheral blood mononuclear cells. *AIDS Res Hum Retroviruses* 1998;14:845–849.
141. Chougnet C, Wynn TA, Clerici M, et al. Molecular analysis of decreased interleukin-12 production in persons infected with human immunodeficiency virus. *J Infect Dis* 1996;174:46–53.
142. Fantuzzi L, Gessani S, Borghi P, et al. Induction of interleukin-12 (IL-12) by recombinant glycoprotein gp120 of human immunodeficiency virus type 1 in human monocytes/macrophages: requirement of γ interferon for IL-12 secretion. *J Virol* 1996;70:4121–4124.
143. Trinchieri G. Cytokines acting on or secreted by macrophages during intracellular infection (IL-10, IL-12, IFN-γ). *Curr Opin Immunol* 1997;9:17–23.
144. Clerici M, Lucey DR, Berzofsky JA, et al. Restoration of HIV-specific cell-mediated immune responses by interleukin-12 in vitro. *Science* 1993;262:1721–1724.
145. Watanabe N, Sypek JP, Mittler S, et al. Administration of recombinant human interleukin 12 to chronically SIVmac-infected rhesus monkeys. *AIDS Res Hum Retroviruses* 1998;14:393–399.
146. Kohl S, Sigaroudinia M, Charlebois ED, et al. Interleukin-12 administered *in vivo* decreases human NK cell cytotoxicity and antibody-dependent cellular cytotoxicity to human immunodeficiency virus-infected cells. *J Infect Dis* 1996;174:1105–1108.
147. Schlaak JF, Tully G, Lohr HF, et al. The presence of high amounts of HBV-DNA in serum is associated with suppressed costimulatory effects of interleukin 12 on HBV-induced immune response. *J Hepatol* 1999;30:353–358.
148. Schlaak JF, Pitz T, Lohr HF, et al. Interleukin 12 enhances deficient HCV-antigen–induced Th1-type immune response of peripheral blood mononuclear cells. *J Med Virol* 1998;56:112–117.
149. Leonard JP, Sherman ML, Fisher GL, et al. Effects of single-dose interleukin-12 exposure on interleukin-12-associated toxicity and interferon-γ production. *Blood* 1997;90:2541–2548.

6
Interleukin-17

Andriani C. Patera and Jeffrey I. Cohen

Medical Virology Section, Laboratory of Clinical Investigation, National Institutes of Health, Bethesda, Maryland

HISTORY

In 1993 Rouvier and colleagues (1) identified a novel mRNA expressed by a hybridoma between a mouse cytotoxic T lymphocyte (CTL) clone and a rat T cell lymphoma. The hybridoma had been stimulated with ionomycin and phorbol myristate acetate (PMA), and the resulting RNA was subtracted with a mixture of RNA from a mouse lymphoma and rat thymoma. This CTL-associated (CTLA) mRNA was named CTLA-8. The CTLA-8 mRNA contains an open reading frame that encodes a predicted protein of 150 amino acids, followed by a 3′ noncoding region containing sequence elements that had been previously identified in cytokines, growth factors, and oncogenes.

In their initial description of CTLA-8, Rouvier and colleagues noted that this gene was homologous to a gene in a lymphotrophic monkey herpesvirus, herpesvirus saimiri (HVS). Comparison of CTLA-8 with gene 13 of HVS showed 57% amino acid identity. Based on these findings, Yao and colleagues (2) constructed fusion proteins containing the HVS protein and its murine homolog. They showed that the purified fusion proteins, as well as supernatants from cells transfected with the native herpesvirus and murine genes, stimulated NF-κB activity and IL-6 secretion by fibroblasts. Based on their cytokine activity, the mouse and monkey proteins were named murine and viral interleukin-17 (mIL-17 and vIL-17), respectively. Subsequent studies (3) showed that the CTLA-8 protein described by Rouvier and colleagues (1) was actually of rat origin and encodes the rat (rIL-17) protein. The sequence of mIL-17 was determined and found to have 88% and 57% amino acid identity with rIL-17 and vIL-17, respectively (Fig. 6.1) (3). Yao and colleagues (4) and Fossiez and coworkers (5) independently cloned human IL-17 (hIL-17) from a human CD4 T cell clone, and from ionomycin and PMA-stimulated peripheral blood mononuclear cell (PBMC) libraries, respectively. The amino acid sequence of hIL-17 was found to be 72% identical to vIL-17 and 63% identical to rIL-17 (Fig. 6.1).

Using a recombinant fusion protein containing the vIL-17 gene fused to the Fc region of human immunoglobulin, Yao and colleagues (2) isolated the receptor for IL-17 (IL-17R) from a murine thymoma cell line. The human IL-17R was subsequently identified (6) and found to have 69% amino acid identity to the mouse receptor.

STRUCTURE AND EXPRESSION OF IL-17 MRNA AND PROTEIN

Using *in situ* hybridization, Rouvier et al. (1) mapped the chromosomal location of hIL-17 to chromosome 2 q31 and rIL-17 (mCTLA8) to the A1-A4 region of chromosome 1.

```
vIL-17   M T F R M T S L V - - - L L L L L S I D C I V K S E I T       25
hIL-17   M T P G K T S L V S - - L L L L L S L E A I V K A G I T       26
rIL-17   M - - - - - - - - - C L M L L L L L N L E A T V K A A V L     20
mIL-17   M S P G R A S S V S L M L L L L L S L A A T V K A A A I       28

vIL-17   S A Q T P R C L A A N - N S F P R S V M V T L S - I R N       51
hIL-17   I P R N P G C P N S E D K N F P R T V M V N L N - I H N       53
rIL-17   I P Q S S V C P N A E A N N F L Q N V K V N L K V I N S       48
mIL-17   I P Q S S A C P N T E A K D F L Q N V K V N L K V F N S       56

vIL-17   W N T - - S S K R A S D Y Y N R S T S P W T L H R N E D       77
hIL-17   R N T N T N P K R S S D Y Y N R S T S P W N L H R N E D       81
rIL-17   L S S K A S S R R P S D Y L N R S T S P W T L S R N E D       76
mIL-17   L G A K V S S R R P S D Y L N R S T S P W T L H R N E D       84

vIL-17   Q D R Y P S V I W E A K C R Y L G C V N A D G N V D Y H      105
hIL-17   P E R Y P S V I W E A K C R H L G C I N A D G N V D Y H      109
rIL-17   P D R Y P S V I W E A Q C R H Q R C V N A E G K L D H H      104
mIL-17   P D R Y P S V I W E A Q C R H Q R C V N A E G K L D H H      112

vIL-17   M N S V P I Q Q E I L V V R K G H Q P C P N S F R L E K      133
hIL-17   M N S V P I Q Q E I L V L R R E P P H C P N S F R L E K      137
rIL-17   M N S V L I Q Q E I L V L K R E P E K C P F T F R V E K      132
mIL-17   M N S V L I Q Q E I L V L K R E P E S C P F T F R V E K      140

vIL-17   M L V T V G C T C V T P I V H N V D                          151
hIL-17   I L V S V G C T C V T P I V H H V A                          155
rIL-17   M L V G V G C T C V S S I V R H A S                          150
mIL-17   M L V G V G C T C V A S I V R Q A A                          158
```

FIG. 6.1. Amino acid sequence alignment of herpesvirus saimiri IL-17 (vIL-17), human IL-17 (hIL-17), rat IL-17 (rIL-17), formerly known as CTLA-8, and mouse IL-17 (mil-17). Boxed amino acids are conserved residues, black boxed amino acids are conserved cysteines, shaded boxed amino acids are conserved potential phosphorylation sites, and hatched boxes are potential N-linked glycosylation sites. Dashes indicate gaps inserted for optimal alignment. Numbers indicate amino acid positions. (From Kennedy J, Rossi DL, Zurawski SM, et al. Mouse IL-17: a cytokine preferentially expressed by αβTCR^{+}CD4^{-} CD8^{-}T cells. *J Interferon Cytokine Res* 1996;16:611–617, with permission.)

hIL-17 is expressed from a 1.2-kb transcript in activated PBMC (5). The 3′ untranslated region of hIL-17 mRNA contains AU-rich instability sequences that are found in mRNAs from other proinflammatory mediators (7) and are predicted to shorten the half-life of mRNAs due to rapid degradation (8) or impaired translation (9). In addition to the instability sequences at its 3′ end, the mIL-17 gene contains an AP-1 (transcription factor binding) site, a glucocorticoid-responsive element, and a binding site for CBP, CTF/NF-1, and NF-Y at its 5′ end.

hIL17 mRNA is predicted to encode a 155–amino acid polypeptide with a 19–amino acid hydrophobic *N*-terminal signal sequence. Amino acid analysis of all four species of IL-17 shows a close relationship between them, with conservation of a number of structural features (Fig. 6.1). hIL-17 has six cysteine residues and an *N*-linked glycosylation site at asparagine 68, which are conserved in mIL-17, rIL-17, and vIL-17. vIL-17 has two additional putative *N*-glycosylation sites.

hIL-17 is secreted as a mixture of homodimeric glycosylated and nonglycosylated polypeptides. Under reducing conditions, 15- and 20-kDa proteins can be detected in the supernatant from IL-17–transfected cells. Treatment of these cells with tunicamycin results in loss of the 20-kDa protein, indicating that the larger species is due to addition of sugar moieties at the single *N*-glycosylation site (4). Similarly, endoglycosidase F digestion yields only the 15-kDa species on reducing gels, with loss of the larger species (5). In contrast, under nonreducing conditions, 30- and 38-kDa proteins are detected, suggesting that hIL-17 forms disulfide linked homodimers. Sequence analysis of the latter two proteins indicates that they have identical amino acid termini beginning at glycine 24 (5).

hIL-17 mRNA has been detected in PMA and ionomycin-activated $CD4^+$ T cells by RT-PCR and Northern blotting, but not in unstimulated T cells, Jurkat T cells, activated peripheral blood B cells, monocytes, or EBV-transformed B cells (4,5). Furthermore, hIL-17 mRNA was found predominantly in the $CD45RO^+$ memory fraction of activated $CD4^+$ T cells (5). IL-17 mRNA was not detected in numerous tissues, including spleen, thymus, and placenta. However, later studies detected the presence of hIL-17 mRNA transcripts in both $CD4^+$ and $CD8^+$ $CD45RO^+$ memory T cells, but not in naive $CD45RA^+$ T cells (10,11). In addition, recent studies by Zhou et al. (12) also detected expression of hIL-17 mRNA by RT-PCR in a B cell line AF10, derived from the human IgE myeloma cell line U266.

At the protein level, hIL-17 was also detected primarily in PMA- and ionomycin-stimulated $CD4^+$ cells, and at much lower levels in $CD8^+$ cells (4). hIL-17 protein was also detected in PBMC stimulated with concanavalin A or anti-CD3 and anti-CD28, but at lower levels than PBMC stimulated with PMA and ionomycin (5).

Both Th1 and Th2 $CD4^+$ T cell clones have been shown to express hIL-17. Aarvak et al. (13) isolated $CD4^+$ T cell clones from synovial membranes or synovial fluid of rheumatoid arthritis patients. Three of 13 Th1 clones, two of four Th0 clones, and zero of 16 Th2 clones produced hIL-17, following stimulation with PHA and anti-CD3 antibody. Furthermore, two Th2 clones that were cultured with IL-2 or IL-12 and anti-IL4 antibody switched to a Th1 phenotype and subsequently produced hIL-17. Scarponi et al. (14) isolated antigen-specific T cell clones from peripheral blood or skin of patients with allergic contact dermatitis. Seventeen of 32 Th1 clones, 16 of 37 Th0 clones, and six of 14 Th2 clones produced hIL-17 after stimulation with PMA and ionomycin or anti-CD3 and anti-CD28 antibody (15).

Expression of hIL-17 is regulated via the protein kinase A pathway (10,11). Ionomycin and PMA stimulation of PBMC in the presence of a cyclic AMP analogue (dibutyryl-cAMP) or prostaglandin E_2 (PGE_2), which results in elevated intracellular cAMP, inhibited expression of hIL-17 mRNA and protein, from total PBMC, or $CD4^+$ and $CD8^+$ T cell fractions purified after stimulation. However, this effect was less evident when $CD8^+$ cells were cultured alone prior to stimulation. Therefore, accessory cells present in the total PBMC population were required for this effect.

In contrast, Kennedy et al. (16) found mIL-17 transcripts exclusively in activated $\alpha\beta TcR^+$ $CD4^-$ $CD8^-$ T cells by Northern blot analysis. While mIL-17 mRNA could be detected by PCR in both activated $CD4^+$ and $CD8^+$ thymocytes, mIL-17 transcripts could not be detected in these cells by Northern blots. Thus, unlike hIL-17, the predominant source of mIL-17 is $\alpha\beta$TcR+ $CD4^-$ $CD8^-$ T cells.

STRUCTURE AND EXPRESSION OF IL-17 RECEPTOR

hIL-17R is located on chromosome 22q11.22-q11.23, whereas mIL-17R is located on chromosome 6 (2). The hIL-17R is predicted to be an 866–amino acid protein. As a type I transmembrane protein, it has a 27–amino acid signal sequence, a 293–amino acid extracellular domain with seven potential *N*-glycosylation sites, a 21–amino acid transmembrane domain, and a 525–amino acid cytoplasmic tail. Transfection of hIL-17R cDNA into cells results in expression of a set of predominantly 128- to 132-kDa proteins. Treatment of the cells with tunicamycin results in a 105- to 107-kDa protein, indicating that the mature hIL-17R contains multiple sugar moieties at its glycosylation sites. The mIL-17 receptor encodes a 120-kDa protein with 864 amino acids. mIL-17R has 82% amino acid similarity to hIL-17R. There are 11 conserved cysteine residues in the two proteins. hIL-17R and mIL-17R are not structurally related to other cytokine receptors, the immunoglobulin superfamily, or the tumor necrosis factor receptor family. Neither hIL-17R nor mIL-17R possess the WSXWS motif common to the hematopoietic receptor family (17), and the unusually large cytoplasmic tail shares no homology with the catalytic domain of other growth factor receptors (18). hIL-17R has a cytoplasmic tail with a IPPPLKPRKVW sequence (2), which is conserved among cytokine receptors (19). IL-17R, however, does not form homodimers in the absence of IL-17 (20).

In contrast to the extremely restricted expression of hIL-17, hIL-17R mRNA was detected by RT-PCR in PBMCs, NK cells, human fibroblasts, and embryonic kidney, lung epithelial, myelomonocytic, and Raji cells. hIL-17R protein was present on the surface of NK, embryonic kidney, myelomonocytic, and Raji cells. mIL-17R was detected by Northern blot analysis in all murine tissues examined, including in spleen, kidney, lung, liver, brain, skeletal muscle, and testes. mIL-17R transcripts were also present in murine splenic B cell lines, pre-B cells, triple negative ($CD3^-4^-8^-$) thymocytes, and various epithelial and fibroblast cell lines (2).

While the interaction of mIL-17 with its receptor induces NF-κB activity, little else is known about the mechanisms used by IL-17R to mediate its activities. The binding affinity of hIL-17 to hIL-17R is relatively low (K_a of 2 to 20×10^7 M^{-1}) (6). Anti–hIL-17R antibody competes with hIL-17R for binding to IL-17 and consequently inhibits the ability of IL-17 to induce IL-6 in human foreskin fibroblasts in a dose-dependent fashion. The relatively weak binding affinity of hIL-17 to its receptor, despite the potent activity of the cytokine *in vitro* (active in the nanogram range) suggests that another IL-17R subunit may exist.

OVERVIEW OF IL-17 ACTIVITY

IL-17 has pleiotropic biological effects, including induction of a number of hematopoietic and inflammatory cytokines from fibroblasts, synoviocytes, epithelial cells, endothelial cells, T cells, and macrophages, represented in Fig. 6.2. The activity of IL-17 is complex and varies depending on the species of origin (human or murine), the cell it is acting on, the activation state of the cell, and whether other cytokines are coexpressed. A summary of IL-17 "cytokine networking" is shown in Table 6.1.

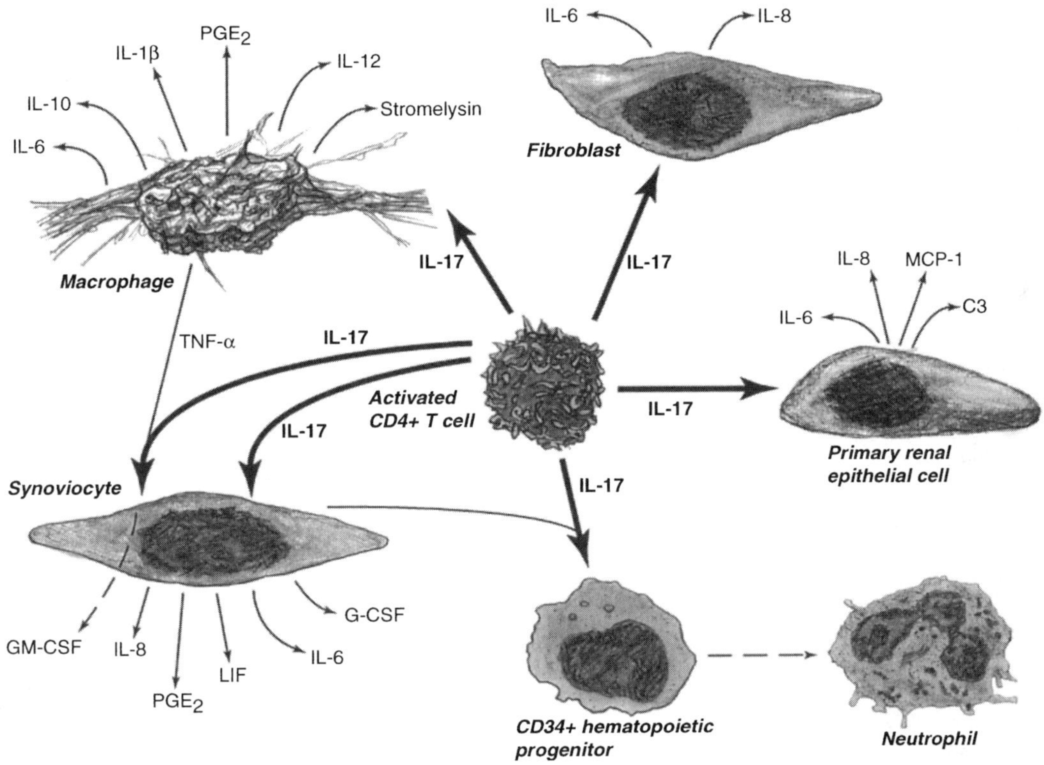

FIG. 6.2. Biological effects of human IL-17 on macrophages, fibroblasts, synoviocytes, CD34+ cells, and primary renal epithelial cells. Dotted arrows indicate the activity requires both IL-17 and a second stimulus. Additional interactions of IL-17 with other cytokines are shown in Table 6.1.

TABLE 6-1. *Biological effect of addition of cytokines to hIL-17 stimulated cells*

Additional stimulus	Cell type	Cytokine produced	Effect
IFN-γ	Synoviocyte	IL-6	Additive
TNF-α	Synoviocyte	IL-6	Additive
TNF-α	Synoviocyte	GM-CSF	Induction
IL-1β low	Synoviocyte	IL-6	Synergistic
IL-1β high	Synoviocyte	IL-6	Additive
IL-1β low	Synoviocyte	LIF	Additive
IL-4 + IL-1β	Synoviocyte	IL-6	Additive
IL-10 + IL-1β	Synoviocyte	IL-6	Additive
IL-13 + IL-1β	Synoviocyte	IL-6	Additive
IL-4	Macrophage	IL-1β, TNF-α	Partial inhibition
IL-10	Macrophage	IL-1β, TNF-α	Complete inhibition
IL-13	Macrophage	IL-1β, TNF-α	Partial inhibition
TGF-β	Macrophage	IL-1β, TNF-α	Partial inhibition
PGE_2	Macrophage	IL-1β	No effect
PGE_2	Macrophage	TNF-α	Inhibition
IFN-γ	Keratinocyte	IL-6, IL-8	Synergistic
TNF-α	Keratinocyte	IL-6, IL-8	Synergistic
IFN-γ	Keratinocyte	RANTES	Inhibition
TNF-α	Keratinocyte	RANTES	Inhibition
IFN-γ	Keratinocyte	MCP-1	No effect
TNF-α	Keratinocyte	MCP-1	No effect

CELL TYPE–SPECIFIC EFFECTS OF IL-17 ON DIFFERENTIATED CELLS

Fibroblasts

Yao et al. (4) showed that addition of hIL-17 to human foreskin fibroblasts (HFF) induced production of IL-6 and IL-8. This activity was blocked by addition of anti–vIL-17 monoclonal antibody. Similarly, mIL-17 and vIL-17 induced production of IL-6 by murine (3T3) fibroblasts (2) in a dose-dependent manner. This could be inhibited by anti–vIL-17 monoclonal antibody. Treatment of HFF cells with hIL-17 increased surface expression of ICAM-1, but not LFA-1, HLA class I or class II molecules. Moreover, Kennedy et al. (16) demonstrated that recombinant hIL-17, mIL-17, and rIL-17 all induced IL-6 production by the murine stromal cell line 30R. Thus, despite sequence homologies of only 60% to 80%, all of these species of IL-17 could bind and activate mIL-17R and induce IL-6 production in a dose-dependent manner. Species specificity was demonstrated, since IL-6 induction in murine cells was five times more effective by mIL-17 than hIL-17 or rIL-17.

Synoviocytes

Both hIL-17 and vIL-17 stimulated human synoviocytes, inducing production of IL-6, IL-8, granulocyte-colony stimulating factor (G-CSF), and prostaglandin E_2 (PGE_2), but not IL-1 or TNF-α. These effects could be blocked by anti–hIL-17 antibody. hIL-17 also induced production of leukemia inhibitory factor (LIF) by synoviocytes (21). Addition of TNF-α and IFN-γ had an additive effect on the ability of IL-17 to induce IL-6 from synoviocytes (5). While IL-17 or TNF-α alone did not induce secretion of GM-CSF, addition of both cytokines together resulted in induction of GM-CSF (5).

Chabaud et al. (21) studied interaction of IL-17 with proinflammatory (IL-1β) and antiinflammatory (IL-4, IL-10, IL-13) cytokines. They showed that hIL-17 interacts with synoviocyte-derived IL-1β to induce IL-6 secretion either additively or synergistically depending on the concentrations used. At low concentrations of IL-17 (1 to 10 ng/mL) and IL-1β (1 to 10 pg/mL), a synergistic effect on IL-6 secretion was observed, but at high levels of IL-17 (>10 ng/mL) and IL-1β (>10 pg/mL) the effect was additive. Low concentrations of IL-17 and IL-1β also had an additive effect in inducing production of LIF by synoviocytes. IL-17 also enhanced the activity of other cytokines to induce IL-6, summarized in Table 6.1. While treatment of synoviocytes with IL-4 and IL-13 resulted in moderate IL-6 induction, costimulation of synoviocytes with IL-17 or IL-1β along with IL-4 or IL-13 enhanced IL-6 production by 30%. In contrast, costimulation of synoviocytes with IL-17 and IL-10 resulted in modest inhibition of IL-6 production. The combination of IL-17 and IL-4 or IL-13 had a stimulatory effect on IL-6; however, these cytokine combinations showed the opposite effect on LIF. While IL-17 stimulated production of LIF, the combination of IL-17 with IL-4 or IL-13 was inhibitory. In contrast, IL-10 in the absence or presence of IL-17 had no effect on LIF production.

Keratinocytes

Similar to its effects on synoviocytes, IL-17 also has synergistic and additive effects on cytokine production by keratinocytes. IL-17 was found to augment IFN-γ–induced ICAM-1 expression, but not HLA-DR expression on keratinocytes (15). hIL-17 alone had no effect on ICAM-1 and did not enhance TNF-α–induced ICAM-1 expression. In addition, hIL-17 induced production of IL-8 by keratinocytes, both directly and synergistically with IFN-γ and TNF-α. In contrast, hIL-17 inhibited IFN-γ and TNF-α–induced production of RANTES, but had no effect on MCP-1. Teunissen et al. (22) also reported that *in vitro* treatment of normal human keratinocytes with rhIL-17 augmented IL-6 and IL-8 secretion, but not IL-1α or IL-15. hIL-17 had a synergistic effect on IFN-γ–induced IL-6 and IL-8 secretion, and in contrast to Albanesi et al. (15), hIL-17 had a slight additive effect on IFN-γ–induced expression of HLA-DR and ICAM-1.

T Cells

Yao et al. (2) showed that increasing amounts of vIL-17 or mIL-17 added to mouse splenic T cells enhanced proliferative responses obtained with suboptimal levels of phytohemagglutinin (PHA). Addition of soluble IL-17R, which neutralizes endogenous IL-17, inhibited IL-2 production by concanavalin A (con A) or PHA-activated murine T cells. Soluble IL-17R also inhibited con A or PHA-induced proliferation of murine T cells. In contrast to the effects observed with mIL-17, recombinant hIL-17 had no significant effect on proliferation or secretion of IFN-γ, IL-4, IL-6, or IL-10 by human T cells or PBMC. hIL-17 also had no significant effect on PBMC or T cell cytotoxicity, or on proliferation and antibody secretion by activated human B cells (5). This may be an important difference in function of IL-17 between species in view of the different tissue sources of IL-17 in humans and mice.

Macrophages

Jovanovic et al. (23) showed that treatment of adherent macrophages with IL-17 induced secretion of IL-1β, IL-6, IL-10, IL-12, TNF-α, PGE_2, and stromelysin. The cytokines were detected 1 to 3 hours after stimulation, peaked at 6 to 9 hours, and plateaued for 24 hours. IL-17 had no effect on nitrite synthesis by macrophages. Addition of either IL-4 or IL-10 with IL-17 reduced the ability of IL-17 to stimulate the release of IL-1β. Addition of IL-13 or TGF-β to IL-17 only partially reduced IL-17 stimulation of IL-1β. Only IL-10 was able to significantly suppress IL-17 induced macrophage release of TNF-α, while IL-4, IL-13, and TGF-β had a partial effect.

Epithelial and Endothelial Cells

Addition of hIL-17 to kidney carcinoma epithelial cell lines, brain endothelial cells, and bronchial epithelial cells resulted in increased levels of IL-6 (5). hIL-17 induced secretion of IL-6, IL-8, and monocyte chemoattractant protein-1 (MCP-1), but not RANTES, by primary renal epithelial cells *in vitro* (24). These cytokines were produced in increasing amounts over a 5-day period and anti–IL-17 antibody abrogated these effects. hIL-17 also induced the production of the complement C3 protein, but not C2 or C4, by renal epithelial cells.

IL-17 EFFECTS ON DIFFERENTIATION OF HEMATOPOIETIC PROGENITOR CELLS

Neutrophils

hIL-17 enhanced the proliferation of $CD34^+$ hematopoietic progenitor cells in the presence of irradiated fibroblasts (5). Culture of the $CD34^+$ cells with hIL-17 and fibroblasts resulted in differentiation of the $CD34^+$ cells to neutrophils after 12 days. This effect was reversed by addition of antibody to G-CSF, indicating that differentiation was probably due to the ability of IL-17 to induce secretion of G-CSF from fibroblasts and not a direct effect of IL-17 on $CD34^+$ cells (25).

Dendritic Cells

hIL-17 has also been found to promote the maturation of bone marrow–derived $CD11c^+$ dendritic cell progenitors (26). rhIL-17 treatment of GM-CSF–stimulated immature mouse bone marrow–derived cells increased surface expression of CD11c, CD40, and MHC class II, and markedly increased expression of CD80 and CD86. However, the expression of these surface molecules on more fully differentiated bone marrow–derived dendritic cells was not significantly affected by exposure to rhIL-17. Since bone marrow–derived dendritic cells are potent antigen-presenting cells for T cell activation and proliferation, the ability of hIL-17 to induce maturation of dendritic cell progenitors may explain the ability of an IL-17 antagonist to inhibit T cell proliferation in mixed leukocyte reactions.

IL-17 EFFECTS ON INNATE IMMUNITY

Recombinant vaccinia viruses expressing cytokines have been used to elucidate the function of several cytokines *in vivo*, including IL-2, IL-4, IL-5, IL-6, IL-10, and IFN-γ (27). We infected mice with recombinant vaccinia virus expressing IL-17. Mice infected with the recombinant virus had increased morbidity and mortality compared to mice infected with control vaccinia virus. Splenocytes obtained from mice infected with vaccinia virus expressing IL-17 showed a significant decrease in lysis of NK-specific target cells compared to cells from mice infected with control vaccinia virus. Therefore, mIL-17 may inhibit the innate immune response *in vivo* (Patera A, Pesnicak L, Berlin I, et al., unpublished data).

SUMMARY OF IL-17 ACTIVITY

Since hIL-17 is produced primarily by activated T cells, the above findings suggest that IL-17 is important as a proinflammatory molecule. Activated T cells recruited to a site of inflammation can secrete IL-17, which in turn induces expression of proinflammatory cytokines (e.g., IL-6, IL-8, PGE_2) by endothelial and epithelial cells, and activated macrophages at these sites. IL-17 also induces production of C3 in epithelial cells, which also can contribute to the local inflammatory response. Upregulation of ICAM-1 by IL-17 on fibroblasts and keratinocytes also may be important for recruiting cells to sites of inflammation. In addition, IL-17 can stimulate differentiation of progenitor cells to neutrophils and dendritic cells. IL-17 also induces secretion of the antiinflammatory cytokine, IL-10, from macrophages, which may limit inflammation to prevent an excessive response and prevent injury to the host.

Like many other cytokines, IL-17 induces secretion of multiple other cytokines. It is not yet known whether the effects of IL-17 are mediated directly or via induction of other cytokines. In addition to inducing secretion of IL-6, IL-8, G-CSF, and PGE_2 from a number of cell types, IL-17 also has additive or synergistic effects on the ability of other cytokines to induce cytokine secretion. For example, TNF-α and IFN-γ enhance IL-17–induced secretion of IL-6 by synoviocytes. Furthermore, IL-17 can interact with another cytokine, TNF-α, to induce secretion of GM-CSF, that neither IL-17 nor TNF-α alone can induce.

IL-17 MECHANISM OF ACTIVITY

IL-17 Activity via NF-κB

Two lines of evidence support activation via NF-κB as a potential mechanism of action of IL-17. First, hIL-17 upregulates NF-κB in human macrophages (23). After treatment with hIL-17, the level of NF-κB decreased for the first hour and then rose over time, peaking at 4 hours. The kinetics of another transcription factor, AP-1, are identical. mIL-17 and vIL-17 also induce NF-κB in murine fibroblasts (2). This effect was specific since antibody to vIL-17 completely inhibited induction of NF-κB. Induction of NF-κB requires the interaction of IL-17 with its receptor since preincubation of cells with anti-IL-17R inhibited NF-κB activity.

Second, the pattern and kinetics of cytokine release by IL-17 is consistent with NF-κB–mediated activation; for a review, see Lenardo and Baltimore (28). NF-κB induces expression of IL-1β, IL-6, and TNF-α. As reviewed above, hIL-17 upregulates secretion of IL-1β, IL-6, and TNF-α in human macrophages, as well as IL-10, IL-12, and PGE_2 (23). The timing of IL-1β and TNF-α release, which have an initial inhibitory phase followed by an increase in levels over 3 hours, parallels the decrease and then subsequent increase of NF-κB in the cell.

Subsequent experiments investigated signaling pathways induced by IL-17 (23). Treatment of macrophages with hIL-17 results in a decrease in intracellular cAMP levels. The kinetics of this decrease correlate with the increase of IL-1β and TNF-α release induced by IL-17. While inhibitors of cyclic AMP (e.g., cholera toxin) inhibited the ability of IL-17 to induce the release of TNF-α, these inhibitors did not reduce the ability of IL-17 to release IL-1β. Similarly, inhibitors of cAMP protein kinase and mitogen-activated protein kinase kinase inhibited the ability of IL-17 to release TNF-α from cells, but did not reduce the ability of IL-17 to release IL-1β. Jovanovic et al. also showed that incubation of macrophages with IL-17 results in an increase in intracellular calcium levels.

Awane et al. (29) further characterized the hIL-17–induced signal transduction and transcriptional activation events in a rat intestinal epithelial cell line, IEC-6. IEC-6 cells stimulated with hIL-17 resulted in induction of NF-κB binding proteins p65 and p50, which form a heterodimeric complex. hIL-17 activated NF-κB to induce expression of two rat chemokines CINC (a CXC chemokine homologous to human GRO-α) and MCP-1 (a CC chemokine). Activation of the CINC chemokine promoter by hIL-17 or IL-1β was dependent on NF-κB–inducing kinase (NIK), IκBα kinase (IKK-α), and TNF receptor–associated factor–6 (TRAF-6). hIL-17 synergized with IL-1β to upregulate the CINC chemokine. Thus, hIL-17 uses the same signaling mediators, NIK and IKK-α, that are used by IL-1β to activate the chemokine promoter.

hIL-17 induced activation of the ERK-1, ERK-2, JNK-1, and p38 MAP kinases, although the pattern of activation varied (29). hIL-17 regulation of ERK-1 and EKR-2 was biphasic, with initial downregulation followed by upregulation of activity. In contrast, hIL-17 induced a gradual activation of p38 and JNK-1, and the latter was dependent on the presence of TRAF-6 but not NIK.

Recent experiments also demonstrate the involvement of hIL-17 in JAK/STAT signal transduction. Stimulation of human U937 monocytic leukemia cells with IL-17 resulted in rapid tyrosine phosphorylation of JAK 1, 2, and 3, Tyk 2, and STAT 1, 2, 3, and 4 (30). Treatment of U937 cells with hIL-17 also induced rapid tyrosine phosphorylation and activation of Raf-1 kinase (31). Thus, hIL-17 induces the phosphorylation of multiple cellular proteins involving both the JAK/STAT and Ras/MAP kinase signaling pathways.

IL-17 Activity by an Alternative Mechanism

IL-17 may also have a posttranscriptional effect by stabilizing cytokine mRNAs (32). mIL-17 increased the half-life of G-CSF mRNA from 1.5 hours in untreated murine 3T3 cells to 4 hours in IL-17–treated cells. The increase in G-CSF mRNA induced by mIL-17 in 3T3 cells was not inhibited by cycloheximide, indicating that this increase does not require new protein synthesis. These results suggest that mIL-17 can increase the levels of certain cytokines in an NF-κB–independent mechanism that does not require protein synthesis for its activation. Instead, mIL-17 may reduce the level of an RNase that normally degrades cytokines.

The increase in G-CSF mRNA by mIL-17 was not affected by a protein tyrosine kinase inhibitor (genistein), indicating that activation of tyrosine kinases may not be required for the effect (32). This finding is supported by the predicted amino acid sequence of mIL-17R. The sequence of the receptor does not have homology with known growth factor receptors that have tyrosine kinase catalytic domains (2). Thus, unlike hIL-17, mIL-17 may not activate the JAK-STAT pathway, which normally requires activation of the JAK tyrosine kinase and phosphorylation of STAT.

ANIMAL MODEL DATA

As noted above, incubation of hIL-17 and irradiated fibroblasts with human $CD34^+$ cells resulted in differentiation of the latter cells into neutrophils. Administration of recombinant IL-17 to C57BL6/N mice resulted in a four- to five-fold increase in peripheral neutrophils on days 3 to 7, and a small increase in the total white blood cell count; for a review, see Fossiez et al. (25). The increase in neutrophils could have been due to differentiation of progenitor cells into neutrophils or mobilization of cells from the bone marrow to the blood. However, IL-17 did not mobilize progenitor cells from the bone marrow to the periphery.

IL-17 increased granulopoiesis in mice when delivered by gene transfer (33). The use of an adenovirus vector to deliver mIL-17 to mice resulted in a five-fold increase in leukocytes, which was primarily due to a granulocytosis. IL-17 resulted in increased colony forming units in the bone marrow and the spleen, and an increase in serum G-CSF levels. The total cellularity of the spleen increased by 50%, but there was no change in overall cellularity of the bone marrow.

To determine whether IL-17–induced neutrophilia has a biologically significant effect, mice were injected with either IL-17 or saline for 3 days and then inoculated with a lethal dose of *E. coli*. Mice receiving IL-17 showed reduced mortality, when compared to those receiving saline alone; for a review, see Fossiez et al. (25). It is uncertain whether this is a direct effect of IL-17, or whether IL-17 induction of IL-6 (a cytokine that also induces neutrophilia) protected the animals (25).

A soluble form of the IL-17 receptor has been shown to inhibit mixed leukocyte responses (MLR) and prolong transplant survival in mice (34). Soluble IL-17 receptor inhibited anti-donor T cell proliferative responses *in vitro*. In nonvascularized allograft transplants, in which cardiac allografts were implanted into the pinna of the ear of mice, survival of the allografts was prolonged from 13 to 20 days in animals receiving soluble IL-17 receptor. In vascularized allografts, in which the heart was transplanted into the abdomen, survival of the allograft increased from 11 to 19 days in animals that received soluble IL-17 receptor. Since IL-17 has been shown to promote the maturation of dendritic cell precursors, with increased surface expression of costimulatory molecules and MHC class II molecules, blocking these activities with soluble IL-17 receptor may thereby enhance allograft survival.

IL-17 has been shown to recruit neutrophils into the airways of rats (35,36). Instillation of IL-17 into the trachea of these animals resulted in increased levels of rat macrophage inflammatory protein–2 (MIP-2), a chemokine, as well as neutrophils in the bronchial lavage fluid. The recruitment of neutrophils was blocked by antibodies to IL-17 or to MIP-2, by dexamethasone, or by a tachykinin receptor antagonist. Similarly, treatment of human bronchial epithelial cells with IL-17 *in vitro* resulted in increased release of IL-8 (a human counterpart of rat MIP-2), and this effect was inhibited by dexamethasone. Furthermore, conditioned medium obtained from IL-17–treated human bronchial epithelial cells increased the migration of neutrophils *in vitro*. In a preliminary study, instillation of lipopolysaccharide into the lungs of rats resulted in increased levels of IL-17 in the bronchoalveolar lavage fluid within 2 hours of the treatment (37).

HVS usually causes asymptomatic infection in squirrel monkeys; however, cottontop tamarins inoculated with the virus develop T cell lymphomas containing the viral genome. The HVS genome contains a functional copy of the IL-17 gene that is expressed during lytic viral infection, but not in virus-transformed T cells. Knappe and colleagues (38) insertionally inactivated the IL-17 gene in HVS. This virus showed no differences in replication or transformation of human or marmoset T cells in vitro when compared to wild-type virus. Intravenous inoculation of cotton tamarins with the IL-17–inactivated virus induced T cell lymphomas similar to those seen with wild-type virus. At present, it is not known whether the HVS IL-17 has a role in infection or persistence of the virus in squirrel monkeys (the natural host of HVS).

Recently an IL-17 receptor "knockout" mice was constructed; for a review, see Spriggs (20). Preliminary results do not show a definite phenotype in these animals. On histopathology and using cell surface markers, their lymphocytes and myeloid cells are unremarkable and are present in normal amounts. Attempts to produce transgenic mice that constitutively overexpress IL-17 have been unsuccessful (33).

Expression of IL-17 in cervical tumor cell lines enhanced tumor growth in mice (39). Human cervical carcinoma cell lines that stably express hIL-17 showed no differences for growth *in vitro* and when implanted into nude mice, the IL-17–transfected cells showed no difference in the incidence of tumor formation when compared to mock transfected cells. However, the IL-17–transfected cells showed a markedly enhanced growth rate compared to the control cells. The tumors derived from IL-17–transfected cells showed expression of hIL-17, increased expression of murine IL-6, and greater infiltration by macrophages when compared to the tumors from mock transfected cells. Analysis of six human cervical carcinomas showed IL-17 mRNA, detected by RT-PCR, in four of the tumors. These four IL-17–positive tumors, unlike the two IL-17–negative tumors, showed infiltration by $CD4^+$ cells.

HUMAN EXPERIENCE

There are no published data on the administration of IL-17 or soluble IL-17 receptor to humans. At present, studies of IL-17 *in vivo* have focused on four areas of research: the role of IL-17 in arthritis, transplant rejection, dermatologic, and neurologic disease.

IL-17 mRNA has been detected in synovial fluid, but not PBMCs, in patients with rheumatoid, psoriatic, or osteoarthritis (40). IL-17 protein was higher in synovial fluid from patients with rheumatoid arthritis than in those with osteoarthritis (41). Immunohistochemical staining of synovial tissues for IL-17 showed the cytokine in a subset of the $CD4^+$ and $CD45RA^+$ cells from patients with rheumatoid arthritis, but not with osteoarthritis. IL-17 inhibited chondrocyte proliferation. IL-17 produced by fragments of synovium, obtained from patients with rheumatoid arthritis, induced production of IL-6 and LIF *in vitro* (21,42). This effect was inhibited by addition of anti-IL-17 monoclonal antibody. Addition of IL-4 and IL-13, but not IL-10, completely blocked the production of IL-17 *in vitro* by synovium from patients with rheumatoid arthritis. Addition of exogenous IL-17 to cultures of synovium from patients with rheumatoid arthritis further increased the production of IL-6. IL-17–induced production of IL-6 was observed less often in synovium from patients with osteoarthritis and was not detected in synovium from normal persons.

IL-17 was shown to stimulate the production of nitric oxide and prostaglandin E_2 in cartilage obtained from patients with osteoarthritis (43,44). This effect was completely inhibited with a protein synthesis inhibitor (cycloheximide), a nitric oxide synthase inhibitor (*N*-monomethyl-L-arginine monoacetate), or a NF-κB inhibitor (pyrrolidine dithiocarbamate), but not by dexamethasone. Similarly, treatment of human articular chondrocytes from persons without joint disease resulted in production of nitric oxide, inducible nitric oxide synthase, cyclooxygenase-2, IL-6, increased NF-κB DNA binding activity, and activation of several mitogen-activated protein kinases (ERK1, ERK2, JNK, p38) (45). Addition of dexamethasone and IL-17 to chondrocytes reduced each of these activities that had been induced by IL-17 alone.

IL-17 resulted in the release of proteoglycans and induced the expression of inducible nitric oxide synthetase, cyclooxygenase, stromelysin, and collagenase from normal human articular cartilage (40). Synovial fluid from patients with rheumatoid arthritis induced osteoclast formation, which was inhibited by antibody to IL-17 (41). Similarly, IL-17 stimulates osteoclast formation in cultures of mouse bone marrow and osteoblasts, which is inhibited by indomethacin. In addition, the combination of IL-17 and TNF-α increased osteoclastic bone resorption when mouse bones were cultured *in vitro* (46). These studies hint that IL-17 might have a role in inflammation and degradation of cartilage seen in rheumatoid arthritis.

IL-17 mRNA has been detected in transplanted human kidneys undergoing rejection by reverse transcription of RNA followed by PCR of the cDNA (24). IL-17 mRNA was not detected in normal human kidneys. IL-17 protein was detected by immunohistochemistry in the cells infiltrating the interstitium or the renal tubules in eight of eight kidneys undergoing rejection from 9 days to 7 years after transplantation. However, IL-17 was not detected in biopsies from normal or pretransplant kidneys or in kidneys with tumors. When cells lines were obtained from the renal biopsies, IL-17 could be detected in the T cells infiltrating the grafts, but not the proximal tubular epithelial cells, after stimulation with PMA and ionomycin. At present, it is unclear whether IL-17 has a causative role in transplant rejection.

Skin biopsies obtained from patients with allergic contact dermatitis and psoriasis showed IL-17 mRNA; however, normal skin did not express IL-17 mRNA (15,22). Antigen-specific T cells obtained from the skin biopsies of patients with allergic contact dermatitis expressed IL-17, interferon-γ and TNF-α mRNAs.

PBMCs from patients with multiple sclerosis and aseptic meningoencephalitis showed higher expression of IL-17 mRNA than cells from normal individuals (47). Furthermore, patients with multiple sclerosis undergoing exacerbation of their disease showed higher levels of mIL-17 mRNA than those in remission. In patients with multiple sclerosis, but not with aseptic meningoencephalitis, IL-17 mRNA was higher in CSF mononuclear cells than in PBMCs.

In a similar study, patients with ischemic stroke showed higher numbers of IL-17 expressing PBMCs during the first 3 days of symptoms compared to healthy persons (48).

The number of PBMCs expressing IL-17 correlated with the degree of neurologic dysfunction. The elevation in IL-17–expressing cells was thought to contribute to the inflammatory process in multiple sclerosis and stroke.

FUTURE DIRECTIONS

The role of IL-17 is unclear in human disease at present. An IL-17–receptor knockout mouse has not shown any phenotypic differences thus far, and attempts to produce transgenic mice that constitutively express IL-17 have been unsuccessful. Injection of IL-17 into mice resulted in neutrophilia, and intratracheal IL-17 caused recruitment of neutrophils into the airway. Detection of elevated levels of IL-17 in synovial fluid from patients with rheumatoid and psoriatic arthritis, in skin biopsies of patients with psoriasis or allergic contact dermatitis, and in the cerebrospinal fluid of patients with multiple sclerosis suggests that this cytokine may have an important role in human inflammation. The observation of IL-17 protein in biopsies of human rejected kidneys and the ability of a soluble IL-17 receptor to delay allograft rejection in mice suggests that this cytokine may have a role in enhancing allograft rejection induced by T cells.

These findings suggest that IL-17 may have a role in other human inflammatory diseases. The ability to block the effects of IL-17 through the use of a soluble IL-17 receptor or monoclonal antibody should provide additional evidence of its activity using animal models and might have potential therapeutic uses in the future.

REFERENCES

1. Rouvier E, Luciani M-F, Mattei M-G, et al. CTLA-8, cloned from an activated T cell, bearing AU-rich messenger RNA instability sequences, and homologous to a herpesvirus saimiri gene. *J Immunol* 1993;15:5445–5456.
2. Yao Z, Fanslow WC, Seldein MF, et al. Herpesvirus saimiri encodes a new cytokine, IL-17, which binds to a novel cytokine receptor. *Immunity* 1995;3:811–821.
3. Yao Z, Timour M, Painter S, et al. Complete nucleotide sequence of the mouse CTLA8 gene. *Gene* 1996;168: 223–225.
4. Yao Z, Painter SL, Fanslow WC, et al. Human IL-17: a novel cytokine derived from T cells. *J Immunol* 1995b; 155:5483–5486.
5. Fossiez F, Djossou O, Chomarat P, et al. T cell interleukin-17 induces stromal cells to produce proinflammatory and hematopoietic cytokines. *J Exp Med* 1996;183:2593–2603.
6. Yao Z, Spriggs MS, Derry JMJ, et al. Molecular characterization of the human interleukin (IL)–17 receptor. *Cytokine* 1997;9:794–800.
7. Caput D, Beutler B, Hartog K, et al. Identification of a common nucleotide sequence in the 3′-untranslated region of mRNA molecules specifying inflammatory mediators. *Proc Natl Acad Sci USA* 1986;83:1670–1674.
8. Shaw G, Kamen R. A conserved UA sequence from the 3′ untranslated region of GM-CSF mediates selective mRNA degradation. *Cell* 1986;46:659–667.
9. Kruys V, Beutler B, Huez G. Translational control mediated by UA-rich sequences. *Enzyme* 1990;44:193–202.
10. Shin HCK, Benbernou N, Fekkar H, et al. Regulation of IL-17, IFN-γ and IL-10 in human CD8$^+$ T cells by cyclic AMP-dependent signal transduction pathway. *Cytokine* 1998;10:841–850.
11. Shin HCK, Benbernou N, Esnault S, et al. Expression of IL-17 in human CD45RO$^+$ T lymphocytes and its regulation by protein kinase A pathway. *Cytokine* 1999;11:257–266.
12. Zhou L, Peng S, Duan J, et al. A human B cell line AF10 expressing hIL-17. *Biochem Mol Biol Int* 1998;45: 1113–1119.
13. Aarvak T, Chabaud M, Miossec P, et al. IL-17 is produced by some proinflammatory Th1/Th0 cells but not by Th2 cells. *J Immunol* 1999;162:1246–1251.
14. Scarponi C, Albanesi C, Federici M, et al. IL-17 is produced by nickel-specific Th1, Th2 and Th0 cells, and cooperates with IFN-γ and IL-4 in amplifying inflammatory responses by humna keratinocytes [Abstract]. *J Invest Dermatol* 1999;113:482.
15. Albanesi C, Cavani A, Girolomoni G. IL-17 is produced by nickel-specific T lymphocytes and regulates ICAM-1 expression and chemokine production in human keratinocytes: Synergistic or antagonistic effects with IFN-γ and TNF-α. *J Immunol* 1999;162:494–502.
16. Kennedy J, Rossi DL, Zurawski SM, et al. Mouse IL-17: a cytokine preferentially expressed by αβTCR$^+$CD4$^-$ CD8$^-$ T cells. *J Interferon Cytokine Res* 1996;16:611–617.

17. Cosman D. The hematopoietin receptor superfamily. *Cytokine* 1993;5:95–106.
18. Hanks SK, Quinn AM, Unter T. The protein kinase family: conserved features and deduced phylogeny of the catalytic domains. *Science* 1988;241:42–52.
19. Murakami M, Narazaki M, Hibi M, et al. Critical cytoplasmic region of the interleukin 6 signal transducer gp130 is conserved in the cytokine receptor family. *Proc Natl Acad Sci USA* 1991;88:11349–11353.
20. Spriggs M.K. Interleukin-17 and its receptor. *J Clin Immunol* 1997;17:366–369.
21. Chaubad M, Fossiez F, Taupin J-L, et al. Enhancing effect of IL-17 on IL-1–induced IL-6 and leukemia inhibitory factor production by rheumatoid arthritis synoviocytes and its regulation by Th2 cytokines. *J Immunol* 1998;161:409–414.
22. Teunissen MBM, Koomen CW, de Waal-Malefyt R, et al. Interleukin-17 and interferon-γ synergize in the enhancement of proinflammatory cytokine production by human keratinocytes. *J Invest Dermatol* 1999;111: 645–649.
23. Jovanovic DV, Di Battista JA, Martel-Pelletier J, et al. IL-17 stimulates the production and expression of proinflammatory cytokines, IL-β and TNF-α, by human macrophages. *J Immunol* 1998;160:3513–3521.
24. van Kooten C, Boonstra JG, Paape ME, et al. Interleukin-17 activates human renal epithelial cells in vitro and is expressed during renal allograft rejection. *J Am Soc Nephrol* 1998;9:1526–1534.
25. Fossiez F, Banchereau J, Murray R, et al. Interleukin-17. *Intern Rev Immunol* 1998;16:541–551.
26. Antonysamy MA, Fanslow WC, Fu F, et al. Evidence for a role of IL-17 in organ allograft rejection: IL-17 promotes the functional differentiation of dendritic cell progenitors. *J Immunol* 1999;162:577–584.
27. Ramshaw I, Ruby J, Ramsey A, et al. Expression of cytokines by recombinant vaccinia viruses: a model for studying cytokines in virus infections in vivo. *Immunol Rev* 1992;127:157–182.
28. Lenardo MJ, Baltimore D. NF-κB: a pleiotropic mediator of inducible and tissue-specific gene control. *Cell* 1989;58:227–229.
29. Awane M, Andres PG, Li DJ, et al. NF-κB–inducing kinase is a common mediator of IL-17–, TNF-α– and IL-1β–induced chemokine promoter activation in intestinal epithelial cells. *J Immunol* 1999;162:5337–5344.
30. Subramaniam SV, Cooper RS, Adunyah SE. Evidence for the involvement of JAK/STAT pathway in the signaling mechanism of interleukin-17. *Biochem Biophys Res Commun* 1999;262:14–19.
31. Subramaniam SV, Pearson LL, Adunyah SE. Interleukin-17 induces rapid phosphorylation and activation of Raf-1 kinase in human monocytic progenitor cell line U937. *Biochem Biophys Res Commun* 1999;259:172–177.
32. Cai X-Y, Gommoll Jr CP, Justice L, et al. Regulation of granulocyte colony-stimulating factor gene expression by interleukin-17. *Immunol Lett* 1998;62:51–58.
33. Schwartzenberger P, La Russa V, Miller A, et al. IL-17 stimulates granulopoiesis in mice: Use of an alternate, novel gene therapy–derived method for in vivo evaluation of cytokines. *J Immunol* 1998;161:6383–6389.
34. Antonysamy MA, Fanslow WC, Fu F, et al. Evidence for a role of IL-17 in alloimmunity: a novel IL-17 antagonist promotes heart graft survival. *Transplant Proc* 1999;31:93.
35. Laan M, Cui Z-H, Hoshino H, et al. Neutrophil recruitment by human IL-17 via C-X-C chemokine release in the airways. *J Immunol* 1999;162:2347–2352.
36. Hoshino H, Lotvall J, Skoogh B-E, et al. Neutrophil recruitment by interleukin-17 into rat airways in vivo. *Am J Respir Crit Care Med* 1999;159:1423–1428.
37. Jordan JA, Yun EC, Sarma VJ, et al. The role of interleukin-17 in LPS-induced inflammatory lung injury [Abstract]. *FASEB J* 1999;13:A1017.
38. Knappe A, Hiller C, Niphus H, et al. The interleukin-17 gene of herpesvirus saimiri. *J Virol* 1998;72:5797–5801.
39. Tartour E, Fossiez F, Joyeux I, et al. Interleukin 17, a T cell derived cytokine, promotes tumorigenicity of human cervical tumors in nude mice. *Cancer Res* 1999;59:3698–3704.
40. Lotz M, Bober L, Narula S, et al. IL-17 promotes cartilage degeneration [Abstract]. *Arthritis Rheum* 1996;39: S120.
41. Kotake S, Udagawa N, Takahashi N, et al. IL-17 in synovial fluids from patients with rheumatoid arthritis is a potent stimulator of osteoclastogenesis. *J Clin Invest* 1999;103:1345–1352.
42. Chabaud M, Durand, J.M, Buchs N, et al. Human interleukin-17: a T cell–derived proinflammatory cytokine produced by the rheumatoid synovium. *Arthritis Rheum* 1999;42:963–970.
43. Attur MG, Patel RN, Abramson SB, et al. Interleukin-17 up-regulation of nitric oxide production in human osteoarthritis cartilage. *Arthritis Rheum* 1997;40:1050–1053.
44. Amin AR, Abramson SB. The role of nitric oxide in articular cartilage breakdown in osteoarthritis. *Curr Opin Rheum* 1998;10:263–268.
45. Shalom-Barak T, Quach J, Lotz M. Interleukin-17–induced gene expression in articular chondrocytes in associated with activation of mitogen-activated protein kinases and NF-κB. *J Biol Chem* 1998;273:27467–27473.
46. van Bezooijen RL, Farih-Sips HCM, Papapoulos SE, et al. Interleukin-17: a new bone acting cytokine in vitro. *J Bone Miner Res* 1999;14:1513–1521.
47. Matusevicius D, Kivisakk P, He B, et al. Interleukin-17 mRNA expression in blood and CSF mononuclear cells is augmented in multiple sclerosis. *Mult Scler* 1999;5:101–104.
48. Kostulas N, Pelidou, S.H, Kivisakk P, et al. Increased IL-1β, IL-8, and IL-17 mRNA expression in blood mononuclear cells observed in a prospective ischemia stroke study. *Stroke* 1999;30:2174–2179.

7
Interleukin-18

*Kenji Nakanishi, *†Tomohiro Yoshimoto, *†Shin-ichiro Kashiwamura, *Hiroko Tsutsui, and †Haruki Okamura

**Department of Immunology and Medical Zoology, †Laboratory of Host Defenses, Institute for Advanced Medical Sciences, Hyogo College of Medicine, Nishinomiya, Hyogo, Japan*

INTRODUCTION

IFN-γ, initially identified by Wheelock (1) in the culture supernatant of mitogen-stimulated T cells, is one of the most well-characterized cytokines that contribute to the host defense against various microbes (2–4). We have been interested in regulation of IFN-γ production *in vivo.* IFN-γ is mainly secreted from $CD8^+$ T cells, Th1 cells, and NK cells. In fact, high levels of IFN-γ production can be obtained *in vivo* by injection of T cell–specific stimuli such as anti-CD3, PPD, or SEA into mice infected with *Bacille Calmette-Guerin* (BCG) (5) or treated with heat-killed *Propionibacterium acnes (P. acnes)* (6). To our surprise, we could also induce high IFN-γ production in the pretreated mice by injection of LPS. Bacterial endotoxin, LPS, can activate macrophages but cannot stimulate T cells or NK cells to produce IFN-γ directly (7). Therefore, we proposed that a novel costimulatory factor for IFN-γ production was produced by LPS-stimulated macrophages *in vivo.*

IL-12 was shown to be produced from activated macrophages and to induce IFN-γ production by T cells and NK cells (8). Indeed, the sera from mice sequentially treated with *P. acnes* and LPS contained high levels of IL-12. However, these sera showed a more striking capacity to induce IFN-γ production than did IL-12 itself, suggesting the presence of other IFN-γ–inducing factors (7,9). Finally, we identified a novel IFN-γ–inducing factor in sera and liver and designated it as IGIF (10,11), which is now designated as IL-18 (12–14). cDNA for human IL-18 was also cloned (15). In principle, human and murine IL-18 are pleiotropic cytokines, and are identical in terms of their structure and functions (11–15). In general, investigators have been seeking novel cytokines using *in vitro* systems. However, the process of IL-18 discovery was unique and resembled that used to find TNF-α. This reminds us of the importance of *in vivo* study for the discovery of unknown factors.

OVERVIEW OF ACTIVITY OF IL-18

As noted above, IL-18 was found in the sera of mice that had been sequentially administered *P. acnes* and LPS (10). IL-18 is synthesized in Kupffer cells and activated macrophages as a precursor form (proIL-18) that requires enzymatic cleavage to become active (16,17). Such cleavage usually occurs intracellularly (16–19), although extracellular processing of pro-IL-18 is also proposed (18). Mature IL-18 is a pleiotropic cytokine that regulates both the innate and acquired immune systems (12–14) (Fig. 7.1). The major

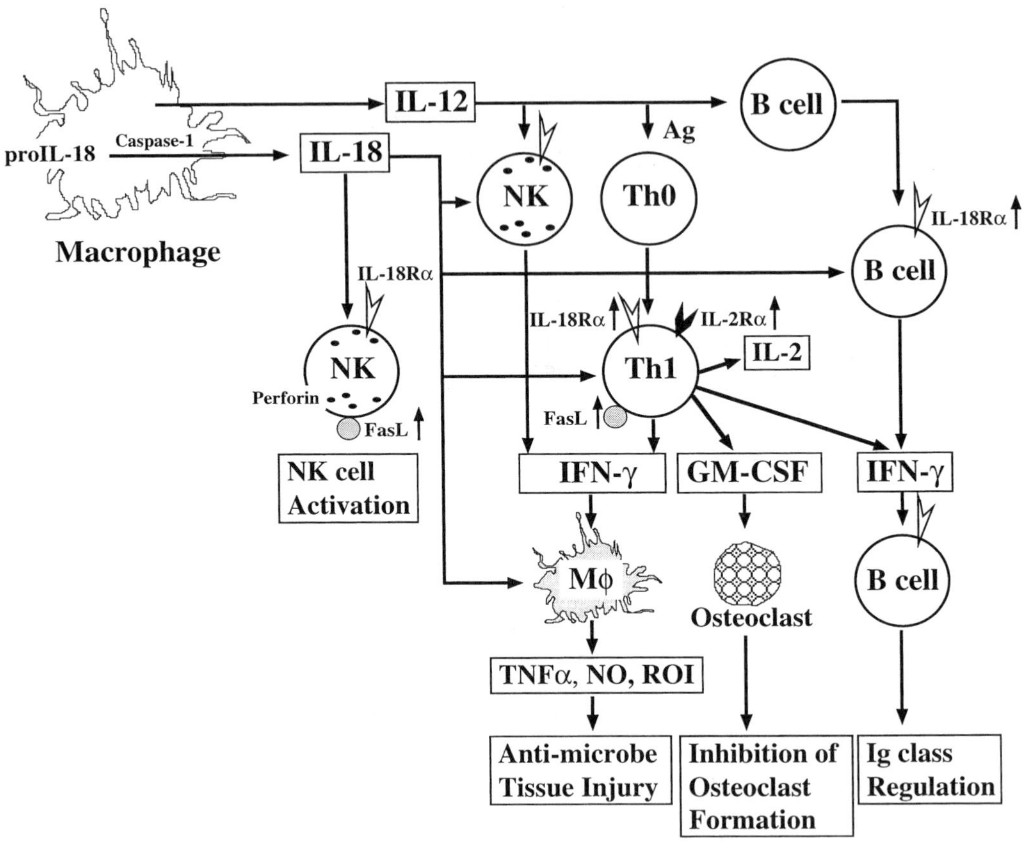

FIG.7.1. Pleiotropic actions of IL-18. IL-18 is a pleiotropic cytokine that regulates both immune cells and nonimmune cells. Both IL-12 and IL-18 are produced by macrophages and synergistically induced IFN-γ production from NK cells, T cells, and B cells. IL-18 stimulates Th1 cells but not Th2 cells, because only Th1 cells express IL-18R. Th1 cells produce ifn-, IL-2, and GM-CSF in response to IL-18. IFN-γ from Th1 and NK cells stimulates macrophages to produce TFNα, nitric oxide, and reactive oxygen intermediates, leading to eradication of intracellular microbes. However, excess production often induces severe tissue injury. Furthermore, IL-18 stimulates NK cells to show NK activity. However, liver NK cells increase FasL when stimulated with IL-18, and kill target cells in a Fas-dependent manner in the liver. GM-CSF from IL-18–stimulated Th1 cells regulates bone metabolism by inhibition of osteoclast formation. Importantly, IFN-γ from IL-18–stimulated Th1 cells and B cells inhibits igE production, suggesting the possibility of a therapeutic use of IL-12 and IL-18 in the treatment of allergic disorders.

activity associated with IL-18 is induction of IFN-γ production from T cells and NK cells, particularly in the presence of IL-12, and enhancement of their cytotoxicity through up-regulation of Fas ligand–mediated mechanisms. Furthermore, IL-18 acts as a costimulant for Th1 cells and augments IFN-γ, IL-2, GM-CSF, and IL-2Rα production, and induces cell proliferation, whereas IL-18 has no effect on IL-4 production or proliferation of Th2 cells. Indeed, the IL-18R is selectively expressed on Th1 cells but not Th2 cells. Thus, expression of IL-18R can be used as a differentiation marker for Th1 cells. Interestingly, IL-18 with IL-12 also induces IFN-γ production from activated B cells, indicating that B cells can also function as a regulatory cell in immune response. The IL-18R consists of IL-1Rrp

(IL-18Rα) and AcPL (IL-18Rβ) (12,14). IL-18Rβ is constitutively expressed on resting T cells, whereas upregulation of IL-18Rα is induced by the action of IL-12. Thus, IL-12 and IL-18 synergistically induce T cells and B cells to develop into IFN-γ–producing cells by induction of IL-18R. In contrast, NK cells constitutively express IL-18R and increase NK activity when stimulated with IL-18 alone. As IFN-γ is a powerful stimulant that acts on macrophages and B cells to produce oxygen radicals and immunoglobulin, respectively, IL-18, an upstream cytokine for IFN-γ, is expected to play an important role in host defenses against various infectious microbes.

MOLECULAR STRUCTURE OF IL-18

The material with IFN-γ–inducing activity was purified either from the sera or the extracts of the liver tissues from *P. acnes*–primed and LPS-challenged mice (10). The samples were sequentially fractionated with ammonium sulfate precipitation, phenyl Sepharose CL-4B, DEAE-Sepharose CL-6B, chromatofocusing Mono P, Superdex-75 and Protein C4 column chromatographies, and preparative SDS-PAGE. Purified IL-18 is a single peptide with a molecular weight of 18,000 and a pI of 4.8 that shows no identity with any other reported proteins (10). Cloned murine and human IL-18 cDNA encode novel proteins consisting of 192 and 193 amino acids, respectively (11,15). The human IL-18 amino acid sequence is 65% homologous to murine IL-18 (15). From these predicted amino acid sequences, it became clear that IL-18 lacks the usual leader sequence necessary for the secretion of IL-18 from the cell membrane, but it does contain an unusual leader sequence, including 35 amino acids at its *N*-terminus. Indeed, like IL-1β, IL-18 is synthesized as a 24-kDa precursor protein, which is then enzymatically cleaved into an 18-kDa biologically active mature protein by IL-1β–converting enzyme (ICE, caspase 1) (11,16–18). Recently, proteinase 3, a serine protease stored in the azurophilic granules of neutrophils and monocytes, has been reported to be an alternative extracellular processing enzyme for IL-1β and IL-18 (18). More recently, we have demonstrated that mature IL-18, like IL-1β, is secreted from macrophages upon stimulation with Fas ligand (FasL) independently of caspase-1 (19). Thus, secretion of mature IL-18 is regulated in several distinct ways.

Although the murine IL-18 peptide shows no apparent similarity to sequences in the databases, it has a 12% homology to murine IL-1α and a 19% homology to murine IL-1β when analyzed by the fold recognition method (20). Homologies between the amino acid sequences for human IL-18 and human IL-1α and those for human IL-18 and human IL-1β are only 15% and 18%, respectively. The conserved protein structure among these cytokines observed in the positions of β-sheets, and IL-1 signature-like sequences, were considered to be important for binding to IL-1 receptor (R), suggesting that IL-18R might have homology to IL-1R. Also, the possibility that IL-18 utilizes the NF-κB signaling strategy was presumed by homology to the IL-1 binding paradigm. Indeed, as lately proven, IL-18 activates NF-κB (21). Although IL-1 failed to inhibit the binding activity of IL-18 to cells (22), the IL-18/IL-18R system is very similar to the IL-1/IL-1R system (14).

GENE AND ITS REGULATION

IL-18 mRNA is constitutively expressed in many cell types. Usually, mRNA for cytokines is not expressed under normal conditions, but is induced after appropriate stimulation. For example, mRNA expression for IL-12 p40, an inducible subunit of IL-12, is strictly regulated. Therefore, IL-12 p40 mRNA expression is not observed in macrophages unless they are activated by stimuli, such as LPS (23,24). This is also the case for IL-1β. In contrast, freshly isolated murine macrophages, human PBMC, and even T cell lines express a substantial amount of IL-18 mRNA without any stimulation (11–14,23–26).

Constitutive expression of IL-18 mRNA in a wide variety of cells is partly due to the particular structure and characteristics of the IL-18 gene. The murine IL-18 gene is composed of seven exons distributed over 26 kb; exons 1 and 2 are considered noncoding (26) (Fig. 7.2). Analysis of the genomic structure to know the mechanism for transcriptional control revealed that there are two distinct promoters identified, one of which is located upstream of exon 1 (5′-flanking region) and the other upstream of exon 2 (intron 1) (26). Interestingly, the promoter activity at the upstream site of exon 2 is constitutively high, while that upstream of exon 1 is upregulatable by activation with LPS, pre-

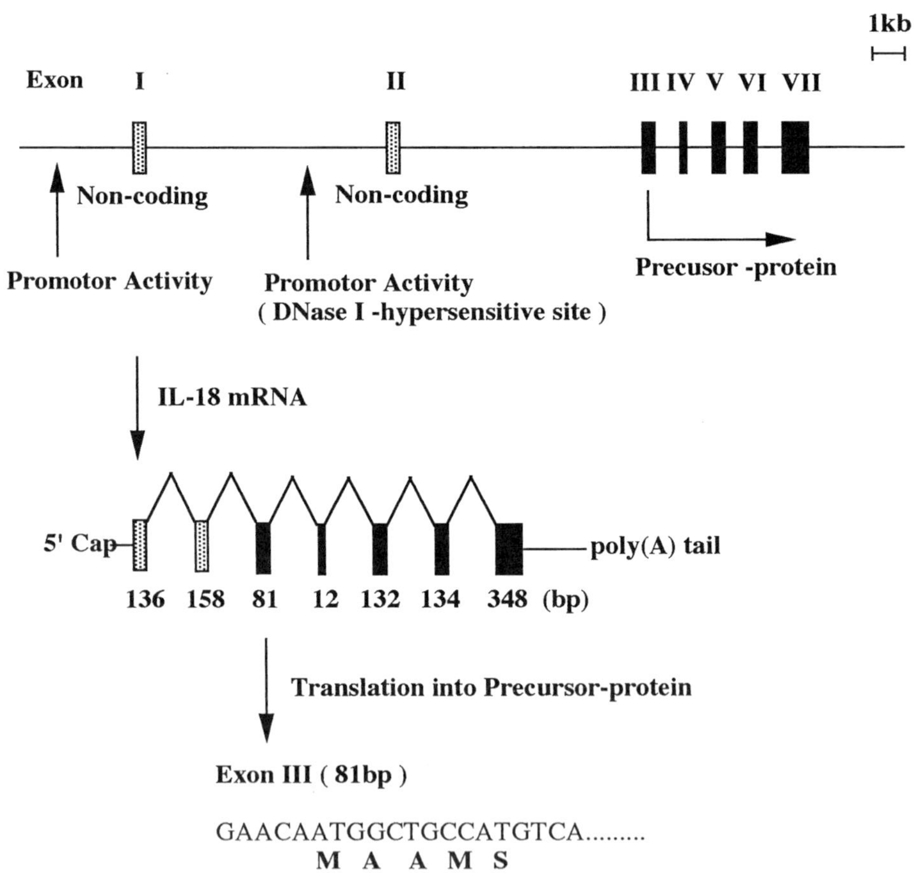

FIG. 7.2. Gene structure of murine IL-18. The murine IL-18 gene comprises seven exons that extend over 26 kb. Exons I and II are considered as 5¹-noncoding exons. Promoter activities are detected in the 5-flanking region and intron 1. Both promoters are TATA-less and not G+C rich. LCSBP (IFN consensus sequence binding protein) and PU.1 bind to promoters in the 5¹-region and intron 1, respectively. The translation initiation site for the IL-18 precursor protein is present in the 5¹-portion of exon iii.

sumably resulting in unusual, constitutive expression of mRNA for IL-18 (11). Recently, IFN consensus sequence binding protein (ICSBP) and PU.1 were shown to bind to the promoters in the 5′-flanking region and intron 1, respectively, suggesting that they are essential for activation of the IL-18 gene (27). These two promoters are TATA-less and non–G+C rich, both of which are used in a wide spectrum of cell types, whereas most other cytokines use a TATA-containing promoter. This may explain why IL-18 is expressed in various cell types including not only macrophages but also nonimmune cells. NF-κB was suggested to be involved in the upregulation of IL-18 gene expression, because a NF-κB recognition sequence is located in the promoter region (26). Moreover, there are also two potential Oct 1 recognition sequences, interacting with the viral transcriptional activator protein VP16, which may also upregulate the expression of the IL-18 gene.

In addition to the spontaneous expression of IL-18 at the transcriptional level, IL-18 mRNA has a long half-life based on the fact that the IL-18 gene has no or only one RNA-destabilizing element (26). Usually, cytokine genes contain so many copies of a RNA-destabilizing element that the cytokine mRNA has a short half-life to exert its action within a restricted period (28). Since the proinflammatory cytokines are responsible for tissue injury, their production may be also downregulated at posttranscriptional levels.

The human IL-18 gene is located on chromosome 11q22.2-22.3, closely linked to the DRD2 (dopamine receptor D2) locus (29). The relative gene order of IL-18 is ATM-IL-18-DRD2-THY1, which is the same as that of murine IL-18 (30). Preliminary experiments on non-obese diabetic (NOD) mice, a mouse model for spontaneous insulin-dependent diabetes mellitus, revealed that the murine IL-18 gene localizes to chromosome 9 within the Idd2 interval, which implicates IL-18 as a NOD susceptibility gene (30).

PROCESSING OF IL-18

As initially predicted by Bazan et al. and by ourselves (11,20), IL-18 has structural similarities to IL-1, particularly IL-1β. Like IL-1β, IL-18 is synthesized as a precursor protein (proIL-18) and is processed by an intracellular cysteine protease, caspase-1. However, recent studies revealed the presence of other processing mechanisms for proIL-18 as described below.

Caspase-1–Dependent Intrinsic IL-18 Processing

Murine IL-18 is produced as a biologically inactive precursor of 24 kDa (proIL-18), which is cleaved into a biologically active mature IL-18 of 18 kDa by caspase-1 (16,17) (Fig. 7.3). Caspase-1 (ICE) is a member of the caspase family, characterized by an intracellular cysteine protease that cleaves after aspartic acid residues in substrates (31,32). Caspase-1 cleaves proIL-18 at Asp^{35}-Asn^{36} (16,17). This was also proven by *in vivo* experiments (16). Serum levels of IL-18 was not elevated in *P. acnes*–primed caspase-1–deficient mice after LPS challenge, whereas they were increased in LPS-challenged *P. acnes*–primed wild-type mice. Elevation of serum IFN-γ, a downstream cytokine induced by IL-18, is also impaired in caspase-1–deficient mice.

Caspase-1 is expressed in many cell types, including T cells, neutrophils, and macrophages (33,34). Like other caspases, caspase-1 is produced in a biologically inactive form. Precursor caspase-1 is a protein of 45 kDa, and is cleaved into a mature form consisting of p10 and p20 subunits by caspase-11 (35) or autoproteolytically (36). LPS has been re-

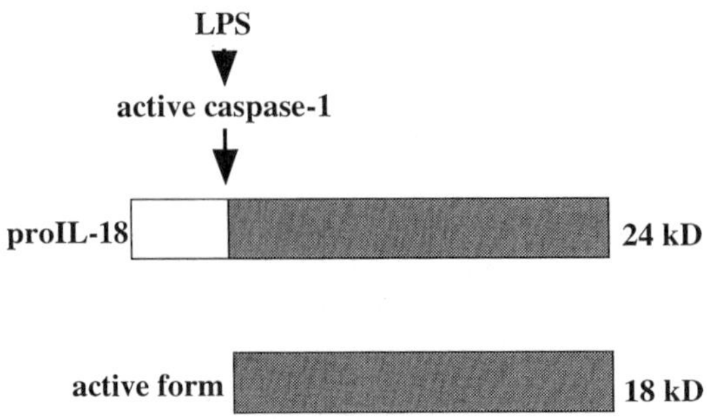

FIG. 7.3. Processing of proIL-18 with caspase-1. IL-18 is synthesized as a 24-kda precursor (proil-18) that is cleaved to the 18-kda mature IL-18 by the active form of caspase-1 induced by stimuli such as LPS.

ported to have the capacity to induce activation of caspase-1 using a human macrophage cell line (37). In fact, caspase-1–dependent IL-18 secretion was observed in murine macrophages upon stimulation with LPS (16). It has also been suggested that caspase-1 is activated by stress, such as reactive oxygen intermediates produced by photooxidative or physical stress (38,39). Interestingly, nitric oxide (NO) directly suppresses the action of caspase-1, resulting in prevention of IL-1β and IL-18 secretion (40). Downregulation of caspase-1 may be important for the protection of the tissues from inflammatory damage and a better strategy for the regulation of biologically active IL-18 production.

Intrinsic Processing of IL-18 by other Proteinases

Caspases other than caspase-1 are involved in cleavage of IL-18. Caspase-4 has the capacity to cleave proIL-18 after ^{35}Asp residue, the same site as caspase-1 does. However, the efficiency of IL-18 processing by caspase-4 is one hundredth or thousandth that of caspase-1 (16). Caspase-3 can also cleave IL-18, either proIL-18 or mature IL-18, but at another site, between Asp^{69} and Ile^{70}, resulting in the accumulation of biologically inactive products (16,41). Therefore, caspase-3 might act as a functional scavenger for mature IL-18 (41). Among caspases, caspase-1 seems to be the authentic processing enzyme for IL-18.

Recently, caspase-1–independent secretion of IL-1β has been demonstrated (42). Thioglycolate-induced murine peritoneal exudate neutrophils secrete IL-1β after stimulation with Fas ligand (FasL). This was observed in the absence of caspase-1. We also observed that both Kupffer cells and splenic macrophages from *P. acnes* –primed caspase-1–deficient mice secreted biologically active IL-18 after stimulation with membrane-associated FasL or soluble FasL (19). This was suppressed by caspase inhibitors, indicating that IL-18 is secreted by FasL-stimulated macrophages using caspases other than caspase-1.

Exogenous Pathway of IL-18 Processing

Recently, proteinase-3, a serine protease, was shown to be able to cleave proIL-18, but presumably at a different cutting site from that of caspase-1 (18). The supernatant of proIL-18 incubated with recombinant proteinase-3 has IFN-γ–inducing activity. Proteinase-3 is a serine protease of 29 kDa localized in the azurophilic granules of neutrophils and monocytes, and in the cytoplasm of endothelial cells (43–45). After being appropriately activated, for example by phagocytosis or stimulation with TNF-α, proteinase-3 is secreted following degranulation and translocates onto the cell surface to exert its enzymatic action (46). This enzyme usually makes a complex in the circulation with α_1-antitrypsin or α_2-macroglobulin, potent protease inhibitors in serum; no free form is found in healthy human serum (46). However, free proteinase-3 appears in some diseases, is elevated in the serum of patients after operation with cardiopulmonary bypass, and appears in inflammatory fluids, such as peritoneal exudate in patients with peritonitis (48–50). Taken together, proteinase-3 may extracellularly exert its enzymatic action to produce biologically active IL-18.

PRODUCING CELLS

Activated macrophages were first shown to produce high levels of IL-18. *P. acnes* –primed and LPS-challenged Kupffer cells showed striking capacity to produce IL-18 (11). Subsequent studies revealed that IL-18 is produced by a wide range of immune competent cells and also by nonimmune cells. Murine macrophages, such as Kupffer cells, splenic macrophages, alveolar macrophages, peritoneal exudate cells, and microglia, secrete functional IL-18 only after activation with appropriate stimuli, such as LPS, phagocytosable substances, and microbial infection (11,24,51–56). In contrast, human peripheral blood mononuclear cells (PBMC) can secrete proIL-18 under normal conditions (25). Thus, human proIL-18 constitutively secreted from PBMC may be cleaved into mature IL-18 extracellularly (18).

Murine dendritic cells, either freshly prepared or derived by culture of bone marrow cells with GM-CSF, in conjunction with IL-4, express IL-18R mRNA (57). Moreover, human dendritic cells derived from human PBMC also constitutively express IL-18 mRNA and produce mature IL-18 (57). A subpopulation of human dendritic cells also express IL-18 mRNA (58). Epidermal cells, particularly keratinocytes, can secrete IL-18, along with IL-12, in response to stimulation with contact allergens (59,60). However, keratinocytes do not have caspase-1 under normal conditions (61) suggesting that contact allergen–induced IL-18 secretion by keratinocytes might be induced in a caspase-1–independent manner, presumably by proteinase-3 extracellularly.

Nonimmune tissues are also sources of IL-18. Intestinal epithelial cells express IL-18 (62). Osteoblastic stromal cells produce IL-18, which inhibits osteoclast-like cell differentiation via induction of GM-CSF but not G-CSF production in lymphocytes (63). Therefore, IL-18 may regulate the balance of bone metabolism. IL-18 is produced by IL-1–stimulated articular chondrocytes (64). IL-18 mRNA is induced in the adrenal cortex, particularly in the zona reticularis and fasciculata that produce glucocorticoid by acute cold stress (65). IL-18 mRNA expression is upregulated in the pancreas of NOD mice after the onset of diabetes mellitus (30). Moreover, IL-18 production is detected in the central nervous system (55,56) as well as the endocrine system (65). These reports allow us to make a hypothesis that IL-18, like IL-1, may play an important role in connecting the immune system to other biosystems, such as endocrine and nervous systems.

IL-18 RECEPTOR

Structure

Human IL-18–binding receptor was purified from L428 cells (human Hodgkin's disease cell line). Scatchard plot analysis of the affinity of IL-18 binding to L428 suggested a single class of low-affinity binding sites for IL-18 (22). A monoclonal antibody that inhibits IL-18 from binding to L428 was used for purification of the human IL-18–binding component (22). The purified protein had a molecular weight between 60 and 100 kDa. Its *N*-terminal and internal amino acid sequences all matched those of human IL-1R–related protein (hIL-1Rrp), which had been published as an orphan receptor belonging to IL-1R family (66,67). COS-1 cells transfected with hIL-1Rrp cDNA showed low-affinity IL-18 binding capacity (K_d 46 nM) (22). Thus, IL-1Rrp is an IL-18–binding component of IL-18R.

A novel member of the IL-1R family, with the highly conserved IL-1R hallmark domains, was recently cloned (68). Based on its homology to IL-1R accessory protein (AcP) (69), a signaling subunit of IL-1R, it is termed an IL-1R AcP–like protein (AcPL). Although AcPL does not directly bind IL-18, coexpression of IL-1Rrp and AcPL is required for mediating IL-18 signaling (68). Since the ligand binding and signaling components of a complex receptor are often termed α and β chains, respectively (14), we have designated IL-1Rrp as IL-18Rα and AcPL as IL-18Rβ in this chapter (Fig. 7.4). However, at this moment, it is uncertain whether the IL-18R composed of IL-18Rα and IL-18Rβ mediates high-affinity IL-18 binding. Recently, a soluble IL-18–binding protein (IL-18 BP) has been cloned (70,71). This protein was purified from human urine. IL-18 BP directly binds to IL-18 and inhibits its IFN-γ–inducing action. IL-18BP may be a soluble decoy receptor, functionally similar to the membrane-associated IL-1R type II. This protein may play a critical role in the regulation of the biological activity of IL-18 *in vivo*.

Murine IL-18Rα is 65 % homologous to human IL-18Rα in overall amino acid sequence. It is related to murine AcP (31% homology), to murine T1/ST2, an orphan receptor of IL-1R family specifically expressed on Th2 cells (30% homology) (72,73), and to murine IL-1R type 1 (27% homology). The cytoplasmic domains exhibit slightly greater sequence homology (36% to 44%) than the extracellular portions (20% to 27%) (66). Murine and human IL-18Rα share 65% identity. Murine IL-18Rβ shows 25% homology to IL-1R type I, 27% to IL-1 AcP, and 26% to IL-18Rα, respectively (68). Murine IL-18 BP is 65.7% identical at the amino acid level with human IL-18BP. There is no apparent homology of IL-18 BP with any other cytokine or cytokine receptor, when examined by the homology research (70).

Human IL-18Rα (IL-1Rrp) maps to chromosome 2q13-21, where genes encoding IL-1β, IL-1β, IL-1R antagonist (IL-1RA), and IL-1 receptors (type 1 and type 2) are located (29,66). On the other hand, human IL-18 maps to chromosome 11q22 closely linked to DRD2 (29). Therefore, genes for IL-18 ligand and IL-18R map to different chromosomes. The gene for IL-18 BP is localized to chromosome 11q13 (70).

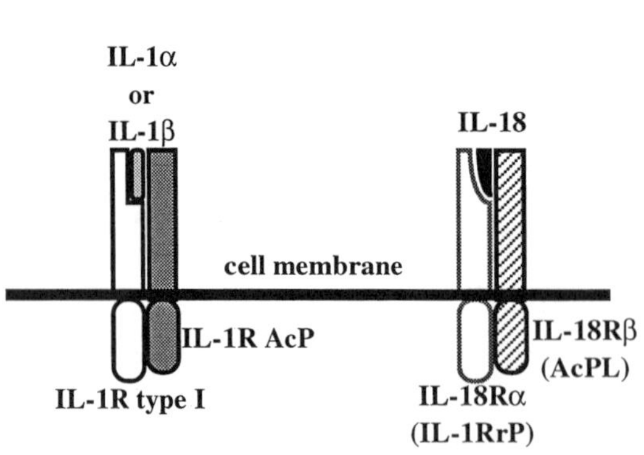

FIG. 7.4. Conformation of IL-1R and IL-18R. Like IL-1R type 1, IL-18Rα has the capacity to bind the ligand IL-18. IL-18Rβ cannot bind IL-18 but with IL-18Rα presumably forms a high-affinity IL-18R that can transduce IL-18 signal into the nucleus.

Regulation of Expression of IL-18R in Lymphoid Cells

Murine splenic T cells only express IL-18Rβ chain, but after stimulation with IL-12 they express the IL-18Rα chain (74–76). Indeed, T cells stimulated with IL-12 have the capacity to specifically bind IL-18 (74,76). The shape of the Scatchard plot is consistent with the presence of both high- and low-affinity IL-18 binding sites. Measurement of ^{125}I-IL-18 bound to IL-12–stimulated T cells revealed that they express 405 high-affinity IL-18R (K_d: 430 pM) and 5,500 low-affinity IL-18R (K_d: 31.4 nM) on each cell (74).

Naive T cells, when stimulated with Ag and IL-12, develop into Th1 cells that express both high- and low-affinity IL-18R (76). Th1 cells from IL-18Rα–deficient mice do not bind IL-18 and do not activate NF-κB or c-jun *N*-terminal kinase (JNK) upon stimulation with IL-18, clearly demonstrating IL-18Rα as an IL-18 binding component (76). IL-18R is not at all expressed on Th2 cells (74,75). In contrast to naïve T cells, NK cells freshly isolated from spleen or liver constitutively express IL-18R, as well as IL-12Rβ2. Both IL-18 and IL-12 augment NK activity independently (77).

IL-18Rα mRNA is detectable in various organs of mice including thymus, spleen, liver, lung, intestine, colon, placenta, prostate, and heart. However, it is not detectable in the brain, kidney, skeletal muscle, or pancreas (66). In addition to the above organs, weak expression of IL-18Rα mRNA is also observed in the testis and ovary. Thus, IL-18Rα mRNA is widely distributed, but not universal. Important questions are as follows: Which cells express the IL-18R? How is the IL-18R expression regulated in these IL-18Rα mRNA–expressing tissues? This may give us some important knowledge to elucidate the physiological roles of IL-18, particularly in nonimmune organs.

IL-18R–MEDIATED SIGNALING PATHWAY

All the members of the IL-1R family are activated in response to infection and contain six distinct, well-conserved domains in their cytoplasmic domains (78). These homologies seem to be important for interactions with signal transducing proteins. IL-18R does not activate JAK/STAT signaling pathways, but shares IL-1R–associated kinase (IRAK) and TNFR-associated factor–6 (TRAF-6) with IL-1R, resulting in nuclear translocation of NF-κB (21,79,80). Indeed, COS cells transfected with a chimeric receptor, in which the IL-18Rα cytoplasmic domain is fused to the extracellular and transmembrane region of type 1 IL-1R, respond to IL-1 by activation of NF-κB (66).

Many cytokines signal through different cell-surface receptors to activate the transcription factor NF-κB to go to the nucleus, where it binds to specific regulatory DNA sequences in the promoters of several cytokine-inducible genes (81). The IFN-γ promoter has consensus sequences for NF-κB, AP-1, a cyclosporin A–sensitive NFAT binding site, an intronic enhancer region (C3), and STAT-4 (82–85). These regions are involved in the regulation of IFN-γ gene expression. Since IL-12 is known to activate STAT-4, and IL-18 as well as IL-12 is shown to activate the binding of c-jun to the AP-1 site (84,85), IL-18 and IL-12 may synergistically induce transcription of the IFN-γ gene through activation of promoter regions of the IFN-γ gene. More importantly, IL-18 utilizes the IRAK/TRAF-6 signaling pathway leading to the activation of NF-κB (22,79), that binds to the NF-κB recognition sequence located at −786 to −776 of the IFN-γ gene regulatory region (designated as KBB site) (86). After activation with IL-18, the IL-18R recruits MyD88, an adapter molecule, providing a platform for IRAK (87,88). IRAK subsequently undergoes phosphorylation and interacts with TRAF-6, leading to nuclear translocation of NF-κB (89) (Fig. 7.5).

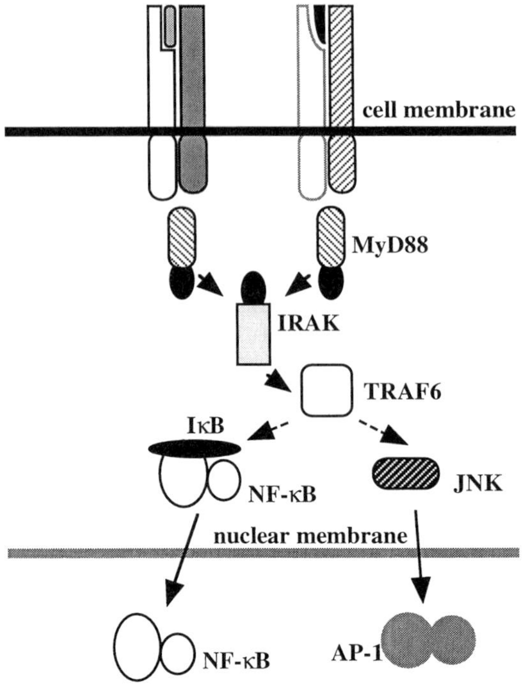

FIG. 7.5. Common signaling pathway shared by IL-1R and IL-18R. When the IL-18R or IL-1R is activated by its corresponding ligand, MyD88 is recruited to the intracellular domain of each receptor, leading to the activation of transcriptional factors.

Targeted disruption of the MyD88 gene resulted in destruction of signaling by both IL-1 and IL-18 (88). T cells from mice with a targeted MyD88 gene are defective in proliferative response as well as induction of acute phase proteins and cytokines in response to IL-1. Increases in IFN-γ production and NK cell activity in response to IL-18 are also abrogated, as is IL-18–induced activation of NF-κB and JNK. Recently, IRAK-deficient mice have been shown to have a defective response to simulation with IL-1 and IL-18 that is similar to that seen in MyD88-deficient mice (90,91). Thus, the IRAK/TRAF6 signaling pathway appears to be a major one. However, there is another distinct signal pathway for IL-18. IL-18 signaling has been suggested to be mediated by mitogen activate protein kinase (MAPK) (92). Protein tyrosine kinase, as well as the *src* kinase LCK, is activated in Th1 cells stimulated with IL-18. Since MAPK pathways are considered to be involved in cell growth, IL-18 may drive proliferation of T and NK cells through this pathway (74,93). Cross-talk between these signaling pathways needs to be further investigated.

BIOLOGICAL FUNCTION *IN VITRO*

IL-18 is a pleiotropic cytokine (Fig.7.1) (12–14). It induces IFN-γ production from T cells, B cells, and NK cells, particularly in the presence of IL-12 (11,84,94–98). Furthermore, IL-18 acts as a costimulant for Th1 cells to augment IFN-γ, IL-2, GM-CSF, and IL-2Rα production, and induces cell proliferation, whereas IL-18 has no effect on Th2 clones (74,76,79,94–97). Indeed, only Th1 clones express IL-18R (74–76,97). Since IFN-γ stimulates macrophages and B cells to produce oxygen radicals and immunoglobulin, respectively, IL-18 is expected to play an important role in host defenses against various infectious microbes. First, we summarize general actions of IL-18 on lymphoid cells *in vitro* and *in vivo*. Then, we demonstrate the potential of IL-18 as a useful therapeutic tool for the treatment of infections that threaten our lives.

Effect of IL-18 on T Cells

IL-18 was originally described as a costimulatory factor for the production of IFN-γ by anti-CD3–stimulated T cells (10–13). However, IL-18 by itself induces only a small amount of IFN-γ in T cells, as is also the case for IL-12. In contrast, combined stimulation of IL-12 and IL-18 is shown to synergistically induce IFN-γ in T cells (10–13,74,79,84,94–97). We found that this action is not enhanced by additional stimulation with immobilized anti-CD3 and that addition of cyclosporin A failed to inhibit it (74). Thus, T cell receptor–mediated T cell activation is not essential for synergistic induction of IFN-γ production by IL-12 and IL-18. However, stimulation with anti-CD3 is a prerequisite condition for induction of Th1 cells. When T cells were stimulated with IL-12 and IL-18 in the presence and absence of anti-CD3, only T cells stimulated under anti-CD3 conditions developed into Th1 cells and increased IFN-γ production in response to IL-18 (74,79). However, T cells stimulated with anti-CD3 and IL-18 did not develop into Th1 cells, showing the cardinal functional difference between IL-12 and IL-18. IL-18 and IL-12 synergize for IFN-γ production from Th1 cells, whereas this combination fails to affect Th2 cells (74,79). Thus, we and others suggested that only Th1 cells express IL-18R and strongly increase IFN-γ production in response to IL-18 (74,75,79). However, mitogenic stimulation such as ConA or PHA induces IFN-γ production from T cells independently of IL-18 (51), suggesting that caspase-1–dependent processing of IL-18 is not needed for IFN-γ production induced by mitogens or antigens.

We compared the number and affinity of IL-18R on fresh T cells, Th1, and Th2 cells. Nonstimulated T cells did not specifically bind ^{125}I-IL-18. In contrast, Th1 cells, which were prepared from freshly isolated T cells followed by incubation with anti-CD3 and IL-12, showed the capacity to specifically bind ^{125}I-IL-18 (76). Furthermore, the Th1 cells increased IL-18Rα mRNA expression as well as protein production (74,75). As expected, IL-18Rα expression was not increased on Th2 cells (74,75), suggesting that the difference of IL-18 responsiveness between Th1 and Th2 cells resulted from their differential expression of IL-18R.

Human T cells also require being stimulated with IL-12 and IL-18 to exhibit their capacity to strongly produce IFN-γ (15,84,99). Human resting CD4$^+$ T cells (CD4$^+$CD45RA$^+$ T cells) express IL-18Rα chain after being stimulated with IL-12 and display dose-dependent production of IFN-γ and proliferation in response to IL-18 (99,100). Thus, increased expression of IL-18R can be used as a differentiation marker for human Th1 cells. Interestingly, simultaneous or ordered stimulation of human T cells with IL-12 and IL-1 induces T cells to produce IFN-γ, suggesting the possibility that IL-1 is also an IFN-γ–inducing factor in human (99).

Effect of IL-18 on CD8$^+$ T Cells

CD8$^+$ T cells are an important source of IFN-γ, and these cells produce high levels of IFN-γ in response to IL-18 (101). CD8$^+$ T cells expressed IL-12Rβ2 but not IL-18R even after exposure to anti-CD3 plus anti-CD28. However, IL-18R expression was induced in $CD8^+$ T cells after additional stimulation with IL-12. Thus, IL-12 stimulation makes $CD8^+$ T cells responsive to IL-18 by induction of the IL-18R (101). The same treatment also induced IL-18R expression on $CD4^+$ T cells, but at a lower level than that in the similarly treated $CD8^+$ T cells. The difference in the level of IL-18R was well correlated to the production of IFN-γ in response to IL-18 (101). Interestingly, IL-18 directly activates the cytoxicity of $CD8^+$ T cells (102), suggesting weak expression of IL-18R on $CD8^+$ T cells.

IL-18 enhances the generation of $CD8^+$ effector T cells in allogeneic mixed lymphocytes culture (103). $CD8^+$ T cells from DBA/2 mice develop into cytotoxic T cells in response to stimulation with mitomycin C–treated splenocytes from BDF1 mice. IL-18 stimulation increases the ratio of $CD8^+/CD4^+$ in the responding cells. Moreover, this stimulation efficiently induced the development of $CD8^+$ effector T cells, that have strong CTL activity against allogeneic target cells and the potential to produce IFN-γ in response to anti-CD3 plus IL-18 or allogeneic cells (C57BL/6 spleen cells) plus IL-18. Thus, IL-18 plays an important role in the development of $CD8^+$ effector T cells.

Effects of IL-18 on B Cells

The activation, proliferation, and differentiation of B cells are highly regulated events in which the action of T cells and their soluble products play a major role (104–108). However, several reports have demonstrated that activated B cells also produce cytokines such as IL-1 (109), IL-6 (110), and IL-10 (111,112). Recently, we showed that a combination of IL-12 and IL-18 induces anti-CD40–activated highly purified murine B cells to produce IFN-γ, which inhibits IL-4–dependent IgE and IgG1 production but enhances IgG2a production without inhibiting the B cell proliferative response (95). Thus, IL-12– and IL-18–stimulated B cells act as regulatory cells that reciprocally regulate IgG1/IgE and IgG2a responses by production of IFN-γ both *in vivo* and *in vitro*. Similarly, these cytokines synergistically induce IFN-γ in B cells from chronic GVHD mice and inhibit Ig production (113). In human PBMC, $CD19^+$ B cells constitutively express IL-18R, and therefore IL-18 may modulate B cells directly (100).

Effects on NK Cells

IL-18, as well as IL-12, was shown to augment functions of NK or NK-T cells (11,15,77,93,114,115). IL-18 acts on NK cells to produce IFN-γ (93,98,114,116). Like its action on T cells, IL-18 alone induces NK cells to produce little IFN-γ, but with IL-12 synergistically induces IFN-γ in NK cells. NK cells constitutively express IL-18R, as well as IL-12Rβ2, and both IL-18 and IL-12 augment NK activity independently of each other (77). IL-18 directly stimulates the cytotoxicity of NK cells, at least independently of IL-2 or IFN-γ (77). This cytotoxicity is exerted through activation of perforin/granzymes. However, as for induction of IFN-γ, stimulation of NK cells with both cytokines induces several hundred-fold more IFN-γ than that induced by either IL-12 or IL-18 alone. Thus, the IFN-γ-inducing activity of IL-18 on NK cells is totally dependent on IL-12. Nuclear run-on analysis revealed that IL-18 in combination with IL-12 enhances transcription of the IFN-γ gene (116). In contrast, its stimulatory activity on cytolysis of NK cells is independent of IL-12. This may indicate that the activation of the signal transducing system for IFN-γ production is not the same as that for perforin- and granzyme-mediated cytotoxicity. IL-18 strongly induces FasL expression in established liver NK cells (114) or Th1 cells (117). However, the physiological meaning of this function remains unknown. Our recent study strongly suggests that FasL might be induced on hepatic NK cells in an IL-18–dependent manner in endotoxin-induced liver injury, in which FasL expressing NK cells might in turn induce IL-18 production by Fas-expressing Kupffer cells, leading to an IL-18–FasL mediated hepatocytotoxicity loop (19). Beside this, IL-18 also acts on NK cells in human PBMCs to produce TNFα, which in turn stimulates IL-1 and IL-8 production from $CD14^+$ cells (118).

Effects on Macrophages

Macrophages and Kupffer cells are major cells that produce IL-12 and IL-18 upon stimulation (11). Interestingly, murine bone-marrow-derived macrophages also produce a large amount of IFN-γ when stimulated with IL-12 and IL-18 (119). Moreover, murine microglial cells not only produce but also respond to IL-18 (56). Thus, the macrophage is a potent inducer of IFN-γ production from T cells, NK cells, and B cells by production of IL-12 and IL-18, but also produces IFN-γ in response to these cytokines (119). IL-18 also stimulates some monocytic cell lines to produce TNFα or ICAM-1 (120,121).

In vitro experiments using the monocytic cell line U1, which contains two copies of HIV-1 in its genome, have demonstrated increased HIV-1 production after stimulation with proinflammatory cytokines, such as IL-1 and TNF-α, or after exposure to IL-6 (122). In these cells, IL-18 increased HIV-1 production 30-fold as measured by synthesis of p24 HIV-1 antigen (120). By gel-shift analysis, binding activity of the transcription factor NF-κB was increased in nuclear extracts from U1 cells 1 h after exposure to IL-18. However, inhibition of TNFα activity by the addition of TNF-binding protein or a neutralizing anti-IL-6 mAb reduced IL-18–stimulated HIV-1 production. In addition, a specific inhibitor of the p38 mitogen-activated protein kinase (MAPK) reduced IL-18–induced HIV-1 replication. These results demonstrate that IL-18–augmented-HIV replication in monocytes is mediated by the induction of TNFα and IL-6, by the activation of p38 MAPK, and by nuclear translocation of NF-κB. These results may suggest a role for IL-18 in HIV-1 pathogenesis. However, at this moment, the production of IL-18 by HIV-infected patients remains unclear. Recently, it was reported that virus infection activates IL-1β and IL-18 production in human macrophages by a caspase-1–dependent pathway (123). Therefore, caspase-1 may represent a target for therapeutic intervention in HIV infection.

BIOLOGICAL FUNCTION *IN VIVO*

Activation of Th1 Cells and NK Cells by IL-18

IL-12 is a major determinant for the development of naïve T cells into IFN-γ–producing Th1 cells *in vitro* (7). The essential role of IL-12 in Th1 cell development *in vivo* has been well established using IL-12– or STAT4–deficient mouse (124,125). IL-18 does not, by itself, induce Th1 cell development but synergizes with IL-12 for IFN-γ production (74,79).Therefore, the requirement of IL-18 for induction of Th1 cells was tested *in vivo* by injecting mice intraperitoneally with heat-killed *P. acnes* (126,127). The hepatic immune system has several unique cells, such as Kupffer cells and hepatic T cells, which are characterized by their expression of intermediate levels of CD3/TCR and IL-2Rβ (128–130). Seven days after injection, splenic T cells and hepatic T cells were purified and stimulated with immobilized anti-CD3 *in vitro*. These T cells strongly produced IFN-γ. Injection of anti–IL-12 Ab totally abrogated these actions of *P. acnes*, while injection of anti–IL-18 Ab did not (130). Furthermore, Kupffer cells prepared from these *P. acnes*–treated mice produced IL-12 and, to a lesser degree, IL-18 *in vitro* (130). To further exclude the possibility of IL-18 as a Th1-inducing factor, we injected *P. acnes* into IL-18–deficient mice (131). Compared to wild-type mice, development of Th1 cells was markedly reduced in *P. acnes*–treated IL-18-deficient mice. We next injected live BCG, which is a much stronger inducer of Th1 cells than heat-killed *P. acnes*, into IL-18–deficienct mice. IL-18–deficient mice showed partial impairment in their Th1 response to BCG infection (131). These results taken together indicate that IL-18 is partially involved in Th1 cell development induced by the action of *P. acnes* or BCG.

Like IL-12 (8), IL-18 is important for the functional development of NK cells (131). IL-18–deficient mice show impaired functional development of NK cells as well as Th1 cells, although the maturation of their T cells or NK cells is intact. IL-18–deficient spleen cells display weaker killing activity than wild-type cells against YAC-1 cells, authentic target cells for the perforin-dependent killing action of NK cells. IL-18-deficient splenocytes as well as IL-12-deficient splenocytes, however, respond like wild-type cells to exogenous IL-12 or IL-18 by augmented NK activity, indicating that the absence of either cytokine does not cause the defect of responsiveness of NK cells to either cytokine. Therefore, IL-12 and IL-18 exert their actions on NK cells independent of each other.

IL-18 as an Inducer of Endotoxin-Induced Liver Injury

IL-18–deficient mice clearly demonstrate that IL-18 is essential for the induction of endotoxin-induced liver injury (132). Mice kept under specific pathogen-free (SPF) conditions compared to humans are relatively resistant to endotoxin, (LPS) (126,127). LPS is a biologically active component localized in the cell wall of gram-negative bacteria that frequently causes severe pathological changes such as septic shock and multiple organ failure. Heat-killed *P. acnes* is one of the sensitizing substances to LPS (126,127). When a small amount of LPS was administered to mice that had been injected with *P. acnes*, most of the mice died of lethal shock, and the mice that survived subsequently suffered from acute liver injury. IL-18 was originally found in the sera of these LPS-challenged *P. acnes*–treated mice (10). The importance of IL-18 in this endotoxin-induced liver injury was suggested by the fact that the administration of neutralizing anti-IL-18 Ab at LPS challenge completely protected *P. acnes*–primed mice from acute liver injury (24). Finally, we know that IL-18–deficient mice are resistant to the endotoxin-induced liver injury (132).

The hepatic immune system has several unique properties based on its anatomical localization. The liver has resident macrophages, Kupffer cells, and resident NK cells. Furthermore, the liver has an abundant number of unique hepatic T cells (128–130). Kupffer cells that have phagocytosed of *P. acnes* produce a small amount of IL-12, which can induce hepatic T cells to develop into Th1 cells and also to express IL-18R (130). After LPS challenge, proinflammatory cytokines are subsequently produced and FasL is eventually induced in the liver (24).

LPS challenge induces rapid secretion of both IL-18 and IL-12 from Kupffer cells, which act on hepatic lymphocytes to produce a huge amount of IFN-γ leading to TNF-α production from Kupffer cells (24). Indeed, neutralizing anti-IL-18 Ab treatment at LPS challenge totally inhibited the induction of IFN-γ mRNA, TNF-α mRNA, and FasL mRNA in the liver, but it does not affect the IL-12 mRNA level. These results indicate that the order of the cytokine activation after LPS challenge is IL-12 and/or IL-18, IFN-γ, TNF-α, and that FasL is a direct product of IL-18 secretion in the liver. Thus, IL-18 is promptly secreted after LPS challenge, and evokes a biohazardous, pro-inflammatory, cytokine network in the liver.

We established liver NK cells from the liver of *P. acnes*–primed mice. These NK cells increase FasL expression in response to IL-18 (114). Transfer of these NK cells after IL-18 stimulation induced liver injury in *P. acnes*–primed mice. Furthermore, NK cell–depleted mice are resistant to the treatment with *P. acnes* and LPS (Tsutsui et al., unpublished data). These results taken together indicate that IL-18 induces Fas-mediated hepatocyte apoptosis by FasL expressing resident NK cells, in addition to the activation of an hepatotoxic cytokine network.

PROTECTIVE ROLE OF IL-18 IN HOST DEFENSE

The principal protective immune response against extracellular microbes consists of specific antibodies and complement. In contrast, intracellular microbes are eliminated by the collaborative actions of phagocytes and T cells. The pattern of T cell cytokine production is pivotal in determining the course of infection (133). Th1 cells are generally associated with resistance to infection with intracellular microbes, whereas Th2 cells are associated with progressive infection. Many pathogenic microbes have evolved to resist innate defense mechanisms. Therefore, protection against such microbes is critically dependent on the function of Th1 cells and NK cells. As noted above, these cells produce IFN-γ in response to IL-12 and IL-18, both of which are produced by macrophages. IFN-γ is a critical factor for NO-dependent killing of microbes by activation of the type 2 isoform of nitric oxide synthase (NOS2) (134,135). IL-18 also directly activates $CD8^+$ T cells (102,103), which play a central role in viral clearance. Additionally, IL-18 as well as IL-12 is accumulated after infection with microbes or microbial products, allowing us to propose the possibility that IL-18 along with IL-12 participates in microbial clearance. Furthermore, exogenous IL-18 might enhance host defense. Along this line, we summarize the roles of IL-18 in host defense.

Bacterial Infection

Mycobacterium avium (M. avium) is an intracellular microorganism that infects and multiplies within macrophages. In a mouse model of disseminated *M. avium* infection, genetically susceptible BALB/c mice show decreased expression of IL-12 and IL-18 in association with a diminished IFN-γ/Th1 response (136). Conversely, resistant DBA/2 mice exhibited increased expression of IL-12, IL-18, and IFN-γ, indicating a good correlation between clearance of *M. avium* and levels of these cytokines (136). To further understand the protective role of endogenous IL-18, IL-18–deficient C57BL/6 mice were infected with *Mycobacterium tuberculosis (M. tuberculosis)* and their capacities to control bacterial growth, granuloma formation, cytokine secretion were examined (137). These mice manifested more marked granulomatous lesions in their lungs and spleens than found in wild-type mice. Furthermore, granulomatous lesion development in IL-18–deficient mice was significantly suppressed by treatment with exogenous IL-18. As compared with the levels in wild-type mice, the splenic IFN-γ levels were low, but the IL-12 levels were equivalent in IL-18–deficient mice. Therefore, IL-18 is important for the generation of protective immunity to mycobacteria, through induction of IFN-γ expression (137).

Leprosy is an infectious disease, in which the balance between Th1 and Th2 cells plays a critical role in determination of disease progression and clinical outcome (138). At one extreme, tuberculoid patients are resistant to infection by virtue of local production of IFN-γ. In contrast, lepromatous leprosy patients have high specific titers but weak cell-mediated immune response because their lesions produce IL-4. In animal models, IL-12 administration resulted in a significant reduction of bacterial counts in mice infected with *M. leprae.* The combination of IL-18 and IL-12 afforded stronger protection in these models (139). Further study using patients infected with *M. leprae* revealed that IL-18 mRNA expression was higher in lesions from resistant tuberculoid as compared with susceptible lepromatous patients, and that monocytes from patients produced IL-18 in response to *M. leprae in vitro* (140). Exogenous IL-18 augmented *M. leprae*–induced IFN-γ in NK cells and T cells from tuberculoid patients, but not those from lepromatous patients *in vitro*, while IL-4 production was not elevated. Moreover, anti-IL-12 Ab partially inhibited *M. leprae*–induced release of IFN-γ in the presence of IL-18, suggesting a combined effect of IL-12 and IL-18 in promoting *M. leprae*–specific Th1 responses, an essential effector weapon for *M. leprae* clearance in the host.

In a model of *Salmonella typhimurium* infection, treatment of mice with anti-IL-18 Ab increased growth of bacteria in the liver and spleen (141). In contrast, administration of IL-18 decreased bacterial numbers in tissue of mice infected with a lethal dose of a virulent strain of salmonella, and protected them from the death in an IFN-γ–dependent manner. Endogenous IL-18 is also involved in defense against infection with *Yersinia enterocolitica* (52). Yersinia-resistant C57BL/6 mice expressed fourfold higher IL-18 mRNA levels than did susceptible BALB/c mice. Administration of anti-IL-18 Ab to infected mice caused a 100- to 1,000-fold increase in bacterial counts in the spleen, indicating that IL-18 is involved in clearance of Yersinia.

Fungal Infection

IL-18 exerts antifungal activity against *Cryptococcus neoformans (C. neoformans).* Peritoneal exudate cells incubated with IL-18, together with IL-12, suppress the growth of *C. neoformans* (142). The effect is dependent on both IFN-γ production by NK cells and NO production by macrophages and is enhanced by TNF-α in an autocrine manner (143), suggesting that IL-18 plays an important role in innate immunity in collaboration with IL-12. Indeed, administration of IL-18 (10 μg/mouse/day) significantly prolonged the survival time of infected mice and reduced their lung and brain loads of organisms by inducing IFN-γ (144). Moreover, IL-12 and IL-18, when used in combination at their individual subtherapeutic, nonprotective doses (0.005 and 2 μg/mouse/day, respectively), showed significant protective effect by upregulation of IFN-γ production but downregulation of IL-4 production (145). The protective effect of these cytokines was mediated by inducing the production of IFN-γ by NK and γδ T cells, but not $CD4^+$ T cells, in the lung during the early period of infection (145).

Viral Infection

The importance of IL-18 is also proved in some vial infections. A protective effect of IL-18 against infection with *Herpes simplex* virus (HSV) was shown in a mouse model (146). Administration of IL-18 to mice before infection remarkably improved survival rates. The effect is also observed in athymic nude mice and SCID mice, suggesting that IL-18 augments innate defensive immunity. The effect is dependent on IFN-γ, but independent of NK cells and NO, leaving the source of IFN-γ obscure. Infection with influenza A virus results in accumulation of IFN-α/β, TNF-α, IL-1β, and IL-18, whereas the production of IL-12 was not detected (147). Supernatants from influenza A virus–infected macrophages induced rapid IFN-γ production in T cells. This was downregulated by the addition of anti–IFN-α/β Abs. Exogenously added IFN-α/β also rapidly stimulated the synthesis of IFN-γ. IL-18 synergized with IFN-α to upregulate IFN-γ production. Therefore, IFN-α/β and IL-18 produced by macrophages during virus infection may act together to induce IFN-γ synthesis and, consequently, may play an important role for both of these cytokines in the development of type 1 immune responses. *In vivo* antiviral effect of IL-18 was also investigated in a mouse model of vaccinia virus infection (148). Intraperitoneal injection of IL-18 significantly suppressed pock formation on the tails of BALB/c mice inoculated intravenously with Vaccinia virus. However, this effect seems to be solely dependent on NK cells or IFN-γ. Participation of various host defense mechanisms including NK cells, CTL and IFN-γ may be important. It has been also revealed that several poxviruses encode putative proteins highly homologous to IL-18BP, which binds IL-18 and blocks its biological activity (70). A remarkable feature of poxvirus infection in humans is multiple small skin lesions, containing a large number of virus particles but lacking inflammatory cell infiltrates. Since IL-18 induces the chemokine IL-8 (118), inhibition of IL-18 by a poxvirus-encoded protein may attenuate the inflammatory antiviral response in host.

Protozoan Infection

Cutaneous inoculation of *Leishmania major (L. major)* induces in most inbred mouse strains a localized lesion that heals spontaneously, resulting in acquisition of resistance to reinfection. However, some susceptible strains develop a fatal visceral illness. Resistance and susceptibility of inbred strain of mice to *L. major* are associated with IFN-γ and IL-4 dominant production by T cells, respectively (133,145,146). $CD4^+$ T cells from regional lymph nodes of infected C57BL/6 mice, a resistant strain, contain high levels of IFN-γ but little IL-4, while $CD4^+$ T cells from infected BALB/c mice, a susceptible one, contain high levels of IL-4 but little IFN-γ (133,149,150). Healing and nonhealing of the infected host can be convertible. Host resistance can be transferred by administration of anti–IL-4 (151) or IL-12 (152) into the susceptible mice. In contrast, host susceptibility can be transferred by the reverse treatments, anti–IFN-γ (153) or anti–IL-12 Ab (154). Healing of lesions caused by *L. major* infection requires the induction and expansion of Th1 cells that produce IFN-γ, a crucial activator of NOS2 (134,135,155). NO production is critical in the killing of intracellular parasites including *L. major* (156). In contrast, IL-4 produced by Th2 cells promotes disease, because IL-4 inhibits the expression of NOS2 (157). The importance of the NO-dependent killing of intracellular parasites was demonstrated by the fact that NOS2-deficient mice developed nonhealing Leishmanial lesions even on a resistant background (158).

IFN-γ plays a pivotal role in protection against *L. major* infection. Since IL-12 and IL-18 synergize for IFN-γ production from T cells, B cells, and NK cells, we investigated whether IL-18 is critically involved in host defense against *L. major* infection (159). We daily administered IL-12 and/or IL-18 into BALB/c mice during the first week after infection. Neither IL-12 (10 ng/mouse) nor IL-18 (1 μg/mouse) solely induced wound healing, while the combination completely protected them from *L. major* infection–induced footpad swelling in a NO-dependent manner (Ohkusu K, Yoshimoto T, Takeda K, et al., unpublished data). Furthermore, these mice acquired protective immunity against *L. major* reinfection. We also investigated a protective role of endogenous IL-18 in *L. major*–resistant C3H/HeN mice. Treatment with neutralizing anti-IL-18 Ab markedly reduced resistance to *L. major* infection by downregulation of IFN-γ production, leading to diminished NO production upon *L. major* infection. Moreover, compared to their wild-type littermates, IL-18–deficient mice on a resistant background (129/SvJ × C57BL/6, C57BL/6) clearly showed reduced resistance to *L. major* infection (160). Thus, IL-18 is critically involved in host immunity to *L. major* infection. Administration of IL-12 and IL-18 provides us with a good therapeutic for *L. major* infection. Furthermore, this combination may also allow us to rationally design *L. major* vaccination.

Vaccination with DNA encoding the immunodominant LACK parasite antigen can elicit prolonged protective immunity to *L. major* in an IL-12/IFN-γ–dependent manner (161). LACK DNA induces IFN-γ from both $CD4^+$ and $CD8^+$ T cells, while LACK protein plus IL-12 induces IFN-γ from only $CD4^+$ T cells. LACK is only processed in the endosome, resulting in binding to class II, while DNA-derived-proteins can bind to both class I and class II depending on their processing pathways. When the proteins are secreted from the transfected cells, they are processed in APC and are presented associated with MHC class II. However, when DNA-derived-proteins are processed in the proteasome without being secreted, they bind to class I. Thus, DNA vaccines may be more a powerful way to protect the host from infection than protein vaccines. Recently, a recombinant leishmania protein, LeIF has been shown to stimulate the Th1 response and to protect BALB/c mice from *L. major* in an IL-12– and IL-18–dependent manner (162). Since the production of IFN-γ by LeIF-stimulated SCID splenocytes is suppressed by the addition of neutralizing antibody to IL-12 or IL-18 in a dose-dependent manner, vaccination with LeIF must stimulate macrophages to produce IL-12 and IL-18 for protection.

IFN-γ is produced after infection with *Trypanosoma cruzi* and has been shown to be crucial in the determination of resistance or susceptibility. IFN-γ was present in high amounts in the serum and in the supernatants of unseparated spleen cells or isolated splenic $CD4^+$ and $CD8^+$ T cells from infected mice when stimulated with *T. cruzi ex vivo.* Using the *in situ* hybridization technique, it has been shown that mRNAs for IL-12 p40 and IL-18 were induced in the spleen by parasitic infection and that these expressions were high during infection with the *T. cruzi* (163). The message for IL-18 was produced earlier during infection and had declined until day 38, when IFN-γ and IL-12 p40 transcripts were optimally expressed. Therefore, *T. cruzi* induces strong IL-12 and IL-18 gene expression *in vivo*, correlating with IFN-γ production.

Malaria is a mosquito-borne infection caused by protozoa of the genus *Plasmodium.* In spite our extensive effort to eradicate this disease, malaria remains one of the most prevalent infectious diseases in tropical and subtropical regions (164). The infection is initiated when sporozoites are injected into the host by the bite of infected mosquitoes *(Anopheles).* Natural infection in the intermediate host, such as mice or humans, consists of two stages corresponding to the life cycle of *Plasmodium*. The sporozoites enter the bloodstream and are rapidly phagocytosed by Kupffer cells and from there pass into hepatocytes, where sporozoites develop into merozoites by an asexual division (165). This is an asymptomatic liver stage. One or two weeks after infection, the infected hepatocytes rupture, releasing thousands of merozoites, thereby initiating the recycling erythrocyte stage of their life cycle (166). This is a blood stage in which the host suffers from systemic illness.

The type of T cell response varies with the stage of infection (167,168). $CD4^+$ T cells mediate immunity against the blood stage, while $CD8^+$ T cells protect against the liver stage (166,169–171). The immune response to extraerythrocytic stages of infection is extensively studied using a murine model system. The protective effects of $CD8^+$ T cells may be mediated by a direct lysis of infected hepatocytes or indirectly by activation of macrophages to produce NO and TNF-α (172,173) that kills parasites.

Resistance to challenge with *P. berghei* sporozoite infection is abrogated by treatment with anti-IFN-γ (167,170), indicating that T-cell– or NK cell–mediated immunity plays a critical role in host defense against infection with *Plasmodium*. We can infect mice by inoculation of the erythrocytic stage. To investigate the symptomatic blood stage of plasmodium infection, we inoculated mice with parasitized erythrocytes. Inoculated mice suffered from liver injury. Histological investigation revealed focal cell necrosis in the liver. Hepatocytes in the lesion were stained with the terminal deoxynucleotidyl transferase (TdT)-mediated dUTP-biotin nick end labeling (TUNEL) method, indicating that they died due to apoptosis (Kashiwamura S, unpublished data). IL-18 was originally found in the serum and the Kupffer cells from the mice sequentially treated with *P. acnes* and LPS (11). We found much higher levels of serum IL-18 in the *P. berghei*–inoculated mice. To determine whether endogenous IL-18 plays a role in defending against *Plasmodium* infection, we administered anti–IL-18. This treatment clearly shortened the survival times of these infected mice (Kashiwamura S, unpublished data). To substantiate further this observation, we injected IL-12 and/or IL-18 into the mice inoculated with *P. berghei*. It has been already reported that injection of IL-12 in sporozoite-infected mice strikingly reduced parasitemia (174). We found that a combination of low doses of IL-12, which by itself shows no toxicity, and relatively high doses of IL-18 diminished mortality of the mice inoculated with *P. berghei* (Kashiwamura S, unpublished observation).

The administration of IL-18, particularly in collaboration with IL-12, seems to be rational for some intractable infections. However, the combination of IL-12 and IL-18 is toxic at relatively high doses. IL-12 has been shown to induce severe pathologic changes in mice (175). In this case, IL-12 causes pulmonary edema and is lethal in IFN-γ–deficient mice. On the other hand, administration of IL-18 (5 μg/day) to mice apparently causes no pathologic changes, but combined administration of IL-12 (0.2 μg/day) and IL-18 (2 μg/day) causes serious diarrhea, notable fatty degeneration in the liver, atrophy of many organs, and even mortality (12). In contrast to the IL-12–induced pathology, IL-18 with IL-12 fails to manifest any pathologic changes in IFN-γ–deficient mice.

CONCLUSION

IL-18 is a pleiotropic cytokine. It induces IFN-γ in T cells, B cells, and NK cells, particularly in the presence of IL-12. IL-18 enhances Fas- or perforin-dependent cytotoxicity of T cells and NK cells. IL-18 acts as a costimulant for Th1 cells, whereas IL-18 has no effect on Th2 cells. However, recent studies indicate that IL-18 without help from IL-12 can stimulate T cells, NK cells, and basophils to produce IL-4 and/or IL-13 (176,177). Thus, the outcome of IL-18 stimulation essentially depends on the presence of IL-12 (Fig. 7.6).

In collaboration with IL-12, IL-18 accelerates inflammatory reaction. IL-18, in some cases, such as host defense and tumor surveillance, protects us, or in other cases, including various tissue injuries, threatens our lives. IL-18 is profoundly involved in the tissue injury in the experimental model of fulminant hepatitis (11). This cytokine seems to be involved in the pathogenesis of some types of inflammatory diseases. However, IL-18 can

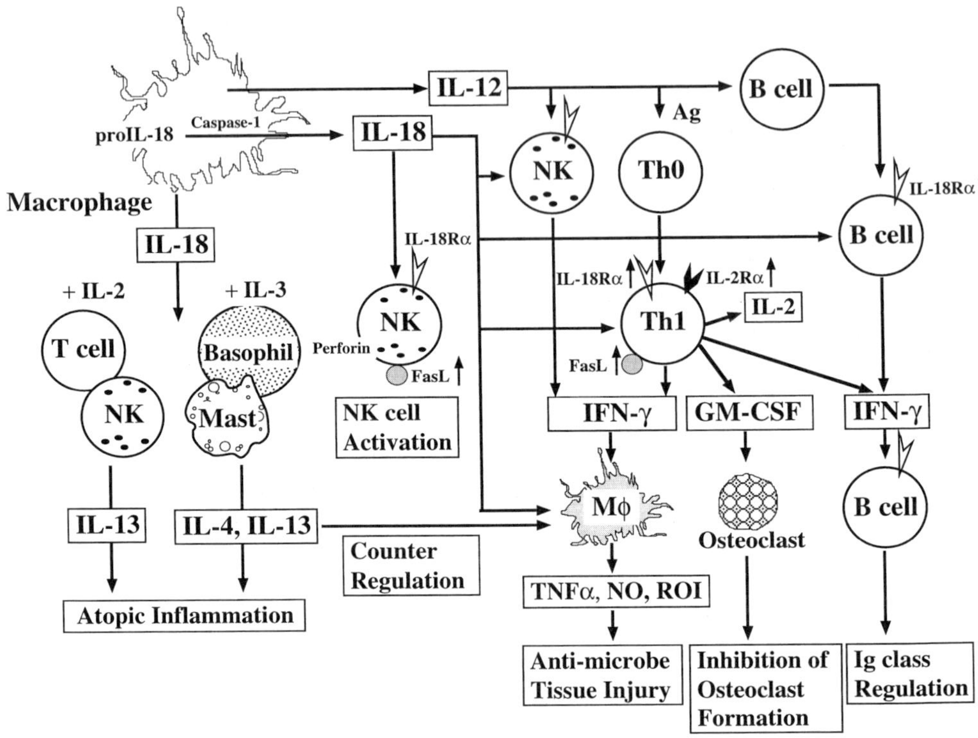

FIG. 7.6. IL-18 stimulates TH1/NK cells along with IL-12, but also acts on T cells, NK cells, and basophils to produce IL-4 and/or IL-13. As shown in the legend of Fig. 7.1, IL-18 stimulates TH1 cells, NK cells, and B cells to produce IFN-γ, which stimulates macrophages to produce cytotoxic factors such as TNF-α, NO, and ROI. IL-18, without help from IL-12, induces TH2 cytokines.

also induce a counter-inflammatory action through induction of IL-4 and IL-13, when IL-12 is not coactivated. This may give a new aspect of possible involvement of IL-18 in atopic responses. In addition to diverse functional features of IL-18 in the immune system, it seems to exert its actions in the nonimmune system because of the expression of IL-18 and/or IL-18R in a wide variety of organs, particularly in tissue parenchymal cells, such as keratinocytes, osteoblasts, chondrocytes, intestinal epithelial cells, microglia, and adrenal cortex cells. This allows us to propose IL-18 as a connecting factor between the immune and other nonimmune systems, including the endocrine and nervous systems. This is an important issue to be elucidated in the following years.

Since IFN-γ plays a pivotal role in host defense, IL-18, an upstream cytokine for IFN-γ, is expected to play an important role against various infectious microbes. Although IL-18 is a potent candidate, therapeutic agent, particularly for intractable infections, we should be reminded that IL-18 gives extremely different effects dependently of the microenvironments. In addition, it should be noted that the administration of overdoses of IL-18, especially in conjunction with IL-12, sometimes results in tissue inflammation. Nevertheless, we hope IL-18 will give us a novel strategy against microbial infection. We believe that upon careful usage IL-18 will be a useful weapon against microbial infections that threaten our lives.

REFERENCES

1. Wheelock E. Interferon-like virus-inhibitor induced in human leukocytes by phytohemagglutinin. *Science* 1965;149:310.
2. Farrar M, Schreiber R. The molecular cell biology of interferon-γ and its receptor. *Annu Rev Immunol* 1993; 11:571.
3. Billiau A. Interferon-γ: biology and role in pathogenesis. *Adv Immunol* 1996;62:61.
4. Boehm U, Klamp T, Groot M, et al. Cellular responses to interferon-γ. *Annu Rev Immunol* 1997;15:749.
5. Wada M, Okamura H, Nagata K, et al. Cellular mechanisms in in vivo production of gamma interferon induced by lipopolysaccharide in mice infected with *Mycobacterium bovis* BCG. *J Interferon Res* 1985;5:431.
6. Okamura H, Kawaguchi K, Shoji K, et al. High-level induction of gamma interferon with various mitogens in mice pretreated with *Propionibacterium acnes*. *Infect Immun* 1982;38:440.
7. Nakamura K, Okamura H, Wada K, et al. Endotoxin-induced serum factor that stimulates gamma interferon production. *Infect Immun* 1989;38:590.
8. Trinchieri G. Interleukin-12: a proinflammatory cytokine with immunoregulatory functions that bridge innate resistance and antigen-specific and adaptive immunity. *Annu Rev Immunol* 1995;13:251.
9. Nakamura K, Okamura H, Nagata K, et al. Purification of a factor which provides a costimulatory signal for gamma interferon production. *Infect Immun* 1993;61:64.
10. Okamura H, Nagata K, Komatsu T, et al. A novel costimulatory factor for gamma interferon induction found in the liver of mice causes endotoxic shock. *Infect Immun* 1995;63:3966.
11. Okamura H, Tsutsi H, Komatsu T, et al. Cloning of a new cytokine that induces IFN-γ production by T cells. *Nature* 1995;378:88.
12. Okamura H, Tsutsui H, Kashiwamura S, et al. Interleukin-18: a novel cytokine that augments both innate and acquired immunity. *Adv Immunol* 1998;70:281.
13. Okamura H, Kashiwamura S, Tsutsui H, et al. Regulation of interferon-γ production by IL-12 and IL-18. *Curr Opin Immunol* 1998;10:259.
14. Dinarello CA. IL-18: A Th1-inducing, proinflammatory cytokine and new member of the IL-1 family. *J Allergy* Clin Immunol 1999;103:11.
15. Ushio S, Namba M, Okura T, et al. Cloning of the cDNA for human IFN-γ-inducing factor, expression in *Escherichia coli*, and studies on the biologic activities of the protein. *J Immunol* 1996;156:4274.
16. Gu Y, Kuida K, Tsutsui H, et al. Activation of interferon-γ inducing factor mediated by interleukin-1β converting enzyme. *Science* 1997;275:206.
17. Ghayur T, Banerjee S, Hugunin M, et al. Caspase-1 processed IFN-γ–inducing factor and regulates LPS-induced IFN-γ production. *Nature* 1997;386:617.
18. Fantuzzi G, Dinarello CA. Interleukin-18 and interleukin-1β: two cytokine substrates for ICE (caspase-1). *J Clin Immunol* 1999;19:1.
19. Tsutsui H, Kayagaki N, Kuida K, et al. Caspase-1–independent, Fas/Fas ligand-mediated IL-18 secretion from macrophages causes acute liver injury in mice. *Immunity* 1999;11:359.
20. Bazan JF, Timans JC, Kastelein. RA. A newly defined interleukin-1. *Nature* 1996;379.
21. Matsumoto S, Tsuji TK, Aizawa Y, et al. Interleukin-18 activates NF-κB in murine T helper type 1 cells. *Biochem Biophys Res Commun* 1997;234:454.
22. Torigoe K, Ushio S, Okura T, et al. Purification and characterization of the human Interleukin-18–receptor. *J Biol Chem* 1997;271:25737.
23. Marshall JD, Aste AM, Chehimi SS, et al. Regulation of human IL-18 mRNA expression. *Clin Immunol* 1999; 90:15.
24. Tsutsui H, Matsui K, Kawada N, et al. IL-18 accounts for both TNF-α- and Fas ligand-mediated hepatotoxic pathways in endotoxin-induced liver injury in mice. *J Immunol* 1997;159:3961.
25. Puren AJ, Fantuzzi G, Dinarello CA. Gene expression, synthesis, and secretion of interleukin 18 and interleukin 1β are differentially regulated in human blood mononuclear cells and mouse spleen cells. *Proc Natl Acad Sci USA* 1999;96:2256.
26. Tone M, Thompson SA, Tone Y, et al. Regulation of IL-18 (IFN-γ–inducing factor) gene expression. *J Immunol* 1997;159:6156.
27. Kim Y-M, Kang T-S, Paik S-G, et al. Roles of IFN consensus sequence binding protein and PU.1 in regulating IL-18 gene expression. *J Immunol* 1999;163:2000.
28. Cosman D. Control of messenger RNA stability. *Immunol Today* 1987;8:16.
29. Nolan KF, Greaves DR, Waldmann H. The human interleukin 18 gene IL-18 maps to 11q22.2-q22.3, closely linked to the DRD2 gene locus and distinct from mapped IDDM loci. *Genomics* 1998;51:161.

30. Rothe H, Jenkins NA, Copeland NG, et al. Active stage of autoimmune diabetes is associated with the expression of a novel cytokine, IGIF, which is located near Idd2. *J Clin Invest* 1997;99:469.
31. Cohen GM. Caspases: the executioners of apoptosis. *Biochem J* 1997;326:1.
32. Alnemri ES, Livingston DJ, Nicholson DW, et al. Human ICE/CED-3 protease nomenclature. *Cell* 1996;87:171.
33. Cerretti DP, Kozlosky CJ, Mosley B, et al. Molecular cloning of the interleukin-1β converting enzyme. *Science* 1992;256:97.
34. Singer II, Scott S, Chin J, et al. The interleukin-1β–converting enzyme (ICE) is localized on the external cell surface membranes and in the cytoplamsic ground substance of human monocytes by immuno-electron microscopy. *J Exp Med* 1995;182:1447.
35. Wang S, Miura M, Jung Y-K, et al. Murine caspase-11, an ICE-interacting protease, is essential for the activation of ICE. *Cell* 1998;92:501.
36. Ramage P, Cheneval D, Chvei M, et al. Expression, refolding, and autocatalytic proteolytic processing of the interleukin-1β–converting enzyme precursor. *J Biol Chem* 1995;270:9378.
37. Schumann RR, Belka C, Reuter D, et al. Lipopolysaccharide activates caspase-1 (interleukin-1–converting enzyme) in cultured monocytic and endothelial cells. *Blood* 1998;91:577.
38. Kirshnamoorthy RR, Crawford MJ, Chaturvedi MM, et al. Photo-oxidative stress down-modulates the activity of nuclear factor-κB via involvement of caspase-1, leading to apoptosis of photoreceptor cells. *J Biol Chem* 1999;274:3734.
39. Clark RSB, Kochanek PM, Chen M, et al. Increases in Bcl-2 and cleavage of caspase-1 and caspase-3 in human brain after head injury. *FASEB J* 1999;13:813.
40. Kim YM, Talanian RV, Li J, et al. Nitric oxide prevents IL-1β and IFN-γ–inducing factor (IL-18) release from macrophages by inhibiting caspase-1 (IL-1β–converting enzyme). *J Immunol* 1998;161:4122.
41. Akita K, Ohtsuki T, Nukada Y, et al. Involvement of caspase-1 and caspase-3 in the production and processing of mature human interleukin 18 in monocytic THP.1 cells. *J Biol Chem* 1997;272:26595.
42. Miwa K, Asano M, Horai R, et al. Caspase-1–independent IL-1β release and inflammation induced by the apoptosis inducer Fas ligand. *Nat Med* 1998;4:1287.
43. Campanelli D, Melchior M, Fu Y, et al. Cloning of cDNA for proteinase 3: A serine protease, antibiotic, and autoantigen from human neutrophils. *J Exp Med* 1990;172:1709.
44. Mayet W-J, Csernok E, Szymkowiak C, et al. Human endothelial cells express proteinase 3, the target antigen aof anticytoplasmic antibodies in Wegener's granulomatosis. *Blood* 1993;82:1221.
45. Csernok E, Lüdemann J, Gross WL, et al. Ultrastructural localization of proteinase 3, the target antigen of anticytoplasmic antibodies circulating in Wegener's granulomatosis. *Am J Pathol* 1990;137:1113.
46. Ernst CM, Schmitt W, Bainton DF, et al. Activated neutrophils express proteinase 3 on their plasma membrane in vitro and in vivo. *Clin Exp Immunol* 1994;95:244.
47. Bergenfeldt M, Axelsson L, Ohlsson K. Release of neutrophil proteinase 4 (3) and leukocyte elastase during phagocytosis and their interaction with proteinase inhibitors. *Scand J Clin Lab Invest* 1992;52:823.
48. Dolman KM, va de Wiel BA, Kam C-M, et al. Determination of proteinase 3-α1-antitrypsin complexes in inflammatory fluids. *FEBS Lett* 1993;314:117.
49. Lundberg E, Bergenfeldt M, Ohlsson K. Release of immunoreactive human neutrophil proteinase 4, normally and in peritonitis. *Scand J Clin Lab Invest* 1991;51:23.
50. Jönsson P. Cardiopulmonary bypass causes release of leukocyte proteinase-3. *Scand J Clin Lab Invest* 1996; 56:721.
51. Fantuzzi G, Puren AJ, Harding MW, et al. Interleukin-18 regulation of interferon γ production and cell proliferation as shown in interleukin-1β–converting enzyme (caspase-1)–deficient mice. *Blood* 1998;91:2118.
52. Bohn E, Sing A, Zumbihl R, et al. IL-18 (IFN-γ–inducing factor) regulates early cytokine production in, and promotes resolution of, bacterial infection in mice. *J Immunol* 1998;160:299.
53. Shibata Y, Foster LA, Kurimoto M, et al. Immunoregulatory roles of IL-10 in innate immunity: IL-10 inhibits macrophage production of IFN-γ–inducing factors but enhances NK cell production of IFN-γ. *J Immunol* 1998;161:4283.
54. Sanchez-Bueno A, Verkhusha V, Tanaka Y, et al. Interferon-γ–dependent expression of inducible nitric oxide synthase, interleukin-12, and interferon-γ–inducing factor in macrophages elicited by allografted tumor cells. *Biochem Biophys Res Commun* 1996;224:555.
55. Conti B, Park LC, Calingasan NY, et al. Cultures of astrocytes and microglia express interleukin 18. *Brain Res Mol Brain Res* 1999;67:46.
56. Prinz M, Hanisch UK. Murine microglial cells produce and respond to interleukin-18. *J Neurochem* 1999;72:2215.
57. Stoll S, Jonuleit H, Schmitt E, et al. Production of functional IL-18 by different subtypes of murine and human dendritic cells (DC): DC-derived IL-18 enhances IL-12–dependent Th1 development. *Eur J Immunol* 1998;28: 3231.
58. de Saint-Vis B, Fugier VI, Massacrier C, et al. The cytokine profile expressed by human dendritic cells is dependent on cell subtype and mode of activation. *J Immunol* 1998;160:1666.
59. Stoll S, Muller G, Kurimoto M, et al. Production of IL-18 (IFN-γ–inducing factor) messenger RNA and functional protein by murine keratinocytes. *J Immunol* 1997;159:298.
60. Aragane Y, Riemann H, Bhardwaj RS, et al. IL-12 is expressed and released by human keratinocytes and epidermoid carcinoma cell lines. *J Immunol* 1994;153:5366.

61. Mizutani H, Black R, Kupper TS. Human keratinocytes produce but do not process pro-interleukin-1 (IL-1) β. *J Clin Invest* 1991;87:1066.
62. Takeuchi M, Nishizaki Y, Sano O, et al. Immunohistochemical and immuno-electron-microscopic detection of interferon-γ-inducing factor ("interleukin-18") in mouse intestinal epithelial cells. *Cell Tissue Res* 1997; 289:499.
63. Udagawa N, Horwood NJ, Elliott J, et al. Interleukin-18 (interferon-γ–inducing factor) is produced by osteoblasts and acts via granulocyte/macrophage colony-stimulating factor and not via interferon-γ to inhibit osteoclast formation. *J Exp Med* 1997;185:1005.
64. Olee T, Hashimoto S, Quach J, et al. IL-18 is produced by articular chondrocytes and induces proinflammatory and catabolic responses. *J Immunol* 1999;162:1096.
65. Conti B, Jahng JW, Tinti C, et al. Induction of interferon-γ–inducing factor in the adrenal cortex. *J Biol Chem* 1997;272:2035.
66. Parnet P, Garka KE, Bonnet TP, et al. IL-1Rrp is a novel receptor-like molecule similar to the type I Interleukin-1 receptor and its homologues T1/ST2 and IL-1R AcP. *J Biol Chem* 1996;271:3967.
67. Sims JE, Gayle MA, Slack JL, et al. Interleukin-1 signaling occurs exclusively via the type I receptor. *Proc Natl Acad Sci USA* 1993;90:6155.
68. Born TL, Thomassen E, Bird TA, et al. Cloning of a novel receptor subunit, AcPL, required for interleukin-18 signaling. *J Biol Chem* 1998;273:29445.
69. Greenfeder SA, Nunes P, Kwee L, et al. Molecular cloning and characterization of a second subunit of the interleuin-1 receptor complex. *J Biol Chem* 1995;270:13757.
70. Novick D, Kim SH, Fantuzzi G, et al. Interleukin-18 binding protein: a novel modulator of the Th1 cytokine response. *Immunity* 1999;10:127.
71. Aizawa Y, Akita K, Taniai M, et al. Cloning and expression of interleukin-18 binding protein. *FEBS Lett* 1999; 445:338.
72. Xu D, Chan WL, Leung BP, et al. Selective expression of a stable cell surface molecule on type 2 but not tpe 1 helper T cells. *J Exp Med* 1998;187:787.
73. Löhning MA, Stroehmann A, Coyle AJ, et al. T1/ST2 is preferentially expressed on murine Th2 cells, independent of interleukin 4, interleukin 5, and interleukin 10, and important for Th2 effector function. *Proc Natl Acad Sci USA* 1998;95:6930.
74. Yoshimoto T, Takeda K, Tanaka T, et al. IL-12 up-regulates IL-18 receptor expression on T cells, Th1 cells, and B cells: synergism with IL-18 for IFN-γ production. *J Immunol* 1998;161:3400.
75. Xu D, Chan WL, Leung BP, et al. Selective expression and functions of interleukin 18 receptor on T helper (Th) type 1 but not Th2 cells. *J Exp Med* 1998;188:1485.
76. Hoshino K, Tsutsui H, Kawai T, et al. Generation of IL-18 receptor–deficient mice: evidence for IL-1 receptor–related protein as an essential IL-18 binding receptor. *J Immunol* 1999;162:5041.
77. Hyodo Y, Matsui K, Hayashi N, et al. IL-18 up-regulates perforin-mediated NK activity without increasing perforin messenger RNA expression by binding to constitutively expressed IL-18 receptor. *J Immunol* 1999;162: 1662.
78. O'Neill LA, Greene C. Signal transduction pathways activated by the IL-1 receptor family: ancient signaling machinery in mammals, insects, and plants. *J Leukoc Biol* 1998;63:650.
79. Robinson D, Shibuya K, Mui A, et al. IGIF does not drive Th1 development but synergizes with IL-12 for interferon-γ production and activates IRAK and NFB. *Immunity* 1997;7:571.
80. Kojima H, Takeuchi M, Ohta T, et al. Interleukin-18 activates the IRAK-TRAF6 pathway in mouse EL-4 cells. *Biochem Biophys Res Commun* 1998;244:183.
81. Baeuerle PA, Henkel T. Function and activation of NF-κB in the immune system. *Annu Rev Immunol* 1994; 12:141.
82. Sica A, Dorman L, Viggiano V, et al. Interaction of NF-κB and NFAT with the interferon-γ promoter. *J Biol Chem* 1997;272:30412.
83. Xu X, Sun YL, Hoey T. Cooperative DNA binding and sequence-selective recognition conferred by the STAT amino-terminal domain. *Science* 1996;273:794.
84. Barbulescu K, Becker C, Schlaak JF, et al. IL-12 and IL-18 differentially regulate the transcriptional activity of the human IFN-γ promoter in primary $CD4^+$ T lymphocytes. *J Immunol* 1998;160:3642.
85. Szabo SJ, Jacobson NG, Dighe AS, et al. Developmental commitment to the Th2 lineage by extinction of IL-12 signaling. *Immunity* 1995;2:665.
86. Kojima H, Aizawa Y, Yanai Y, et al. An essential role for NF-κB in IL-18–induced IFN-γ expression in KG-1 cells. *J Immunol* 1999;162:5063.
87. Croston GE, Cao A, Goeddel DV. NFκB activation by interleukin-1 requires an IL-1 receptor–associated protein kinase activity. *J Biol Chem* 1995;270:16514.
88. Adachi O, Kawai T, Takeda K, et al. Targeted disruption of the MyD88 gene results in loss of IL-1– and IL-18–mediated function. *Immunity* 1998;9:143.
89. Cao Z, Xiong J, Takeuchi M, et al. IRAK TRAF-6. *Nature* 1996;383:443.
90. Thomas JA, Allen JL, Tsen M, et al. Impaired cytokine signaling in mice lacking the IL-1 receptor–associated kinase. *J Immunol* 1999;163:978.
91. Kanakaraj P, Ngo K, Wu Y, et al. Defective interleukin (IL)-18–mediated natural killer and T helper cell type 1 responses in IL-1 receptor–associated kinase (IRAK)–deficient mice. *J Exp Med* 1999;189:1129.

92. Tsuji TK, Matsumoto S, Koide K, et al. Interleukin-18 induces activation and association of p56(lck) and MAPK in a murine TH1 clone. *Biochem Biophys Res Commun* 1997;237:126.
93. Tomura M, Zhou XY, Maruo S, et al. A critical role for IL-18 in the proliferation and activation of NK1.1$^+$ CD3$^-$ cells. *J Immunol* 1998;160:4738.
94. Micallef MJ, Ohtsuki T, Kohno K, et al. Interferon-γ–inducing factor enhances T helper 1 cytokine production by stimulated human T cells: synergism with interleukin-12 for interferon-γ production. *Eur J Immunol* 1996; 26:1647.
95. Yoshimoto T, Okamura H, Tagawa Y, et al. Interleukin 18 together with interleukin 12 inhibits IgE production by induction of interferon-γ production from activated B cells. *Proc Natl Acad Sci USA* 1997;94:3948.
96. Kohno K, Kataoka J, Ohtsuki T, et al. IFN-γ–inducing factor (IGIF) is a costimulatory factor on the activation of Th1 but not Th2 cells and exerts its effect independently of IL-12. *J Immunol* 1997;158:1541.
97. Ahn H-J, Maruo S, Tomura M, et al. A mechanism underlying synergy between IL-12 and IFN-γ–inducing factor in enhanced production of IFN-γ. *J Immunol* 1997;
98. Hunter CA, Timans J, Pisacane P, et al. Comparison of the effects of interleukin-1α, interleukin-1β and interferon-γ–inducing factor on the production of interferon-γ by natural killer. *Eur J Immunol* 1997;27:2787.
99. Tominaga K, Yoshimoto T, Torigoe K, et al. IL-12 synergizes with IL-18 or IL-1β for IFN-γ production from human T cell. *Int Immunol* (in press).
100. Kunikata T, Torigoe K, Ushio S, et al. Constitutive and induced IL-18 receptor expression by various peripheral blood cell subsets as determined by anti-hIL-18R monoclonal antibody. *Cell Immunol* 1998;189:135.
101. Tomura M, Maruo S, Mu J, et al. Differential capacities of CD4$^+$, CD8$^+$, and CD4$^-$CD8$^-$ T cell subsets to express IL-18 receptor and produce IFN-γ in response to IL-18. *J Immunol* 1998;160:3759.
102. Kohyama M, Saijyo K, Hayasida M, et al. Direct activation of human CD8$^+$ cytotoxic T lymphocytes by interleukin-18. *Jpn J Cancer Res* 1998;89:1041.
103. Okamoto I, Kohno K, Tanimoto T, et al. Development of CD8$^+$ effector T cells is differentially regulated by IL-18 and IL-12. *J Immunol* 1999;162:3202.
104. Nakanishi K, Cohen DI, Blackman M, et al. Ig RNA expression in normal B cells stimulated with anti-IgM antibody and T cell–derived growth and differentiation factors. *J Exp Med* 1984;160:1736.
105. Nakanishi K, Malek T, Smith K, et al. Both interleukin 2 and a second T cell–derived factor in EL-4 supernatant have activity as differentiation factor in IgM synthesis. *J Exp Med* 1984;160:1605.
106. Howard M, Nakanishi K, Paul WE. B cell growth and differentiation factors. *Immunol Rev* 1984;78:185.
107. Howard M, Paul WE. Regulation of B-cell growth and differentiation by soluble factors. *Annu Rev Immunol* 1983;1:307.
108. Kishimoto T. Factors affecting B cell growth and differentiation. *Annu Rev Immunol* 1985;3:133.
109. Pistoia V, Cozzolino F, Rubartelli A, et al. In vitro production of interleukin 1 by normal and malignant human B lymphocytes. *J Immunol* 1986;136:1688.
110. Smeland EB, Blomhoff HK, Funderud S, et al. Interleukin 4 induces selective production of interleukin 6 from normal human B lymphocytes. *J Exp Med* 1989;170:1463.
111. Gerard C, Bruyns C, Marchant A, et al. Interleukin 10 reduces the release of tumor necrosis factor and prevents lethality in experimental endotoxemia. *J Exp Med* 1993;177:547.
112. Velupillai P, Harn DA. Oligosaccharide-specific induction of interleukin 10 production by B220$^+$ cells from schistosome-infected mice: a mechanism for regulation of CD4$^+$ T-cell subsets. *Proc Natl Acad Sci USA* 1994; 91, 18.
113. Lauwerys BR, Renauld JC, Houssiau FA. Inhibition of in vitro immunoglobulin production by IL-12 in murine chronic graft-vs.-host disease: synergism with IL-18. *Eur J Immunol* 1998;28:2017.
114. Tsutsui H, Nakanishi K, Matsui K, et al. Interferon-γ–inducing factor up- regulates Fas ligand–mediated cytotoxic activity of murine natural killer cell clones. *J Immunol* 1996;157:3967.
115. Dao T, Mehal WZ, Crispe IN. IL-18 augments perforin-dependent cytotoxicity of liver NK-T cells. *J Immunol* 1998;161:2217.
116. Walker W, Aste-Amezaga M, Kastelein RA, et al. IL-18 and CD28 use distinct molecular mechanism to enhance NK cell production of IL-12–induced IFN-γ. *J Immunol* 1999;162:5894.
117. Dao T, Ohashi K, Kayano T, et al. Interferon-γ–inducing factor, a novel cytokine, enhances Fas ligand–mediated cytotoxicity of murine T helper 1 cells. *Cell Immunol* 1996;173:230.
118. Puren AJ, Fantuzzi G, Gu Y, et al. Interleukin-18 (IFN γ–inducing factor) induces IL-8 and IL-1β via TNF-α production from non-CD14$^+$ human blood mononuclear cells. *J Clin Invest* 1998;101:711.
119. Munder M, Mallo M, Eichmann K, et al. Murine macrophages secrete interferon γ upon combined stimulation with interleukin (IL)-12 and IL-18: a novel pathway of autocrine macrophage activation. *J Exp Med* 1998; 187:2103.
120. Shapiro L, Puren AJ, Barton HA, et al. Interleukin 18 stimulates HIV type 1 in monocytic cells. *Proc Natl Acad Sci USA* 1998;95:12550.
121. Kohka H, Yoshino T, Iwagaki H, et al. Interleukin-18/interferon γ–inducing factor, a novel cytokine, up-regulates ICAM-1 (CD54) expression in KG-1 cells. *J Leukoc Biol* 1998;64:519.
122. Poli G, Kinter AL, Justement JS, et al. Retinoic acid mimics transforming growth factor β in the regulation of human immunodeficiency virus expression in monocytic cells. *Proc Natl Acad Sci USA* 1992;89:2689.
123. Pirhonen J, Sareneva T, Kurimoto M, et al. Virus infection activates IL-1β and IL-18 production in human macrophages by a caspase-1–dependent pathway. *J Immunol* 1999;162:7322.

124. Magram J, Connaughton SE, Warrier RR, et al. IL-12–deficient mice are defective in IFN γ production and type 1 cytokine responses. *Immunity* 1996;4:471.
125. Kaplan MH, Sun YL, Hoey T, et al. Impaired IL-12 responses and enhanced development of Th2 cells in Stat4-deficient mice. *Nature* 1996;382:174.
126. Tsutsui H, Mizoguchi Y, Morisawa. S. Importance of direct hepatocytolysis by liver macrophages in experimental fulminant hepatitis. *Hepato-Gastroenterology* 1992;39:553.
127. Yoshimoto T, Nakanishi K, Hirose K, et al. High serum IL-6 level reflects susceptible status of the host to endotoxin and IL-1/tumor necrosis factor. *J Immunol* 1992;148:3596.
128. Abo T, Ohteki T, Seki S, et al. The appearance of T cells bearing self-reactive T cell receptor in the livers of mice injected with bacteria. *J Exp Med* 1991;174:417.
129. Bendelac A, Rivera MN, Park SH, et al. Mouse CD1-specific NK1 T cells: development, specificity, and function. *Annu Rev Immunol* 1997;15:535.
130. Matsui K, Yoshimoto T, Tsutsui H, et al. *Propionibacterium acnes* treatment diminishes CD4$^+$NK1.1+ T cells but induces type 1 T cells in the liver by induction of IL-12 and IL-18 production from Kupffer cells. *J Immunol* 1997;159:97.
131. Takeda K, Tsutsui H, Yoshimoto T, et al. Defective NK cell activity and Th1 response in IL-18–deficient mice. *Immunity* 1998;8:383.
132. Sakao Y, Takeda K, Tsutsui H, et al. IL-18–deficient mice are resistant to endotoxin-induced liver injury but highly susceptible to endotoxin shock. *Int Immunol* 1999;11:471.
133. Sher A, Coffman R. Regulation of immunity to parasites by T cells and T-cell–derived cytokines. *Annu Rev Immunol* 1992;10:385.
134. Dalton DK, Pitts-Meek S, Keshav S, et al. Multiple defects of immune cell function in mice with disrupted interferon-γ genes. *Science* 1993;259:1739.
135. Huang S, Hendriks W, Althage A, et al. Immune response in mice that lack the interferon-γ receptor. *Science* 1993;259:1742.
136. Kobayashi K, Nakata N, Kai M, et al. Decreased expression of cytokines that induce type 1 helper T cell/interferon-γ responses in genetically susceptible mice infected with *Mycobacterium avium*. *Clin Immunol Immunopathol* 1997;85:112.
137. Sugawara I, Yamada H, Kaneko H, et al. Role of interleukin-18 (IL-18) in mycobacterial infection in IL-18-gene- disrupted mice. *Infect Immun* 1999;67:2585.
138. Salgame P, Abrams JS, Clayberger C, et al. Differing lymphokine profiles of functional subsets of human CD4 and CD8 T cell clones. *Science* 1991;254:279.
139. Kobayashi K, Kai M, Gidoh M, et al. The possible role of interleukin (IL)-12 and interferon-γ–inducing factor/IL-18 in protection against experimental *Mycobacterium leprae* infection in mice. *Clin Immunol Immunopathol* 1998;88:226.
140. Garcia VE, Uyemura K, Sieling PA, et al. IL-18 promotes type 1 cytokine production from NK cells and T cells in human intracellular infection. *J Immunol* 1999;162:6114.
141. Mastroeni P, Clare S, Khan S, et al. Interleukin 18 contributes to host resistance and gamma interferon production in mice infected with virulent *Salmonella typhimurium*. *Infect Immun* 1999;67:478.
142. Zhang T, Kawakami K, Qureshi MH, et al. Interleukin-12 (IL-12) and IL-18 synergistically induce the fungicidal activity of murine peritoneal exudate cells against *Cryptococcus neoformans* through production of γ interferon by natural killer cells. *Infect Immun* 1997;65:3594.
143. Kawakami K, Qureshi MH, Koguchi Y, et al. Role of TNF-α in the induction of fungicidal activity of mouse peritoneal exudate cells against cryptococcus neoformans by IL-12 and IL-18. *Cell Immunol* 1999;193:9.
144. Kawakami K, Qureshi MH, Zhang T, et al. IL-18 protects mice against pulmonary and disseminated infection with *Cryptococcus neoformans* by inducing IFN-γ production. *J Immunol* 1997;159:5528.
145. Qureshi MH, Zhang T, Koguchi Y, et al. Combined effects of IL-12 and IL-18 on the clinical course and local cytokine production in murine pulmonary infection with *Cryptococcus neoformans*. *Eur J Immunol* 1999;29:643.
146. Fujioka N, Akazawa R, Ohashi K, et al. Interleukin-18 protects mice against acute *Herpes simplex* virus type 1 infection. *J Virol* 1999;73:2401.
147. Sareneva T, Matikainen S, Kurimoto M, et al. Influenza A virus–induced IFN-α/β and IL-18 synergistically enhance IFN-γ gene expression in human T cells. *J Immunol* 1998;160:6032.
148. Tanaka-Kataoka M, Kunikata T, Takayama S, et al. In vivo antiviral effect of interleukin 18 in a mouse model of Vaccinia virus infection. *Cytokine* 1999;11.
149. Reiner SL, Locksley RM. The regulation of immunity to *Leishmania major*. *Annu Rev Immunol* 1995;13:151.
150. Heinzel FP, Sadick MD, Mutha S, et al. Production of interferon-γ, IL-2, IL-4, and IL-10 by CD4$^+$ lymphocytes in vivo during healing and progression of murine leishmaniasis. *Proc Natl Acad Sci USA* 1991;88:7011.
151. Sadick MD, Heinzel FP, Holaday BJ, et al. Cure of murine leishmaniasis with anti-interleukin 4 monoclonal antibody. Evidence for a T cell–dependent, interferon γ–independent mechanism. *J Exp Med* 1990;171:115.
152. Heinzel FP, Schoenhaut DS, Rerko RM, et al. Recombinant interleukin 12 cures mice infected with *Leishmania major*. *J Exp Med* 1993;177:1505.
153. Belosevic M, Finbloom DS, Van der Medide PH, et al. Administration of monoclonal anti-IFN γ antibodies in vivo abrogates natural resistance of C3H/HeN mice to infection with *Leishmania major*. *J Immunol* 1989;143:266.

154. Heinzel FP, Rerko RM, Ahmed F, et al. Endogenous IL-12 is required for control of Th2 cytokine responses capable of exacerbating leishmaniasis in normally resistant mice. *J Immunol* 1995;155:730.
155. Diefenbach A, Schindler H, Donhauser N, et al. Type 1 interferon (IFNα/β) and type 2 nitric oxide synthase regulate the innate immune response to a protozoan parasite. *Immunity* 1998;8:77.
156. Liew FY, Li Y, Moss D, et al. Resistance to *Leishmania major* infection correlates with the induction of nitric oxide synthase in murine macrophages. *Eur J Immunol* 1991;21:3009.
157. Liew FY, Li Y, Severn A, et al. A possible novel pathway of regulation by murine T helper type-2 (Th2) cells of a Th1 cell activity via the modulation of the induction of nitric oxide synthase in macrophages. *Eur J Immunol* 1991;21:2489.
158. Wei XQ, Charles IG, Smith A, et al. Altered immune response in mice lacking inducible nitric oxide synthase. *Nature* 1995;375:408.
159. Nakanishi K, Ohkusu K, Okamura H, et al. Molecular mechanism of host resistance induced by IL-12 and IL-18 against infection with *Leishmania major*. *Int Parasitol* 1998;9:269.
160. Wei X-Q, Leung BP, Niedbala W, et al. Altered immune responses and susceptibility to *Leishmania major* and *Staphylococcus aureus* infection in IL-18–deficient mice. *J Immunol* 1999;163:2821.
161. Gurunathan S, Prussin C, Sacks DL, et al. Vaccine requirements for sustained cellular immunity to an intracellular parasitic infection. *Nat Med* 1998;4:1409.
162. Skeiky YA, Kennedy M, Kaufman D, et al. LeIF: a recombinant Leishmania protein that induces an IL-12–mediated Th1 cytokine profile. *J Immunol* 1998;161:6171.
163. Meyer Zum, Buschenfelde C, Cramer S, et al. *Trypanosoma cruzi* induces strong IL-12 and IL-18 gene expression in vivo: correlation with interferon-γ (IFN-γ) production. *Clin Exp Immunol* 1997;110:378.
164. Nussenzweig V, Nussenzweig R. Rationale for the development of an engineered oporozoite malaria vaccine. *Adv Immunol* 1989;45:283.
165. Meis JEGM, Verhave JP, Jap PHK, et al. An ultrastructual study on the role of Kuppfer cells in the process of infection by *Plasmodium berghei* in rats. *Parasitology*1983;86:231.
166. Hollingdale MR. Malaria and the liver. *Hepatology* 1983;5:327.
167. Schofield L, Villaquiran J, Ferreira A, et al. Gamma interferon, CD8+ T cells and antibodies are required for immunity to malaria sporozoites. *Nature* 1987;330:664.
168. Podoba JE, Stevenson MM. CD4+ and CD8+ T cells both contribute to acquired immunity to blood-stage *Plasmodium chabaudi* AS. *Infect Immun* 1991;59:51.
169. Hoffman S, Isenbarger D, Long G, et al. Sporozoite vaccine induces genetically restricted T cell elimination of malaria from hepatocytes. *Science* 1989;244:1078.
170. Mellouk S, Green SJ, Nacy CA, et al. IFN-γ inhibits development of *Plasmodium berghei* exoerythrocytic stages in hepatocytes by an L-arginine–dependent effector mechanism. *J Immunol* 1991;146:3971.
171. Taylor-Robinson AW, Philips RS. Protective CD4+ T cell lines raised against *Plasmodium chabaudi* show characteristics of either Th1 or Th2 cells. *Parasite Immunol* 1993;15:301.
172. Stevenson MM, Tam MF, Wolf SF, et al. IL-12–induced protection against blood-stage *Plasmodium chabaudi* AS requires IFN-γ and TNF-α and occurs via a nitric oxide-dependent mechanism. *J Immunol* 1995;155:2545.
173. Doolan D, Sedegah M, Hedstrom R, et al. Circumventing genetic restriction of protection against malaria with multigene DNA immunization: CD8+ T cell–, interferon γ–, and nitric oxide–dependent immunity. *J Exp Med* 1996;183:1739.
174. Sedegah MS, Finkelman F, Hoffman SL. Interleukin 12 induction of intereron γ–dependent protection against malaria. *Proc Natl Acad Sci USA* 1994;91:10700.
175. Car BD, Eng VM, Schnyder B, et al. Role of interferon-γ in interleukin 12–induced pathology in mice. *Am J Pathol* 1995;147:1693.
176. Hoshino T, Wiltrout RH, Young H. IL-18 is a potent coinducer of IL-13 in NK and T cells: a new potential role for IL-18 in modulating the immune response. *J Immunol* 1999;162:5070.
177. Yoshimoto T, Tsutsui H, Tominaga K, et al. IL-18, although antiallergic when administered with IL-12, stimulates IL-4 and histamine release by basophils. *Proc Natl Acad Sci USA* In press.

8

Chemokines in Infectious Disease

Philip E. Tarr and *Daniel R. Lucey

Albert Einstein College of Medicine, Bronx, New York, and
**Division of Infectious Diseases, Department of Medicine, Washington Hospital Center, Washington, DC*

"The endothelial cells which allow the passage of leukocytes, and the leukocytes themselves which escape from the vessels in order to reach the point of entrance of the micro-organisms, all must be influenced in a special fashion. . . . [T]he phagocytes exhibit a positive chemiotaxis [sic], . . .That is to say, a perception of the chemical composition of the surrounding medium . . . And this form of sensitiveness is a condition indispensable to a state of immunity and to the disappearance of the micro-organisms."—Elie Metchnikoff (1)

INTRODUCTION

Ever since Metchnikoff's observations on the role of phagocytes in immunity over 100 years ago, the existence of leukocyte-specific attractant signals has intrigued scientists in infectious disease and immunology. Chemokines, a contraction of the terms "chemotaxis" and "cytokines," have now emerged as key intercellular mediators in the regulation of inflammatory processes, by means of their selective effects on leukocyte migration (reviewed in 2–9). Chemokines are by far the largest described cytokine subfamily. Since the identification in 1987 of interleukin (IL)–8 as the first chemoattractant specific for a subset of leukocytes, over 40 human chemokines and at least 16 chemokine receptors have been described.

Chemokines are separated from other cytokines and chemoattractant molecules by distinctive features: (a) The definition of a protein as a chemokine is based on structure, namely the presence of conserved cysteines at the *N*-terminus. (b) Chemokines are the only cytokines that bind to specific G-protein–coupled, seven-transmembrane (7-TM) spanning receptors on target cells. (c) Chemokines are specific leukocyte attractants. Although there are many other chemoattractants, such as leukotriene B_4 and complement component C_{5a}, that signal through 7-TM receptors, they lack the defining structural characteristics and the target cell specificity of chemokines.

In this chapter, we first summarize the biology of the chemokines and then review four major infectious disease topics that provide the background for therapeutic approaches to infectious diseases involving the chemokine system: (a) the role of chemokines in the regulation of the immune response; (b) entry of host cells by microbes by using chemokine receptors. It is well established that chemokine receptors are used by the malaria pathogen *Plasmodium vivax* and by the human immunodeficiency virus (HIV) to enter host cells]; (c) interference with the chemokine system as a microbial strategy to subvert the host immune response; (d) involvement of the chemokine system in clinical infectious disease syndromes. Recently, the functional spectrum of chemokines has been extended well beyond infection. Chemokines are now believed to be important in the regulation of tissue differentiation, hematopoiesis, atherosclerosis, allergy, and autoimmunity. At present, to write a therapeutically oriented review of chemokines must recognize that the literature is rapidly evolving, and that many experimental findings await confirmation and extension by other groups. The first pharmacologic agents based on the chemokine system are only now entering clinical trials.

CHEMOKINES

Chemokines are small soluble proteins (7–10 kDa in molecular size of the monomeric chemokines) consisting of a single polypeptide chain 68 to 120 amino acids in length with 20% to 95% sequence identity among each other. Most chemokines have four conserved cysteines forming two essential disulfide bonds near the *N*-terminus. At present, all but two chemokines fall into two of four subfamilies, the CXC (or α) and the CC (or β) subfamilies, according to the position of the first two cysteines, which are either adjacent (CC) or separated by a nonconserved amino acid (CXC) (2–5). Lymphotactin, which has two conserved cysteines but only one in the *N*-terminal domain, currently is the only member of the C (or γ) subfamily. Fractalkine has three amino acids between the first two cysteines at the *N*-terminal end of a mucin-like structure and represents the only chemokine in the CX3C (or δ) subfamily. Fractalkine exists both as a soluble chemokine and as an adhesion molecule on endothelial cells. The chemokine abbreviations used here are listed in the Glossary to this chapter (p. 173). As will be discussed below (p. 148), chemokine receptors are subfamily-restricted and are classified as CXC, CC, XC, and CX3C receptors.

The CXC chemokines have been further subdivided according to the presence of an *N*-terminal ELR (glutamate-leucine-arginine) motif preceding the first cysteine. The ELR motif identifies neutrophil-targeted CXC chemokines. The non-ELR CXC chemokines are a functionally heterogeneous group but have little or no activity on neutrophils. The CC chemokines are also functionally diverse, but have been primarily considered attractants of mononuclear cells, eosinophils, and basophils, but not neutrophils. There are T-lymphocyte–specific chemokines in both the CC and CXC subfamilies (10), and the functional distinction between CXC and CC chemokines by cell targets is not absolute (11–15), underscoring the biologic complexity of the chemokine network.

Many of the genes that encode chemokines have been localized. CC chemokine genes cluster on human chromosome 17, except for TARC, LARC, ELC, and SLC (See Glossary for definitions), whose genes map to chromosomes 16, 2, 9, and 9, respectively (16). The CXC genes cluster on human chromosome 4 except for the stromal-derived factor–1 (SDF-1) gene which is on chromosome 10. The lymphotactin gene is localized on chromosome 1, and the fractalkine gene on chromosome 16. Chemokine gene expression is in part regulated by the NFκB family of transcription factors (17,18), a concept based on correlations between chemokine gene expression and NFκB transcriptional activation, shared NFκB binding motifs among the promoter sequences of several chemokine genes, and reduced chemokine expression after inhibition of NFκB.

The recent rapid discovery of novel chemokines is mainly a result of bioinformatics, based on the screening of databases of expressed sequence tags (EST) generated by randomly sequencing cDNA libraries (19). This process is facilitated by the characteristically short coding sequence (usually about 300 base pairs) of chemokines. To address the expanding chemokine aliases that accompanied the discovery of chemokines by multiple groups at the same time, a systematic classification was developed in 1999 (20). The new chemokine nomenclature uses the letters "L" (for "ligand") and "R" (for "receptor") to identify the standardized chemokine subclass roots (CC, CXC, XC, CX3C) (20). The new nomenclature and the chemokine names that are commonly used today are shown in Table 8.1.

TABLE 8-1. *Chemokine classification*

New nomenclature	Common names	Main receptors[a]	Main target cells[a]
CXC α chemokines			
CXCL1	MGSA/GROα	CXCR2, Duffy	Neutrophils, red blood cells
CXCL2	MIP2a/GROβ	CXCR2	Neutrophils
CXCL3	MIP2b/GROγ	CXCR2	Neutrophils
CXCL4	PF-4	No GPCR binding known	No known leukocyte attractant activity
CXCL5	ENA-78	CXCR2	Neutrophils
CXCL6	GCP-2	CXCR1, CXCR2	Neutrophils
CXCL7	NAP-2	CXCR2, Duffy	Neutrophils
CXCL8	IL-8	CXCR1, Duffy	Neutrophils
CXCL9	Mig	CXCR3	Th1 cells
CXCL10	IP-10	CXCR3	Th1 cells
CXCL11	I-TAC	CXCR3	Th1 cells
CXCL12	SDF-1	CXCR4	Neutrophils, naive T cells, B cells, macrophages, immature and mature dendritic cells
CXCL13	BCA-1/BLC	CXCR5	B cells
CC β chemokines			
CCL1	I-309	CCR8	Macrophages, Th2 cells, thymocytes
CCL2	MCP-1	CCR1, CCR2, Duffy	Monocytes, basophils, immature dendritic cells, Th1/Th2 cells, NK cells, red blood cells
CCL3	MIP-1α	CCR1, CCR5	Macrophages, eosinophils, basophils, immature dendritic cells, Th1/Th2 cells, NK cells, thymocytes
CCL4	MIP-1β	CCR1, CCR5, CCR8	Macrophages, basophils, immature dendritic cells, Th1/Th2 cells, NK cells, thymocytes
CCL5	RANTES	CCR1, CCR3, CCR5, Duffy	Macrophages, eosinophils, basophils, immature dendritic cells, Th1/Th2 cells, NK cells, thymocytes
CCL7	MCP-3	CCR1, CCR2, CCR3	Macrophages, eosinophils, basophils, immature dendritic cells, Th1/Th2 cells, NK cells, thymocytes
CCL8	MCP-2	CCR1, CCR2, CCR3, CCR5	Macrophages, eosinophils, basophils, immature dendritic cells, Th1/Th2 cells, NK cells, thymocytes
CCL11	Eotaxin	CCR3	Eosinophils, basophils, Th2 cells
CCL13	MCP-4	CCR1, CCR2, CCR3	Macrophages, eosinophils, basophils, immature dendritic cells, Th1/Th2 cells, NK cells, thymocytes
CCL14	HCC-1, NCC-2	CCR1	Monocytes, eosinophils, basophils, immature dendritic cells, Th1/Th2 cells, NK cells

Continued

TABLE 8-1. *Continued*

New nomenclature	Common names	Main receptors[a]	Main target cells[a]
CCL15	HCC-2, Leukotactin (Lcn)-1, MIP-5	CCR1, CCR3	Neutrophils, monocytes, eosinophils, basophils, immature dendritic cells, Th1/Th2 cells
CCL16	HCC-4, LEC, monotactin-1	Not identified	—
CCL17	TARC, STCP-1	CCR4	Immature dendritic cells, Th2 cells, NK cells, thymocytes
CCL18	PARC, DC-CK-1, MIP-4	Not identified	Naive (CD45A+) T cells
CCL19	ELC, MIP-3β, exodus-3	CCR7	Mature dendritic cells, naive T (Th2?) cells
CCL20	LARC, MIP-3α, exodus-1	CCR6	Immature dendritic cells; T cells in secondary lymphoid tissue, CD34+ cells
CCL21	SLC, 6Ckine, Exodus-2, TCA4	CCR7	Mature dendritic cells, naive T(Th2?) cells
CCL22	MDC, STCP-1	CCR4	Immature dendritic cells, Th2 cells, NK cells, thymocytes
CCL23	MPIF-1, MIP-3	CCR1	Monocytes, eosinophils, basophils, immature dendritic cells, Th1/Th2 cells, NK cells; inhibits hematopoiesis
CCL24	Eotaxin-2, MPIF-2	CCR3	Eosinophils, basophils, Th2 cells
CCL25	TECK	CCR9	Thymocytes, T cells
CCL26	MIP-4α	Not identified	—
C chemokines			
XCL1	Lymphotactin	XCR1	T cells, NK cells
CX_3C chemokines			
CX_3CL1	Fractalkine/ neurotactin	CX_3CR1	Macrophages, T cells, NK cells

[a]Note that chemokine receptor distribution on leukocytes and target cells of chemokines are based mainly on *in vitro* studies, which have, in some cases, conflicted.
NK cell, natural killer cell; Th1 cell, T helper 1 cell; Th2 cell, T helper 2 cell.

CHEMOKINE RECEPTORS

Many chemokines ligate multiple chemokine receptors, and many chemokine receptors are ligated by multiple chemokines *in vitro*. This promiscuity of chemokines is reflected in redundant biologic effects on target cells *in vitro*. Nonetheless, leukocyte recruitment and activation occur *in vivo* with some degree of selectivity, which is at least in part derived from the temporally and spatially regulated expression of both chemokines and receptors (8,21–23). As displayed in Table 8.2, chemokine receptors have restricted specificities to leukocyte subtypes. Five receptors specific for CXC chemokines, nine receptors specific for CC chemokines, and the receptors for lymphotactin (XCR1 subfamily) and fractalkine (CX3CR1 subfamily) have been cloned to date. Thus, the classification of chemokine receptors into subgroups is based on ligand specificity, which in part is determined by the presence of certain shared amino acid motifs (20).

Chemokine receptors belong to the rhodopsin family of G-protein–coupled receptors (GPCR) with 7-TM domains (reviewed in 8, 20, 24, and 25), which makes the chemokine family unique among cytokines. β-adrenergic receptors and histamine receptors are additional examples of GPCRs. Other chemoattractants, such as leukotriene B_4 and C_{5a} (26,27), also ligate GPCRs, but their biologic effects are not target cell specific. Chemokine receptors are expressed in leukocytes; they are single polypeptide chain re-

TABLE 8-2. *Chemokine receptor classification*

Receptor	Other names	Cellular expression[a]	Ligands
CXCR1	IL-8R type 1, IL-8RA	Neutrophils	IL-8, GCP-2, ENA-78
CXCR2	IL-8R type 2, IL-8RB	Neutrophils, eosinophils	IL-8, GRO-α, -β, -γ; NAP-2, ENA-78
CXCR3	GPR9	Activated Th1 cells	Mig, IP-10, I-TAC
CXCR4	Fusin, LESTR, HUMSTR, HM89, LCR-1, NPYRL	Neutrophils, naive T cells, B cells macrophages, immature and mature dendritic cells	SDF-1α, -1β
CXCR5	BLR-1, MDR15	B lymphocytes	BCA-1/BLC
CCR1	CC-CCR1, HM145, MIP-1(αR)	Neutrophils, monocytes, eosinophils, basophils, immature dendritic cells, Th1/Th2 cells, NK cells	RANTES, MIP-1α, MIP-1β, MCP-1, MCP-2, MCP-3, MCP-4, MPIF-1, MIP-5, HCC-1, Lkn-1
CCR2	CC-CCR2-A, CC-CCR2-B, MCP-1RA, MCP-1RB	Monocytes, Th1/Th2 cells, NK cells	MCP-1, MCP-2, MCP-3, MCP-4
CCR3	Eotaxin receptor, CC-CCR3, CCR3, CMKBR-3	Eosinophils, basophils, Th2 cells	Eotaxin, eotaxin-2, RANTES, MCP-2, MCP-3, MCP-4, MCP-5
CCR4	CC-CCR4, K5-5	Immature dendritic cells, Th2 cells, NK cells, thymocytes, memory T cells with skin homing phenotype	MDC, TARC
CCR5	CC-CCR5, Chem-R13, CMKBR-5	Monocytes, Th1 cells, immature dendritic cells, thymocytes	RANTES, MIP-1α, MIP-1β, MCP-2
CCR6	CCRL3, KRY-6, GPR-CY-4, STRL-22	Immature dendritic cells; T cells in secondary lymphoid tissue, CD34+ cells	LARC
CCR7	BLR-2, EBI-I	Mature dendritic cells, naive T(Th2?) cells	ELC, SLC
CCR8	ChemR-I, CCRL-I, GPR-CY-6, TER-I	Macrophages, Th2 cells, thymocytes	I-309, MIP-1β, TARC
CCR9	—	Thymocytes, memory T cells with gastrointestinal homing phenotype	TECK
CX_3CR1	CMKBRL-I, V28	Natural killer (NK) cells, T cells, monocytes	Fractalkine/Neurotactin
XCR1	GPR-5	T cells, NK cells	Lymphotactin
Duffy	DARC	Red blood cells, endothelial cells	MGSA, IL-8, RANTES, MCP-1, NAP-2

[a]Note that chemokine receptor distribution on leukocytes is based mainly on *in vitro* studies, which have, in some cases, conflicted.

ceptors with 25% to 80% amino acid similarity to each other. While their three-dimensional structure is unknown, chemokine receptors contain four conserved, disulfide-bond forming cysteines (one in each of the four extracellular domains) that appear critical for the conformation of the ligand binding site. A schematic representation of a chemokine receptor is given in Fig. 8.1. Ligand binding domains of chemokine receptors are coupled to phospholipase signal transduction pathways via pertussis toxin–inhibited, heterotrimeric G_i proteins. Activation of G_i proteins may be regulated *in vivo* by the RGS (regulators of G protein signaling) family of proteins (28), providing additional flexibility to chemokine receptor–mediated effector programs. The diverse signal transduction pathways activated by chemokine receptor ligation have been reviewed (5,10,24). These

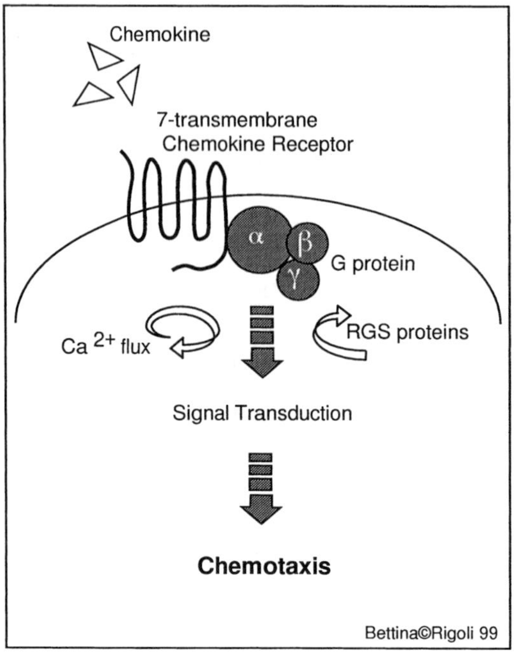

FIG. 8.1. Diagram of a chemokine receptor. Chemokine receptors belong to the family of seven transmembrane (7-TM) receptors. 7-TM receptors are single-chain receptors that span the plasma membrane seven times. They are coupled to intracellular signal transduction pathways through heterotrimeric G_i proteins. G protein signaling is regulated by RGS proteins. Ca^{2+} flux is a commonly reported readout of chemokine receptor signaling. [From Rigoli B (b.rigoli@dplanet.ch), with permission.]

include activation of protein kinase C and phospholipase, and the generation of diacylglycerol and inositol triphosphate (IP_3): IP_3 mobilizes Ca^{2+} from intracellular stores. Ca^{2+} flux is a standard readout of signaling through chemokine receptors. Ligand-induced dimer formation of chemokine receptors may be required for functional responses, i.e., Ca^{2+} flux and chemotaxis (29). Further insight into the factors that underlie the selectivity of chemokine effects *in vivo* may emerge from the biochemical characterization of chemokine receptors and the diverse signaling programs that may control diverse functional outcomes in individual leukocyte subsets (30).

A unique niche in the chemokine receptor universe is occupied by Duffy, the Duffy antigen receptor complex (DARC). Duffy is the only known mammalian chemokine receptor that binds multiple subclasses of chemokines. While its exact function is unknown, Duffy is a nonsignaling molecule on red blood cells that may scavenge CC and CXC chemokines and thereby regulate blood chemokine levels and leukocyte traffic to inflammatory sites (31). However, the majority of persons of West African descent lack Duffy on their red cells (they are "Duffy negative") (32), but they may express Duffy in nonerythroid tissues. These findings suggest the potential for extravascular chemokine scavenging by Duffy (32,33). As Duffy is required for the entry of human red cells by *P. vivax*, Duffy-negative individuals are resistant to infection by this malaria-causing protozoal pathogen (34).

CHEMOKINES AND THE IMMUNE RESPONSE

Regulation of Chemokine Secretion

Chemokines can be divided by their secretion pattern into constitutively secreted and inducible chemokines. Constitutively secreted chemokines include SLC, ELC, TARC, monocyte-derived chemokine (MDC), SDF-1, dendritic cell chemokine–1 (DC-CK-1), and B cell–activating chemokine–1 (BCA-1), and they signal through CCR4, CCR7, CXCR4, and CXCR5. Most constitutive chemokines are highly expressed in lymphoid organs and attract naive B and T cells as well as maturing dendritic cells to lymphoid organs for antigen presentation, as discussed below.

In contrast to this secretion pattern are the inducible chemokines, such as IL-8, IP-10, Mig, MCP family, MIP-1α, MIP-1β, and RANTES (see Glossary for all definitions), and eotaxin. Most cell types can produce chemokines in response to cytokines and inflammatory stimuli, such as LPS/endotoxin and other bacterial cell wall components, radiation, hypoxia, free oxygen radicals, and viral infection (35–43). Secretion of chemokines by resident cells, such as endothelial cells (17), epithelial cells (39,44,45), and fibroblasts (46), is among the earliest tissue responses to injury, and serves as a link connecting innate and adaptive immunity (18,46). Overlap exists between inducable versus constitutive activity of chemokines. As an example, eotaxin regulates both the traffic of eosinophils and Th2 cells during allergic inflammation and the baseline homing of eosinophils into nonhematopoietic tissues during healthy states (47).

Chemokines may function *in vivo* in a network-like fashion together with cytokines and other leukocyte attractants that signal through 7-TM receptors, including leukotriene B_4 (27), some prostaglandins, and the complement component C5a (26). C5a may stimulate chemokine production directly (48) or via the influx of leukocytes to inflammatory sites. The depletion of active C5 leads to reduced IL-8 and MIP-2 expression (49), as well as the attenuation of experimental glomerulonephritis *in vivo* (50,51). Chemokines may function as an amplifying link between complement activation, which is very rapid, and leukocyte migration, which occurs slowly (over hours) (49).

Regulation of Leukocyte Traffic

By virtue of their target cell specificity, chemokines have the potential to selectively recruit and activate subsets of leukocytes to and at sites of antigenic challenge.

In the multistep model of leukocyte trafficking proposed by Springer (52), extravascular migration of leukocytes occurs in response to a concentration gradient of chemotactic factors. This occurs in a stepwise fashion and includes (a) weak adhesion and leukocyte rolling along the endothelium, (b) activation and firm adhesion, and then (c) leukocyte migration across the endothelium. Chemokines act predominantly at the second and third step in this process by activating integrins and fibronectin to mediate firm adhesion of leukocytes to endothelial cells as a prerequisite for transendothelial migration (52–54). The immobilization of IL-8 on the endothelial surface has been shown to be required for neutrophil adhesion and emigration and is mediated by the C-terminal domain of IL-8 (55). Chemokines can also be immobilized via their C-terminus by binding to proteoglycans on endothelial surfaces and in the extracellular matrix (56–59). This has been suggested to retain chemokines, enhance concentration gradients, and prolong their local functional activity. While the importance of chemokines in leukocyte migration is now well established, their role in leukocyte activation is less clear (60). Chemokine blockade has led to reduced macrophage microbicidal activity *in vitro* (61). Phagocytosis and microbial killing *in vivo* is likely to depend on interactions of chemokines with inflammatory cytokines.

Chemokines are emerging as key regulators of the function of Langerhans cells and dendritic cells (DCs), the sentinel cells of the immune system, and the most potent inducers of primary T cell responses (62–65). The current model of how chemokines may regulate the generation of primary immune responses (reviewed in 66) is shown in Fig.

8.2. It is suggested that immature DCs migrate to peripheral sites of tissue damage/antigen challenge in response to inflammatory chemokine signals through CCR1, -2, -5, and -6, and CXCR1 (67,68). After antigen capture, DCs mature, as reflected in the upregulation of molecules involved in antigen presentation and costimulation, and migrate to lymphoid tissues. Migration is accompanied by downregulation of receptors for inflammatory chemokines, and upregulation of receptors for constitutive chemokines, including CCR7, the receptor for both SLC and ELC (69). These chemokines attract maturing DCs and are produced constitutively by lymphatic endothelial cells, stromal cells, and mature DCs in secondary lymphoid tissues. SLC and ELC also attract naive T and B cells (which also express CCR7) for antigen presentation by DCs. Moreover, maturing DCs upregulate chemokines that attract T cells, such as TARC and DC-CK-1 (65,70), as well as MDC, which may mediate T cell/B cell interactions. Another chemokine produced in

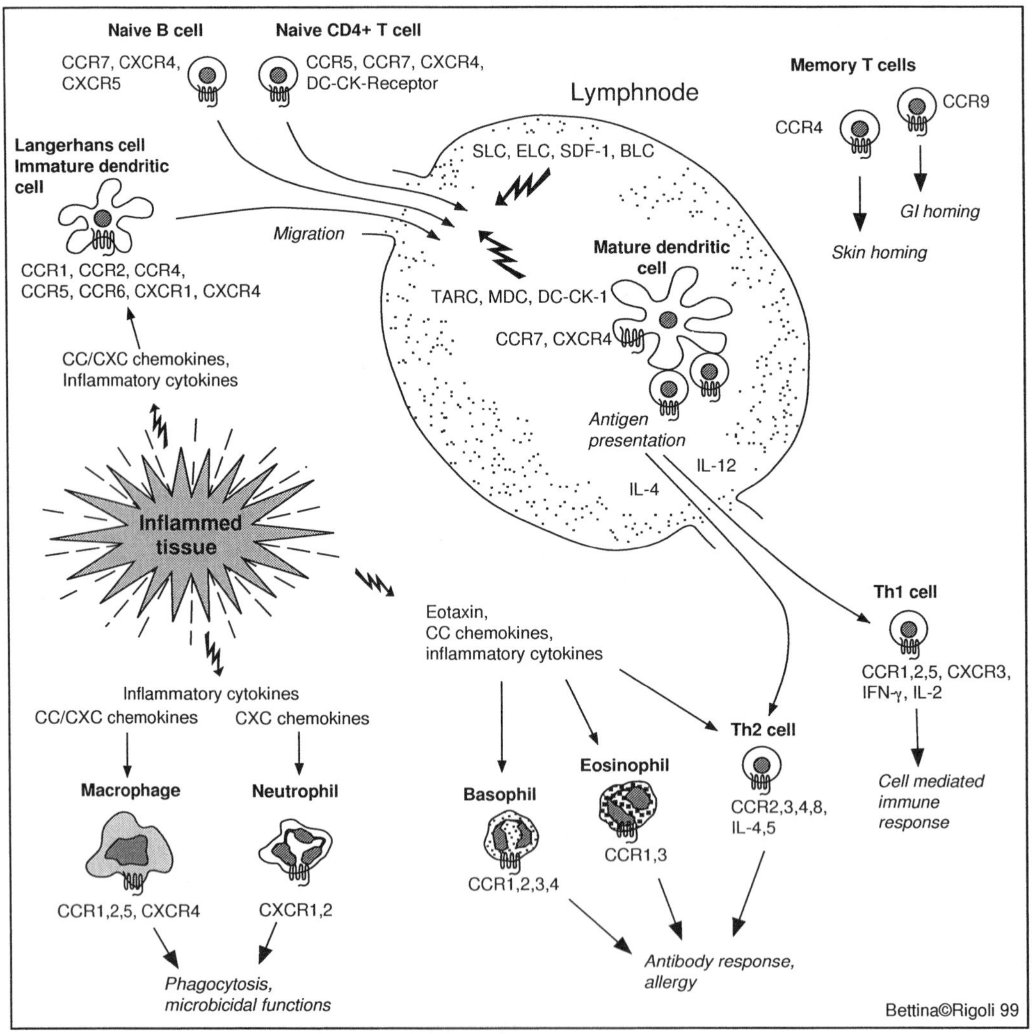

FIG. 8.2. Regulation of the migration and differentiation of dendritic cells, B cells, and T cells by chemokines and chemokine receptors. [From Rigoli B (b.rigoli@dplanet.ch), with permission.]

lymphoid tissue is SDF-1, which is important for the attraction of maturing DCs and naive T and B cells, all of which express the SDF-1 receptor CXCR4 (71,72). Naive B cells also express CXCR5, which ligates BLC/BCA-1, a constitutive chemokine produced in B cell zones of secondary lymphoid organs (73,74).

Regulation of Th1/Th2 Responses

Chemokine receptors may be differentially expressed in T cells in relation to their state of activation and differentiation (3,66). When activated via their T cell receptor, T cells switch from expressing receptors for constitutive to receptors for inflammatory chemokines (75). For example, naive T cells express CCR7 and CXCR4, and are attracted to lymphoid organs where antigen is presented. Activation by proinflammatory cytokines induces expression of most chemokine receptors, including CCR1, -2, -3, and -5, and CX3CR-1 (38,76–78), consistent with the induction of an effector phenotype and migration to sites of inflammation.

An intriguing role has been suggested for chemokine receptors in the polarization of $CD4^+$ T cell helper immune responses. Naïve $CD4^+$ T cells develop into either T helper 1–like (Th1) or T helper 2–like (Th2) effector cells, depending on the cytokine microenvironment present during priming of the naive T cells (79,80). IL-12 induces a Th1 response, characterized by $CD4^+$ T cell secretion of IFN-γ, IL-2, and TNF-β. IL-4 induces a Th2 cytokine secretion profile, which includes IL-4, IL-5, IL-6, IL-10, and IL-13. The predominance of Th1 immunity has been linked not only to cell-mediated immunity and the clearance of intracellular infections, but also to chronic inflammatory states such as Crohn's disease and psoriasis. In contrast, Th2 predominance may correlate with impaired cellular immunity, an increase in B cell activity, and the presence of allergic and helminthic parasitic diseases (79–82).

Some (83–88, reviewed in 66), but not other (89,90) investigators have reported Th1- and Th2-specific chemokine receptor expression patterns (as summarized in Fig. 8.2). Th2 cells may selectively express CCR3, CCR4, and CCR8. CXCR3, CCR5, and perhaps CCR1 and CCR2 have been found preferentially on Th1 cells. The corresponding chemokines may selectively regulate the migration and homing of Th1 and Th2 cells. Th1 cells appear to preferentially chemotax to RANTES, MIP-1α, and MIP-1β. In contrast, Th2 cells express CCR3 and respond to eotaxin (85). CCR3 is also expressed on basophils and eosinophils, the eotaxin-responsive cell types that are synergistically induced by Th2 cytokines (IL-4, IL-5) during allergic inflammation. Th2 cells have also been characterized by the expression of CCR4 and responsiveness to MDC and TARC (87,88), although the hallmark of the Th2 phenotype, IL-4 production, was more strongly associated with CCR3 expression. It has been suggested that CCR4 and CCR9 mediate the selective skin versus intestinal homing behavior of lymphocytes, along with the differential expression of the integrin α4β7, but not in a Th1- or Th2-specific manner (90,91). Thus, chemokine/receptor expression patterns on T cells *in vivo* are complex. While the precise role of chemokines in the regulation of Th1/Th2 responses is still undetermined, they appear to represent a regulatory mechanism for the induction and fine-tuning of effector immune responses.

Chemokine secretion may also be linked to the cytolytic activity of cytotoxic T cells (CTL) (56,77,92,93). Whereas most inflammatory chemokines are *de novo* synthesized following adequate stimulation, CC chemokines such as RANTES, MIP-1α, and MIP-1β may be prestored in cytolytic granules of CTL, and are secreted upon T cell receptor mediated activation. Chemokines may also be involved in the termination of the immune response. This process may be mediated in part by cytokines such as transforming growth factor (TGF)–β and IL-10, which downregulates most chemokines but induces HCC-4 (94); chemokine-complexing antibodies (95); endogenous corticosteroids; and, possibly, chemokine scavenging through Duffy (31–33). It might be speculated that inadequate inhibition of such local chemokine production is involved in the pathogenesis of chronic inflammation.

Morphogenesis, Hematopoiesis, and Tumor Growth

The same diversity of chemokine signals that regulates the specificity of leukocyte recruitment during inflammation may also govern cell migration during development and normal homeostasis. For example, mice with homozygous deletions of either SDF-1 or its receptor CXCR4 have impaired hematopoiesis, abnormal cerebellar development and gastrointestinal vascularization, and die perinatally in association with a defective ventricular septum of the heart (96–98). The exact role of chemokines during such developmental events is currently unknown. Chemokines may act in bringing and keeping cells together as a functional unit (3,5), as exemplified by chemokine mediation of the encounter between dendritic cells and lymphocytes for antigen presentation (70), and between stromal cells and B cells during early myelopoiesis (71). Chemokines and receptors may also be involved in the regulation of early lymphopoiesis (99) and hematopoiesis (13,22,100,101). The interaction with CXCR2 on endothelial cells has been postulated to mediate angiogenic effects of ELR-CXC chemokines, and the expression of CXCR3 on malignant B cells might indicate a potential effect of chemokines on tumor cell migration (102). However, the exact function of chemokines in angiogenesis and tumor growth presently remains unresolved (97,103–105).

ROLE OF CHEMOKINES IN INFECTIOUS DISEASE

Many infectious and inflammatory diseases are characterized by elevated levels of distinct chemokines. Evidence for the involvement of chemokines in these conditions is derived from (a) *in vitro* studies showing upregulation of chemokine mRNA and chemokine secretion in damaged tissues; (b) upregulation of local chemokines during experimental injury or infection *in vivo*, and increased chemokine levels at sites of disease in human patients compared to controls; and (c) *in vivo* chemokine neutralization experiments indicating reduced leukocyte migration to the site of infection/inflammation and reduction of pathology in various animal models.

Direct evidence for a role of chemokines in the pathogenesis of infectious disease has been recorded in animals, based on chemokine and receptor gene knockout experiments (21–23, reviewed in 8). In humans, the most robust evidence for a role of chemokines is derived from (a) the innate resistance to infection by *P. vivax* in Duffy negative individuals (34); and (b) the individuals with mutations and polymorphisms in chemokine receptor genes who have either an altered susceptibility to HIV infection or who have an alteration in the clinical course of the disease (106–108). Such evidence is currently unavailable for other human diseases.

Correlation of Chemokines with Type of Inflammation and Pathology

Local induction of chemokines at sites of infection is now well documented in the literature. The specificity of leukocyte infiltrates during infection with different pathogens may be mediated by specific chemokines, observed as inducing predominantly mononuclear or predominantly neutrophil effects (CC versus ELR-CXC subfamilies, respectively). For example, IL-8 expression correlates with neutrophilic inflammation in the bronchoalveolar lavage (BAL) fluid from patients with pulmonary tuberculosis (38). *In vitro*, *Mycobacterium tuberculosis* and its cell wall components cause cytokine (IL-1, TNF-α) and IL-8 release from alveolar macrophages (38). IL-8 is also increased in the BAL fluid of patients with cystic fibrosis, and *Pseudomonas aeruginosa* adhesins and exoenzymes induce IL-8 production in respiratory epithelial cells *in vitro* (39). This suggests a mechanism contributing to the chronic neutrophilic airway inflammation associated with the persistence of this organism in patients with cystic fibrosis. During infection with respiratory syncytial virus (RSV), increased numbers of neutrophils are found in the BAL and nasal wash fluid, along with eosinophil degranulation products (42,109). Infection of upper airway cells with RSV *in vitro* has variably been associated with the release of IL-8 (109–111), or RANTES and MIP-1α (42,109). Levels of different CXC and CC chemokines have been shown to be elevated in the cerebrospinal fluid during bacterial and viral meningitis (reviewed in 112). Selective elevations of MCP-1 and mononuclear inflammation have been correlated during AIDS-related cytomegalovirus encephalitis (113). CC chemokines and mononuclear inflammation have been found in the vesicles of recurrent orolabial *Herpes simplex* virus (HSV)–1 infection lesions and are induced in HSV-infected keratinocytes *in vitro* (41). Selective expression of MCP-1 and MIP-1α has been taken to explain the recruitment of T cells and macrophages in the lesions of cutaneous leishmaniasis (114). Each of these studies highlights the local presence of different chemokines after infection with various pathogens and serves to emphasize the key role of chemokines in the recruitment of specific subsets of leukocytes.

High cytokine levels, such as TNF-α and IL-6, and high chemokine levels, including IL-8, MCP-1, and MCP-2, have been correlated with a poor outcome in patients with bacterial pneumonia, sepsis, or the adult respiratory distress syndrome (ARDS) (115–117). The clinical usefulness of chemokine measurements during febrile states is currently unclear due to the complexity of factors that influence their concentrations in body fluids (118). Chemokine levels often correlate with the levels of inflammatory cytokines and acute phase reactants such as the erythrocyte sedimentation rate and C-reactive protein (119).

The contribution of chemokines to the pathophysiology of infectious diseases is suggested by neutralization studies in animals (120,121). As an example, in mice with experimental pneumonia due to *Cryptococcus neoformans* or *Klebsiella pneumoniae*, prior chemokine neutralization (MCP-1, MIP-2) with monoclonal antibodies was linked to reduced leukocyte recruitment and an approximately threefold increase in the pathogen burden (120,121). A recent area of investigation is the role of chemokines in the genetic susceptibility/resistance of different mouse strains to certain pathogens, such as *Leishmania major* (122). Whereas associations of chemokines and their receptors with Th1 versus Th2 cytokine profiles are now emerging (83–88), a direct role in the differential induction of these responses has not yet been shown.

The most striking evidence for chemokine mediation of pathology in infectious diseases was generated by findings in MIP-1α knockout mice. These mice failed to develop myocarditis after infection with the noncytopathic Coxsackievirus B3 (CVB3) (23). Since MIP-1α knockout mice had normal numbers of functioning lymphocytes, and no difference in CVB3 viral titers, the dramatic reduction in pathology may be linked to deficient recruitment of T cells to the CVB3-infected tissues. MIP-1α knockout mice also had a reduction in the severity of pneumonitis after inoculation with influenza A virus, even though increased viral titers and delayed (but complete) clearance of the virus was recorded. These findings suggest that the effects of chemokine blockade *in vivo* likely depend on viral (such as inoculum and cytopathogenicity) and host (type and strength/duration of immune response) parameters that govern the outcome of a given infection (123).

In humans, a role for chemokines as direct mediators of pathologic processes is not as clear. As an example, in experimental human rhinovirus infection, no tissue damage was demonstrable in biopsy specimens, but levels of IL-8 (as well as IL-1β and IL-6) in nasal secretions correlated with symptom score. The infected subjects with no symptoms showed the same low nasal IL-8 levels as the uninfected control subjects (124). These findings suggest that the host response, rather than direct cytopathic effects of the virus, was responsible for the symptoms. In other experiments, CC chemokine levels correlated with both pathologic changes in tissue and symptoms. In subjects with experimental influenza A, viral titers and symptom score correlated with the nasal levels of IL-6, interferon (IFN)–α, and CC chemokines, but not IL-8 (125–127). The presence, early in the disease course, of symptoms and elevated CC chemokine levels is consistent with the mononuclear inflammation generally associated with the first stage of influenza virus infection. IL-8 appeared only after symptoms had already improved, at a time when migration of neutrophils into the infected mucosa was recorded.

A role for chemokines in linking chronic inflammation and persistent bacterial infection is an area of active investigation and is now documented at least indirectly in two settings (128,129). Persistent infection with invasive *Porphyromonas gingivalis*, a major pathogen in chronic periodontal disease, may relate to the inhibition by this pathogen of IL-8 secretion by gingival epithelial cell cultures *in vitro*; noninvasive strains did not inhibit IL-8 secretion (128). By inhibiting IL-8, this pathogen might subvert neutrophil infiltration and phagocytosis. In contrast, the virulence of cytotoxin-producing, cytotoxin-associated gene A (cagA)–positive *Helicobacter pylori* strains as agents of chronic inflammatory gastritis may be at least partially reflected in their induction of IL-8 and other chemokines and attraction of neutrophils. The less virulent cagA-negative strains stimulate far less chemokine production in gastric mucosal cells (129,130). The cagA protein is, however, not a direct chemokine inducer. Additional mechanisms likely mediate the persistence in the host of cagA+ *H. pylori* strains and the associated chronic gastritis.

Exploitation of the Chemokine System by Microorganisms

Subversion of the immune response is a major mechanism of persistence of pathogens in the host (131). As shown in Table 8.3, the expression and/or secretion of chemokine or chemokine receptor homologues is now recognized as a strategy of an expanding number of pathogens to interfere with chemokine/receptor interactions, thereby modifying the host immune response (132). Chemokine receptors on leukocytes may make ideal targets for utilization by infectious agents, essentially converting a host defense cell into an important vector for replication and spread of the microbe (24). As mentioned previously, chemokine receptors are identified as coreceptors for two important human pathogens, *P. vivax* which binds to Duffy on red blood cells (32,34), and HIV which requires both CD4 and a chemokine receptor to enter cells (133). In addition, cell entry of *Streptococcus pneumoniae* is mediated by the receptor for platelet activating factor, a lipid chemoattractant receptor that is structurally related to chemokine receptors (134).

Chemokine modulation is also emerging as an extensively utilized survival strategy of many classes of viruses.

TABLE 8-3. *Methods by which human microbial pathogens use chemokines and chemokine receptors*

Method	Microorganism	Chemokine/chemokine receptor
Microbial exploitation of the chemokine system		
Use of chemokine receptors for cell entry	HIV-1	See Table 8-4
	Plasmodium Vivax	DARC
Use of receptor encoded by other virus for cell entry	HIV-1	CMV US28
Virally encoded chemokine receptor for cell signaling	HHV-8/KSHV	ORF74 GPCR
Use of viral chemokines for angiogenesis	HHV-8/KSHV	vMIP-I, vMIP-II
Use of viral chemokines to ? attract cells and spread virus	HHV-6	U83 ?
	HIV-1	nef, tat
Microbial immune evasion by subversion of chemokine signaling		
Virally encoded chemokine antagonists	Molluscum Contagiosum virus	MC148
	HHV-8/KSHV	vMIP-I, vMIP-II
Virally encoded chemokine scavengers	CMV	US28
	HHV-6 (?)	US12 (?)
	Poxviruses	multiple
Virally encoded chemokines that modify Th1/Th2 balance	HHV-8	vMIP-I, -II

Cytomegalovirus

Human cytomegalovirus (CMV) encodes US28, a functional receptor for several CC chemokines that is most related in sequence to CCR1 (135,136). In response to CMV infection *in vitro*, fibroblasts secrete RANTES and MCP-1. CMV-infected cells also express US28, which binds these chemokines, leading to their functional inactivation via intracellular sequestering, suggesting a mechanism utilized by CMV to prevent the recruitment of immune cells to the environment of infected cells (137). In addition, US28 may function as an HIV-1 entry coreceptor, suggesting a mechanism to explain the upregulation of HIV replication that has been recorded in CMV-infected patients in some studies (135). CMV also encodes a CXC chemokine that binds to CXCR2 and has IL-8–like agonist activity. This might play a role in the attraction of leukocytes that, once infected, allow for systemic dissemination of CMV (138).

Human Herpesvirus 8

Human herpesvirus 8 [HHV-8/Kaposi sarcoma–associated herpesvirus (KSHV)] encodes two proteins (vMIP-I and -II) that block multiple chemokine receptors (CCR1, CCR2, CCR3, CCR5, CCR8, CXCR4) and potently inhibit monocyte migration in response to CC chemokines (139,140). vMIP-I and -II attract Th2 cells, and vMIP-II also may antagonize Th1 cell chemotaxis, suggesting a potential role for these proteins in immune evasion by HHV-8 (141). Both vMIPs are angiogenic *in vitro* and may play a role in the vascular proliferation associated with Kaposi's Sarcoma. Moreover, the binding of vMIP-II to CCR3 and CCR5 may inhibit binding of HIV-1. Since CCR3 is an HIV coreceptor on microglia (142), infection with HHV-8 may reduce the infection of microglial cells with HIV and, possibly, the occurrence of HIV-associated brain disease, including HIV-associated dementia (139,143,144). vMIP-II has already been found to be a therapeutically useful chemokine blocker in a rat glomerulonephritis model, where it reduced leukocyte influx and proteinuria (145).

HHV-8 also encodes a GPCR, the product of open reading frame (ORF) 74 (146,147). HHV-8 GPCR is most related in sequence to CXCR1 and CXCR2, but is the only currently known chemokine receptor that signals constitutively. Signaling through HHV-8 GPCR is associated with cell transformation and angiogenesis (148). These findings suggest that HHV-8 GPCR is a viral oncogene that may drive the cellular proliferation that accompanies HHV-8 associated malignancies, i.e., Kaposi's sarcoma, primary-effusion lymphoma, and Castleman's disease (146,148,149).

Human Herpesvirus 6

Human herpesvirus 6 (HHV-6) replicates mainly in $CD4^+$ T cells and may persist in a latent state in monocytes and macrophages. The U83 gene of HHV-6 encodes a functional chemokine that might play a role in the spread of HHV-6 by attracting mononuclear cells to sites of viral replication (150). Furthermore, the HHV-6 gene U12 encodes a functional CC-chemokine receptor whose biological role at present is unknown (151). Infection of $CD4^+$ T cells with HHV-6 is associated with downregulation of CXCR4 expression but upregulation of CD4, suggesting complex interactions of HHV-6 with the pathogenesis of HIV disease (152).

Human Immunodeficiency Virus

Utilization of the chemokine system is now increasingly recognized as a crucial component of the intercellular spread and replication of HIV. The Tat protein of HIV is a potent monocyte attractant. This activity may be related to a region in the Tat gene that encodes a peptide (*CysL24-51*) with functional CC chemokine activity mediated via CCR2 and CCR3 (153). Secreted Tat may attract monocytes towards HIV-producing cells and facilitate spread of the virus. A recent report highlights yet another crucial role for the HIV Nef protein in the pathogenesis of HIV disease. *In vitro*, Nef was shown to induce in macrophages the production of MIP-1α and MIP-1β, associated with the chemotaxis of lymphocytes to the infected macrophages. These chemokines and an additional, unidentified soluble factor may activate the attracted lymphocytes, suggesting a crucial role for infected macrophages in the spread of HIV (154). The role of chemokines in HIV infection will be further summarized in the next section.

Molluscum Contagiosum *Virus*

Molluscum contagiosum virus (MCV) encodes MC148, a secreted CC chemokine homologue with broad-spectrum (CC and CXC) chemokine-blocking activity. This might explain the absence of an inflammatory response in molluscum lesions and virus persistence (155). Other nonhuman poxviruses also encode chemokine-scavenging proteins (156).

These viral chemokine and chemokine receptor homologues highlight strategies that may allow viral persistence in the host through avoidance of an effective immune response.

Human Immunodeficiency Virus

The evolving understanding of the role of chemokines and chemokine receptors in the pathogenesis of HIV disease has been thoroughly reviewed (108,157–160). Three major areas relevant to the context of therapeutic strategies will be summarized here: (a) use of chemokine receptors as coreceptors by HIV for entry into target cells; (b) impact of chemokine receptor expression on the risk of HIV transmission and disease progression; and (c) chemokine levels *in vivo* and *in vitro* at different stages of HIV disease.

Chemokine Receptors as Coreceptors for Human Immunodeficiency Virus Infection

Since the landmark discovery in 1996 that chemokine receptors serve as coreceptors for HIV binding, membrane fusion, and entry into target cells (14,15,161–164), there has been rapid progress in the understanding of HIV disease pathogenesis, and novel therapeutic approaches are being developed based on modulation of the chemokine system. The physical association between a chemokine coreceptor and the complex of the HIV envelope glycoprotein and the primary receptor CD4 is necessary for cellular infection by HIV (230,324,325; reviewed in 24). Currently, at least 11 chemokine receptors have been reported to serve as coreceptors for HIV and/or simian immunodeficiency virus (SIV) *in vitro*, as summarized in Table 8.4. How many of these 11 receptors are operative *in vivo* as coreceptors for HIV is uncertain, as is their exact biology and tissue distribution. The current consensus is that CCR5 and CXCR4 are the two most important HIV coreceptors. The nomenclature for distinctive phenotypic HIV strains changed in 1998 and is now based on chemokine receptor usage rather than their target cell type (Fig. 8.3). In the old, potentially confusing nomenclature, non–syncytium-inducing (NSI) HIV strains that were able to infect monocyte-macrophages and primary T cells *in vitro*, but not T cell lines were called macrophage-tropic ("M-tropic"). In the new nomenclature, such M-tropic strains of HIV are termed "R5" to indicate that they enter target cells by means of CCR5. Similarly, in the old nomenclature, syncytium-inducing (SI) strains of HIV that could infect T cell lines and primary T cells *in vitro*, but not monocyte-macrophages, were defined as T cell line–tropic (T-tropic) strains. In the new nomencla-

TABLE 8-4. *Chemokine receptors used by HIV and SIV as co-receptors for cell entry* in vitro

Chemokine receptor	Ligands	Cellular expression	Virus
CXCR4	SDF-1α, SDF-1β	Lymphocytes, macrophages, brain	X4, R5X4
CCR2	MCP-1, MCP-2, MCP-3, MCP-4, MCP-5	Monocytes, T cells	R5X4
CCR3	Eotaxin-1, eotaxin-2, RANTES, MCP-2, MCP-3, MCP-4, MCP-5	Eosinophils, microglia, Th2 cells	R5X4
CCR5	RANTES, MIP-1α, MIP-1β	Monocytes, T cells	R5, R5X4, HIV-2, SIV
CCR8	I-309	Monocytes, thymocytes	R5X4, HIV-2, SIV
STRL33/Bonzo/TYMSTR	Unknown	T cells, monocytes, placenta	R5X4, SIV
BOB/GPR-15	Unknown	T cells, colon	R5X4, SIV
GPR-1	Unknown	Macrophages, lymphocytes, brain	SIV, some HIV strains
CX_3CR-1/V28	Fractalkine	Lymphocytes, brain	R5X4, HIV-2, SIV
APJ	Unknown	?	X4, R5X4, SIV
Cytomegalovirus (CMV) US28	RANTES, MIP-1(, MCP-1	CMV-infected cells	R5X4

R5, CCR5 using ("M-tropic") virus; X4, CXCR4 using ("T-tropic") virus; R5X4, CCR5 and/or CXCR4 using ("dual tropic") virus.

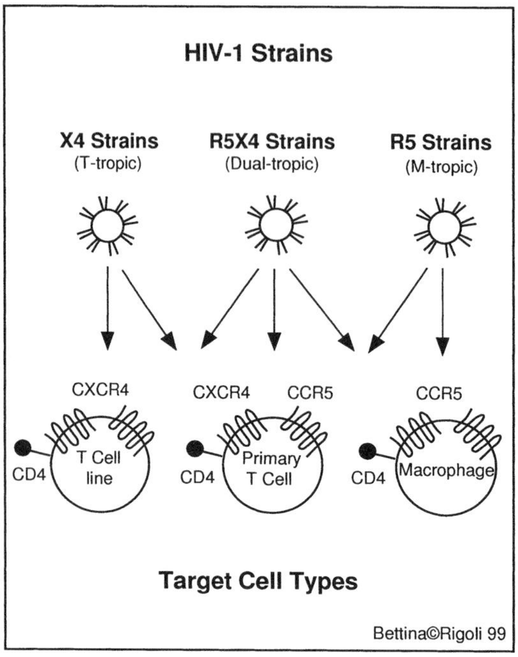

FIG. 8.3. Current model for chemokine coreceptor usage and target cell types of HIV-1. Chemokine receptor usage rather than the target cell type is the basis for the new nomenclature of HIV phenotypes. T cell line–tropic (T-tropic) hiv strains are now referred to as x4 strains. Dual-tropic hiv strains (with tropism for T cell lines, primary T cells, and macrophages) are now designated as R5X4 strains. Macrophage-tropic (m-tropic) strains are now referred to as r5 strains. [From Berger EA, Murphy PM, Farber JM. Chemokine receptors as HIV-1 coreceptors: roles in viral entry, tropism, and disease. *Annu Rev Immunol* 1999;17:657–700, and Rigoli B (b.rigoli@planet.ch), with permission.]

ture, these T-tropic/SI strains of HIV are termed "X4" strains to signify that they use CXCR4 to infect cells. HIV strains that were previously called "dual-tropic" are now termed "R5X4" to reflect the fact that they enter cells using either CCR5 or CXCR4.

Impact of Chemokine Receptor Expression on the Risk of Human Immunodeficiency Virus Transmission and Disease Progression

Epidemiologic evidence that chemokine receptor expression has clinical relevance to HIV transmission and disease progression (reviewed in 106 and 157) was initially derived from the observation that persons lacking expression of CCR5 are almost completely resistant to infection with HIV and appear to suffer no adverse consequences from the absence of CCR5 expression (107). Rarely, when such persons do become infected with HIV, it is with X4 strains that, overall, account for less than 10% of transmitted strains of HIV (168).

A homozygous mutation in CCR5 associated with the absence of cellular expression of CCR5 is a 32–base pair deletion in the CCR5 gene ("CCR5Δ32") (107). This homozygous genotype is present in about 1% of Caucasians, while up to 20% of Caucasians are heterozygous for the mutation. Subjects with a heterozygous CCR5Δ32 mutation are not protected against transmission of HIV, but may have a modestly delayed rate of HIV disease progression (169,170) and, perhaps, lower rates of HIV-associated dementia (171). This genotype might result in lower levels of R5 HIV strains in the brain and therefore less infection of microglial and other CCR5-expressing cells. In addition, the onset of toxoplasmosis as the initial AIDS-defining illness may be delayed in HIV-infected patients who are heterozygous for the CCR5Δ32 mutation (172). The CCR5Δ32 mutation is rare in individuals of African or Asian descent (173). A case report describes an additional CCR5 mutation termed CCR5-m303 (174), also associated with absent cellular expression of CCR5.

Furthermore, a homozygous polymorphism in the CCR5 promoter (base pair 59029-G/G) that is detectable among all ethnic groups has a substantially greater effect on disease progression than the above mentioned mutations (175). Additional chemokine receptor mutations that are associated with delayed disease progression in HIV-infected persons include a mutation in CCR2b, termed CCR2-64I (176,177), and a homozygous mutation in the 3′-untranslated region (SDF1-3′A) of the SDF-1 mRNA (178). The protective mechanism of the CCR2-64I mutation may lie in the heterodimerization of the mutant CCR2 with CCR5 and CXCR4, which may reduce the availability of functional HIV coreceptors on the cell surface (29,179).

Differential chemokine receptor expression due to genetic polymorphisms is likely responsible for a part of the host determinants of HIV disease progression. It must be noted, however, that other host factors contribute in important ways to HIV disease, including the HLA haplotype (180,181), the activity of HIV-specific cytotoxic T lymphocytes (182), and as yet unidentified mechanisms. A unique mode of protection may be operative in hematopoietic stem cells, which were recently found to be resistant to infection with HIV *in vitro*, despite the expression of CD4 and functional CCR5 and CXCR4 (183). Novel therapeutic strategies may emerge from the elucidation of the mechanism of stem cell protection from HIV infection.

Over 90% of HIV strains transmitted person-to-person and via blood transfusion are R5 strains, even if the transmitting source is infected with both R5 and X4 strains. Therefore, CCR5 and CXCR4 expression by different cell types is an area of intense investigation (184), in an attempt to define the initial cell types infected after transmission. For example, freshly isolated macrophages and T cells from human genital mucosal surfaces expressed both CCR5 and CXCR4, thus appearing as the likely primary targets for sexually transmitted HIV. The majority of DCs expressed CXCR4 but not CCR5, although indirect infection of DCs from T cells via DC-T cell interactions may be responsible for HIV spread to the lymph nodes and the circulation (185). DC-T cell interaction was also necessary for T cell activation and HIV production, since HIV may replicate less well in resting T cells. DCs in the peripheral blood express both CXCR4 and CCR5, and can be infected with both R5 and X4 strains of HIV *in vitro* (186,187). The selective transmission of R5 strains remains unexplained in this experimental system, but a possible mechanism was suggested by a recent report of the biochemical characteristics of chemokine receptors (136). These may be present on the macrophage surface as either monomers or higher molecular weight forms. The presence of CXCR4 mainly in the high molecular weight form was associated in this experiment with inefficient association of CXCR4, CD4, and X4 strains of HIV (188). To date, however, no conclusive explanation has emerged for the selective transmission of R5 strains of HIV.

In approximately 50% of patients initially infected with R5 strains of HIV, there eventually is a transition to either X4 or R5X4 strains, associated with a more rapid disease progression and decline in $CD4^+$ T cell counts (158). Why this change occurs in only 50% of patients is currently unknown. A recently described polymorphism in the CCR5 promoter (175) may affect the transcription of the CCR5 gene and govern the infectability of $CD4^+$ T cells by R5 strains, and hence, disease progression. Since only a small fraction of $CD4^+$ T cells express CCR5, R5 strains induce a less rapid depletion of $CD4^+$T cells than do X4 strains, even though their cytopathogenicity may be the same (189). Explanations for the R5 to X4 transition have focused intensively on the levels of CCR5 and CXCR4 expression in lymph nodes, antigen presenting cells, and T cells (184). Even though there is clear evidence for persistent immune activation even in asymptomatic individuals, the upregulation of chemokine receptor expression by inflammatory cytokines induced by opportunistic infections appears to play a major role in the associated high levels of viral replication and accelerated disease progression (158). As an example, IL-2 *in vivo* upregulates CCR5 (but not CXCR4) expression and likely enhances HIV replication and the infectability of target cells in the absence of antiretroviral therapy (190). In addition, HIV envelope proteins not only bind to, but also signal through, CCR5 and CXCR4. This signaling may be associated with activation and chemoattraction of $CD4^+$ T cells as well as with increased viral replication and spread (191–193), even though signaling through chemokine receptors is not required for membrane fusion and target cell entry *in vitro*.

Finally, inflammation at the site of initial HIV inoculation (e.g., genital ulcer disease) likely results not only in skin breaks conducive to HIV infection but also to increased chemokine receptor expression. The association between inflammation and chemokine receptor expression may be a further factor to explain the increased risk of HIV transmission in such settings.

Chemokine Levels **in Vivo** *and* **in Vitro** *at Different Stages of Human Immunodeficiency Virus Disease*

The first reports in 1995 of the potential HIV blocking activity of $CD8^+$ T cell secreted CC chemokines on activated $CD4^+$T cells *in vitro* (92) identified CC chemokines as possible endogenous antiviral factors active *in vivo* and stimulated attempts to correlate circulating CC chemokine levels with HIV disease progression. Subsequent observations led to a more complex picture: (a) a part of the *in vitro* HIV suppressive activity ascribed to CC chemokines is derived from other unidentified soluble products of $CD8^+$ T cells (194); (b) CC chemokines have little, if any, effect on HIV infection of macrophages and dendritic cells *in vitro*; and (c) CC chemokines only block infection with R5 strains and may potentially enhance the replication of X4 strains *in vitro* (192,193,195,196).

Multiple reports have attempted to correlate disease progression with low circulating CC chemokine levels, but the results have been conflicting (160,197,198). Recently, the converse was reported, namely that high serum RANTES levels were a marker of rapidly progressive disease (199). Possible explanations for the diverging results include the difference in CC chemokines evaluated, failure to take into account the time span since HIV seroconversion, the patients selected for comparison, fluctuations in RANTES levels due to platelet release of RANTES, and whether chemokine levels were measured *in vivo* (especially in serum) or *in vitro* after antigenic or mitogenic stimulation. CC chemokine levels have also been suggested to correlate with successful therapeutic intervention, such as vaccination (see below), and antiviral therapy. For example, one study recorded that three-agent antiretroviral therapy that included a protease inhibitor was more effective than two-agent antiretroviral therapy in suppressing viral replication and in restoring *in vitro* T cell immunoreactivity to microbial antigens in HIV-infected subjects, and these findings correlated with higher serum CC chemokine levels (200). At present, however, the clinical value of measuring serum chemokine levels in HIV-infected patients remains unclear (197).

Chemokines in Inflammatory and "Idiopathic" Diseases

While a full discussion of the involvement of chemokines in these diseases is beyond the scope of this chapter, a brief synopsis follows in light of the rapidly expanding literature in this area. The local upregulation of chemokine receptors and attraction of leukocytes has suggested a role for chemokines in multiple chronic inflammatory diseases (11). Chemokines may contribute to disease expression in schistosomiasis and tuberculosis (201), as well as sarcoidosis (202), inflammatory bowel disease (203,204), atherosclerosis (205–208), psoriasis (209,210), inflammatory arthritis (36), and experimental autoimmune encephalomyelitis (211,212).

TGF-β is a cytokine that may play an important role in regulating tissue repair following inflammation (213). Chemokines may cooperate with TGF-β in this process (214). Fibrosis may develop when persistent activation of macrophages and fibroblasts occurs. These cells secrete a variety of chemokines and upregulate chemokine receptors (46,213–215). Moreover, activated macrophages can be directly activated to release IL-8 (40,216) by free radical injury to the extracellular matrix as a result of neutrophil degranulation. Thus, IL-8 may be a key mediator in the "vicious cycle" of neutrophil attraction, tissue damage, chronic inflammation, and fibrosis (104,216).

Chemokines may be involved in the pathogenesis of inflammatory renal diseases (217). Neutralization experiments with antibodies against a single chemokine in animal models of glomerulonephritis (49,215,218,219) have demonstrated significant reductions of proteinuria and renal injury. It has been shown that certain urinary chemokines levels are elevated in human patients with active glomerulonephritis (MCP-1 and IL-8) (221), lupus nephritis (MCP-1) (222), and as a favorable prognostic indicator after *Bacille Calmette-Guerin* (BCG) therapy of bladder cancer (IL-8) (223). These observations suggest that one may be able to use chemokines in novel disease monitoring strategies.

Ischemia and reperfusion injury have been associated with increased local production of chemokines (224–226). In a rabbit model of ARDS, significant local production of IL-8 occurred during the reperfusion phase, in conjunction with neutrophil influx and lung injury. This injury was prevented by an anti-IL-8 mAb (225). Chemokines are emerging tools to study the mechanisms involved in allograft rejection (227–228, reviewed in 229). In renal transplant recipients with rejection who improved with steroid administration, urinary MCP-1 fell, but increased in those with no response to steroids (228).

The concept that chemokines exert their immunoregulatory role by attracting effector cells in functional units (1,66,85,230) is reflected in current models of allergic inflammation (231). Activated Th2 cells secrete IL-4 and IL-5 and attract the pathophysiologically related eosinophils and basophils. Th2 cells, eosinophils and basophils all share CCR3 and are attracted concomitantly by eotaxin and other chemokines that target CCR3, such as RANTES and MCP-2, -3, and -4 (203,231,232). T cells expressing CCR3 are found with eosinophils in atopic dermatitis and nasal polyps, whereas the lymphocytes in nonallergic inflammation are generally CCR3 negative (230). CC chemokines may thus mediate the influx of eosinophils and other inflammatory cells into the airways of patients with asthma (233), and into nasal secretions in patients with allergic rhinitis (234). In addition, CC chemokines may mediate eosinophil degranulation and much of the non–IgE-dependent histamine and leukotriene release by basophils (231). Finally, RANTES and MIP-1α may augment the effects of IL-4 on the activation of B-cells expressing surface IgE, whereas IL-8 has an inhibitory effect (235).

POTENTIAL THERAPIES INVOLVING THE CHEMOKINE SYSTEM

As the *in vivo* function of chemokines and chemokine receptors is becoming more clearly defined, interest in the chemokine system as a target for immune modulation is rapidly expanding. Attention initially centered on identifying chemokine receptor antagonists as novel antiinflammatory agents, but has increasingly focused on HIV following the identification of chemokine receptors as HIV entry coreceptors. The first phase I trial of AMD3100, a CXCR4 blocker, has recently been completed (236). Chemokine applications are also being pursued in the vaccine field, and BB-10010, a modified MIP-1α was evaluated in phase II trials as a stem cell protector during cancer chemotherapy (237,238).

Some antiinflammatory agents that are already in clinical use are now known to have effects on the chemokine system. For example, the inhibition by corticosteroids of NF-κB is associated with reduced transcription of several cytokine and chemokine genes, including IL-8, MCP-1, and RANTES (234,239,240). Cyclophosphamide may also suppress chemokine production (241), and thalidomide may inhibit IL-8 production, via the inhibition of NF-κB (242). An intriguing role as chemokine suppressants has recently emerged for angiotensin-converting enzyme (ACE) inhibitors. Angiotensin II has been shown to increase MCP-1 and RANTES expression by smooth muscle cells and endothelial cells, respectively, associated with monocyte influx into blood vessel walls (207,208). The ACE inhibitor quinapril and two angiotensin II receptor blockers reduced such chemokine expression via blockade of the NF-κB pathway, associated with a reduction of macrophage infiltration and a trend towards reduced atheroma formation in rabbits (207,208).

Chemokines

Blockade of chemokine receptors with chemokines would appear to be an appealing therapeutic strategy. That, however, is not being investigated for numerous reasons. All chemokines are proteins, making parenteral injection necessary, and they have short half lives *in vivo*. Potential pro-inflammatory adverse effects, however, might be the most prominent drawback to the use of chemokines in human patients, including the possibility of inducing or worsening preexisting inflammation/ autoimmunity, as has occasionally been observed with the use of proinflammatory cytokines such as IL-2 and IL-12. Additional concerns regarding exposure to high systemic chemokine levels are immunosuppression and increased susceptibility to infection. For example, rabbits that received intravenous IL-8 developed rapid and transient neutropenia, followed by sustained leukocytosis and inhibition of neutrophil migration (243). Transgenic mice that overexpressed IL-8 or MCP-1 at high levels did not develop leukocyte infiltrates in response to local IL-8 administration (244). High MCP-1 expression in mice was associated with a several-fold increased susceptibility to infection with *M. tuberculosis* and *Listeria monocytogenes* (245). These reports suggest that consistently high chemokine levels may lead to leukocyte desensitization and/or the ablation of a physiologically active chemokine gradient, receptor overstimulation or downregulation. Nonetheless, one report indicated clinical benefit when MCP-1 was given for 2 days after experimental endotoxemia in mice (246). In contrast to observations made in settings of high chemokine levels, the relatively low level expression of chemokines in transgenic animals usually has induced the expected focal leukocyte infiltrates, consistent with the concept that chemokines function *in vivo* at low concentrations at the local level (247).

As the human trials of chemokines have only recently been initiated, these safety issues are currently unresolved. A partial solution to these concerns may be derived from the evaluation in patients of the effects on the chemokine network of already licensed proinflammatory cytokines, such as IL-2 and granulocyte-macrophage colony-stimulating factor (GM-CSF). GM-CSF may cause transient leukopenia before it induces leukocytosis, with no discernible adverse consequences. GM-CSF is well tolerated and may prove useful as a vaccine adjuvant (248,249). *In vitro*, it increases the resistance of uninfected $CD4^+$ T cells to HIV infection and enhances the activity of several antiretroviral agents (250–252). GM-CSF may reduce HIV replication and increase CD4⁺ T cell counts in patients receiving antiretroviral therapy (248,253). These effects appear to be, at least in part, mediated through its effects on the downregulation of CCR5 and CXCR4 expression on macrophages and CD4⁺ cells (250,252). IL-2, when given to HIV-infected patients with CD4⁺ T cell counts substantially increases CD4⁺ T cell counts (254) (see Chapter 2). *In vitro,* it also upregulates CD4⁺ T cell expression of CCR5, which could enhance HIV replication. However, this was not seen when IL-2 was coadministered with antiretroviral therapy (190). Other cytokines and their antagonists, such as IL-1 receptor antagonists, may also function in part through actions on chemokine expression (255).

Elucidation of the immune mechanisms to be modified in a particular setting is crucial in rationally designing chemokine intervention strategies, as exemplified in the potential effects of CC chemokines during HIV infection (suppressive activity versus enhanced replication) (192,193,196). Thus, safety concerns currently make it unlikely that native CC chemokines soon will be used therapeutically against HIV.

Chemically Modified Chemokines

Chemokines are essential for host defense, but they potentially could cause tissue pathology and enhance HIV infection through their proinflammatory effects. Thus, the concept of chemokines as double-edged swords has stimulated modifications of chemokines that block chemokine receptors but lack signaling chemotactic activity. A number of such chemokine derivatives have now been generated (256). The functional domains of several chemokines are localized within the N-terminus, but the chemokine receptor binding domains are outside the N-terminus. By deletion or substitution of one or several N-terminal amino acid residues, functional chemokine receptor antagonists have been constructed. These agents bind to their original receptor, do not signal, and prevent the binding of the native chemokine to the blocked receptor. Examples include derivatives of RANTES, MCP-1, GRO-α, PF-4, and MCP-3 (256–261). Some of these agents have had relevant effects in animal models.

In other instances, N-terminal truncation has been associated with a change in receptor specificity rather than functionality (262). This may represent a biological mechanism that is active *in vivo* to reduce redundant chemokine effects on target cells, and is mediated in part by CD26, an enzyme with peptidase activity that is expressed on activated T cells and macrophages. As an example, truncated RANTES (3-68) was found to signal through CCR5, and no longer through CCR1, in contrast to the native RANTES(1-68) (262). Other chemokine derivatives are based on single amino acid substitutions.

Modified chemokines are promising agents for chemokine receptors blockade in several settings. The best assessment at present is that their therapeutic potential is limited by their peptide nature, likely requiring frequent parenteral administration. Since small-molecule, chemically synthesized GPCR antagonists with high oral bioavailability have been discovered in the past, such compounds are likely also to be developed for chemokine receptors.

RANTES Derivatives

The first reports of nonsignaling RANTES derivatives generated considerable enthusiasm. As outlined above, these are RANTES molecules with N-terminal chemical modifications, and are termed RANTES(9-68), aminooxypentane (AOP)–RANTES, N-nonanoyl (NNY)–RANTES, and Met-RANTES (which has an additional methionine at the N-terminus) (263–265). Met-RANTES is chemotactically inactive *in vitro*, and antagonizes the effects of both RANTES and, to a lesser degree, MIP-1α (264). AOP-RANTES and NNY-RANTES (265–267) are partial antagonists. They inhibit CCR5 binding and infection of peripheral blood mononuclear cells by R5 HIV-1 strains in a concentration dependent manner (267,268). Chemokine receptor internalization and inhibition of receptor recycling is also observed (266), similar to the events following interaction of the native ligands SDF-1α and RANTES with their respective receptors (266,269). The role *in vivo* of receptor internalization in the pathogenesis of HIV infection, and the possible functional activity of intracellular chemokine receptors are under investigation.

Another area of study that may shed light on the exact mechanism of receptor antagonism of modified chemokines are their effects, compared to the native chemokine, on triggering different signaling pathways. As an example, AOP-RANTES, like native RANTES, induces Ca^{2+} flux, the traditional readout of functional chemokine receptor ligation. However, AOP-RANTES does not induce chemotaxis, and this has now been linked to differential signaling (307).

While these *in vitro* reports of RANTES derivatives as CCR5 blockers are encouraging, their effects *in vivo* are not yet known. The potential of RANTES to enhance HIV replication has stimulated efforts to identify CCR5 blockers lacking this potential safety concern. Preliminary data suggests that RANTES variants that are unable to form high molecular mass aggregates do not stimulate HIV infection *in vitro*, in contrast to native RANTES. Further evaluation of these compounds is ongoing (270).

MIP-1α Derivatives

The first chemokine derivative to be tested in human trials is BB-10010 (237,238). This is a modified MIP-1α with a single amino acid substitution that has a reduced tendency, compared to the native MIP-1α molecule, to form high molecular weight aggregates. BB-10010 appears to mimic MIP-1α in its signaling activity. Aside from minor injection site reactions, no inflammatory, adverse effects accompanied the administration of BB-10010 to human volunteers and patients with advanced breast cancer (237). BB-10010 was investigated in phase II clinical trials for its potential myeloprotective properties during cancer chemotherapy, based on the effects of MIP-1α on stem cell cycling (238). In a phase I study of BB-10010 in HIV-infected patients, no effects on viral load, CD4-T cell count or chemokine receptor usage were seen, likely due to the suboptimal serum levels of BB-10010 achieved (171; L. Czaplewski, personal communication, 1999).

A recently described signaling variant of MIP-1α, termed MIP-1αP/LD78β, appears to be as potent as AOP-RANTES in blocking entry of R5 HIV strains *in vitro*. Amino-terminal variants of this protein, such as AOP-MIP-1αP are under evaluation (272).

MCP-1 Derivatives

N-terminal modification has also been performed on the native MCP-1, which has 76 residues, hence its designation MCP-1(1-76) (273). N-terminal truncation of MCP-1 has generated MCP-1(2-76) with increased activity on eosinophils but reduced activity on basophils. Further truncation generated MCP-1 variants with retained activity on both cell types [e.g., MCP-1(4-76) and (5-76)] or no activity on either cell type [(MCP-1(6-76 through 10-76)] (273). The opposite strategy, i.e., N-terminal amino acid addition, might also prove useful to identify chemokine variants with antagonistic properties (274). *In vivo* testing of these MCP-1 derivatives has not yet been reported.

Melanoma Growth Stimulatory Activity (MGSA) Derivatives

An attractive antimalarial treatment strategy involving the chemokine system was first suggested when Duffy was identified as the receptor on red blood cells for *P. vivax* (34). The natural ligands of Duffy, IL-8 and melanoma growth stimulatory activity (MGSA), were found to be efficient blockers of red cell invasion by *Plasmodium knowlesi in vitro.* However, they had the undesirable effect of activating neutrophils by also binding to CXCR2. Based on the distinct binding regions of MGSA for Duffy and CXCR2, two single–amino acid mutants of MGSA have been constructed. One of them, H19A, is a nonsignaling CXCR2 blocker *in vitro* (275). The other mutant, E6A, binds inefficiently to CXCR2 but binds to Duffy, thereby blocking red cell infection by *P. vivax in vitro* (276). Animal testing of these MGSA derivatives has not yet been reported.

Chemokine Antagonists

Chemokine receptor blockade is at present one of the most attractive investigational targets of anti-inflammatory therapy. Most of the modified versions of chemokines that were mentioned above are chemokine receptor blockers, and a large scale effort is currently ongoing to screen natural and synthetic compounds for potential chemokine receptor antagonism. For example, hymenialdisine, a natural derivative of a marine sponge, inhibits NF-κB, reduces IL-8 secretion, and has antiinflammatory activity in animals (277). Most attractive for human use would be the development of small molecule, orally absorbed chemokine receptor blockers. AMD3100 is the first small molecule chemokine receptor antagonist to enter clinical development (see below). Additional such compounds have already been identified (reviewed in 278), consistent with the success in developing antagonists of other GPCR in the past (e.g., β-adrenergic blockers, antihistamines).

A crucial and currently unresolved question is whether blocking of a single chemokine will be of benefit in light of the redundancy of chemokine functions. Knockout experiments (22,23,279) and therapeutic chemokine receptor blockade in mice (256,280) have revealed that chemokine redundancy, as defined *in vitro*, may not be relevant *in vivo* where chemokines display specificity with regards to the timing, site and levels of expression. Indeed, intervention aimed at a single receptor has already been found effective in several animal models (50,281). Blockade of a single chemokine receptor may "break the chain" of inflammatory events without other chemokines substituting for the blocked one (280). For example, in an animal model of glomerulonephritis, treatment with anti–IL-8 antibodies decreased recruitment of neutrophils by only 40%, but completely abolished proteinuria (218). Other examples include the complete abrogation of myocarditis in the MIP-1α knockout mouse after experimental coxsackievirus B3 infection (23), and the complete prevention of reperfusion associated lung injury with anti–IL-8 mAbs (225).

In other models, the effects of chemokine blockade have not been as dramatic, emphasizing the emerging perspective that the outcome of chemokine blockade depends on both the specific pathogen and the particular organ involved (162). Finally, in one rat study of experimental glomerulonephritis, MCP-1 blockade with twice daily mAbs was found effective at day 4 but reduced neither proteinuria nor glomerular crescent formation at day 8. Blockade of additional chemokines or receptors might be essential for sustained effects in specific diseases (220).

Safety Issues

An unresolved concern regarding the use of chemokine antagonists is the potential impairment of the host response towards infectious pathogens. For example, mice pretreated with anti–MCP-1 prior to the induction of endotoxemia had a higher mortality than control animals (246), and MIP-1α knockout mice had an increased pathogen burden after experimental Influenza virus infection (23). The associated clinical effects need to be carefully evaluated in each setting, since, depending on the pathogen, chemokine blockade in animals has been either beneficial (e.g., infection with noncytopathic organisms where disease expression is a consequence of immunopathology) or detrimental (e.g., infection with cytopathic organisms) (23,120). The absence of increased risk of spontaneous infections in individuals with the homozygous CCR5Δ32 mutation appears to support the concept that redundancy governs some aspect of chemokine regulation of immunity. More subtle immune defects may be revealed by further infection challenge studies in mice treated with chemokine blockers or in receptor knockout mice (8). Preliminary observations indicate that mice pretreated with the CCR5 antagonist Met-RANTES had decreased chemotaxis of dendritic cells in response to microbial challenge (282). Another concern about chemokine receptor blockade is interference with key events during morphogenesis by blocking receptors for constitutively expressed chemokines, such as SDF-1/CXCR4 (283). It is currently unclear if such blockade will have any adverse effects in adults (283).

Antichemokine Monoclonal Antibodies (mAbs)

Chemokine blockade with mAbs is another promising approach that is relatively well studied in experimental animals. mAbs have already proven to be valuable tools for the study of the effects of chemokines in animal models after using them for neutralization. The effects seen with mAbs against IL-8, MIP-1α, and MCP-1 have been significant (210,212,219,225). A single dose of an anti-MCP-1 mAb prevented experimental glomerulonephritis and was associated with a 40% reduction in proteinuria (284). Anti-CCR5 mAbs are being evaluated as CCR5 blockers in HIV and may be useful to dissect the molecular details of HIV coreceptor binding and fusion/entry events (184,285). Clinical use of mAbs for various indications has consistently revealed certain general disadvantages of mAbs. These include the need to give mAbs by injection, high cost, and the development of anti–mAb-neutralizing antibodies.

Chemokine Receptor Blockade and HIV Infection

The evidently healthy state of individuals with homozygous CCR5Δ32 mutations suggests that therapeutic CCR5 blockade should be well tolerated and that further modifications of CCR5 blockers may lead to more active compounds. Strategies to block chemokine receptors or to prevent receptor expression have several advantages (108), including the blockade of HIV entry rather than inhibition of events that follow infection of cells, the interference with steps in the HIV life cycle that complement current antiretroviral drug targets, and the prospect of developing a strategy that might prevent expression of multiple chemokine receptors.

A major safety concern is that CCR5 blockade may drive HIV evolution towards the use of CXCR4 (265,286). Since it appears that other coreceptors are less important, at least *in vitro* (286,87), combination blockade of CCR5 and CXCR4 may be a feasible receptor based treatment strategy for established HIV infection, undoubtedly in combination with antiretroviral drug therapy. In addition to the potential use of native and chemically modified SDF-1 (269,288), strategies for blocking X4 using HIV-1 strains are already being developed. One approach has involved the construction of T22 and ALX40-4C (283,289), two peptide inhibitors of SDF-1 binding to CXCR4 and X4 HIV-1 strains *in vitro*. *In vivo* results are not yet available. A disadvantage of current peptide approaches in general is their high cost and the need for parenteral administration.

Intrakines

Another strategy to functionally inhibit CXCR4 is the use of a so-called intrakine (a term derived from "intracellular chemokine"). This is a gene therapy approach involving the retroviral delivery of the SDF-1 gene with a signal sequence attached to it that targets the expressed protein to the endoplasmic reticulum (ER). In the ER, this modified SDF-1 protein binds newly synthesized CXCR4 and prevents its transport to the cell surface (290). By this approach, lymphocytes have essentially been converted *in vitro* into CXCR4 knockout variants that were resistant to infection with X4 HIV strains. Potential limitations to the clinical applicability of this strategy include the need to remove large numbers of lymphocytes from patients, the technical obstacles involved with gene therapy, concerns about the viability and immunologic competence of the transduced lymphocytes, and the evolutionary pressure generated by the intrakine on HIV to use other chemokine receptors for cell entry (291). RANTES and MIP-1α intrakines to block cell surface expression of CCR5 have also been constructed by the same group (292).

Small Molecule Chemokine Receptor Antagonists

AMD3100 is a small, chemically synthesized molecule of the bicyclam family (293). Bicyclams are potent inhibitors of early events in the life cycle of X4 HIV isolates (294,295). AMD3100 selectively binds to CXCR4 and thereby inhibits binding and signaling of SDF-1, as well as HIV-1 and 12G5, a CXCR4 specific monoclonal antibody. AMD3100 does not interact with the principal neutralizing determinant in the third variable (V3) region of the HIV-1 glycoprotein envelope. AMD3100 does not signal and does not seem to cause CXCR4 downregulation (293). AMD3100 was relatively nontoxic in SCID hu mice and caused a dose-dependent decrease in HIV viremia, an effect that was potentiated by antiretroviral drugs (296). Potential disadvantages of AMD3100 include the emergence of resistant HIV strains (297), and reduced efficacy against X4 strains that use alternative coreceptors (133,299,300). Of note, AMD3100 may redirect X4 and R5X4 HIV strains to the R5 phenotype (301). Intravenous dose escalating studies of AMD3100 have recently been completed in twelve healthy volunteers (236). AMD-3100 was well tolerated. A major limitation of AMD3100 is its low oral bioavailability. No drug was detected in the blood of six subjects after oral dosing. Clinical evaluation of AMD3100 is currently ongoing in HIV-infected subjects.

The molecular delineation of the extracellular domains of CCR5 and CXCR4 that are involved in HIV *env*–mediated membrane fusion and viral entry (302,303) has proven extremely complex. Thus, rational drug development based on such knowledge is not anticipated to occur soon. The *in vitro* anti-HIV activity of a small-molecule antagonist of

CCR5, TAK-779, was recently reported, and animal studies of this compound are underway (304–306). A small molecule CXCR2 antagonist (SB225002) (307), a CCR3 antagonist, and several CCR1 antagonists of the 4-hydroxypiperidine class (308) are also in preclinical development for diseases other than HIV.

Ex Vivo Modification of Lymphocytes to Downregulate Chemokine Receptors or Upregulate Chemokine Expression

Additional approaches to immune therapy of HIV infection that may rely on chemokine modulation involve infusions of autologous lymphocytes. One approach has been to induce HIV-1 resistance in $CD4^+$ T cells of HIV-infected patients by the *ex vivo* stimulation of these cells with immobilized mAbs to both CD3 and CD28 (309–312). CD3/CD28 stimulation may induce a R5-HIV-1–resistant T cell state via downregulated CCR5 expression, independent of the proliferative effects that CD28 ligation induces in T cells (10,310,311). This has led to the expansion (10^9-fold to 10^{11}-fold) of CD4+ T cells *ex vivo* in the absence of exogenous cytokines. The CD3/CD28 stimulated CD4 cells remained, however, permissive to infection with X4 strains of HIV, possibly due to incomplete downregulation of CXCR4. This *ex vivo* approach to immune reconstitution for HIV infection is technically difficult and labor intensive.

In another approach (313), 11 patients with advanced HIV disease who were all receiving antiretroviral drugs were given infusions of lymphocytes that were harvested from the patients' own lymph nodes and then expanded *ex vivo* with anti-CD3 antibodies and IL-2. The infusions were associated with a twofold, transient increase in serum MIP-1α levels in most subjects, as well as elevated $CD4^+$T cell counts, reductions in viral load, and reversal of skin test anergy in some subjects. The mechanisms by which the lymphocyte infusions mediated the immunomodulatory and antiviral effects are not known, but the process might have involved increases in CD8-mediated cytotoxicity, HIV modulating factors such as CC chemokines, IL-16, and other yet unidentified CD8+ T cell derived antiviral factors (313). Even though this strategy is technically cumbersome and was complicated by seroma formation at the site of lymph node resection in four of 11 subjects, it suggests a potential immunotherapeutic approach to HIV disease that involves modulation of the chemokine system.

Chemokines and Vaccines

Cytokines are already in clinical evaluation as vaccine adjuvants (249,314), that is, for the augmentation of the immunogenicity of vaccine antigens, and to induce the desired immune mechanism (Th1 versus Th2) for the antigen in question. Attempts to immunize against cancer are associated with additional issues, including the need to induce and maintain an immune response after established disease. Cancer cells may evade an effective immune response by the downregulation of MHC molecules, and by the lack of tumor-specific antigens and/or costimulatory molecules (reviewed in 315). Recent reports suggest that chemokines might be useful to improve the suboptimal efficacy of cancer vaccines. In an effort to further augment the adjuvant activity of IL-2 and GM-CSF, poorly immunogenic murine leukemia cells were transduced with the respective cytokine genes with or without the additional insertion of the lymphotactin gene (316). The cancer cells secreting both the cytokine (especially IL-2) and lymphotactin were more effective than the vaccine expressing the cytokine or lymphotactin alone in suppressing the growth of established tumor in a $CD4^+$ and $CD8^+$ T cell–dependent manner, and in prolonging the survival of the tumor bearing mice.

Chemokines have also been fused to lymphoma-specific variable immunoglobulin domains. Such idiotype antigens generally are poorly immunogenic, but they were able to protect mice against subsequent challenge with wild-type lymphoma cells when the antigen was fused with IP-10 or MCP-3 (317). Analogous effects were obtained using a DNA vaccination approach, which relied upon DNA constructs encoding the antigen and chemokine. While the protective mechanism of such chemokine-fusion vaccines is currently unclear, $CD4^+$–mediated and $CD8^+$–mediated immunity appear to be involved, and the interaction of the chemokine with its receptor might potentially facilitate uptake and presentation of the attached antigen by dendritic cells (317). Chemokine DNA has also been coadministered as an adjuvant with HIV *env*-DNA vaccines to mice, and was found to enhance antigen-specific responses in a Th1 or Th2 biased fashion (318).

In addition to their use as adjuvants, chemokines have also been used as vaccine antigens. In a DNA vaccine strategy, rats were protected against the subsequent induction of experimental autoimmune encephalomyelitis (EAE), possibly based on the induction of neutralizing antibodies to the chemokines involved in the trafficking to the brain of EAE-associated leukocytes (319). While anti-MIP-1α and anti-MCP-1 antibodies were associated with protection from subsequent EAE induction, anti-MIP-1β antibodies aggravated the severity of the disease, highlighting both the potential relevance of antichemokine vaccination strategies in the autoimmune setting as well as the need for careful elucidation of the mediators involved in the disease under study.

Chemokines and HIV Vaccines

In general, efforts to develop preventive HIV vaccines are now increasingly focusing on antigens derived from R5 strains of the virus. In contrast, the first decade of HIV vaccine development used almost exclusively X4 HIV strains as vaccine antigens, in part because X4 strains were initially more easily grown *in vitro* in large quantities. A theoretical concern, however, is that an HIV vaccine that prevents transmission of R5 strains might allow X4 strains to be transmitted in vaccinees protected from infection with R5 strains. Such a concern is unlikely to delay efforts to develop the first preventive HIV vaccine.

The sites of interaction between chemokine coreceptors and the HIV-envelope gp120-CD4 complex are being pursued as immunization targets, in an effort to inhibit the binding and cell entry of HIV. A key determinant of this interaction appears to be localized, at least in part, in the third hypervariable domain (V3) of gp120 (165,320). Neutralizing antibodies against such binding epitopes on gp120 have already been constructed (165). The suboptimal immunogenicity of gp120-V3 peptides as vaccine antigens likely will mandate the use of immunologic adjuvants (314,321). The high mutation rate of HIV envelope proteins may limit the efficacy of vaccines directed against V3 regions. A recent report suggests, however, that during the process of HIV binding and fusion, highly conserved, immunogenic envelope regions may transiently be exposed (298). Cells expressing envelope protein were cocultured with cells expressing CD4 and CCR5. The putative fusion-associated epitopes were "captured" by treating the cultured cells with formaldehyde during different stages of the fusion process of the two cell types. Such inactivated whole cell vaccine preparations were injected into transgenic mice that express human CD4 and CCR5 which were are tolerant to the human components of the vaccine. The immunized mice developed antibodies that neutralized 23 of 24 primary HIV-1 isolates, including X4 strains to which the mice had not been exposed, suggesting that the neutralization target does not lie in the CCR5 component of the vaccine. These findings have led to ongoing efforts to dissect the molecular mechanisms involved in the apparent efficacy of this HIV vaccine in mice (298).

The induction of the CC chemokines RANTES, MIP-1α and -β has been used as a readout of the immunogenicity of several HIV vaccines, including a gp120-V3 vaccine *ex vivo* (321). CC chemokines were surrogate markers of protection associated with the use of HIV-ISCOM (immunostimulating complex) preparations with subsequent intravenous chimeric simian-HIV (SHIV) challenge (322). High CC chemokine levels and CD8+ T cell derived suppressive factors have also been shown to be markers of protection when an envelope subunit SIV vaccine was given intradermally, intramuscularly, or targeted to the iliac lymph nodes in macaques, with subsequent rectal SIV challenge (323,324). In contrast, when a live attenuated SIV vaccine was used in macaques, CC chemokines were of minor importance compared to the CD8+ T cell–derived suppressive factors (325). In a report that is relevant to the HIV vaccine field (326), it was noted that women with recurrent spontaneous abortions who were alloimmunized with their partner's mononuclear cells may develop relative resistance to infection with HIV. *In vitro*, these women's mononuclear cells show long lasting reductions in CCR5 and CXCR4 expression, along with increases in plasma CC chemokines and CD8+ T cell–derived suppressive factors (326). These reports emphasize that the protective mechanisms elicited by candidate HIV vaccines are likely to be complex (327), but may include the induction of CC chemokines and/or reductions in chemokine receptor expression.

Selective Targeting of HIV-Infected Cells Employing Chemokine Receptor Strategies

A therapeutic approach to HIV infection that selectively eliminates HIV-infected cells has been tested *in vitro* using two rhabdoviruses: rabies and vesicular stomatitis virus (VSV) (328,329). After the deletion of their G glycoprotein (responsible for membrane fusion and viral entry), the rhabdoviruses were engineered to express CXCR4. The CXCR4-expressing rhabdoviruses were able to bind to HIV-infected cells expressing HIVgp120 on the cell surface, followed by entry into the cells, rapid replication, direct cytopathic effect, and cell killing. Since HIV-uninfected cells do not express HIVgp120, they were not targeted. A G glycoprotein–deleted VSV transduced with envelope genes from R5 or X4 HIV has been suggested as a novel HIV vaccination strategy. In theory, such a live hybrid virus carrying HIV antigens would specifically target CD4 expressing cells, including dendritic cells, and induce effective cellular and humoral immunity to HIV (330).

Obvious safety concerns remain regarding the clinical use and the transmissibility of live, replicating rhabdoviruses, particularly in immunosuppressed patients, and the potential toxicity to HIV-infected tissues (e.g., brain) in individuals with a wide tissue distribution of HIV. However, these reports introduce novel therapeutic strategies (331), for example, the targeted delivery to HIV-infected cells of antiviral drugs packaged in novel liposomal delivery devices that express chemokine receptors (332).

FUTURE CONSIDERATIONS

The discovery of new chemokines is rapidly progressing along with the screening of ESTs through bioinformatics. On the background of chemokine selectivity versus redundancy, novel disease mechanisms and treatment targets undoubtedly will be identified. In the near future, studies of the clinical safety and efficacy of several pharmacologic agents involving the chemokine system will be reported. Prominent among these efforts is the development of potent and selective chemokine receptor antagonists against HIV. Other critical areas of active study include cancer, atherosclerosis, and novel anti-inflammatory strategies involving chemokine blockade. New drug targets may emerge from further biochemical characterization of chemokine receptors and their signaling pathways. Much remains to be learned about the exact functioning of chemokines in the human body. Proof of their clinical relevance will be provided by novel therapies and vaccines based on chemokine and chemokine receptor research. For infectious diseases where therapeutic intervention today is limited, elucidation of the unique biology of the chemokine system will be crucial in determining how it can be modified to fullest advantage.

GLOSSARY

BCA-1 B cell–activating chemokine–1
BLC B lymphocyte chemoattractant
BLR Burkitt's lymphoma receptor
DARC Duffy antigen receptor complex
DC-CK-1 Dendritic cell chemokine–1
ELC EBI-1 ligand chemokine/Epstein-Barr virus–induced ligand chemokine
ENA-78 Epithelial cell–derived neutrophil attractant 78
GCP-2 Granulocyte chemotactic protein–2
GPCR G protein coupled receptor
GRO Growth-related oncogene
HCC-1,2 Hemofiltrate CC chemokine–1,2
IL-8 Interleukin-8
IL-8RA Interleukin-8 receptor A
γIP-10 Interferon-inducible protein–10
I-TAC Interferon-inducible T cell alpha chemoattractant
LARC Liver and activation-regulated chemokine
LEK Liver-expressed chemokine
Lkn-1 Leukotactin-1
MCP Monocyte chemoattractant protein
MDC Monocyte-derived chemokine
MGSA Melanoma growth stimulatory activity
Mig Monokine induced by interferon gamma
MIP Macrophage inflammatory protein
MPIF-1,2 Myeloid progenitor inhibitory factor–1,2
NAP-2 Neutrophil-activating peptide–2
PARC Pulmonary and activation-regulated chemokine (identical to DC-CK-1)
PF-4 Platelet factor–4
RANTES Regulated on activation, normal T expressed, and secreted
SDF Stromal-derived factor
SLC Secondary lymphoid tissue chemokine
STCP-1 Stimulated T cell chemotactic protein
TARC Thymus and activation-regulated chemokine
TCA-4 T cell activation protein–4
TECK Thymus-expressed chemokine

ACKNOWLEDGMENTS

We wish to thank Dr. Philip Murphy for sharing unpublished data and many helpful discussions, Drs. Craig Hendrix and Lloyd Czaplewski for sharing unpublished data, Bettina Rigoli for preparation of Figs. 8.2 and 8.3, and Drs. Julio Aliberti, Brian Kelsall, Thomas Jones, and Steven M. Holland for critical review of the manuscript.

REFERENCES

1. Metchnikoff E. The mechanism of natural immunity against micro-organisms. In: Metchnikoff E. *Immunity in infectious diseases.* Cambridge: Cambridge University Press, 1905.
2. Rollins BJ. Chemokines. *Blood* 1997;90:909–928.
3. Baggiolini M. Chemokines and leukocyte traffic. *Nature* 1998;392:565–568.
4. Luster AD. Chemokines-chemotactic cytokines that mediate inflammation. *N Engl J Med* 1998;338:436–445.
5. Baggiolini M, Dewald B, Moser B. Human chemokines: an update. *Annu Rev Immunol* 1997;15:675–705.
6. Wuyts A, Proost P, Van Damme J. Interleukin-8 and other CXC chemokines. In: Thomson A, ed. *The cytokine handbook,* 3rd ed. San Diego: Academic Press, 1998:271–312.
7. Bacon KB, Greaves DR, Dairaghi DJ, et al. The expanding universe of C, CX3C, and CC chemokines. In: Thomson A, ed. *The cytokine handbook*, 3rd ed. San Diego: Academic Press, 1998:753–776.
8. Locati M, Murphy PM. Chemokines and chemokine receptors: biology and clinical relevance in inflammation and AIDS. *Annu Rev Med* 1999;50:425–440.
9. Zlotnik A, Morales J, Hedrick JA. Recent advances in chemokines and chemokine receptors. *Crit Rev Immunol* 1999;19:1–47.
10. Ward SG, Bacon K, Westwick J. Chemokines and T lymphocytes: more than an attraction. *Immunity* 1998;9:1–11.
11. Johnston B, Burns AR, Suematsu M, et al. Chronic inflammation upregulates chemokine receptors and induces neutrophil migration to monocyte chemoattractant protein–1. *J Clin Invest* 1999;103:1269–1276
12. Gerszten RE, Garcia-Zepeda EA, Lim YC, et al. MCP-1 and IL-8 trigger firm adhesion of monocytes to vascular endothelium under flow conditions. *Nature* 1999;398:718–723.
13. Broxmeyer HE, Cooper S, Hangoc G, et al. Dominant myeloprotective effector functions mediated by chemokine receptor CCR1. *J Exp Med* 1999;189:1987–1992.
14. Bleul CC, Farzan M, Choe H, et al. The lymphocyte chemoattractant SDF-1 is a ligand for LESTR/FUSIN and blocks HIV-1 entry. *Nature* 1996;382:829–833.
15. Oberlin E, Amara A, Bachelerie F, et al. The CXC chemokine SDF1 is the ligand for LESTR/fusin and prevents infection by T cell line adapted HIV1. *Nature* 1996;382:833–835.
16. Yoshie O, Imai T, Nomiyama H. Novel lymphocyte-specific CC chemokines and their receptors. *J Leuckoc Biol* 1997;62:634–644.
17. Karakurum M, Shreeniwas R, Chen J, et al. Hypoxic induction of interleukin-8 gene expression in human endothelial cells. *J Clin Invest* 1994;93:1564–1570.
18. Xia Y, Pauza ME, Feng L, et al. RelB regulation of chemokine expression modulates local inflammation. *Am J Pathol* 1997;151:375–387.
19. Wells TNC, Peitsch MC. The chemokine information source: Identification and characterization of novel chemokines using the WorldWideWeb and expressed sequence tag databases. *J Leukoc Biol* 1997;61:545–550.
20. Murphy PM, Baggiolini M, Charo IF. International union of pharmacology nomenclature for chemokine receptors. *Pharmacol Rev* 2000;52:145–176.
21. Lu B, Rutledge BJ, Gu L, et al. Abnormalities in monocyte recruitment and cytokine expression in monocyte chemoattractant protein 1–deficient mice. *J Exp Med* 1998;187:601–608.
22. Gao J-L, Wynn TA, Chang Y, et al. Impaired host defense, hematopoiesis, granulomatous inflammation and type 1–type 2 cytokine balance in mice lacking CC chemokine receptor 1. *J Exp Med* 1997;185:1959–1968.
23. Cook DN, Beck MA, Coffman TM, et al. Requirement of MIP-1α for an inflammatory response to viral infection. *Science* 1995;269:1583–1585.
24. Premack BA, Schall TJ. Chemokine receptors: gateways to inflammation and infection. *Nat Med* 1996;2: 1174–1178.
25. Murphy PM. Chemokine receptors: Structure, function and role in microbial pathogenesis. *Cytokine Growth Factor Rev* 1996;7:47–64.
26. Höpken UE, Lu B, Gerard NP, et al. The C_{5a} chemoattractant receptor mediates mucosal defence to infection. *Nature* 1996;383:86–89.
27. Huang W-W, Garcia-Zepeda EA, Sauty A, et al. Molecular and biological characterization of the murine leukotriene B_4 receptor expressed on eosinophils. *J Exp Med* 1998;188:1063–1074.
28. Bowman EP, Campbell JJ, Druey KM, et al. Regulation of chemotactic and proadhesive responses to chemoattractant receptors by RGS (regulator of G-protein signaling) family members. *J Biol Chem* 1998;23: 28040–28048.
29. Rodriguez-Frade JM, Vila-Coro AJ, Martin de Ana A, et al. The chemokine monocyte chemoattractant protein–1 induces functional responses through dimerization of its receptor CCR2. *Proc Natl Acad Sci USA* 1999; 96:3628–2633.
30. Rodriguez-Frade JM, Vila-Coro AJV, Martin A, et al. Similarities and differences in RANTES- and (AOP)-RANTES-triggered signals: implications for chemotaxis. *J Cell Biol* 1999;144:755–765.
31. Darbonne WC, Rice GC, Mohler MA, et al. Red blood cells are a sink for interleukin 8, a leukocyte chemotaxin. *J Clin Invest* 1991;88:1362–1369.
32. Neote K, Mak JY, Kolakowski LF, et al. Functional and biochemical analysis of the cloned Duffy antigen: identity with the red blood cell chemokine receptor. *Blood* 1994;84:44–52.
33. Chaudhuri A, Nielsen S, Elkjaer ML, et al. Detection of Duffy antigen in the plasma membranes and caveolae of vascular endothelial and epithelial cells of nonerythroid organs. *Blood* 1997;89:701–712.

34. Horuk R, Chitnis CE, Darbonne WC, et al. A receptor for the malarial parasite *Plasmodium vivax:* the erythrocyte chemokine receptor. *Science* 1993;261:1182–1184.
35. Furie MB, Randolph GJ. Chemokines and tissue injury. *Am J Pathol* 1995;146:1287–1301.
36. Koch AE, Kunkel SL, Harlow LA, et al. Macrophage inflammatory protein-1 α. A novel chemotactic cytokine for macrophages in rheumatoid arthritis. *J Clin Invest* 1994;93:921–928.
37. O'Grady NP, Tropea M, Preas II HL, et al. Detection of macrophage inflammatory proetin (MIP)-1α and MIP-1β during experimental endotoxemia and human sepsis. *J Infect Dis* 1999;179:136–141.
38. Zhang YH, Broser M, Cohen H, et al. Enhanced interleukin-8 release and gene expression in macrophages after exposure to mycobacterium tuberculosis and its components. *J Clin Invest* 1995;95:586–592.
39. DiMango E, Zar HJ, Bryan R, et al. Diverse Pseudomonas aeruginosa gene products stimulate respiratory epithelial cells to produce interleukin-8. *J Clin Invest* 1995;96:2204–2210.
40. McKee CM, Penno MB, Cowman M, et al. Hyaluronan (HA) fragments induce chemokine gene expression in alveolar macrophages. The role of HA size and CD44. *J Clin Invest* 1996;98:2403–2413.
41. Mikloska Z, Danis VA, Adams S, et al. In vivo production of cytokines and β (C-C) chemokines in human recurrent *Herpes simplex* lesions—do *Herpes simplex* virus–infected keratinocytes contribute to their production? *J Infect Dis* 1998;177:827–838.
42. Saito T, Deskin RW, Casola A, et al. Respiratory syncytial virus induces selective production of the chemokine RANTES by upper airway epithelial cells. *J Infect Dis* 1997;175:497–504.
43. Sprenger H, Meyer RG, Kaufmann A, et al. Selective induction of monocyte and not neutrophil-attracting chemokines after influenza A virus infection. *J Exp Med* 1996;184:1191–1196.
44. Lilly CM, Nakamura H, Kesselman H, et al. Expression of eotaxin by human lung epithelial cells: induction by cytokines and inhibition by glucocorticoids. *J Clin Invest* 1997;99:1767–1773.
45. Kagnoff MF, Eckmann L. Epithelial cells as sensors for microbial infection. *J Clin Invest* 1997;100:6–10.
46. Smith RS, Smith TJ, Blieden TM, et al. Fibroblasts as sentinel cells. Synthesis of chemokines and regulation of inflammation. *Am J Pathol* 1997;151:317–322.
47. Matthews AN, Friend DS, Zimmermann N, et al. Eotaxin is required for the baseline level of tissue eosinophils. *Proc Natl Acad Sci USA* 1998;95:6273–6278.
48. Ember JA, Sanderson SD, Hugli TE, et al. Induction of interleukin-8 synthesis from monocytes by human C_{5a} anaphylatoxin. *Am J Pathol* 1994;144:393–403.
49. Wu, X, Dolecki GJ, Lefkowith JB. GRO chemokines: a transduction, integration, and amplification mechanism in acute renal inflammation. *Am J Physiol* 1995;269:F248–F256.
50. Wu X, Dolecki GJ, Sherry B, et al. Chemokines are expressed in a myeloid cell–dependent fashion and mediate distinct functions in immune complex glomerulonephritis in rat. *J Immunol* 1997;158:3917–3924.
51. Wang Y, Hu Q, Madri JA, et al. Amelioration of lupus-like autoimmune disease in NZB/WF1 mice after treatment with a blocking monoclonal antibody specific for complement component C5. *Proc Natl Acad Sci USA* 1996;93:8563–8568.
52. Springer TA. Traffic signals for lymphocyte recirculation and leukocyte migration: the multistep paradigm. *Cell* 1994;76:301–314.
53. Foxman EF, Campbell JJ, Butcher EC. Multistep navigation and the combinatorial control of leukocyte chemotaxis. *J Cell Biol* 1997;5:1349–1360.
54. Woldemar Carr M, Alon R, Springer TA. The CC chemokine MCP-1 differentially modulates the avidity of β1 and β2 integrins on T lymphocytes. *Immunity* 1996;4:179–187.
55. Middleton J, Neil S, Wintle J, et al. Transcytosis and surface presentation of IL-8 by venular endothelial cells. *Cell* 1997;91:385–395
56. Wagner L, Yang OO, Garcia-Zepeda EA, et al. Beta-chemokines are released from HIV1 specific cytolytic T cell granules complexed to proteoglycans. *Nature* 1998;391:908–911.
57. Tanaka Y, Adams DH, Hubscher S, et al. T cell adhesion induced by proteoglycan-immobilized cytokine MIP-1. *Nature* 1993;361:79–82.
58. McFadden G, Kelvin D. New strategies for chemokine inhibition and modulation. *Biochem Pharmacol* 1997; 54:1271–1280.
59. Webb LMC, Ehrengruber MU, Clark-Lewis I, et al. Binding to heparan sulfate or heparin enhances neutrophil responses to interleukin-8. *Proc Natl Acad Sci USA* 1993;90:7158–7162.
60. Lira SA, Zalamea P, Heinrich JN, et al. Expression of the chemokine N51/KC in the thymus and epidermis of transgenic mice results in marked infiltration of a single class of inflammatory cells. *J Exp Med* 1994; 180:2039–2048.
61. Aliberti JCS, Machado FS, Souto JT, et al. (-chemokines enhance parasite uptake and promote nitric oxide–dependent microbiostatic activity in murine inflammatory macrophages infected with *Trypanosoma cruzi*. *Infect Immun* 1999;67:4819–4826.
62. Banchereau J, Steinman RM. Dendritic cells and the control of immunity. *Nature* 1998;392:245–252.
63. Sallusto F, Palermo, Lenig D, et al. Distinct patterns and kinetics of chemokine production regulate dendritic cell production. *Eur J Immunol* 1999;29:1617–1625.
64. Cyster JG. Chemokines and the homing of dendritic cells to the T cell areas of lymphoid organs. *J Exp Med* 1999;189:447–450.
65. Tang HL, Cyster JG. Chemokine up-regulation and activated T cell attraction by maturing dendritic cells. *Science* 1999;284:819–822.

66. Sallusto F, Lanzavecchia A, Mackay CR. Chemokines and chemokine receptors in T-cell priming and Th1/Th2-mediated responses. *Immunol Today* 1998;19:568–574.
67. Dieu MC, Vanbervliet B, Vicari A, et al. Selective recruitment of immature and mature dendritic cells by distinct chemokines expressed in different anatomic sites. *J Exp Med* 1998;188:373–386.
68. Sozzani S, Luini W, Borsatti A, et al. Receptor expression and responsiveness of human dendritic cells to a defined set of CC and CXC chemokines. *J Immunol* 1997;157:1993–2000.
69. Saeki H, Moore AM, Brown MJ, et al. Secondary lymphoid tissue chemokine (SLC) and CC chemokine receptor 7 (CCR7) participate in the emigration pathway of mature dendritic cells from the skin to regional lymph nodes. *J Immunol* 1999;162:2472–2475.
70. Adema GJ, Hartgers F, Verstraten R, et al. A dendritic cell derived CC chemokine that preferentially attracts naive T cells. *Nature* 1997;387:713–717.
71. D'Apuzzo M, Rolink A, Loetscher M, et al. The chemokine SDF-1, stromal derived factor 1, attracts early stage B cell precursors via the chemokine receptor CXCR-4. *Eur J Immunol* 1997;27:1788–1793.
72. Bleul CC, Schultze JL, Springer TA. B lymphocyte chemotaxis regulated in association with microanatomic localization, differentiation state, and B cell receptor engagement. *J Exp Med* 1998;187:753–762.
73. Förster R, Mattis AE, Kremmer E, et al. A putative chemokine receptor, BLR-1, directs B cell migration to defined lymphoid organs and specific anatomic compartments of the spleen. *Cell* 1996;87:1037–1047.
74. Gunn MD, Ngo VN, Ansel KM, et al. A B-cell homing chemokine made in lymphoid follicles activated Burkitt's lymphoma receptor 1. *Nature* 1998;391:799–803.
75. Sallusto F, Kremmer E, Palermo B, et al. Switch in chemokine receptor expression upon TCR stimulation reveals novel homing potential for recently activated T cells. *Eur J Immunol* 1999;29:2037–2045.
76. Lauw FN, Dekkers PEP, te Velde AA, et al. Interleukin-12 induces sustained activation of multiple host inflammatory mediator systems in chimpanzees. *J Infect Dis* 1999;179:646–652.
77. Price DA, Klenerman P, Booth BL, et al. Cytotoxic T lymphocytes, chemokines and antiviral immunity. *Immunol Today* 1999;20:212–216.
78. Loetscher P, Seitz M, Baggiolini M, et al. Interleukin-2 regulates CC chemokine receptor expression and chemotactic responsiveness in T lymphocytes. *J Exp Med* 1996;184:569–577.
79. Mosmann TR, Coffman RL. Th1 and Th2 cells: Different patterns of lymphokine selection lead to different functional properties. *Annu Rev Immunol* 1989;7:145–173.
80. Romagnani S. Human Th1 and Th2 subsets: doubt no more. *Immunol Today* 1991;12:256–259.
81. Lucey DR, Clerici M, Shearer GM. Type 1 and type 2 cytokine dysregulation in human infectious, neoplastic, and inflammatory diseases. *Clin Microbiol Rev* 1996;9:532–562.
82. Lucey DR. Evolution of the type 1 (Th1)–type 2 (Th2) cytokine paradigm. *Infect Dis Clin North Am* 1999; 13:1–9.
83. D'Ambrosio D, Iellem A, Bonecchi R, et al. Selective upregulation of chemokine receptors CCR4 and CCR8 upon activation of polarized human T type 2 Th cells. *J Immunol* 1999;161:5111–5115.
84. Zingoni A, Soto H, Hedrick JA. The chemokine receptor CCR8 is preferentially expressed in Th2 but not Th1 cells. *J Immunol* 1998;161:547–551.
85. Sallusto F, Mackay CR, Lanzavecchia A. Selective expression of the eotaxin receptor CCR3 by human T helper 2 cells. *Science* 1997;277:2005–2007.
86. Loetscher P, Uguccioni M, Bordoli L, et al. CCR5 is characteristic for Th1 lymphocytes. *Nature* 1998;391:344–345.
87. Bonecchi R, Bianchi G, Bordignon PP, et al. Differential expression of chemokine receptors and chemotactic responsiveness of type 1 T helper cells (Th1s) and Th2s. *J Exp Med* 1998;187:129–134.
88. Sallusto F, Lenig D, Mackay CR, et al. Flexible programs of chemokine receptor expression on human polarized T helper 1 and T helper 2 lymphocytes. *J Exp Med* 1998;187:875–883.
89. Annunziato F, Cosmi L, Galli G, et al. Assessment of chemokine receptor expression by human Th1 and Th2 cells in vitro and in vivo. *J Leukoc Biol* 1999;65:691–699.
90. Campbell JJ, Heraldsen G, Pan J, et al. The chemokine receptor CCR4 in vascular recognition by cutaneous but not intestinal memory T cells. *Nature* 1999;400:776–780.
91. Zabel BA, Agace WW, and Campbell JJ. Human G-protein coupled receptor GPR-9-6/cc chemokine receptor 9 is selectively expressed on intestinal homing T lymphocytes, mucosal lymphocytes, and thymocytes, and is required for thymus expressed chemokine-mediated chemotaxis. *J Exp Med* 1999;190:1241–1255.
92. Cocchi F, DeVico AL, Garzino-Demo A, et al. Identification of RANTES, MIP-1α, and MIP-1β as the major HIV-suppressive factors produced by CD8+ T cells. *Science* 1995;270:1811–1815.
93. Hadida F, Vieillard V, Autran B, et al. HIV-specific T cell cytotoxicity mediated by RANTES via the chemokine receptor CCR3. *J Exp Med* 1998;188:609–614.
94. Hedrick JA, Helms A, Vicari A, et al. Characterization of a novel CC chemokine, HCC-4, whose expression is increased by interleukin-10. *Blood* 1998;91:4242–4247.
95. Sylvester I, Suffredini AF, Boujoukos AJ, et al. Neutrophil attractant protein–1 and monocyte chemoattractant protein–1 in human serum. Effects of intravenous lipopolysaccharide on free attractants, specific IgG autoantibodies and immune complexes. *J Immunol* 1993;151:3292–3298.
96. Nagasawa T, Hirota S, Tachibana, et al. Defects of B cell lymphopoiesis and bone marrow myelopoiesis in mice lacking the CXC chemokine PBSF/SDF-1. *Nature* 1996;382:635–638.
97. Tachibana K, Hirota S, Iizasa H, et al. The chemokine receptor CXCR-4 is essential for vascularization of the gastrointestinal tract. *Nature* 1998;393:591–594.

98. Zou YR, Kottman AH, Kuroda M, et al. Function of the chemokine receptor CXCR4 in hematopoiesis and in cerebellar development. *Nature* 1998;393:595–599.
99. Vicari AP, Figueroa DJ, Hedrick JA, et al. TECK: a novel CC chemokine specifically expressed by thymic dendritic cells and potentially involved in T cell development. *Immunity* 1997;7:291–301.
100. Aiuti A, Webb IJ, Bleul C, Springer T, et al. The chemokine SDF-1 is a chemoattractant for human CD34$^+$ hematopoietic progenitor cells and provides a new mechanism to explain the mobilization of CD34$^+$ progenitors to peripheral blood. *J Exp Med* 1997;185:111–120.
101. Broxmeyer HA, Sherry B, Cooper S. Comparative analysis of the human macrophage inflammatory protein family of cytokines (chemokines) on proliferation of human myeloid progenitor cells. Interacting effects involving suppression, synergistic suppression, and blocking of suppression. *J Immunol* 1993;150:3448–3458.
102. Trentin L, Agostini C, Facco M, et al. The chemokine receptor CXCR-3 is expressed on malignant B cells and mediates chemotaxis. *J Clin Invest* 1999;104:115–121.
103. Koch AE, Polverini PJ, Kunkel SL, et al. Interleukin-8 as a macrophage-derived mediator of angiogenesis. *Science* 1992;258:1798–1801.
104. Keane MP, Arenberg DA, Lynch III JP, et al. The CXC chemokines, IL-8 and IP-10, regulate angiogenic activity in idiopathic pulmonary fibrosis. *J Immunol* 1997;159:1437–1443.
105. Luster AD, Leder P. IP-10, a CXC chemokine, elicits a potent thymus-dependent antitumor response in vivo. *J Exp Med* 1993;178:1057–1065.
106. Stewart G. Chemokine genes—beating the odds. *Nat Med* 1998;4:275–277.
107. Liu R, Paxton WA, Choe S, et al. Homozygous defect in HIV1 co-receptors accounts for resistance for some multiply exposed individuals to HIV1 infection. *Cell* 1996;86:367–377.
108. Cairns JS, D'Souza MP. Chemokines and HIV-1 second receptors: the therapeutic connection. *Nat Med* 1998;5:563–568.
109. Harrison AM, Bonville CA, Rosenberg HF, et al. Respiratory syncytial virus–induced chemokine expression in the lower airways. *Am J Respir Crit Care Med* 1999;159:1918–1924.
110. König B, Krusat T, Streckert HJ, et al. IL-8 release from human neutrophils by the respiratory syncytial virus is independent of viral replication. *J Leukoc Biol* 1996;60:253–260.
111. Fiedler MA, Wernke-Dollries K, Stark JM. Respiratory syncytial virus increases IL-8 gene expression and protein release in A549 cells. *Am J Physiol* 1995;269:K865–K872.
112. Täuber MG, Moser B. Cytokines and chemokines in meningeal inflammation: Biology and clinical implications. *Clin Infect Dis* 1999;28:1–12.
113. Bernasconi S, Cinque P, Peri G, et al. Selective elevation of monocyte chemotactic protein–1 in the cerebrospinal fluid of AIDS patients with cytomegalovirus encephalitis. *J Infect Dis* 1996;174:1098–1101.
114. Ritter U, Moll H, Laskay T, et al. Differential expression of chemokines in patients with localized and diffuse cutaneous *American leishmaniasis*. *J Infect Dis* 1996;173:699–709.
115. Hack CE, Hart M, Strack RJM, et al. Interleukin-8 in sepsis: relation to shock and inflammatory mediators. *Infect Immun* 1992;60:2835–2842.
116. Chollet-Martin S, Montravers P, Gibert C, et al. High levels of interleukin-8 in the blood and alveolar spaces of patients with pneumonia and adult respiratory distress syndrome. *Infect Immun*ol 1993;61:4553–4559.
117. Hack CE, DeGroot ER, Felt-Bersma RJF, et al. Increased plasma levels of interleukin-6 in sepsis. *Blood* 1989; 74:1704–1710.
118. Matuschak GM. Circulating cytokine concentrations and outcome prediction in intensive care unit patients: still the tip of the iceberg? *Crit Care Med* 1996;24:1769–1771.
119. Benson M, Jodal U, Agace W, et al. Interleukin-6 and IL-8 in children with febrile urinary tract infection and asymptomatic bacteriuria. *J Infect Dis* 1996;174:1080–1084.
120. Huffnagle GB, Strieter RM, Standiford TJ, et al. The role of monocyte chemotactic protein–1 (MCP-1) in the recruitment of monocytes and CD4$^+$ T cells during pulmonary *Cryptococcus neoformans* infection. *J Immunol* 1995;155:4790–4797.
121. Greenberger MJ, Strieter RM, Kunkel SL, et al. Neutralization of macrophage inflammatory protein–2 attenuates neutrophil recruitment and bacterial clearance in murine *Klebsiella pneumonia*. *J Infect Dis* 1996;173: 159–165.
122. Vester B, Müller W, Solbach W, et al. Early gene expression of NK cell–activating chemokines in mice resistant to *Leishmania major*. *Infect Immun* 1999;67:3155–3159.
123. Zinkernagel RM. Immunology taught by viruses. *Science* 1996;271:173–178.
124. Turner RB, Weingand KW, Chyon-Hwa L, et al. Association between interleukin-8 concentration in nasal secretions and severity of symptoms of experimental rhinovirus colds. *Clin Infect Dis* 1998;26:840–846.
125. Skoner DP, Gentile DA, Patel A, et al. Evidence for cytokine mediation of disease expression in adults experimentally infected with influenza A virus. *J Infect Dis* 1999;180:10–14.
126. Hayden FG, Fritz RS, Lobo MC, et al. Local and systemic cytokine responses during experimental human influenza A virus infection. *J Clin Invest* 1998;101:643–649.
127. Fritz RS, Hayden FG, Calfee DP, et al. Nasal cytokine and chemokine responses in experimental influenza A virus infection: results of a placebo-controlled trial of intravenous zanamivir treatment. *J Infect Dis* 1999; 180:586–593.
128. Darveau RP, Belton CM, Reife RA, et al. Local chemokine paralysis, a novel pathogenic mechanism for *Porphyromonas gingivalis*. *Infect Immun* 1998;66:1660–1665.

129. Shimoyama T, Everett SM, Dixon MF, et al. Chemokine mRNA expression in gastric mucosa is associated with *Helicobacter pylori* cagA positivity and severity of gastritis. *J Clin Pathol* 1998;51, 765–770.
130. Peek Jr RM, Blaser MJ. Pathophysiology of *Helicobacter pylori*–induced gastritis and peptic ulcer disease. *Am J Med* 1996;102:200–207.
131. Marrack P, Kappler J. Subversion of the immune system by pathogens. *Cell* 1994;76:323–332.
132. Pease JE, Murphy PM. Microbial corruption of the chemokine system: an expanding paradigm. *Semin Immunol* 1998;10:169–178.
133. Clapham PR, Weiss RA. Spoilt for choice of co-receptors. *Nature* 1997;388:230–231.
134. Cundell DR, Gerard NP, Gerard C, et al. Streptococcus pneumoniae anchor to activated human cells by the receptor for platelet-activating factor. *Nature* 1995;377:435–438.
135. Pleskoff O, Tréboute C, Brelot A, et al. Identification of a chemokine receptor encoded by human cytomegalovirus as a cofactor for HIV1 entry. *Science* 1997;276:1874–1878.
136. Gao J-L, Murphy PM. Human cytomegalovirus open reading frame US28 encodes a functional β chemokine receptor. *J Biol Chem* 1994;269:28539–28542.
137. Bodaghi B, Jones TR, Zipeto D, et al. Chemokine sequestration by viral chemoreceptors as a novel viral escape strategy: Withdrawal of chemokines from the environment of cytomegalovirus-infected cells. *J Exp Med* 1998;188:855–866.
138. Penfold MET, Dairaghi DJ, Duke GM, et al. Cytomegalovirus encodes a potent alpha chemokine. *Proc Natl Acad Sci USA* 1999;96:9839–9844.
139. Boshoff C, Endo Y, Collins PD, et al. Angiogenic and HIV-inhibitory functions of KSHV-encoded chemokines. *Science* 1997;278:290–294.
140. Kledal TN, Rosenkilde MM, Coulin F, et al. A broad-spectrum chemokine antagonist encoded by Kaposi's sarcoma-associated herpesvirus. *Science* 1997;277:1656–1659.
141. Endres MJ, Garlisi CG, Xiao H, et al. The Kaposi's sarcoma-related herpesvirus (KSHV.-encoded chemokine vMIP-I is a specific agonist for the CC chemokine receptor CCR8. *J Exp Med* 1999;189:1993–1998.
142. He J, Chen Y, Farzan M, et al. CCR3 and CCR5 are co-receptors for HIV-1 infection of microglia. *Nature* 1997; 385:645–649.
143. Liestoel K, Goplen AK, Dunlop O, et al. Kaposi's sarcoma and protection from HIV dementia [Letter]. *Science* 1998;280:361–362.
144. Baldeweg T, Catalan J, Gazzard BG, et al. Kaposi's sarcoma and protection from HIV dementia [Letter]. *Science* 1998;280:362.
145. Chen S, Bacon KB, Li L, et al. In vivo inhibition of CC and CX3C chemokine-induced leukocyte infiltration and attenuation of glomerulonephritis in Wistar-Kyoto (WKY) rats by vMIP-II. *J Exp Med* 1998;188: 193–198.
146. Arvanitakis L, Geras-Raaka E, Varma A, et al. Human herpesvirus KSHV encodes a constitutively active G-protein–coupled receptor linked to cell proliferation. *Nature* 1997;385:347–350.
147. Gershengorn MC, Geras-Raaka E, Varma A, et al. Chemokines activate Kaposi's sarcoma–associated herpesvirus G protein–coupled receptor in mammalian cells in culture. *J Clin Invest* 1998;102:1469–1472.
148. Bais C, Santomasso B, Coso O, et al. G-protein–coupled receptor of Kaposi's sarcoma–associated herpesvirus is a viral oncogene and angiogenesis activator. *Nature* 1998;391:86–89.
149. Murphy PM. Pirated genes in Kaposi's sarcoma. *Nature* 1997;385:296–299.
150. Zou P, Isegawa Y, Nakano K, et al. Human herpesvirus 6 open reading frame U83 encodes a functional chemokine. *J Virol* 1999;73:5926–5933.
151. Isegawa Y, Ping Z, Nakano K, et al. Human herpesvirus 6 open reading frame U12 encodes a functional βchemokine receptor. *J Virol* 1998;72:6104–6112.
152. Yasukawa M, Hasegawa A, Sakai I, et al. Downregulation of CXCR-4 by human herpesvirus 6 (HHV-6) and HHV-7. *J Immunol* 1999;162:5417–5422.
153. Albini A, Ferrini S, Benelli R, et al. HIV-1 tat protein mimicry of chemokines. *Proc Natl Acad Sci USA* 1998; 95:13153–13158.
154. Swingler S, Mann A, Jacqué J-M, et al. HIV-1 Nef mediates lymphocyte chemotaxis and activation by infected macrophages. *Nat Med* 1999;5:997–1003.
155. Krathwohl MD, Hromas R, Brown DR, et al. Functional characterization of the CC chemokine-like molecules encoded by molluscum contagiosum virus types 1 and 2. *Proc Natl Acad Sci USA* 1997;94:9875–9880.
156. Smith CA, Smith TD, Smolak PJ, et al. Poxvirus genomes encode a secreted, soluble protein that preferentially inhibits βchemokine activity yet lacks sequence homology to known chemokine receptors. *Virology* 1997;236:316–327.
157. Berger EA, Murphy PM, Farber JM. Chemokine receptors as HIV-1 coreceptors: roles in viral entry, tropism, and disease. *Annu Rev Immunol* 1999;17:657–700.
158. Cohen O, Weissman D, Fauci AS. The immunopathogenesis of HIV infection. In: Paul WE, ed. *Fundamental immunology.* Philadelphia: Lippincott–Raven Publishers, 1999:1455–1509.
159. Horuk R. Chemokine receptors and HIV-1: the fusion of two major research fields. *Immunol Today* 1999;20:89–94.
160. Lee B, Montaner LJ. Chemokine immunobiology in HIV-1 pathogenesis. *J Leukoc Biol* 1999;65:552–565.
161. Feng Y, Broder CC, Kennedy PE, et al. HIV-1 entry cofactor: functional cDNA cloning of a seven-transmembrane G protein–coupled receptor. *Science* 1996;272:872–877.

162. Dragic T, Litwin V, Allaway GP, et al. HIV-1 entry into CD4+ cells is mediated by the chemokine receptor CC-CKR-5. *Nature* 1996;381:667–673.
163. Deng H, Liu R, Ellmeier W, et al. Identification of a major co-receptor for primary isolates of HIV-1. *Nature* 1996;381:661–666.
164. Alkhatib G, Combadiere C, Broder CC, et al. CC CKR5: a RANTES, MIP-1α, MIP-1βreceptor as a fusion co-factor for macrophage-tropic HIV-1. *Science* 1996;272:1955–1958.
165. Trkola A, Dragic T, Arthos J, et al. CD4 dependent, antibody sensitive interactions between HIV1 and its core-ceptor CCR5. *Nature* 1996;384:184–187.
166. Wu L, Gerard NP, Wyatt R, et al. CD4-induced interaction of primary HIV-1 gp120 glycoproteins with the chemokine receptor CCR5. *Nature* 1996;384:179–183.
167. Lapham CK, Ouyang J, Chandrasekhar B, et al. Evidence for cell-surface association between fusin and the CD4-gp120 complex in human cell lines. *Science* 1996;274:602–605.
168. Michael NL, Nelson JAE, Kewalramani VN, et al. Exclusive and persistent use of entry coreceptor CXCR4 by human immunodeficiency virus type 1 from a subject homozygous for CCR5 Δ32. *J Virol* 1998;72:6040–6047.
169. Dean M, Carrington M, Winkler C, et al. Genetic restriction of HIV-1 infection and progression to AIDS by a deletion allele of the CKR5 structural gene. *Science* 1996;273:1856–1862.
170. Misrahi M, Teglas JP, N'Go N, et al. CCR5 chemokine receptor variant in HIV1 mother to child transmission and disease progression in children. *JAMA* 1998;279:277–280.
171. Van Rij RP, Portegies P, Hallaby T, et al. Reduced prevalence of the CCR5 Δ32 heterozygous genotype in human immunodeficiency virus–infected individuals with AIDS dementia complex. *J Infect Dis* 1999;180:854–857.
172. Meyer L, Magierowska M, Hubert J-B, et al. CCR5 Δ32 deletion and reduced risk of toxoplasmosis in persons infected with human immunodeficiency virus type 1. *J Infect Dis* 1999;180:920–924.
173. Husain S, Goila R, Shahi S, et al. First report of a healthy Indian heterozygous for Δ32 mutant of HIV-1 co-re-ceptor CCR5 gene. *Gene* 1998;207:141–147.
174. Quillent C, Oberlin E, Braun J, et al. HIV-1 resistance phenotype conferred by combination of two separate in-herited mutations of CCR5 gene. *Lancet* 1998;351:14–18.
175. McDermott DH, Zimmermann PA, Guignard F, et al. CCR5 promoter polymorphism and HIV-1 disease pro-gression. *Lancet* 1998;352:866–870.
176. Kostrikis LG, Huang Y, Moore JP, et al. A chemokine receptor CCR2 allele delays HIV1 disease progression and is associated with a CCR5 promoter mutation. *Nat Med* 1998;4:350–353.
177. Michael NL, Louie LG, Rohrbaugh AL, et al. The role of CCR5 and CCR2 polymorphisms in HIV1 transmis-sion and disease progression. *Nat Med* 1997;3:1160–1162.
178. Winkler C, Modi W, Smith MW, et al. *Gene*tic restriction of AIDS pathogenesis by an SDF-1 chemokine gene variant. *Science* 1998;279:389–393.
179. Mellado M, Rodriguez-Frade JM, Vila-Coro AJ, et al. Chemokine control of HIV-1 infection. *Nature* 1999; 400:723–724.
180. Kaslow RA, Carrington M, Apple R, et al. Influence of combinations of human major histocompatibility com-plex genes on the course of HIV1 infection. *Nat Med* 1996;2:405–411.
181. Beyrer C, Artenstein AW, Rugpao S, et al. Epidemiologic and biologic characterization of a cohort of human immunodeficiency virus type 1 highly exposed, persistently seronegative female sex workers in Northern Thai-land. *J Infect Dis* 1999;179:59–67.
182. Bernard NF, Yannakis CM, Lee JS, et al. Human immunodeficiency virus (HIV)–specific cytotoxic T lymph-cyte activity in HIV-exposed seronegative persons. *J Infect Dis* 1999;179:538–547.
183. Shen H, Cheng T, Preffer FI, et al. Intrinsic human immunodeficiency virus type 1 resistance of hematopoietic stem cells despite coreceptor expression. *J Virol* 1999;73:728–737.
184. Wu L, Paxton WA, Kassam N, et al. CCR5 levels and expression pattern correlate with infectability by macrophage-tropic HIV-1, in vitro. *J Exp Med* 1997;185:1681–1691.
185. Hladik F, Lentz G, Akridge RE, et al. Dendritic cell–T-cell interactions support coreceptor-independent human immunodeficiency virus type 1 transmission in the human genital tract. *J Virol* 1999;73:5833–5842.
186. Granelli-Piperno A, Moser B, Pope M, et al. Efficient interaction of HIV1 with purified dendritic cells via mul-tiple chemokine receptors. *J Exp Med* 1996;184:2433–2438.
187. Ayehunie S, Garcia-Zepeda EA, Hoxie JA, et al. Human immunodeficiency virus–1 entry into purified blood dendritic cells through CC and CXC chemokine receptors. *Blood* 1997;90:1379–1386.
188. Lapham CK, Zaitseva M, Lee S, et al. Fusion of monocytes and macrophages with HIV-1 correlates with bio-chemical properties of CXCR-4 and CCR5. *Nat Med* 1999;5:303–308.
189. Grivel J-C, Margolis LB. CCR5 and CXCR4 tropic HIV-1 are equally cytopathic for their T cell targets in hu-man lymphoid tissue. *Nat Med* 1999;5:344–346.
190. Zou W, Foussat A, Houhou S, et al. Acute upregulation of CCR5 expression by CD4+ T lymphocytes in HIV infected patients treated with IL-2. *AIDS* 1999;13:455–463.
191. Weissman D, Rabin RL, Arthos J, et al. Macrophage-tropic HIV and SIV envelope proteins induce a signal through the CCR5 chemokine receptor. *Nature* 1997;389:981–985.
192. Kinter A, Catanzaro A, Monaco J, et al. CC-chemokines enhance the replication of T-tropic strains of HIV-1 in CD4+ T cells: Role of signal transduction. *Proc Natl Acad Sci USA* 1998;95:11880–11885.
193. Trkola A, Gordon C, Matthews J, et al. The CC-chemokine RANTES increases the attachment of human im-

munodeficiency virus type 1 to target cells via glycosaminoglycans and also activates a signal transduction pathway that enhances viral infectivity. *J Virol* 1999;73:6370–6379.
194. Moriuchi H, Moriuchi M, Combadiere C, et al. CD8+ T cell derived soluble factor(s), but not β-chemokines RANTES, MIP-1α, and MIP-β, suppress HIV-1 replication in monocyte/macrophages. *Proc Natl Acad Sci USA* 1996;93:15341–15345.
195. Schmidtmayerova H, Sherry B, Bukrinsky M. Chemokines and HIV replication. *Nature* 1996;382:767.
196. Gordon CJ, Muesing MA, Proudfoot AEI, et al. Enhancement of human immunodeficiency virus type 1 infection by the CC-chemokine RANTES is independent of the mechanism of virus-cell fusion. *J Virol* 1999;73:684–694.
197. Garzino-Demo A, DeVico AL, Cocchi F, et al. Beta chemokines and protection from HIV type 1 disease. *AIDS Res Hum Retroviruses* 1998;14(suppl 2):S177–S184.
198. Saha K, Volsky DJ. Are β chemokines innocent bystanders in HIV type 1 disease progression? *AIDS Res Hum Retroviruses* 1998;14:1–2.
199. Polo S, Veglia F, Malnati MS, et al. Longitudinal analysis of serum chemokine levels in the course of HIV-1 infection. *AIDS*1999;13:447–454.
200. Rinaldo Jr CR, Liebmann JM, Huang XL, et al. Prolonged suppression of human immunodeficiency virus type 1 (HIV-1) viremia in persons with advanced disease results in enhancement of CD4 T cell reactivity to microbial antigens but not to HIV-1 antigens. *J Infect Dis* 1999;179:326–336.
201. Chensue SW, Warmington KS, Ruth JH, et al. Role of monocyte chemoattractant protein–1 (MCP-1) in Th1 (mycobacterial) and Th2 (schistosomal) antigen-induced granuloma formation. *J Immunol* 1996;157:4602–4608.
202. Agostini C, Cassatella M, Zambello R, et al. Involvement of the IP-10 chemokine in sarcoid granulomatous reactions. *J Immunol* 1998;161:6413–6420.
203. Garcia-Zepeda EA, Rothenberg ME, Ownbey RT, et al. Human eotaxin is a specific chemoattractant for eosinophil cells and provides a new mechanism to explain tissue eosinophilia. *Nat Med* 1996;2:449–456.
204. Reinecker HC, Loh EY, Ringler DJ, et al. Monocyte-chemoattractant protein 1 gene expression in intestinal epithelial cells and inflammatory bowel disease mucosa. *Gastroenterology* 1995;108:40–50.
205. Boring L, Gosling J, Cleary M, et al. Decreased lesion formation in CCR2–/– mice reveals a role for chemokines in the initiation of atherosclerosis. *Nature* 1998;394:894–897.
206. Boisvert WA, Santiago R, Curtiss LK, et al. A leukocyte homologue of the IL-8 receptor CXCR2 mediates the accumulation of macrophages in atherosclerotic lesions of LKL receptor-deficient mice. *J Clin Invest* 1998; 101:353–363.
207. Hernandez-Presa M, Bustos C, Ortego M, et al. Angiotensin-converting enzyme inhibition prevents arterial nuclear factor-κB activation, monocyte chemoattractant protein–1 expression, and macrophage infiltration in a rabbit model of early accelerated atherosclerosis. *Circulation* 1997;95:1532–1541.
208. Wolf G, Ziyadeh FN, Thaiss F, et al. Angiotensin II stimulates expression of the chemokine RANTES in rat glomerular endothelial cells. Role of the angiotensin type 2 receptor. *J Clin Invest* 1997;100:1047–1058.
209. Gillitzer R, Wolff K, Tong D, et al. MCP-1 mRNA expression in basal keratinocytes of psoriatic lesions. *J Invest Dermatol* 1993;101:127–131.
210. Gottlieb AB, Luster AD, Posnett DN, et al. Detection of a (interferon-induced protein IP-10 in psoriatic plaques. *J Exp Med* 1988;168:941–948.
211. Karpus WJ, Ransohoff RM. Chemokine regulation of experimental autoimmune encephalomyelitis: Temporal and Spatial expression patterns governs disease pathogenesis. *J Immunol* 1998;161:2667–2671.
212. Karpus WJ, Kennedy KJ. MIP-1(and MCP-1 differentially regulate acute and relapsing autoimmune encephalomyelitis as well as Th1/Th2 lymphocyte differentiation. *J Leukoc Biol* 1997;62:681–687.
213. Hogaboam CM, Steinhauser ML, Chensue SW, et al. Novel roles for chemokines and fibroblasts in interstitial fibrosis. *Kidney Int* 1998;54:2152–2159.
214. Gharaee-Kermani M, Denholm EM, Phan SH. Costimulation of fibroblast collagen and transforming growth factor (1 expression by monocyte chemoattractant protein–1 via specific receptors. *J Biol Chem* 1996;271: 17779–17784.
215. Lloyd CM, Minto AM, Dorf ME, et al. RANTES and monocyte chemoattractant protein–1 (MCP-1) play an important role in the inflammatory phase of crescentic nephritis, but only MCP-1 is involved in crescent formation and interstitial fibrosis. *J Exp Med* 1997;185:1371–1380.
216. Carré PC, Mortenson RL, King Jr TE, et al. Increased expression of the interleukin-8 gene by alveolar macrophages in idiopathic pulmonary fibrosis. *J Clin Invest* 1991;88:1802–1810.
217. Rovin BH, Phan LT. Chemotactic factors and renal inflammation. *Am J Kidney Dis* 1998;31:1065–1084.
218. Feng L, Xia Y, Yoshimura T, et al. Modulation of neutrophil influx in the rat with anti–macrophage inflammatory protein–2 (MIP-2) antibody. *J Clin Invest* 1995;95:1009–1017.
219. Wada T, Tomosugi N, Naito T, et al. Prevention of proteinuria by the administration of anti–interleukin-8 antibody in experimental acute immune complex–induced glomerulonephritis. *J Exp Med* 1994;180:1135–1140.
220. Fujinaka H, Yamamoto T, Takeya M, et al. Suppression of anti-glomerular basement membrane nephritis by administration of anti-monocyte chemoattractant protein–1 antibody in WKY rats. *J Am Soc Nephrol* 1997;8: 1174–1178.
221. Noris M, Bernasconi S, Casiraghi, et al. Monocyte chemoattractant protein–1 is excreted in excessive amounts in the urine of patients with lupus nephritis. *Lab Invest* 1995;73:804–809
222. Wada T, Yokoyama H, Su SB, et al. Monitoring urinary levels of monocyte chemotactic and activating factor reflects disease activity of lupus nephritis. *Kidney Int* 1996;49:761–767.

223. Thalmann GN, Dewald B, Baggiolini M, et al. Interleukin-8 expression in the urine after Bacillus Calmette Guerin therapy: a potential prognostic factor of tumor recurrence and progression. *J Urol* 1997;158:1340–1344.
224. Colletti LM, Kunkel SL, Walz A, et al. Chemokine expression during hepatic ischemia reperfusion-induced lung injury in the rat. *J Clin Invest* 1995;95:134–141.
225. Sekido N, Mukaida N, Harada A, et al. Prevention of lung reperfusion injury in rabbits by a monoclonal antibody against interleukin-8. *Nature* 1993;365:654–657.
226. Matsumoto T, Yokoi K, Mukaida N, et al. Pivotal role of interleukin-8 in the acute respiratory distress syndrome and cerebral reperfusion injury. *J Leukoc Biol* 1997;62:581–587.
227. Adams DH, Afford SA, Fear J, et al. Hepatic expression of macrophage inflammatory protein 1(after liver transplantation. *Transplantation* 1996;61:817–825.
228. Grandaliano G, Gesualdo L, Ranieri E, et al. Monocyte chemotactic peptide–1 expression and monocyte infiltration in acute renal transplant rejection. *Transplantation* 1997;63:414–420.
229. Melter M, McMahon G, Fang J, et al. Current understanding of chemokine involvement in allograft transplantation. *Pediatr Transplant* 1999;3:10–21.
230. Gerber BO, Zanni MP, Uguccioni M, et al. Functional expression of the eotaxin receptor CCR3 in T lymphocytes co-localizing with eosinophils. *Curr Biol* 1997;7:836–843.
231. Kita H, Gleich GJ. Chemokines active on eosinophils: potential roles in allergic inflammation. *J Exp Med* 1996; 183:2421–2426.
232. Collins PD, Marleau S, Griffiths-Johnson DA, et al. Cooperation between interleukin-5 and eotaxin to induce eosinophil accumulation in vivo. *J Exp Med* 1995;182:1169–1174.
233. Alam R, York J, Boyars M, et al. Increased MCP-1, RANTES, and MIP-1(in bronchoalveolar lavage fluid of allergic asthmatic patients. *Am J Respir Crit Care Med* 1996;153:1398–1404.
234. Sim TC, Reece LM, Hilsmeier KA, et al. Secretion of chemokines and other cytokines in allergen-induced nasal responses: inhibition by topical steroid treatment. *Am J Respir Crit Care Med* 1995;152:927–933
235. Kimata H, Yoshida A, Ishioka C, et al. RANTES and macrophage inflammatory protein 1(selectively enhance immunoglobulin (IgE) and IgG4 production by human B cells. *J Exp Med* 1996;183:2397–2402.
236. Hendrix CW, Flexner CW, MacFarland RT, et al. Pharmacokinetics and safety of AMD-3100, a novel antagonist of the CXCR4 chemokine receptor, in human volunteers. *Antimicrob Agents Chemother* 2000;44: 1667–1673.
237. Marshall E, Howell AH, Powles R, et al. Clinical effects of human macrophage inflammatory protein–1 alpha MIP-1((LD78) administration to humans: a phase I study in cancer patients and normal healthy volunteers with the genetically engineered variant, BB-10010. *Eur J Cancer* 1998;7:1023–1029.
238. Clemons MJ, Marshall E, Dürig J, et al. A randomized phase II study of BB-10010 (macrophage inflammatory protein–1() in patients with advanced breast cancer receiving 5-fluorouracil, adriamycin, and cyclophosphamide chemotherapy. *Blood* 1998;92:1532–1540.
239. Mukaida N, Morita M, Ishikawa Y, et al. Novel mechanism of glucocorticoid-mediated gene repression. Nuclear factor-κB is target for glucocorticoid-mediated interleukin 8 gene repression. *J Biol Chem* 1994;269: 13289–13295.
240. Mukaida N, Zachariae CCO, Gusella GL, et al. Dexamethasone inhibits the induction of monocyte chemotactic-activating factor production by IL-1 or tumor necrosis factor. *J Immunol* 1991;146:1212–1215.
241. Seitz M, Loetscher P, Dewald B, et al. In vitro modulation of cytokine, cytokine inhibitor, and prostaglandin E release from bold mononuclear cells and synovial fibroblasts by antirheumatic drugs. *J Rheumatol* 1997;24: 1471–1476.
242. van Fenema EM, Hu S, Sheng WS, et al. Thalidomide inhibits IL-8 production by human microglia [Abstract]. Presented at the First International Congress on Cytokines/Chemokines in Infectious Diseases, Bethesda, MD, September 8–10, 1999.
243. Hechtman DH, Cybulsky MI, Fuchs HJ, et al. Intravascular IL-8: inhibitor of polymorphonuclear leukocyte accumulation at sites of acute inflammation. *J Immunol* 1991;147:883–892
244. Simonet WS, Hughes TM, Nguyen HQ, et al. Long term impairment of neutrophil migration in mice overexpressing human interleukin-8. *J Clin Invest* 1994;94:1310–1318.
245. Rutledge BJ, Rayburn H, Rosenberg R, et al. High level monocyte chemoattractant protein–1 expression in transgenic mice increases their susceptibility to intracellular pathogens. *J Immunol* 1995;155:4838–4843.
246. Zisman DA, Kunkel SL, Strieter RM, et al. MCP-1 protects mice in lethal endotoxemia. *J Clin Invest* 1997;99: 2832–2836.
247. Fuentes ME, Durham SK, Swerdel MR, et al. Controlled recruitment of monocytes and macrophages to specific organs through transgenic expression of monocyte chemoattractant protein–1. *J Immunol* 1995;155:5769–5776.
248. Skowron G, Stein D, Drusano G, et al. The safety and efficacy of granulocyte-macrophage colony-stimulating factor (Sargramostim) added to indinavir- or ritonavir-based antiretroviral therapy: a randomized double-blind, placebo-controlled trial. *J Infect Dis* 1999;180:1064–1071.
249. Tarr PE, Lin R, Mueller EA, et al. Evaluation of tolerability and antibody response after recombinant human granulocyte-macrophage colony-stimulating factor (rhGM-CSF) and a single dose of recombinant hepatitis B vaccine. *Vaccine* 1996;14:1199–1204.
250. Matsuda S, Akagawa K, Honda M, et al. Suppression of HIV replication in human monocyte-derived macrophages induced by granulocyte-macrophage colony-stimulating factor. *AIDS Res Hum Retroviruses* 1995;11:1031–1038.

251. Hammer SM, Gillis JM, Pinkston P, et al. Effect of zidovudine and granulocyte-macrophage colony-stimulating factor on human immunodeficiency virus replication in alveolar macrophages. *Blood* 1990;75: 1215–1219.
252. DiMarzio P, Tse J, Landau NR. Chemokine receptor regulation and HIV type 1 tropism in monocytes-macrophages. *AIDS Res Hum Retroviruses* 1998;14:129–137.
253. Brites C, Gilbert MJ, Pedral-Sampaio D, et al. A randomized, placebo-controlled trial of granulocyte-macrophage colony stimulating factor and nucleotide analogue therapy in AIDS. *J Infect Dis* 2000;182: 1531–1535.
254. Davey Jr RT, Chaitt DG, Albert JM, et al. A randomized trial of high- versus low-dose subcutaneous interleukin-2 outpatient therapy for early human immunodeficiency virus type 1 infection. *J Infect Dis* 1999; 179:849–858.
255. Brown Z, Strieter RM, Neild GH, et al. IL-1 receptor antagonist inhibits monocyte chemotactic peptide 1 generation by human mesangial cells. *Kidney Int* 1992;42:95–101.
256. Baggiolini M, Moser B. Blocking chemokine receptors. *J Exp Med* 1997;186:1189–1191.
257. Moser B, Dewald B, Barella L, et al. Interleukin-8 antagonists generated by *N*-terminal modification. *J Biol Chem* 1993;268:7125–7128.
258. Jones SA, Dewald B, Clark-Lewis I, et al. Chemokine antagonists that discriminate beween interleukin-8 receptors. Selective blockers of CXCR2. *J Biol Chem* 1997;272:16166–16169.
259. Gong JH, Uguccioni M, Dewald B, et al. RANTES and MCP-3 antagonists bind multiple chemokine receptors. *J Biol Chem* 1996;271:10521–10527.
260. Gong JH, Clark-Lewis I. Antagonists of monocyte chemoattractant protein 1 identified by modification of functionally critical NH2-terminal residues. *J Exp Med* 1995;181:631–640.
261. Hayashi S, Kurdowska A, Miller EJ, et al. Synthetic hexa- and heptapeptides that inhibit IL-8 from binding to and activating human blood neutrophils. *J Immunol* 1995;154:814–824.
262. Oravecz T, Pall M, Roderiquez G, et al. Regulation of the receptor specificity and function of the chemokine RANTES by dipeptidyl peptidase IV (CD26)–mediated cleavage. *J Exp Med* 1997;186:1865–1872.
263. Wells TNC, Power CA, Lusti-Narasimhan M, et al. Selectivity and antagonism of chemokine receptors. *J Leukocyte Biol* 1996;53–60.
264. Proudfoot AEI, Power CA, Hoogewerf AJ, et al. Extension of recombinant human RANTES by the retention of the initiating methionine produces a potent antagonist. *J Biol Chem* 1996;271:2599–2603.
265. Mosier DE, Piccio GR, Gulizia RJ, et al. Highly potent RANTES analogues either prevent CCR5 using human immunodeficiency virus type 1 infection in vivo or rapidly select for CXCR4 using variants. *J Virol* 1999; 73:3544–3550.
266. Mack M, Luckow B, Nelson PJ, et al. Aminooxypentane-RANTES induces CCR5 internalization but inhibits recycling: a novel mechanism of HIV infectivity. *J Exp Med* 1998;187:1215–1224.
267. Simmons G, Clapham PR, Picard L, et al. Potent inhibition of HIV1 infectivity in macrophages and lymphocytes by a novel CCR5 antagonist. *Science* 1997;276:276–279.
268. Arenzana-Seisdedos F, Virelizier JL, Rousset D, et al. HIV blocked by chemokine antagonist. *Nature* 1996;383:400.
269. Amara A, Le Gall S, Schwartz O, et al. HIV coreceptor downregulation as antiviral principle: SDF-1 alpha dependent internalization of the chemokine receptor CXCR4 contributes to inhibition of HIV replication. *J Exp Med* 1997;186:139–146.
270. Czaplewski LG, McKeating J, Craven CJ, et al. Identification of amino acid residues critical for aggreggation of human CC chemokines macrophage inflammatory protein (MIP)-1α MIP-1β, and RANTES. *J Biol Chem* 1999;274:16077–16084.
271. Czaplewski L. Preclinical and clinical evaluation of the therapeutic potential of hMIP-1α, hMIP-1β and RANTES. [Abstract]. Presented at the IBC's International Industry Conference on HIV Co-receptors. Washington, DC: 20-21 November, 1997.
272. Nibbs RJB, Yang J, Landau NR, et al. LD78(, a non-allelic variant of human MIP-1((LD78(), has enhanced receptor interactions and potent HIV suppressive activity. *J Biol Chem* 1999;274:17478–17483.
273. Weber M, Uguccioni M, Baggiolini M, et al. Deletion of the NH2-terminal residue converts monocyte chemotactic protein 1 from an activator of basophil mediator release to an eosinophil chemoattractant. *J Exp Med* 1996;183:681–685.
274. Masure S, Paemen L, Proost P, et al. Expression of a human mutant monocyte chemotactic protein 3 in pichia pastoris and characterization as an MCP-3 receptor antagonist. *J Interferon Cytokine Res* 1995;15:955–963.
275. Baly DL, Horuk R, Yansura DG, et al. A His19 to Ala mutant of melanoma growth stimulatory activity is a partial antagonist of the CXCR2 receptor. *J Immunol* 1998;161:4944–4949.
276. Hesselgesser J, Chitnis CE, Miller LH, et al. A mutant of melanoma growth stimulating activity does not activate neutrophils but blocks erythrocyte invasion by malaria. *J Biol Chem* 1995;270:11472–11476.
277. Breton JJ, Chabot-Fletcher MC. The natural product hymenialdisine inhibits interleukin-8 production in U937 cells by inhibition of nuclear factor–κB. *J Pharmacol Exp Ther* 1997;282:459–466.
278. Schwarz MK, Wells TNC. Interfering with chemokine networks—the hope for new therapeutics. *Curr Opin Chem Biol* 1999;3:407–417.
279. Lu B, Rutledge BJ, Gu L, et al. Abnormalities in monocyte recruitment and cytokine expression in monocyte chemoattractant protein 1–deficient mice. *J Exp Med* 1998;187:601–608.

280. Gong JH, Ratkay LG, Waterfield JD, et al. An antagonist of monocyte chemoattractant protein 1 (MCP-1) inhibits arthritis in the MFL-/pr mouse model. *J Exp Med* 1997;186:131–137.
281. Strieter RM, Standiford TJ, Huffnagle GB, et al. "The good, the bad, and the ugly": the role of chemokines in models of human disease. *J Immunol* 1996;156:3583–3586.
282. Aliberti J, Schito M, Wells T, et al. In vivo inhibition of CCR5/ligand interaction suppresses microbial induced activation and mobilization of splenic dendritic cells [Abstract]. Presented at the First International Congress on Cytokines/Chemokines in Infectious Diseases, Bethesda, MD, September 8–10, 1999.
283. Murakami T, Nakajima T, Koyanagi Y, et al. A small molecule CXCR4 inhibitor that blocks T cell line–tropic HIV-1 infection. *J Exp Med* 1997;186:1389–1393.
284. Tang WW, Qi M, Warren JS. The role of monocyte chemoattractant protein–1 (MCP-1) in anti-GBM Ab GN [Abstract]. *J Am Soc Nephrol* 1995;6:855.
285. Olson WC, Rabut GEE, Nagashima KA, et al. Differential inhibition of human immunodeficiency virus type 1 fusion, gp120 binding, and CC-chemokine activity by monoclonal antibodies to CCR5. *J Virol* 1999;73:4145–4155.
286. Michael NL, Moore JP. HIV-1 entry inhibitors: evading the issue. *Nat Med* 1999;5:740–742.
287. Zhang Y-J, Moore JP. Will multiple coreceptors need to be targeted by inhibitors of human immunodeficiency virus type 1 entry? *J Virol* 1999;73:3443–3448.
288. Yang OO, Swanberg SL, Lu Z, et al. Enhanced inhibition of human immunodeficiency virus type 1 by Met-stromal derived factor-1(correlates with downmodulation of CXCR4. *J Virol* 1999;73:4582–4589.
289. Doranz BJ, Grovit-Ferbas K, Sharron MP, et al. A small molecule inhibitor directed against the chemokine receptor CXCR4 prevents its use as an HIV-1 coreceptor. *J Exp Med* 1997;186:1395–1400.
290. Chen JD, Bai X, Yang AG, et al. Inactivation of HIV-1 chemokine coreceptor CXCR4 by a novel intrakine strategy. *Nat Med* 1997;3:1110–1116.
291. Lusso P. A chemokine trap for HIV co-receptors. *Nat Med* 1997;3:1074–1075
292. Yang AG, Bai X, Huang XF, et al. Phenotypic knockout of HIV type 1 chemokine coreceptor CCR5 by intrakines as potential therapeutic approach for HIV-1 infection. *Proc Natl Acad Sci USA* 1997;94:11567–11572.
293. Donzella GA, Schols D, Lin SW, et al. AMD3100, a small molecule inhibitor of HIV1 entry via the CXCR4 co-receptor. *Nat Med* 1998;4:72–77.
294. De Vreese K, Reymen D, Griffin P, et al. The bicyclams, a new class of potent human immunodeficiency virus inhibitors, block viral entry after binding. *Antiviral Res* 1996;29:209–219.
295. Schols D, Struyf S, Van Damme J, et al. Inhibition of T-tropic HIV strains by selective antagonization of the chemokine receptor CXCR4. *J Exp Med* 1997;186:1383–1388.
296. Datema R, Rabin L, Hincenbergs M, et al. Antiviral efficacy in vivo of the anti-human immunodeficiency virus bicyclam SDZ SID 791 (JM 3100), an inhibitor of infectious cell entry. *Antimicrob Agents Chemother* 1996;40:750–754.
297. DeVreese K, Kofler-Mongold V, Leutgeb C, et al. The molecular target of bicyclams, potent inhibitors of human immunodeficiency virus replication. *J Virol* 1996;70:689–696.
298. LaCasse RA, Follis KE, Trahey M, et al. Fusion-competent vaccines: broad neutralization of primary isolates of HIV. *Science* 1999;283:357–362.
299. Liao F, Alkhatib G, Peden KWC, et al. STRL33, a novel chemokine receptor-like protein, functions as a fusion cofactor for both macrophage-tropic and T cell line–tropic HIV-1. *J Exp Med* 1997;185:2015–2123.
300. Deng H, Unutmaz D, KewalRamani VN, et al. Expression cloning of new receptors used by simian and human immunodeficiency viruses. *Nature* 1997;388:296–300.
301. Esté JA, Cabrera C, Blanco J, et al. Shift of clinical human immunodeficiency virus type 1 isolates from X4 to R5 and prevention of emergence of the syncytium-inducing phenotype by blockade of CXCR4. *J Virol* 1999;73:5577–5585.
302. Chabot DJ, Zhang P-F, Quinnan GV, et al. Mutagenesis of CXCR4 identifies important domains for human immunodeficiency virus type 1 X4 isolate envelope-mediated membrane fusion and virus entry and reveals cryptic coreceptor activity for R5 isolates. *J Virol* 1999;73:6598–6609.
303. Farzan M, Mirzabekov T, Kolchinsky P, et al. Tyrosine sulfation of the amino terminus of CCR5 facilitates HIV-1 entry. *Cell* 1999;96:667–676.
304. Baba M, Nishimura O, Kanzaki N, et al. A small-molecule nonpeptide CCR5 antagonist with highly potent and selective anti–HIV-1 activity. *Proc Natl Acad Sci USA* 1999;96:5698–5703.
305. Kanzaki N, Kuroshima K, Shiraishi M, et al. Tak-779, a small molecule CCR5 antagonist: receptor binding properties [Abstract]. Presented at the 39th Interscience Conference on Antimicrobial Agents and Chemotherapy (ICAAC), San Francisco, September 26–29, 1999.
306. Baba M, Okamoto M, Ino M, et al. Tak-779, a small molecule CCR5 antagonist: anti–HIV-1 activity and pharmacokinetic properties [Abstract]. Presented at the 39th Interscience Conference on Antimicrobial Agents and Chemotherapy (ICAAC), San Francisco, September 26–29, 1999.
307. White JR, Lee JM, Young PR, et al. Identification of a potent, selective non-peptide CXCR2 antagonist that inhibits interleukin-8–induced neutrophil migration. *J Biol Chem* 1998;273:10095–10098.
308. Hesselgesser J, Ng HP, Liang M, et al. Identification and characterization of small molecule functional antagonists of the CCR1 chemokine receptor. *J Biol Chem* 1998;273:15687–15692.
309. Carroll RG, Riley JL, Levine BL, et al. Differential regulation of HIV-1 fusion cofactor expression by CD28 costimulation of $CD4^+$ T cells. *Science* 1997;276:273–276.

310. Riley JL, Carroll RG, Levine BL, et al. Intrinsic resistance to T cell infection with HIV type 1 induced by CD28 costimulation. *J Immunol* 1997;158:5545–5553.
311. Carroll RG, Riley JL, Levine BL, et al. The role of co-stimulation in regulation of chemokine receptor expression and HIV-1 infection in primary T lymphocytes. *Semin Immunol* 1998;10:195–202.
312. Riley JL, Levine BL, Craighead N, et al. Naive and memory CD4 T cells differ in their susceptibilities to human immunodeficiency virus type 1 infection following CD28 costimulation: Implications for transmission and pathogenesis. *J Virol* 1998;72:8273–8280.
313. Triozzi PL, Aldrich W, Bresler HS, et al. Cellular immunotherapy of advanced human immunodeficiency virus type 1 using autologous lymph node lymphocytes: effects on chemokine production. *J Infect Dis* 1999;179: 245–248.
314. Lin R, Tarr PE, Jones TC. Present status of the use of cytokines as adjuvants with vaccines to protect against infectious diseases. *Clin Infect Dis* 1995;21:1439–1449.
315. Pardoll DM. Cancer vaccines. *Nat Med* 1998;4:525–531.
316. Dilloo D, Bacon K, Holden W, et al. Combined chemokine and cytokine gene transfer enhances antitumor immunity. *Nat Med* 1996;2:1090–1095.
317. Biragyn A, Tani K, Grimm MC, et al. Genetic fusion of chemokines to a self tumor antigen induces protective, T-cell dependent antitumor immunity. *Nat Biotechnol* 1999;17:253–258.
318. Kim JJ, Nottingham LK, Sin JI, et al. CD8 positive T cells influence antigen-specific immune responses through the expression of chemokines. *J Clin Invest* 1998;102:1112–1124.
319. Youssef S, Wildbaum G, Maor G, et al. Long-lasting protective immunity to experimental autoimmune encephalomyelitis following vaccination with naked DNA encoding CC chemokines. *J Immunol* 1998;161: 3870–3879.
320. Cocchi F, DeVico AL, Garzino-Demo A, et al. The V3 domain of the HIV-1 gp120 envelope glycoprotein is critical for chemokine-mediated blockade of infection. *Nat Med* 1996;2:1244–1247.
321. Jones GJ, van Hoegen P, Weber J, et al. Immunization with human immunodeficiency virus type 1 rgp120 w61d in QS21/MPL adjuvant primes T cell proliferation and CC chemokine production to multiple epitopes within variable and conserved domains of gp120 w61d. *J Infect Dis* 1999;179:558–566.
322. Heeney JL, Teeuwsen VJP, Van Gils M, et al.(-chemokines and neutralizing antibody titers correlate with sterilizing immunity generated in HIV-1 vaccinated macaques. *Proc Natl Acad Sci USA* 1998;95:10803–10808.
323. Wang Y, Tao L, Mitchell E, et al. The effect of immunization on chemokines and CCR5 and CXCR4 coreceptor functions in SIV binding and chemotaxis. *Vaccine* 1999;17:1826–1836.
324. Lehner T, Wang Y, Cranage M, et al. Protective mucosal immunity elicited by targeted iliac lymph node immunization with a subunit SIV envelope and core vaccine in macaques. *Nat Med* 1996;2:767–775.
325. Gauduin M-C, Glickman RL, Means R, et al. Inhibition of simian immunodeficiency virus (SIV) replication by $CD8^+$ T lymphocytes from macaques immunized with live attenuated SIV. *J Virol* 1998;72:6315–6324.
326. Wang Y, Tao L, Mitchell E, et al. Allo-immunization elicits $CD8^+$ T cell–derived chemokines, HIV suppressor factors and resistance to HIV infection in women. *Nat Med* 1999;5:1004–1009.
327. Heeney J, Akerblom L, Barnett S, et al. HIV-1 vaccine–induced immune responses which correlate with protection from SHIV infection: compiled preclinical efficacy data from trials with ten different HIV-1 vaccine candidates. *Immunol Lett* 1999;66:189–195.
328. Mebatsion T, Finke S, Weiland F, et al. A CXCR4/CD4 pseudotype rhabdovirus that selectively infects HIV-1 envelope protein-expressing cells. *Cell* 1997;90:841–847.
329. Schnell MJ, Johnson JE, Buonocore L, et al. Construction of a novel virus that targets HIV-1 infected cells and controls HIV-1 infection. *Cell* 1997;90:849–857.
330. Boritz E, Gerlach J, Johnson JE, et al. Replication-competent rhabdoviruses with human immunodeficiency virus type 1 coats and green fluorescent protein: entry by a pH-independent pathway. *J Virol* 1999;73: 6937–6945.
331. Nolan GP. Harnessing viral devices as pharmaceuticals: fighting HIV's fire with fire. *Cell* 1997;90:821–824.
332. Endres MJ, Jaffer S, Haggarty B, et al. Targeting of HIV- and SIV-infected cells by CD4-chemokine receptor pseudotypes. *Science* 1997;278:1462–1464.
333. Reproduced from ref. 157. With permission, from the *Annual Reviews of Immunology,* Vol. 17, © 1999, by Annual Reviews http://www.AnnualReviews.org.

9
G-CSF and GM-CSF

Thomas Hartung, *J. Milton Gaviria, †Sara M. Garrido, and ‡Richard K. Root

*Department of Biological Pharmacology, University of Konstanz, Konstanz, Germany; *In Internal Medicine, Infectious Diseases, Mid-Columbia Medical Associates, Kennewick, Washington, †Columbia Basin Hematology and Oncology, Kennewick, Washington; and ‡Harborview Medical Center, Infectious Diseases, Seattle, Washington*

INTRODUCTION

Acute host defenses against infection depend upon phagocytic leukocyte responses. These cells, in particular granulocytes, are often consumed in this process. Therefore, the maintenance of cell formation by the bone marrow and an increased recruitment of leukocytes are mandatory for coping effectively with the infectious challenge. The importance of hematopoiesis for antibacterial defense becomes evident in myelosuppressed patients who are severely prone to all types of infection. A direct correlation between absolute neutrophil (PMN, or polymorphonuclear neutrophil) count and risk of infection has been demonstrated (1).

The signaling molecules controlling in large part the formation of these cells have been identified and cloned: granulocyte colony-stimulating factor (G-CSF) and granulocyte-macrophage colony-stimulating factor (GM-CSF) represent the key mediators of granulocyte hematopoiesis. Not surprisingly, the production of both factors is increased during bacterial infection. Interestingly, G-CSF is frequently detected in high levels in the circulation of these patients, while GM-CSF appears to be produced only locally (2).

Recombinant G-CSF and GM-CSF have been available clinically, to treat neutropenia for almost one decade (Table 9.1). Despite ongoing discussions about the cost/benefit relationships for these supportive treatments, their overall efficacy in reducing infectious episodes in neutropenic patients has been clearly demonstrated. Only recently has the potential of these drugs for the therapy of nonneutropenic infection been addressed. Due to the rapid endogenous production of the cytokines, there is only a limited therapeutic window in the nonneutropenic subject, either as prophylactic treatment or substitution for insufficient endogenous production. Both indications have to be carefully defined since amplification of immune reactions may not only improve host defense but might also promote harmful inflammatory reactions, which represent the adverse side of the nonspecific response.

G-CSF and GM-CSF not only modify host responses by increasing the number of leukocytes, but can have direct effects on immune cell functions (3). Some effects can be explained by further maturation of granulocytes, but both hematopoietic factors also specifically prime granulocyte functional responses. Furthermore, both mediators modulate the inflammatory response—however, in opposite directions. Overall GM-CSF has

TABLE 9-1. *Commercially available formulations of G-CSF and GM-CSF*

	Generic name	Trade name	Country
G-CSF	Filgrastim	Neupogen	Europe, U.S., Canada, Australia
		Gran	Japan, Taiwan, Korea, China
	Lenograstim	Neutrogin	Japan, China
		Granocyte	Europe, Australia
	Nartograstim	Neu-Up	Japan
GM-CSF	Molgramostim	Leukomax	Europe, Canada
	Sargramostim	Leukine	U.S.

From Root RK, Dale DC. Granulocyte colony-stimulating factor and granulocyte-macrophage colony-stimulating factor: comparisons and potential for use in the treatment of infections in nonneutropenic patients. *J Infect Dis* 1999;179 Suppl 2:S342–S352, with permission.

proven to be a proinflammatory and G-CSF an antiinflammatory immunomodulator. These unique pharmacodynamic profiles that combine hematopoietic/antiinfectious effects with either anti- or proinflammatory capabilities now offer new clinical options in the treatment of infectious diseases.

ISOLATION, CHARACTERIZATION, AND PHARMACOLOGY OF THE MYELOPOIETIC CYTOKINES

G-CSF

Metcalf and coworkers were the first to define the myelopoietic properties of serum or urine obtained from neutropenic patients or those infected or treated with endotoxins. In later work, many of the bioactivities described (Table 9.2). were traced back to a single molecule that was named G-CSF. Human G-CSF was first purified from the bladder carcinoma cell line 5637 in 1985 (4), and subsequently cloned and expressed in *Escherichia coli* (5), and monkey COS cells (6,7). The single copy of the gene encoding G-CSF is situated on the long arm of chromosome 17. It codes for a protein of 174 amino acids with a molecular mass of 18 kDa, which is O-glycosylated in its native form (apparent relative weight is approximately 19.6 kDa). Murine and human G-CSF share 73% homology at the amino acid level, explaining the significant species cross-reactivity (4).

TABLE 9-2. *Common abbreviations of the names used for G-CSF and GM-CSF*

Abbreviation	Name
G-CSF; CSF-G	Granulocyte colony-stimulating factor
CSF-β; CSF-3	Colony-stimulating factor β or 3, respectively
MGI-1G; MGI-2	Macrophage-granulocyte inducer 1G or 2 respectively
G/M-CSA	Granulocyte-macrophage colony-stimulating activity
DF	Differentiation factor
	Pluripoietin
pCSF	Pluripotent CSF
GM-CSF; CSF-GM	Granulocyte-macrophage colony-stimulating factor
CSF-α; CSF-2	Colony-stimulating factor α or 2, respectively
MGI-1GM	Macrophage-granulocyte inducer 1GM
Eo-CSF	Eosinophil CSF
HCGF	Hematopoietic cell growth factor
KTGF	Keratinocyte-derived T-cell growth factor
NIF-T	T cell-derived neutrophil migration inhibition factor

From Ibelgaufts H. *Lexikon der Zytokine.* Munich: Medikon Verlag, 1992, with permission.

Pharmaceutical forms of recombinant G-CSF (Table 9.1) approved for clinical use include a nonglycosylated protein expressed in *E. coli* (filgrastim) and a glycosylated form expressed in Chinese hamster ovary cells (lenograstim) or yeast (nartograstim). Both forms share practically the same pharmacodynamic properties (8), though their pharmacokinetics differ (9). It seems that the differences between the glycosylated and nonglycosylated forms of G-CSF are not clinically important (10).

Hematopoietic growth factors (CSFs) are produced continuously in some tissues such as bone marrow. They are also produced readily at the focus of infectious or inflammatory disorders. The endogenous production of a CSF is often overlooked when treating patients with recombinant material. Logically it might be assumed that therapeutic efficacy can only be reached if there is an absolute or relative CSF deficiency. Therefore, the endogenous production and its regulation deserve careful attention with regard to putative indications.

The production of G-CSF is initiated by a number of factors (Table 9.3) in various cell populations, i.e., monocytes and macrophages as major producers, bone marrow stromal cells, endothelial cells, fibroblasts, PMN, and a number of tumor cell lines, e.g., derived from squamous cell carcinoma and hepatoma (11-28).

Some factors are known to modulate the extent of G-CSF formation induced by these stimuli: G-CSF production by human monocytes was increased by IFN-γ, prostaglandin E_2 (PGE_2), and calcium ionophore A23187 (12,29–31), but suppressed by dexamethasone, indomethacin, IL-10, and IL-4 (12,29–32).

G-CSF was detectable in rodent serum after challenge with *Pseudomonas aeruginosa* (26), *Listeria monocytogenes* (33), or feces (34) and in murine endotoxic shock (21). The G-CSF serum levels of dogs injected with endotoxin (LPS) increased within 2 hours, peaked at 4 hours, and had not returned to normal 24 hours after challenge (35).

TABLE 9-3. *Stimuli for G-CSF and GM-CSF formation*

Stimulus type	Stimulus	G-CSF	GM-CSF
Bacterial	Endotoxin, lipopolysaccharide	+	+
	Lipoteichoic acid	+	
	SEA (*S. aureus* enterotoxin)		+
	Heat-killed *S. aureus*	+	
	Mycobacterium avium	+	+
Inflammatory mediators	Interleukin-1 (IL-1)	+	+
	Tumor necrosis factor (TNF)	+	+
	Interferon-γ (IFNγ)	+	+
	Interleukin-2 (IL-2)		+
	Interleukin-4 (IL-4)	+	+
	Interleukin-13 (IL-13)		+
Hematopoietic growth factors	GM-CSF	+	
	G-CSF		+
	M-CSF	+	+
	Interleukin-3 (IL-3)	+	+
Other	Phorbol ester, PMA	+	+
	Phytohemagglutinin	+	+
	Concanavalin A		+
	Ionomycin		+
	Immunoglobulin E, IgE		+

From Hartung T, Wendel A. Immunomodulatory properties of filgrastim (r-met-HuG-CSF) in preclinical models. In: Morstyn G, Dexter M, Foote M, et al., eds. *Filgrastim in clinical practice.* New York: Marcel Dekker, 1998:397–427, and Hartung T. Anti-flammatory effects of GCSF. *Curr Opin Hematol* 1998;5:221–225, with permission.

Detectable G-CSF serum levels are rarely found in healthy donors (36,37), but the factor is extractable from all major organs at levels higher than those present in the circulation; tissue production levels can be elevated rapidly (within minutes or hours) after stimulation (38). In febrile patients (39,40), especially in the acute phase of infection (37), and in a variety of neutropenic disorders (13,36,41,42), endogenous G-CSF serum levels are elevated. The level of G-CSF in the serum peaks within 3 hours of injury in trauma patients and rapidly decreases again during the following 7 days, whereas patients with sepsis retain high plasma levels (43).

After injection of 10 μg/kg G-CSF subcutaneously (SC) into humans, serum G-CSF levels remained above 10 ng/mL for 10 to 16 hours (44). In general, pharmacological doses of G-CSF raised the serum levels of the factor to ranges attained by endogenous production during infection. Administration of exogenous G-CSF could either substitute for inadequate endogenous production or initiate its actions more rapidly.

GM-CSF

GM-CSF was first purified from mouse lung-conditioned medium in 1977 and from the supernatant of a HTLV I–infected T-cell line (Mo) in 1984 (45). Murine GM-CSF was cloned in 1984 (46) and human GM-CSF in 1985 (47,48). A number of bioactivities were later traced back to this molecule (Table 9.2).

The single copy of the gene encoding human GM-CSF is localized on chromosome 5, region 5q21-5q32 (49), close to the genes for IL-3, IL-4, IL-5, M-CSF, the M-CSF receptor, and an early growth response factor (EGR-1). The gene for GM-CSF encodes a protein of 144 amino acids, which undergoes cleavage of a 17–amino acid segment from the amino terminus; this results in a mature protein of 127 amino acids (50), with four α-helices and two β-sheets, stabilized in a bilobed configuration by two disulfide bridges. The apparent range of molecular mass lies between 14,500 and 35,000 (51). This heterogeneity is due to the variable N-linked addition of complex carbohydrates at two sites and the glycosylation of two serine residues near the amino terminus.

Nonglycosylated GM-CSF expressed in *E. coli* (molgramostim) and glycosylated GM-CSF expressed in Chinese hamster ovary (CHO) carcinoma cells (sargramostim), have comparable effects on the induction of leukocytosis in monkeys *in vivo* (52). Their pharmacokinetics, as studied in healthy volunteers, were quite different: the nonglycosylated form more rapidly reached a higher peak and had a shorter half-life than the glycosylated form (53). The two forms may also be distributed differently in the body.

Preclinical studies with recombinant human GM-CSF are limited by the lack of cross-species reactivity in mice (54). The protein sequence homology between human and murine GM-CSF is only 60% (47). Human GM-CSF does not appear to activate canine PMN *in vitro* and may actually downregulate their inflammatory responses (55). Even in monkeys, only short-term studies can be undertaken because antibodies develop toward human GM-CSF (56).

The expression of GM-CSF by T-lymphocytes (57), B lymphocytes (58), fibroblasts (58), mast cells (59), endothelial cells (60), epithelial cells (61,62), macrophages (63), and NK cells (64) is controlled by either transcriptional or posttranscriptional regulation.

Apart from the cells of the immune system, various other tissues also have the ability to produce GM-CSF: human endothelial cells (65,66), human mesothelial cells (67), mammary artery and aortic smooth muscle (68), fibroblasts (66), astrocytes (69), the colon epithelial cell lines T84, HT29, and Caco-2 (70), as well as human thymic epithelia (61). This broad variety of cellular sources distinguishes GM-CSF from G-CSF.

Table 9.3 provides an overview of the factors involved in initiating the production of GM-CSF. Notably, GM-CSF has rarely been found in the circulation at detectable levels, but is extractable from all major organs at higher concentrations (38). It usually acts locally in a paracrine manner (2).

OVERVIEW OF ACTIVITY

Hematopoiesis

G-CSF

G-CSF directly stimulates the initial proliferation of a large proportion of granulocyte-macrophage progenitors in bone marrow and supports the survival and proliferation of some multipotential erythroid and eosinophil progenitors. G-CSF acts in synergy with IL-3 to support lineages, such as megakaryocytes, resulting in platelet production (71) as well as early pluripotent stem cells (4) and pre–B-cells (71). Low concentrations of G-CSF predominantly stimulate pure PMN colonies, while high concentrations of G-CSF result in the development of macrophage-containing colonies (4,72).

Injection of G-CSF results in neutrophilia by increasing the production of PMN in the bone marrow and hastening the release of less mature forms into the circulation (73–76). Human volunteers injected with G-CSF also developed monocytosis (77–81). G-CSF treatment also can increase lymphocyte counts (78,82). Treatment with high doses of G-CSF (10 or 100 μg/kg/day) led to a 1.5- to 2.5-fold increase in absolute lymphocyte counts (27). Volunteers treated repeatedly with G-CSF responded with a maximal lymphocyte count on day 8 (83). Lymphocyte subtyping—CD4, CD8, and CD16 (i.e., natural killer cells) and CD19 (i.e., B cells)— revealed that all subpopulations increased during treatment, without major changes in the proportions. Another study on nine healthy volunteers reported an increase in absolute lymphocytes ($CD3^+$, $CD19^+$, NK cells, as well as activated T-lymphocytes) after 4 days of G-CSF administration (81).

GM-CSF

GM-CSF was originally identified as a growth factor capable of supporting the clonal proliferation of granulocyte-macrophage progenitors in culture (reviewed in 51). *In vitro* granulocyte and monocyte progenitor cells die by apoptosis within a few hours in the absence of GM-CSF (50,84), whereas they become irreversibly committed to the production of neutrophils, eosinophils and monocytes if the factor is present (50). When bipotential granulocyte-macrophage progenitors were treated with high concentrations of GM-CSF *in vitro*, many cells were forced to enter the granulocytic pathway, whereas low concentrations resulted in the formation of pure macrophage progeny (85). This phenomenon may be explained in part by the observation that GM-CSF downregulates M-CSF receptor expression (86).

GM-CSF can also stimulate megakaryocyte colony-formation and can act in synergy with erythropoietin to further the growth of erythrocyte precursors *in vitro* (50,87,88). *In vitro* GM-CSF supported the growth and function of Langerhans' cells (50) and osteoclasts (89). GM-CSF is also involved in the proliferation and differentiation of murine dendritic cells (90).

Primates administered GM-CSF showed an increase in leukocytes (PMN fivefold, lymphocytes twofold to fourfold, monocytes threefold to fourfold, platelets and erythrocytes unaffected) during 7 days of treatment. SC administration was found to be more effective than intravenous (IV) infusion (52,91). The leukocytosis initiated by administration of GM-CSF was dose dependent (92). Phase I studies in humans have found that route and schedule are also important: SC or continuous IV administration of lower doses elicit responses similar to those achieved with short IV infusion of higher doses (92). Peripheral blood progenitor cells increase after GM-CSF treatment, but little increase in bone marrow progenitors has been documented (92).

Many primary myeloid leukemias and leukemic cell lines as well as several T-cell acute lymphocytic leukemias depend on or respond to GM-CSF to grow in culture (51). Although there has been concern that the hematopoietic growth factors such as GM-CSF might stimulate the growth of solid tumors or leukemias, such stimulation has not been observed to date *in vivo* (93,94).

Immunomodulation

G-CSF and GM-CSF affect immune functions beyond mere changes in absolute and relative numbers of leukocyte subpopulations (Table 9.4). PMN are a prime target of this immunomodulation by both agents.

G-CSF

G-CSF appears to induce directly only minor alterations in PMN functions. More important is its ability to modify the response of these cells to subsequent stimulation. While phagocytosis and oxidative burst are augmented, G-CSF barely affects degranulation and chemotaxis. PMN exposed *in vitro* to G-CSF improved their killing of *E. coli* (95,96) and *Staphylococcus aureus* (97). G-CSF also primed PMN for an enhanced oxidative burst triggered by the bacterial chemotactic peptide fMLP (98), ionomycin (99), complement factor

TABLE 9-4. *Immunomodulatory effects of G-CSF and GM-CSF*

Leukocyte type	Function	G-CSF	GM-CSF
Neutrophilic granulocyte	Blood count	↑	↑
	Oxidative burst	↑	↑
	Phagocytosis	↑	↑
	Cytokine release		↑
	Soluble TNF receptors	↑	
	IL-1 receptor antagonist	↑	
	Cytotoxicity		↑
	Degranulation		↑
	Adherence		↑
	Apoptosis	↓	↓
Basophilic granulocyte	Histamine release		↑
	Apoptosis		↓
Eosinophilic granulocyte	Blood count		↑
	Phagocytosis		↑
	Adhesion		↑
	Degranulation		↑
	Leukotriene C_4 formation		↑
Monocyte	Blood count	(↑)	↑
	Phagocytosis		↑
	Adhesion, chemokinesis		↑
	Cytotoxicity		↑
	Pro-inflammatory cytokines	↓	↑
	Prostaglandin E_2	↑	
Lymphocytes	Blood count	(↑)	
	Plasma cell formation		↑

C5a (100), or opsonized zymosan (101). *De novo* expression of PMN CD64 in G-CSF–treated patients was associated with increased antibody-dependent cellular toxicity (ADCC) (102). G-CSF treatment increases release of anti-inflammatory mediators, i.e., enhanced release of IL-1 receptor antagonist (IL-1ra) (103) and IFN-α (104) and decreased formation of the chemotactic leukotriene B_4 (Hartung, unpublished observations).

A number of studies demonstrate effects of G-CSF on mononuclear cells. Mononuclear cells play a primary role in controlling systemic inflammatory reactions. The inflammatory response is driven primarily by the cytokines TNF-α, IL-1, and IFN-γ, which are produced by monocytes/macrophages and lymphocytes. Counterregulatory measures include a reduction in their production or secretion, as well as the release of their respective antagonists, e.g., soluble TNF receptors (sTNF-R) or IL-1ra.

G-CSF modifies the response of rodent and human mononuclear cells to immunostimulatory agents, such as the Gram-negative cell wall component lipopolysaccharide (LPS), by causing a decrease in the production of proinflammatory cytokines and an increase in anti-inflammatory cytokine release (105–108). These effects have been attributed to a G-CSF receptor on human monocytes (109). These findings have been replicated in a series of *ex vivo* human volunteer studies. Whole blood from G-CSF–treated volunteers responded to a variety of immunostimuli (e.g., LPS, preparations from Gram-positive bacteria, superantigens, phorbol esters) with reduced TNF and IL-1 activity in comparison to blood from placebo-treated controls (77,83,103,109). Neutrophils from these G-CSF–treated volunteers showed increased *ex vivo* LPS-inducible IL-1ra release. The shedding of soluble TNF receptors was unaffected when calculated on a per PMN basis. The release of the chemoattractant leukotriene B_4, when expressed per neutrophil, was decreased significantly (Hartung, unpublished observations). In addition, IFN-γ production by lymphocytes from G-CSF–treated volunteers was attenuated in LPS-stimulated whole blood.

The effects of daily G-CSF treatment for 12 days in 24 healthy volunteers were examined. Compared to a placebo group, TNF-α, IL-12, and IFN-γ release in whole blood samples in response to *ex vivo* stimulation by LPS was reduced compared with the control group throughout the entire treatment period (83). The *in vitro* addition of IL-12 to LPS-stimulated blood from G-CSF–treated donors reversed the attenuation of IFN-γ and TNF-α release. This suggests that suppression of IL-12 release may be pivotal in the antiinflammatory activity of G-CSF (83).

To assess the time window in which treatment with exogenous G-CSF might alter the course of an infection, a volunteer trial was held in which G-CSF was injected either 2 hours or 24 hours before challenge with LPS *in vivo* (110). Administration of G-CSF shortly before LPS boosted the levels of TNF, IL-6, IL-8, IL-1ra, and both forms of sTNF-R. In contrast, G-CSF injection 1 day prior to challenge significantly decreased the levels of IL-8 and moderately attenuated the release of TNF and IL-6. IL-1ra and sTNF-R levels were already increased prior to LPS injection. Administration of LPS resulted in a further increase in the levels of sTNF-R I and II while IL-1ra release remained unaltered. Despite the different effects on cytokine release patterns, both treatment regimens resulted in similar positive effects on neutrophil activation and similar changes in surface molecule expression. In addition, both G-CSF pretreatments blocked LPS-induced granulocyte accumulation in the lung.

GM-CSF

GM-CSF has both direct and indirect actions on neutrophils. The indirect action is a priming effect leading to enhanced responsiveness to physiologically relevant agents (chemotactic factors, leukotrienes, PAF, IL-8), which may be released locally at sites of inflammation (111). These secondary stimuli can directly activate chemotaxis, the respiratory burst, arachidonic acid metabolism, calcium fluxes, phagocytosis, and degranulation, but their effects are dramatically potentiated by preexposure to GM-CSF. GM-CSF appears to prime PMN for enhanced functions in a sequence of time-dependent physiologic events corresponding to chemotaxis (5 to 15 min), immobilization (30 min), phagocytosis (1 to 2 hours), and enhanced oxidative metabolism (2 hours) (112).

GM-CSF was found to potentiate the LPS-induced TNF-α and IL-1 production of murine and human monocytic cells (113–115). GM-CSF is also a potent enhancer of LPS-induced TNF-α production *in vivo* in normal as well as in experimentally immunocompromised (LPS-desensitized) mice (116). Furthermore, *in vitro* and *ex vivo* experiments revealed that LPS-induced IL-1 release from bone marrow or spleen cells was also enhanced in GM-CSF–treated mice (117). However, in low doses GM-CSF exerted anti-inflammatory rather than proinflammatory effects in patients (118).

MECHANISM OF ACTION/SIGNAL TRANSDUCTION/GENE REGULATION

G-CSF

The gene for the G-CSF receptor (G-CSF-R, CD114) is located on the short arm of chromosome 1. Three distinct human G-CSF receptor cDNAs have been obtained. The major human G-CSF receptor has a calculated molecular weight of 90 kDa, but an apparent molecular mass of 150 kDa due to extensive glycosylation. It is an 813–amino acid polypeptide with a single transmembrane domain, a small cytoplasmic domain, and a large extracellular domain with the tryptophan-serine-x-tryptophan-serine (WSXWS) motif (86). One of the three cDNAs isolated from human cells lacked most of the transmembrane sequence, suggesting that it encodes a soluble, secreted form of the receptor. The physiological role of such a receptor is unclear; it may serve as a "sink" to eliminate excess cytokines and thus modulate their activities. The mouse and human G-CSF receptor cDNA share more than 60% homology at the amino acid level, consistent with the ability of both human and murine G-CSF to bind to both species' G-CSF receptors (86). PMNs display about 300 to 1,000 G-CSF high-affinity receptors per cell, depending on their level of differentiation; this can effect biological responses at low levels of occupancy (4,27,119). When G-CSF binds to its receptor, the complex is internalized, a mechanism necessary for G-CSF to perform its functional activity (120). Myeloid progenitor cells, monocytes, macrophages, platelets, some T and B lymphoid cell lines, endothelial cells, placenta, and trophoblastic cells also all express G-CSF receptors in varying numbers, but eosinophils and erythroid cells do not (4,110,121–123). Furthermore, the cell lines KG-1, H128, H69, NFS-60, and HL-60 have high-affinity binding sites for G-CSF (124–126).

The precise second messenger pathways used by G-CSF have not yet been identified. G-CSF has no direct effect on membrane depolarization, Ca^{2+} flux, or intracellular free Ca^{2+} concentrations (86). Prior to the proliferative response induced by G-CSF binding to murine myeloblastic NFS-60 cells, a time-dependent activation of guanosine triphosphate-binding proteins and adenylate cyclase occurs (126).

GM-CSF

GM-CSF receptors are expressed on human neutrophils, eosinophils, and monocytes, on purified CFU-GM, and on some nonhematopoietic cells (127). Neutrophils display only a single class of high-affinity receptors, while monocytes and myeloid leukemic cell lines have two classes of binding sites, one with high and one with lower affinity (4). The cDNAs for two receptor subunits, designated α and β, have been cloned (128,129). The α-subunit cDNA encodes a low-affinity binding protein for GM-CSF, but cotransfection of this subunit with the β-subunit cDNA reconstituted the high-affinity GM-CSF-R (129). Isolated expression of the β-subunit, which is shared with the receptors for IL-3 and IL-5 (130), did not generate any binding capacity for human GM-CSF. The high-affinity receptor has a molecular weight of 84 kDa (127) with an affinity of approximately 30 pM (112). It is expressed in low numbers (50 to 1,000 sites per cell) (86). GM-CSF receptors are expressed as soluble forms as well as membrane-anchored proteins (131); the soluble isoforms arise from translation of specific mRNA and are the product of differential splicing.

GM-CSF had no direct effect on membrane depolarization, Ca^{2+} flux or intracellular free Ca^{2+} concentration (86,132) and produced no detectable increase in neutrophilic inositol-triphosphate or diacylglycerol levels, making phospholipase C activation an unlikely second messenger system (86). Though there is no region on the low-affinity human GM-CSF receptor that would be expected to have tyrosine kinase activity (86), it was found that p42 and p44 MAP kinases are prominently tyrosine-phosphorylated in response to GM-CSF in a temperature-dependent fashion *in vitro*, even in non-proliferating neutrophils (133,134). The guanylate cyclase system is another possible pathway for GM-CSF–induced signal transduction in neutrophils. GM-CSF raised cGMP levels (86), an effect that was abrogated by pertussis toxin, which inactivates certain G proteins. Some of the effects of GM-CSF on human PMN were attenuated by a guanylate cyclase inhibitor (135). Lastly, the direct stimulation of arachidonic acid, LTB_4 and platelet activating factor (PAF) synthesis and release may play a role in signal transduction (86). An inhibitor of 5-lipoxygenase attenuated some of the effects of GM-CSF on human neutrophils (135).

SUMMARY OF ANIMAL MODEL DATA

G-CSF

Endogenous formation of G-CSF has a major impact on hematopoiesis as well as on defense against infection: G-CSF knockout mice or animals treated with anti–G-CSF-antibodies exhibited chronic neutropenia and impaired ability to control infection with *L. monocytogenes* (136), *P. aeruginosa* (26), or fecal peritonitis (34).These findings indicate that G-CSF is a major player in the regulation of granulocytopoiesis, both in normal baseline and emergency situations.

Improved neutrophil counts and functions through treatment with G-CSF were beneficial in a variety of infection models with absolute or functional neutropenia. Mice made neutropenic with cyclophosphamide and challenged with *P. aeruginosa, Serratia marcescens,* or *S. aureus* (137,138) had a higher survival rate when treated with G-CSF. G-CSF also improved recovery in a *P. aeruginosa* burn wound infection model in mice (139–141), especially in combination therapy with gentamicin (140). G-CSF treatment was further beneficial to mice challenged with *P. aeruginosa* pneumonia after hemorrhage (142). Newborn rats are known to have impaired PMN functions. They were protected from challenge with group B streptococci when G-CSF was given simultaneously (143–145). When G-CSF was given prenatally, 6 days before an LD_{90} challenge with group B streptococci at birth, the survival of the pups was increased dramatically (146). However, in another study, pretreatment with G-CSF had no effect on the survival of newborn rats challenged intraperitoneally (IP) with the same pathogen (147).

In comparison to the information available on infections in neutropenic animals, infection in non-neutropenic hosts has been studied and reviewed even more extensively (26,38,97,148,149). Only a few model examples will be quoted here.

LPS is a building block of the Gram-negative bacterial outer membrane. Therefore, injection of LPS is considered a model for the nonspecific inflammatory response to bacterial infection. When endotoxic shock was induced in mice and rats by injection of high doses of LPS, G-CSF–pretreated animals' survival was significantly improved in comparison to controls (105). Similarly, G-CSF prevented LPS-induced liver injury in galactosamine-sensitized rodents. In both cases, TNF activity was decreased in the serum. In LPS-challenged pigs and guinea pigs, lung injury was partially attenuated after G-CSF pretreatment (150,151).

G-CSF also offered protection in a variety of peritonitis models. As little as 2 μg/kg G-CSF administered to mice after the onset of peritonitis brought about by cecal ligation and puncture (CLP) was beneficial and synergized with antibiotics (152,153). A dose of 15 μg/kg G-CSF decreased lethality, improved renal and hepatic functions compared to controls, and attenuated histopathology in the lung (154). Similarly, in a rat CLP model, G-CSF decreased mortality and serum TNF levels (155). When a human stool suspension was inoculated into the peritoneum of rats, they were protected by G-CSF in combination with antibiotics (156). Here, a correlation between TNF levels and mortality was observed: G-CSF–treated animals had total suppression of TNF serum levels. Benefits were obtained in analogous mouse and rat models without concurrent antibiotic therapy (34,157). Sepsis after IP implantation of an *E. coli*–infected clot in dogs was improved by G-CSF (158).

In pneumonia models, G-CSF effects were more variable. G-CSF pretreatment protected rats against pneumococcal pneumonia (159). No effect was noted in rats fed a chronic ethanol diet, a model for the immunosuppression experienced by alcohol abusers. However, in a *Klebsiella pneumoniae* experimental infection model G-CSF protected both control and ethanol-treated animals (160). Rabbits inoculated transtracheally with *Pasteurella multocida* and administered G-CSF at 24 hours postchallenge tended towards improved survival (77 versus 67%), but showed a slight increase in inflammation of liver, spleen and lung (161). Detrimental effects of G-CSF were described in rats treated before, during and after intrabronchial application of *E. coli* with or without hyperoxia (162). In a splenectomized mouse model of pneumococcal pneumonia, pretreatment with G-CSF at 24 hours before challenge and continuation for 3 days postchallenge was found to improve survival.

In mice, G-CSF administered for two days after infection significantly improved the survival rate in a lethal model of soft tissue infection with *P. aeruginosa* (163). Mice pretreated daily with a combination of clarithromycin and G-CSF for 3 days before and after IV challenge with *Mycobacterium avium* complex had significantly decreased levels of infection in spleen and lungs (164). Severe combined immunodeficient (SCID) mice, which are devoid of B and T lymphocytes, as well as normal mice, inoculated IV with *L. monocytogenes* followed by G-CSF for 5 days, had lower counts of viable bacteria in the liver than nontreated mice (165).

In non-bacterial murine infections, G-CSF stimulated nonspecific protection against Sendai virus infection (166). Mice made neutropenic with cyclophosphamide were protected against challenge with *Candida albicans, Cryptococcus neoformans,* or *Aspergillus fumigatus* by G-CSF (137,138,167,168). Others, however, noted no beneficial effect in another model of neutropenic murine cryptococcosis (169) and local candidosis (170).

In summary, G-CSF treatment has been found to be beneficial in a broad variety of infection models. In general, the best responses were noted when G-CSF was given concurrent with the infectious challenge or as pretreatment. Results with G-CSF treatment after infection has been established have been inconsistent. Very few adverse effects of G-CSF treatment have been recorded.

GM-CSF

GM-CSF pretreatment of neutropenic mice given usually lethal doses of *P. aeruginosa, S. aureus,* or *C. albicans* resulted in a significant dose-dependent improvement of survival (171,172). GM-CSF given with IL-6 or leukemia inhibitory factor (LIF) protected myelosuppressed mice from fatal *P. aeruginosa* infection (172).

Canturk et al. (173) evaluated the effect of GM-CSF on wound healing in an experimental diabetic rat model. Forty rats were randomly divided into three groups: group I, healthy rats receiving saline as control; group II, diabetic rats receiving saline; and group III, diabetic rats receiving GM-CSF. Neutrophil counts and phagocytosis were significantly increased in group III compare to group II. Wound healing was significantly impaired in group II compared to groups I and III (173).

GM-CSF was protective in animal models of impaired PMN function. In a murine model of 20% surface burn followed by CLP on day 10 after injury, survival was significantly better in animals treated with GM-CSF (174). Neonatal rats have been found to have deficient PMN production and function. Prophylactic rmuGM-CSF given IP at 6 hours before a 90% lethal dose challenge of *S. aureus* significantly improved the survival in neonatal rats (175). Similar results were reported for streptococcal sepsis (176,177).

The survival in two mouse models of gut-derived sepsis was also improved by GM-CSF (178). However, the prophylactic administration of rmuGM-CSF neither augmented leukocyte numbers nor protected mice from lethal fecal peritonitis in another set of investigations (34). Rats given rmuGM-CSF with sepsis-induced organ injury by CLP showed earlier mortality and a lower survival rate (179). In addition to the mild hepatic injuries observed from shock, the livers of GM-CSF–treated rats showed centrilobular degeneration, ALT elevations, and necrotic changes. Therefore, the systemic application of GM-CSF, as opposed to its natural local production, might be dangerous when infection is already present.

Administering neutralizing monoclonal antibody specific for GM-CSF to *C. neoformans*–infected mice increased mortality and induced more rapid progression of the disease (180). Endogenous GM-CSF also appears to play a role in the initial host defense response to *Leishmania donovani*. GM-CSF mRNA was upregulated in infected mouse livers and the infection exacerbated when the animals were treated with anti–GM-CSF antibody (181). GM-CSF was also found to reduce the proportion of cultured peritoneal macrophages infected with *Leishmania tropicana* collected from mice (92). However, GM-CSF may also play a role in the pathogenesis of Leishmania infection itself: murine lung-conditioned medium has colony-stimulating activity on bone marrow cells and on promastigotes of *Leishmania mexicana* amazonensis. Both activities are abrogated by immunoprecipitation with an anti–mu-GM-CSF antibody (45). Antibodies against both GM-CSF and IL-3 were also protective in mice infected with *Plasmodium berghei* (182). However, antibodies against GM-CSF or IL-3 alone had no effect.

Mice chronically infected with *Trypanosoma cruzi* (Chagas disease) have a defect in their cellular immune response, which was corrected by the administration of GM-CSF *in vivo* (183).

RmuGM-CSF has been found to protect mice against Sendai virus and herpes simplex virus infection (42,166).

In summary, GM-CSF administered prophylactically seems to be beneficial in several animal infection models. However, when severe infections are already present and active, it has detrimental effects when administered alone, though it may be a useful adjuvant to antibiotic therapy. In contrast to G-CSF, GM-CSF appears to act as a proinflammatory factor. A further indication for GM-CSF may be to increase eosinophil cell counts to combat parasitic infection. Here, GM-CSF has an advantage over G-CSF, as it also activates monocytes and macrophages. If enhanced macrophage activation, including the production of IL-1 and TNF is desired, GM-CSF may again be indicated (71). To date, too little is known about a possible benefit of GM-CSF in the treatment of viral infections.

CLINICAL APPLICATIONS OF G-CSF AND GM-CSF

Clinical Use in Myelosuppressive Chemotherapy and Neutropenic Fever

Neutropenia is often seen in many chemotherapeutic regimens used to treat patients with cancer. In fact, myelosuppression is often the dose-limiting factor of such drugs. Besides this quantitative effect, intensive chemotherapy has been shown to induce qualitative defects in neutrophil function, including decreased chemotaxis, production of radical oxygen species (ROS), and microbicidal activity (184,185). *In vitro* and *in vivo* studies in patients with cancer undergoing intensive chemotherapy have shown that G-CSF improves and often restores the impaired production of ROS, microbicidal activity, and antibody-dependent cellular cytotoxicity (ADCC) by neutrophils (186–188). *In vivo* studies in patients with cancer have shown that GM-CSF effectively enhances neutrophil production of ROS and degranulation (188,189, reviewed in 190).

Bodey et al. (1) noted that the clinical risk of severe infectious complications in patients receiving chemotherapy for cancer is directly related to the severity and length of neutropenia. The risk of infection increases as the absolute neutrophil count (ANC; neutrophils and bands) falls below 1,000/mm^3 and is greatest below 100/mm^3. Despite advances in antimicrobial therapy and critical care management, infections continue to be a leading cause of morbidity and mortality in patients with profound and prolonged neutropenia. However, patients with neutropenia are not a homogeneous group; that is, not all neutropenic patients have the same risk of developing serious complications and dying during a febrile episode. Based on the severity and duration of neutropenia these patients can be categorized as “low risk” or “high risk” (191). Usually, low-risk patients have a duration of neutropenia of less than 7 days and tend to do well even when they develop moderate to severe myelosuppression (patients with sarcomas, testicular cancer, or breast cancer). High-risk patients are those who typically develop profound neutropenia for more than 10 to 14 days (patients with hematologic malignancies, lymphomas, or hematopoietic stem cell recipients). As a result, high-risk patients often develop serious infections during febrile episodes, which may lead to prolonged stays in the intensive care unit or to death (191). Other factors implicated in higher risk for infections and other serious complications during febrile episodes include severe mucositis and penetration of the skin by vascular devices.

Clinical studies have been performed to evaluate the effects of myeloid growth factors along with antibiotics on the outcomes of febrile neutropenic episodes. Maher et al. (192) conducted a multicenter, double-blind, randomized trial that included 218 patients over 4 years. Of 216 evaluable patients, 109 received G-CSF and 107 received placebo. In comparison to placebo, G-CSF significantly reduced the median number of days of severe neutropenia (ANC < 500/mm^3) from 4 to 3 and of ANC < 1,000/mm^3 from 5 to 3. The median number of days with fever were the same in both groups, but fewer patients receiving G-CSF had prolonged fever. No significant differences in the length of hospital stay were observed. In addition, the number of days of treatment and total dose of antibiotics were almost identical in the two groups. In a subgroup analysis, G-CSF decreased the number of days of neutropenia and accelerated neutrophil recovery regardless of baseline neutrophil count. Statistically significant differences occurred in patients who had moderate to severe neutropenia at baseline. G-CSF resulted in reduction of time to resolution of fever only in patients with baseline ANC of <100/mm^3 (192).

Aviles et al. (193) conducted a prospective clinical trial of 119 patients with microbiologically proven infections and severe neutropenia after intensive chemotherapy to investigate the effectiveness and toxicity of G-CSF. Patients treated for lymphoma, Hodgkin's disease, or myeloma received antibiotics (ceftazidime and amikacin) without G-CSF (control group), or with G-CSF (treatment group). The response rate for bacteremias in the control group was 53%, while in the treatment group it was 80%. In patients with Gram-negative bacterial infections, administration of G-CSF in addition to antibiotics significantly improved neutrophil recovery and decreased duration of fever and hospital stay. No significant differences in response rates for patients with Gram-positive infections were documented.

GM-CSF has also been used to ameliorate the neutropenia seen during dose-intensive chemotherapy. Yau et al. (194) performed a prospective, double-blind, randomized, placebo-controlled, phase III trial that included 56 patients with lymphoma or breast cancer to evaluate the effect of GM-CSF in neutropenic fever. Patients received submyeloablative doses of cyclophosphamide, etoposide, and cisplatin, and were randomized to receive GM-CSF (sargramostim 250 μg/m^2) or placebo SC every 12 hours. GM-CSF–treated patients had a significant decrease in duration of neutropenia after the first course of chemotherapy compared to patients who received placebo (10 days and 12 days, respectively, $p = 0.01$). No significant difference in the duration of neutropenia was achieved after the second and third courses of chemotherapy. There was no difference between the two groups in the number of hospitalizations for febrile neutropenia nor incidence of bacteremia (194).

Mayordomo et al. (195) compared the effect of adding G-CSF or GM-CSF to standard antibiotic therapy in cancer patients with fever and chemotherapy-induced neutropenia. This study involved 121 patients; 39 patients were randomized to the G-CSF arm, 39 to the GM-CSF arm, and 43 to receive antibiotics alone. The initial empiric antibiotic treatment consisted of ceftazidime 2 gm IV every 6 hours and amikacin 500 mg IV every 12 hours. Antibiotics were modified in patients with significant blood cultures or clinical findings. Treatment was initiated within 8 hours of the onset of neutropenic fever. The mean duration of grade IV neutropenia was significantly shorter for patients receiving CSFs (2 days, range 1 to 6) than that for patients receiving placebo (3 days, range 1 to 16) ($p < 0.001$). The mean duration of neutropenia (ANC < 1,000/mm^3) was also significantly shorter for patients receiving CSFs compared to those receiving placebo. Duration of fever was not significantly different in the three arms of the study. The number of patients who required a change in antibiotics was also not significantly different in the three groups. Median hospital stay was shorter in patients receiving CSFs compared to the ones on placebo, but this was mainly a function of protocol policy that required patients to stay on antibiotics for 2 days after recovery of neutropenia. There were eight deaths: four due to infection and four due to tumor progression. All deaths occurred in patients with severe neutropenia and positive blood cultures (195). Although the duration of neutropenia end points were shorter in the groups that received CSFs, there was little, if any, evidence that this led to clinical benefit.

In summary, the high cost of CSFs in the setting of chemotherapy-induced neutropenic fever has led to the conclusion that their use for primary prophylaxis is more cost-effective when the expected risk of neutropenic fever is more than 40% (191,196). It is possible that primary CSF administration may be warranted in patients at higher risk for chemotherapy-induced infectious complications such as in those with preexisting neutropenia due to disease, poor performance status, and more advanced cancer, decreased immune function, open wounds, or already active tissue infections. After an episode of neutropenic fever or severe or prolonged neutropenia, chemotherapy dose reduction should be considered as a primary therapeutic option instead of secondary prophylaxis with CSFs. CSFs should not be routinely used for patients with neutropenia who are afebrile.

Therapy with CSFs should be considered for those patients with neutropenia and fever who are at higher risk for infection-associated complications, including profound neutropenia (ANC < 100/mm^3), uncontrolled primary disease, pneumonia, hypotension, sepsis syndrome, and invasive fungal infection (191). Currently, there is no justification for the use of CSFs to increase chemotherapy dose-intensity, or schedule, or both, outside of a clinical trial. Both G-CSF and GM-CSF shorten the duration of neutropenia and reduce infectious complications in patients undergoing high-dose cytotoxic chemotherapy sup-

TABLE 9-5. *Clinical uses of CSFs in febrile neutropenia, myelosuppressive chemotherapy, stem cell transplantation (SCT)*[a]

Recommendations	Considerations
For primary prophylaxis of febrile neutropenia	
CSF is recommended with chemotherapy expected to produce FN in ≥ 40% of the cases.	CSF may be considered in patients with preexisting neutropenia, poor performance status, advanced cancer, prior immunosuppression, open wounds or active infections
CSF can be used in acute leukemia patients 55 years of age or older, after completion of chemotherapy.	Intermittent use of CSF may be considered in a subset of patients with myelodysplastic syndromes with severe neutropenia and recurrent infections
For secondary prophylaxis of febrile neutropenia	
CSF is not routinely recommended to maintain the same chemotherapy dose-intensity.	Consider chemotherapy dose reduction after FN or severe or prolonged neutropenia after previous chemotherapy treatment
For patients with febrile neutropenia	
CSF is not routinely recommended for the majority of patients with uncomplicated FN (fever ≤ 10 days duration; no evidence of active infection, hypotension, multiorgan dysfunction or invasive fungal infection; and no uncontrolled malignancies.	CSF use may be reasonable in patients with FN at higher risk for infection-associated complications (ANC <100/μL), uncontrolled primary disease, pneumonia, hypotension, multiorgan dysfunction or invasive fungal infection
For patients undergoing SCT	
CSF is routinely used for mobilization of peripheral blood stem cells (PBSC) for transplantation	CSF may be used to accelerate hematopoietic reconstitution after either bone marrow or PBSC transplantation
CSF is recommended in the event of graft failure	

[a]Based on the American Society of Clinical Oncology Guidelines for the use of hematopoietic colony-stimulating factors (191).

CSF, hematopoietic colony-stimulating factors; FN, febrile neutropenia; SCT, stem cell transplantation.

ported by hematopoietic stem cell transplantation (HSCT). Currently, use of CSFs is routinely recommended as adjunct to allogeneic or autologous peripheral-blood progenitor cell (PBPC) transplantation, both for mobilization of PBPCs and as a means to accelerate hematopoietic reconstitution after bone marrow transplantation (BMT) or PBPC transplantation (191). CSFs might be considered in patients treated for hematologic malignancies, especially acute myelogenous leukemia (AML) and acute lymphoblastic leukemia (ALL). Patients 55 years of age or older undergoing chemotherapy for AML are the most likely to benefit from CSFs. Although much concern has been raised about the potentially dangerous effect of CSFs stimulating myeloid leukemia cells, randomized trials have not shown this to be clinically relevant. Nevertheless, caution should be exercised when CSFs are used in patients with myeloid malignancies. Table 9.5 depicts the current recommendations and suggested considerations for the use of CSFs in patients with cancer.

Clinical Use in HIV Infection

Hematologic cytopenias occur in 10% to 20% of individuals in the early stages of infection with the human immunodeficiency virus (HIV) and in 75% to 90% of those with advanced disease not receiving highly active antiretroviral therapy (HAART) (197). Several factors account for the cytopenias seen in this patient population, including ineffective hematopoiesis, premature destruction of circulating blood cells (increased apoptosis, autoimmunity, infections), malignancies, and myelosuppression (antimicrobial and chemotherapeutic agents).

HIV-infected patients not only develop neutropenia but also have abnormal neutrophil function, including decreased production of ROS, abnormal microbicidal activity, and impaired ADCC. Increased apoptosis has been found in HIV-infected patients, especially when the CD4 count was below 200/mm^3 (198). In addition, dysregulation of cytokine production by macrophages infected with HIV-1 can be demonstrated *in vitro*. Increased secretion of proinflammatory cytokines (i.e., IL-1β, IL-6, IL-8, and TNF-α) and reduced secretion of G-CSF and GM-CSF by monocyte-derived macrophages has been documented after stimulation with LPS (199). *In vitro* and *ex vivo* studies have shown that G-CSF effectively decreases the rate of neutrophil apoptosis, enhances production of ROS, and improves the abnormal microbicidal activity and ADCC in HIV-infected patients (198,200–202). Enhanced production of ROS, phagocytosis, and ADCC has been observed when GM-CSF is administered to HIV-infected patients (203).

Although the relationship between low neutrophil counts and infectious complications has not been as well documented in HIV patients as it has been in cancer patients with chemotherapy-induced neutropenia, recent data indicate that neutropenia is an independent risk factor for bacterial infection in patients with advanced HIV infection, with increased risk of infection when the ANC is less than 1,000/mm^3, and further increased risk when the ANC is less than 500/mm^3 (204). As a result, neutropenia often leads to dose reduction or discontinuation of important myelosuppressive medications, many of which are key to the treatment of HIV and associated infections. Kuritzkes et al. (205) showed that G-CSF is safe and effective in correcting moderately severe neutropenia in patients with advanced HIV infection. This 24-week, randomized, controlled, open-label, multicenter study enrolled 258 HIV-infected patients with CD4 counts less than 200/mm^3 and ANC between 750 and 1,000/mm^3. Patients were randomized to receive daily or intermittent SC doses of G-CSF or placebo. Patients in the treatment groups received either daily G-CSF (starting at 1 µg/kg/day, adjusted up to 10 µg/kg/day) or intermittent G-CSF (starting at 300 μg/day 1 to 3 days per week, adjusted up to 600 μg/day, 7 days per week) necessary to achieve an ANC between 2,000 and 10,000/mm^3. Patients in the control group received G-CSF only if severe neutropenia developed. Severe neutropenia was less frequent in patients who received daily (12.8%) or intermittent (8.2%) G-CSF in comparison to patients in the control group (34.1%; $p < 0.002$ and $p < 0.0001$, respectively). G-CSF–treated patients had fewer bacterial infections, shorter hospital stay, and fewer days of antimicrobial therapy. G-CSF did not increase plasma HIV RNA level and did not produce unexpected adverse effects. Although death rates were slightly lower in the G-CSF–treated groups, no significant difference in survival was shown (205).

Hermans et al. (206), in an open-label, noncomparative, multicenter study of 171 HIV-infected patients with neutropenia, showed that G-CSF (median dose 1 μg/kg/day) reversed neutropenia (ANC more than 2,000/mm^3) within 2 days in 60% of the patients. After reversal of neutropenia, a median dose of G-CSF 300 μg thrice weekly was needed to sustain an appropriate ANC during the study period. The ability to administer medications that induce neutropenia (i.e., ganciclovir, zidovudine, and cotrimoxazole) increased by 20% during G-CSF therapy. In this study, G-CSF was well tolerated. In addition, a slight increase in CD4, CD8, and total lymphocyte counts was observed with no changes in HIV p24 antigen levels (206).

Retrospective studies of HIV-infected patients have shown increased survival when G-CSF has been administered for neutropenia in the setting of a concurrent infection (198,201). In a retrospective analysis of 91 HIV-infected patients with disseminated *Mycobacterium avium* complex (MAC) infection, patients received G-CSF (300 μg SC 5 days a week) when the ANC was lower than 500/mm^3 until the ANC was stable between 1,000 and 2,000/mm^3. Subjects treated with G-CSF lived longer than those who did not receive G-CSF (355 days and 211 days, respectively; $p < 0.01$). Increased survival was also seen in the group of patients who received clarithromycin and G-CSF versus clarithromycin alone (377 days and 252 days, respectively; $p < 0.01$) (207).

When whole blood cytokine release was studied in blood drawn from HIV-infected patients stratified according to CD4 counts, a significant reduction in IL-2 production was found in advanced stages. Notably, IL-2 production was restored in the presence of G-CSF *in vitro* (208), suggesting that G-CSF might reconstitute endogenous IL-2 production, which is critical in maintaining CD8 control of viral replication.

GM-CSF has been studied in AIDS patients undergoing myelosuppressive chemotherapeutic or antiviral regimens. A prospective, randomized, phase III trial evaluated the efficacy of GM-CSF in conjunction with ganciclovir in the treatment of cytomegalovirus (CMV) retinitis (209). Fifty-one AIDS patients were randomized to receive standard ganciclovir therapy or ganciclovir and GM-CSF administered by daily SC injections. Of 36 evaluable patients, 21 received ganciclovir alone and 15 ganciclovir and GM-CSF. Fewer patients on GM-CSF became neutropenic (ANC < 750/mm^3), 40% compared to 59% of patients in the non–GM-CSF group. The overall incidence of neutropenic episodes was lower in the GM-CSF group than in the non–GM-CSF group (20 and 68, respectively). There was also a trend toward a lower rate of CMV retinitis relapses and improved maintenance of appropriate ganciclovir dose (209).

Kaplan et al. (210) evaluated the clinical and virologic effects of GM-CSF administered to patients with HIV-associated non-Hodgkin's lymphoma (NHL) receiving chemotherapy with cyclophosphamide, doxorubicin, vincristine, and prednisone (CHOP). Five patients were randomized to receive GM-CSF (10 to 20 μg/kg/day) on days 1 through 10 of each chemotherapy cycle (early GM-CSF), 11 patients received the same dose on days 4 through 13 of each chemotherapy cycle (delayed GM-CSF), and 10 patients did not receive GM-CSF. Compared with the control group, the delayed GM-CSF group had shorter mean durations of neutropenia (13 and 4.9 days, respectively; p = 0.02), higher mean nadirs of the ANC (360/mm^3 and 890/mm^3, respectively; p = 0.009), fewer chemotherapy cycles complicated by neutropenic fever (67% and 27%, respectively; p = 0.001), fewer days of hospitalization for neutropenic fever (4.9 and 1.8 days, respectively; p = 0.004), and fewer reductions in chemotherapy dosages. In the third week after chemotherapy, median HIV-1 p24 antigen levels remained below baseline in the control group, but rose to 243% of baseline values in the GM-CSF group (p = 0.01), suggesting stimulation of HIV-1 replication; the clinical significance of this finding is unclear. GM-CSF did not have any impact on survival or tumor relapse rate (210).

Angel et al. (211) evaluated the effect of GM-CSF in advanced HIV disease (effect on opportunistic infections and CD4 cell counts). This phase III randomized, double-blind, placebo-controlled trial enrolled subjects with CD4 cell counts less than or equal to 100/mm^3 with a prior AIDS-defining illness on stable antiretroviral therapy. Subjects were stratified by baseline HIV RNA level (less than, equal to, or more than 30,000 copies/mL), and randomized to receive SC injections of GM-CSF 250 μg or placebo thrice weekly for 24 weeks. Three hundred and nine subjects received at least one dose of study drug; 70% completed 24 weeks of therapy. Groups were well balanced at baseline. Significant increases in the neutrophil and CD4 cell counts were observed at 1, 3, and 6 months in the GM-CSF groups. GM-CSF significantly reduced the incidence of overall infections (78% placebo and 67% GM-CSF; p = 0.03) and delayed time to first infection (56 days placebo and 97 days GM-CSF; p = 0.04). No statistical difference in cumulative opportunistic infections was observed among groups. Change in HIV-RNA was not significantly different among groups. In patients with HIV-RNA levels below the limit of detection at baseline, more GM-CSF patients maintained an undetectable viral load at 24 weeks (54% placebo and 83% GM-CSF; p = 0.02). GM-CSF was well tolerated (211).

Ex vivo studies with monocyte and monocyte-derived macrophages (MDM) from HIV-infected patients have shown defective phagocytosis and killing of different opportunistic pathogens, including MAC (212, reviewed in 213). Addition of GM-CSF *ex vivo* was able to restore the impaired phagocytosis of MAC (212). In addition, administration of GM-CSF to a patient with a multidrug resistant MAC infection delayed culture positivity (212). The clinical significance of this still needs to be evaluated.

In conclusion, G-CSF and GM-CSF shorten neutropenia in HIV-infected patients, lower the rate of bacterial infections, and shorten antimicrobial use and hospital stay. *In vitro* studies suggest that GM-CSF stimulates the replication of HIV-1 in monocytes, but the antiviral effect of zidovudine is enhanced by GM-CSF (reviewed in 214). As GM-CSF is able to modulate several functions of lymphocytes and monocytes, this might affect HIV replication. The clinical significance of these modulatory effects needs to be evaluated further. G-CSF can be used safely in HIV-infected patients and allows for the use of other myelosuppressive medications. Despite these beneficial effects, prospective studies have not shown longer survival rate for HIV-infected patients treated with CSFs. Consideration for the use of a CSF should be given for HIV-infected patients with ANC less than 1,000/mm^3. When possible, dose reduction of myelotoxic medications or change to a less myelotoxic therapy should be considered. Adjunctive use of a CSF should be also considered in the management of multidrug resistant mycobacterial infections. Table 9.6 offers a practical approach to the use of CSFs in HIV-infected patients.

TABLE 9-6. *Suggested approach to the use of CSFs in HIV-infected patients*

Consider CSF use in patients with persistent and significant neutropenia (ANC <1,000/μL)
Use the lowest effective dose of CSF to maintain ANC ≥ 1,000/mL
Identify potential myelosuppressive drugs
Change to less myelotoxic medications whenever possible
Evaluate the patient for underlying opportunistic infections that may contribute to neutropenia
Consider CSF use in the management of multidrug resistant mycobacterial infections

CSF, hematopoietic colony-stimulating factor; ANC, absolute neutrophil count.

Clinical Use in Diabetes Mellitus

Patients with poorly controlled diabetes mellitus (DM) are known to have abnormal neutrophil function manifested by decreased adhesion, migration, phagocytosis, microbicidal activity, and production of ROS (215–218). Greater neutrophil dysfunction has been seen in patients with higher levels of HbA_{1c} (215). Improvement or restoration of neutrophil function is generally seen with adequate glycemic control. Infections aggravate abnormal glucose metabolism in diabetic patients. This, in turn, leads to further derangement of the nonspecific and specific host defense mechanisms creating a vicious circle of worsening infection and metabolic abnormalities.

In vitro G-CSF is able to correct the abnormal production of ROS and the impaired myeloperoxidase (MPO) activity seen in neutrophils of patients with poorly controlled DM. Furthermore, a direct correlation between the levels of HbA_{1c} and G-CSF enhancement of neutrophil function has been demonstrated, with a greater improvement in PMN function seen in patients with the worst glycemic control (215).

In a prospective, randomized, double-blinded placebo-controlled trial, Gough et al. (219) assessed the ability of G-CSF to improve neutrophil function and clinical outcomes in 40 diabetic patients with foot infections . Twenty patients received G-CSF (5 μg/kg/day for 7 days), and 20 patients received placebo; both groups also received standard antimicrobial therapy. G-CSF therapy was associated with earlier bacterial eradication from the infected ulcer (4 versus 8 days, respectively), faster resolution of cellulitis (7 versus 12 days), shorter hospital stay (10 versus 17.5 days), and a shorter duration of intravenous antimicrobial therapy (8.5 versus 14.5 days). Furthermore, after 7 days of G-CSF therapy, neutrophil production of ROS was significantly higher in the treatment group than in the placebo group (219).

In a case report, two insulin-dependent diabetic patients with chronic nonhealing leg ulcers due to necrobiosis lipoidica diabeticorum were treated by repetitive topical application of GM-CSF on the ulcer over a 10-week period. Topical GM-CSF apparently healed the ulcers of both patients in 10 weeks. During follow-up, the ulcers remained healed for more than 3 years (220).

Larger prospective, randomized, placebo-controlled studies will be necessary to validate the efficacy and to further characterize the indications of G-CSF use in the setting of diabetic foot infections. Human trials evaluating the effects of GM-CSF in diabetic patients are still pending.

Clinical Use in Sepsis and Trauma

Acute neutropenia may occur as the initial response to many systemic bacterial and fungal infections, and is often seen immediately after endotoxin challenge in healthy volunteers. The pathogenesis of neutropenia in sepsis is not completely understood. The initial drop in neutrophil counts might be related to increased neutrophil adherence to the endothelium in response to endotoxin and other microbial products leading to upregulation of selectins on neutrophils (LAM-1) and on endothelial cells [intercellular adhesion molecule (ICAM), and endothelial leukocyte adhesion molecule (ELAM)] (reviewed in 221). Bone marrow suppression by prostaglandin E_2 (PGE_2) released from macrophages activated by endotoxin has been postulated as another factor contributing to sepsis associated neutropenia (222). In most subjects, neutropenia is followed by a rise in neutrophil count over the next several hours. Endotoxin actively stimulates the release of neutrophils from marrow reserves through release of cytokines (e.g., TNF-α, GM-CSF, and G-CSF), and through C3a (reviewed in 221).

Documentation of neutrophil functional abnormalities in sepsis or trauma has been inconsistent. Some studies have found decreased neutrophil function, while others have found normal or increased neutrophil function (i.e., chemotaxis, phagocytosis, production of ROS, and microbicidal activity) in this clinical setting. The variability of these results might be related in part to the different techniques and experimental conditions used in these studies (reviewed in 221).

TNF-α and IL-1, released in response to LPS and to other immune stimulatory products of microorganisms, have been identified as major mediators of the initial organ and metabolic abnormalities seen in trauma and sepsis. Patients with severe trauma or infections had increased levels of TNF-α, IL-1, IL-6, and IL-8. Although these inflammatory cytokines are essential in combating infections, their expression could contribute to endothelial and organ damage when excessively up-regulated leading to what is clinically known as the systemic inflammatory response syndrome (SIRS) (223). On the other hand, a number of clinical and experimental studies have shown that in parallel to the proinflammatory cytokines, anti-inflammatory cytokines are also produced (224,225). Substantially elevated levels of circulating IL-10 have been detected in sepsis patients (225). Moreover, monocytes from patients in the later stages of sepsis had decreased HLA-DR antigen expression when compare to normal individuals (226).

Several clinical trials of patients with sepsis and/or trauma have shown a direct correlation between the levels of TNF-α, IL-6, IL-8, and G-CSF and active illness, with the highest levels seen in patients with severe sepsis and septic shock. Persistent high levels of TNF-α, IL-6, and IL-8 have been associated with poor outcome (43,227–229). Animal models of sepsis have shown that pretreatment with G-CSF enhances LPS clearance, lowers TNF-α, and improves survival. G-CSF interferes with the synthesis and/or release of TNF-α, but not with the effects of TNF-α. In addition, G-CSF did not induce multiorgan failure (105,230).

Presneill et al. (231) performed a prospective observational cohort study in critically ill patients with sepsis and septic shock to evaluate the circulating levels of G-CSF and GM-CSF and their relationship to the development of multiorgan dysfunction and mortality. A total of 82 critically ill adult patients were enrolled (29 with septic shock, 17 with sepsis without shock, 22 with shock without sepsis, and 14 without sepsis or shock). The groups were well balanced, and the shock and septic shock groups had similar degrees of physiologic disturbances. IL-6 levels were elevated in all subjects, with almost logarithmic incremental increases; the highest levels were observed in patients with septic shock followed by those with sepsis. In general, levels of IL-6, G-CSF, and leukemia inhibitor factor (LIF) were significantly higher in patients with sepsis and septic shock than in control or other shock patients. However, they were not independently predictive of mortality, or the development of multiorgan dysfunction. GM-CSF was rarely elevated (231).

Arslan et al. (232) evaluated TNF-α levels and the impact of G-CSF on survival of burn patients with sepsis. Seventy-eight patients with burn-related sepsis were enrolled prospectively: 51 patients received standard treatment with G-CSF 5 μg/kg/day on the first 3 days, 4 μg/kg/day on days 4 through 6, and 3 μg/kg/day on days 7 through 9. Twenty-seven burn patients received only standard treatment without G-CSF. A marked decline in the TNF-α level by day 7 was observed in patients who survived in both groups, while TNF-α levels were persistently high in patients who did not survive. The survival rate was 42 of 51 (82.3%) in the G-CSF group and nine of 27 (33.3%) in the non–G-CSF group (232).

Studies in leukopenic patients with sepsis have shown that G-CSF (0.5 to 2 μg/kg/day SC) in addition to antimicrobial therapy, corrected the low neutrophil count, reduced the number of failing organs, and led to increased survival. Administration of G-CSF attenuated the inflammatory immune response and did not induce tissue injury (233,234). Use of G-CSF (0.5 to 2 μg/kg/day SC) in non-neutropenic patients with trauma or sepsis may reduce the number of bacteremias and ameliorate life-threatening infections, but had no beneficial effects on length of hospital stay or mortality. G-CSF resulted in improved generation and function of neutrophils and appeared to counterregulate increase of proinflammatory cytokines. G-CSF administration was safe and did not induce lung injury or multiorgan failure (MOF) (235,236).

Flohe et al. (237) evaluated the *ex vivo* modulatory effect of GM-CSF on TNF-α production after stimulation with LPS in healthy donors and patients with multiple injury, sepsis, and cardiac surgery. *Ex vivo* GM-CSF pretreatment of whole blood from healthy volunteers resulted in a marked increase of LPS-induced TNF-α production in a dose-dependent manner. GM-CSF also increased HLA-DR expression on monocytes but not on T- or B-cells. TNF-α production was mildly impaired after cardiac surgery, moderately impaired after injury, and severely impaired in sepsis. GM-CSF *ex vivo* was able to increase TNF-α production with the least effect observed in blood from septic patients. GM-CSF also enhanced the impaired HLA-DR expression in monocytes of patients. Further, GM-CSF incubation *in vitro* elevated TNF-α synthesis in normal monocytes and whole blood treated with a combination of anti-inflammatory mediators, such as IL-10, TGF-β, and PGE_2 (237).

Fanning et al. (238) studied cytokine production in seven patients with SIRS. Various proinflammatory mediators (IL-6, GM-CSF, IL-1β, TNF-α), known to modulate neutrophil apoptosis *in vitro*, were elevated in the plasma of SIRS patients compared with those of controls. The antiinflammatory cytokine, IL-10, was also elevated in the SIRS patients. Neutrophils isolated from patients with SIRS showed significantly delayed spontaneous apoptosis when compared with those of the control group. The antiapoptotic effect of SIRS plasma was specifically attenuated by neutralizing GM-CSF in SIRS plasma, but not IL-6, IL-1β, or TNF-α. Suppression of neutrophil apoptosis was correlated with inhibition of production of ROS, quantified as peroxide production. Suppression of neutrophil apoptosis was reversed by addition of neutralizing antibodies to GM-CSF or addition of recombinant human IL-10 (238).

The timing of G-CSF administration seems to affect its biologic effects. *In vivo* experiments in healthy volunteers challenged with LPS have shown that G-CSF given 2 hours before the challenge increased the release of TNF, IL-6, IL-8, IL-1ra and sTNFr I and II. In contrast, administration of G-CSF at 24 hours before LPS challenge significantly reduced the release of IL-8 and slightly reduced release of TNF and IL-6. However, the release of IL-1ra and sTNFr I and II were increased (110). This showed that timing of G-CSF administration in relation to LPS challenge might be an important determinant of its anti-inflammatory effects. In general, SIRS is characterized by an imbalance among proinflammatory and anti-inflammatory factors. At the present time, it is unknown what favors one or the other in a given patient. G-CSF, with its anti-inflammatory effect, and GM-CSF, with its proinflammatory effect, might be potentially of use in correcting that imbalance.

Clinical Use in Fungal Infections

Invasive fungal infections are a significant cause of morbidity and mortality among immunocompromised patients. The clinical outcome of these infections remains poor despite the development of new formulations and new antifungal agents. *Candida* spp and *Aspergillus* spp remain the most common pathogens implicated in systemic fungal infections.

In vitro studies in healthy volunteers have shown that G-CSF enhances neutrophil antifungal activity toward *Candida* blastoconidia and *pseudohyphae*, and *Aspergillus* hyphae. This modulatory effect is based on increased neutrophil production of ROS (239–241). *In vitro* studies with GM-CSF in healthy volunteers have also demonstrated its ability to enhance the antifungal activity of neutrophils and monocytes against *C. albicans, A. fumigatus,* and *F. solani* (242,243). In addition, *in vitro* G-CSF has also been shown to improve the abnormal neutrophil fungicidal activity against *A. fumigatus* seen in neutrophils of HIV-infected patients and in neutrophils exposed to corticosteroids *in vitro* (244,245). *In vitro* GM-CSF significantly enhanced monocyte fungicidal activity against *A. fumigatus,* even when monocyte antifungal activity was depressed as a result of prior treatment with dexamethasone (246).

Clinical reports have suggested a beneficial effect of CSFs as adjunctive therapy for treatment of systemic mycosis. Published case reports have suggested favorable results with the administration of G-CSF (247-249), and GM-CSF (250), in addition to antifungals for the treatment of zygomycosis in diabetic and cancer patients.

A small study looked at the effect of G-CSF on neutrophil fungicidal activity in neutropenic HIV-infected patients and in healthy volunteers (251). Nine HIV-infected patients with ANC less than 1,000/mm^3 received G-CSF (5 μg/kg SC single dose), and nine healthy volunteers who did not receive G-CSF served as controls. Neutrophil counts increased threefold to 11-fold within 24 hours and returned to baseline within 96 hours. While phagocytic activity was preserved in HIV-infected patients, fungicidal activity of neutrophils from HIV-infected patients was significantly impaired compared to that of non-HIV-infected subjects. Neutrophils from HIV-infected patients had abnormal production of ROS that was corrected by *in vivo* administration of G-CSF leading to improvement of neutrophil fungicidal activity against *C. albicans* and *C. neoformans* (251).

Recently, a randomized multicenter trial in Europe compared the clinical outcomes of non–HIV-infected, nonneutropenic patients with systemic candidiasis treated with fluconazole versus fluconazole and G-CSF. Although patients treated with G-CSF experienced a faster resolution of the infection, there was no significant difference in the mortality rate between the two groups. Increasing neutrophil counts were correlated with faster clearance of candida from the bloodstream and improved clinical outcome (252).

Cytokines are a promising tool for the treatment of disseminated or refractory fungal infections due to candida or molds. However, until more data are available, their use should be limited to clinical trials. Future randomized clinical studies should evaluate the immunomodulatory effects of CSFs alone or in combination with IFN-γ, and further explore the benefits of combination immunotherapy and antimicrobial chemotherapy.

Clinical Use in Pneumonia

Pneumonia continues to be a leading cause of death in the United States, and resolution of infection seems to be dependent on neutrophil number and function (253). Therefore, considerable interest has emerged on the use of CSFs in the setting of complicated pneumonia. Use of G-CSF in a murine model of pneumococcal pneumonia showed that pretreatment at 24 hours or 10 minutes before initiation of infection significantly improved survival in animals given an LD_{50} dose of bacteria. G-CSF also significantly increased myeloperoxidase (MPO) activity and ANC up to 72 hours postinfection. Reductions in bacterial counts in the lungs at 48 and 72 hours postinfection were observed but did not reach statistical significance. In contrast, G-CSF did not increase survival of animals infected with the LD_{100} inoculum (254). This suggests that the efficacy of G-CSF in pneumonia is therefore optimal when given very early after the onset of infection.

Several studies have been conducted using G-CSF in patients with pneumonia. In a phase I study, 31 patients with community-acquired bacterial pneumonia (CAP) were treated with G-CSF in dosages up to 600 μg/day SC for 10 days. Doses of G-CSF above 150 μg/day increased neutrophil counts by as much as three times the normal values without being associated with adverse effects. Duration of fever, length of antibiotic therapy, and length of hospitalization were not adversely affected in the G-CSF treatment group (255).

A phase III multicenter, multinational, double-blind placebo-controlled trial was carried out to evaluate if adjunctive G-CSF therapy would reduce the morbidity and hasten the resolution of bacterial pneumonia (256). A total of 756 patients were enrolled, 380 received G-CSF 300 μg/day SC, until resolution of the pneumonia or for a maximum of 10 days, and 376 received placebo. The death rate was low in both groups (6%), and the time to resolution of clinical signs, improved oxygenation, and length of hospitalization were similar. However, treatment with G-CSF hastened radiologic improvement and seemed to reduce serious complications such as empyema, adult respiratory distress syndrome (ARDS), and disseminated intravasculars coagulation (DIC). The clinical effects of G-CSF treatment were more pronounced in a subgroup of patients with multilobar pneumonia. G-CSF therapy was well tolerated in patients with pneumonia (256).

In another placebo-controlled study, Wunderink et al. (257) examined the safety and efficacy of G-CSF in patients with severe CAP or nosocomial pneumonia and sepsis. Twelve patients received G-CSF (300 μg/day SC), and six patients received placebo. Although the study group was small, mortality at days 15 and 29 was significantly lower in the G-CSF–treated group (2/12 and 3/12) than in the placebo group (4/6 and 4/6) ($p = 0.04$ and $p = 0.01$, respectively) (257).

These two prior studies in humans suggested that G-CSF might be beneficial in the setting of severe and complicated pneumonia (e.g., ARDS, empyema). This led to two recent phase III trials of G-CSF adjunctive therapy in patients with either multilobar CAP, or pneumonia complicated by sepsis and organ failure. In the multilobar CAP study, G-CSF administration was associated with a modest reduction in mortality overall that was significant only in the subgroup of patients with pneumococcal bacteremia. There was no reduction in the development of organ failure, such as ARDS (258). In the sepsis study, which enrolled patients with either CAP or nosocomial pneumonia, administration of G-CSF 300 μg/day did not have an effect on mortality or secondary organ failure (259). In both studies, G-CSF was only given at least 24 hours after hospitalization and after initiation of antibiotic therapy, in order to meet both clinical and microbiologic entry criteria. More studies are needed to determine whether this delay in G-CSF administration missed a window of opportunity to positively affect the clinical outcomes of patients with severe CAP or nosocomial pneumonia. Since many patients who develop sepsis as a complication of severe infection often develop systemic immune suppression (221,225,226,260), it seems possible that the immune suppressive actions of exogenous G-CSF given at this relatively late time may add to this condition. Therefore, G-CSF administration after multiorgan failure has occurred may not be beneficial.

Clinical Use in Other Various Conditions

The observed beneficial effects of CSFs in animal and human studies and their relatively low incidence of adverse effects have stimulated interest in clinical trials aimed at evaluating the safety and efficacy of CSFs combined with antimicrobial therapy for the management of infections in non-neutropenic patients.

G-CSF has been studied in the prevention of postoperative infections. A phase II, open-label, nonrandomized, single-center trial evaluated the rate of infectious complications in patients undergoing esophagectomy for esophageal cancer. Nineteen evaluable patients were treated with G-CSF at 300 μg/day or 480 μg/day SC for 2 days prior and up to 7 days after surgery. Neutrophil function (phagocytosis and ROS production) was enhanced after G-CSF treatment. No infection occurred in the treatment group within the first 10 days after esophagectomy. In comparison, in a historical control group of 77 patients treated at the same center, 23 patients (29.9%) developed infections within the first 10 days after esophagectomy. In addition, no postoperative deaths occurred in the treatment group compared to 9.1% in the historical control group (261). Another randomized, placebo-control study evaluated the efficacy of G-CSF prophylaxis in postoperative infections in patients undergoing surgery for head and neck cancer. Twenty four patients were randomized to received G-CSF (5 μg/kg) or placebo 12 hours before surgery. G-CSF administration was associated with enhanced neutrophil phagocytosis and ROS production. In the G-CSF–treated group, two of 12 (17%) patients developed postoperative infections compared to nine of 12 (75%) patients in the placebo group ($p < 0.001$) (262).

GM-CSF has also been evaluated in surgical infection prophylaxis. A pilot, intention to treat study was performed in cancer patients undergoing elective surgery for the diagnosis or treatment of malignancy. Patients were chosen based upon a preoperative assessment of high postoperative infection risk. GM-CSF was administered perioperatively at two doses, 125 μg/m^2/day (12 patients), or 250 μg/m^2/day (11 patients), for a total of 10 days in both groups. GM-CSF was well tolerated and caused no severe or life-threatening adverse reactions. A dose dependent leukocytosis was observed in both groups. Only one wound infection was diagnosed during the study period (263).

These studies suggest that, in certain high-risk settings, CSF administration might reduce postoperative infections. The clinical relevance and application of these findings needs further evaluation.

Preparations and Adverse Effects

In the United States, G-CSF has been approved for four different indications. In patients with cancer receiving myelosuppressive chemotherapy G-CSF should be given starting at 5 μg/kg/day SC for up to 2 weeks, or until the ANC has reached 10,000/mm^3 following the expected chemotherapy-induced neutrophil nadir. G-CSF should not be administered in the 24-hour period before the administration of chemotherapy and no earlier than 24 hours after the administration of cytotoxic chemotherapy. In bone marrow transplant recipients, the recommended dose of G-CSF is 5 to 10 μg/kg/day given SC or IV. The recommended dose of G-CSF for the mobilization of PBPC is 10 to 15 μg/kg/day SC at least 4 days before the first leukapheresis procedure and continued until the last one. G-CSF should be administered to those patients in whom the diagnosis of congenital, cyclic, or idiopathic neutropenia has been confirmed. For congenital neutropenia, the recommended daily starting dose is 6 μg/kg twice a day SC. For idiopathic or cyclic neutropenia, the recommended daily starting dose is 5 μg/kg/day SC. In patients with severe chronic neutropenia, chronic administration is required to maintain clinical benefit. The dose should be individually adjusted based on the clinical course and ANC (264). Pharmacokinetic analysis favors SC administration over IV use for all indications.

In the United States, GM-CSF has been approved for five different indications. In patients with acute nonlymphocytic leukemia (ANLL) following induction chemotherapy GM-GSF should be given at a dose of 250 μg/m^2/day SC until neutrophil recovery. The safety and efficacy of GM-CSF has not been assessed in patients with ANLL under 55 years of age. In PBPC collection and autologous transplantation, the recommended dose of GM-CSF is 250 μg/m^2/day IV or SC at least 4 days before the first leukapheresis procedure and continued until the last one. GM-CSF has also been approved for acceleration of myeloid recovery in patients with NHL, ALL, and Hodgkin's disease undergoing autologous BMT or PBPC transplantation, and in patients undergoing allogeneic BMT or PBPC transplantation from HLA-matched related donors. GM-CSF is also indicated in patients who have undergone allogeneic or autologous BMT or PBPC transplantation in whom engraftment is delayed or has failed (265). The preferred route of administration is SC.

In general, the effects of physiologically active proteins such as CSFs are short lived due to their rapid clearance in the body. The covalent attachment of polyethylene glycol (PEG) to some of these proteins is currently being investigated to extend their half lives. A single PEG group attached to the *N*-terminal residue of rhG-CSF increases its circulation time and has no effect on its activity. A single SC injection of PEG–rhG-CSF leads to prolonged elevation of the ANC starting within 24 hours of administration, and lasting up to 7 days after the injection (266).

Recently, the efficacy and toxicity of SD/01 (a PEG-conjugated filgrastim) were compared to those of G-CSF. Thirteen patients with non–small-cell lung cancer were randomized to receive daily G-CSF (5 μg/kg/day) for 5 days starting 2 weeks before chemotherapy and again 24 hours after chemotherapy until neutrophil recovery or a single injection of SD/01 (30, 100, or 300 μg/kg) at 2 weeks before chemotherapy and again 24 hours after administration of carboplatin and paclitaxel. Postchemotherapy median nadirs were similar in the G-CSF group and the group receiving SD/01 30 μg/kg, with higher nadirs seen in the groups receiving SD/01 100 or 300 μg/kg. Dose limiting toxicities were not noted and the toxicity profile of SD/01was similar to that of daily G-CSF. CD34$^+$ cells were mobilized in all groups (267). Animal studies aimed to evaluate the effect of PEG-modified GM-CSF on different hematopoietic cell lines are underway. Currently, clinical trials are in progress to further clarify the pharmacology and clinical applications of PEG-CSFs.

The most common adverse effect reported with G-CSF administration is mild to moderate bone and musculoskeletal pain, seen in 20% to 30% of recipients depending on the dose administered (149). Although the etiology of bone pain remains poorly understood, it is usually attributed to the rapid proliferation of myeloid cells within the bone marrow. The pain is usually worse at higher doses of G-CSF and with more vigorous bone marrow recovery. Aside from this effect, G-CSF seems to be fairly innocuous and no dose-limiting toxicities (other than bone pain) have been reported after years of its use. Besides

TABLE 9-7. *Approved and experimental indications of G-CSF and GM-CSF*

Indication	G-CSF	GM-CSF
Aplastic anemia	Approved in some countries	
Acute leukemia	Approved in some countries	Approved in some countries
Bone marrow transplantation	Approved	Approved
Chemotherapy-induced neutropenia	Approved	Approved
Diabetic foot infection	Experimental (phase II)	
Fungal infection, candedemia	Experimental (phase II)	
Myelodysplastic syndrome	Approved in some countries	
Nonneutropenic infection	Experimental (phase II–III)	
Neutropenia in HIV infection	Approved in some countries	Approved in some countries
Peripheral blood progenitor cell transplantation	Approved in most countries	Approved in some countries
Severe chronic neutropenia	Approved	

From Frumkin LR, Dale DC. The role of colony-stimulating factors in HIV disease. *AIDS Reader* 1996;6: 185–193, with permission.

bone pain, other adverse effects seen include fatigue, fever, anorexia, and arthralgia. These are usually mild and easily controlled with symptomatic therapy. Laboratory abnormalities observed have included anemia and thrombocytopenia. Allergic reactions have been rarely reported (less than one in 200,000), and rhG-CSF is generally regarded as nonantigenic. Cutaneous vasculitis resembling Sweet's syndrome has been described rarely, especially after prolonged G-CSF treatment (268).

GM-CSF treatment has been associated with a slightly higher frequency of adverse reactions. The most frequent reported side effect is fever, which occurs in more than 20% of patients. The presence of fever may affect the evaluation of responses to the treatment of infection (269). Fever is often accompanied by myalgias and flu-like symptoms. First-dose reactions, consisting of flushing, tachycardia, hypotension, musculoskeletal pain, dyspnea, nausea, vomiting, and arterial oxygen desaturation, have been reported in up to 5% of recipients (270). These appear to be most pronounced when bacterially derived recombinant GM-CSFs (e.g., molgramostim) are used and given IV.

In summary, CSFs are able to increase neutrophil counts and upregulate phagocyte function. CSFs play a critical role in host defense response during infection. As suggested by experimental animal models of infection, CSFs may potentially be administered prophylactically or therapeutically in different infectious processes. Currently, more controlled clinical trials are required to define the proper role of G-CSF and GM-CSF in the clinical management of specific infections. Table 9.7 depicts some of the approved and experimental uses of G-CSF and GM-CSF.

REFERENCES

1. Bodey GP, Buckley M, Sathe YS, et al. Quantitative relationships between circulating leukocytes and infections in patients with acute leukemia. *Ann Intern Med* 1996;64:328–340.
2. Gasson JC. Molecular physiology of granulocyte-macrophage colony-stimulating factor. *Blood* 1991;77: 1131–1145.
3. Hartung T. Immunomodulation by colony-stimulating factors. *Rev Physiol Biochem Pharmacol* 1993;136: 1–164.
4. Moore MA. The clinical use of colony stimulating factors. *Annu Rev Immunol* 1991;9:159–191.
5. Souza LM, Boone TC, Gabrilove J, et al. Recombinant human granulocyte colony-stimulating factor: effects on normal and leukemic myeloid cells. *Science* 1986;232:61–65.
6. Tsuchiya M, Asano S, Kaziro Y, et al. Isolation and characterization of the cDNA for murine granulocyte colony-stimulating factor. *Proc Natl Acad Sci USA* 1986;83:7633–7637.
7. Nagata S, Tsuchiya M, Asano S, et al. Molecular cloning and expression of cDNA for human granulocyte colony-stimulating factor. *Nature* 1986;319:415–418.

8. Yuo A, Kitagawa S, Ohsaka A, et al. Stimulation and priming of human neutrophils by granulocyte colony-stimulating factor and granulocyte-macrophage colony-stimulating factor: qualitative and quantitative differences. *Biochem Biophys Res Commun* 1990;171:491–497.
9. Nissen C, Carbonare VD, Moser Y. *In vitro* comparison of the biological potency of glycosylated versus nonglycosylated rG-GSF. *Drug Invest* 1994;7:346–352.
10. Frampton JE, Yarker YE, Goa KL. Lenograstim. A review of its pharmacological properties and therapeutic efficacy in neutropenia and related clinical settings. *Drugs* 1995;49:767–793.
11. Vellenga E, Rambaldi A, Ernst TJ, et al. Independent regulation of M-CSF and G-CSF gene expression in human monocytes. *Blood* 1988;71:1529–1532.
12. Hamilton JA, Whitty GA, Royston AK, et al. Interleukin-4 suppresses granulocyte colony-stimulating factor and granulocyte-macrophage colony-stimulating factor levels in stimulated human monocytes. *Immunology* 1992;76:566–571.
13. Sallerfors B, Olofsson T. Granulocyte-macrophage colony-stimulating factor (GM-CSF) and granulocyte colony-stimulating factor (G-CSF) secretion by adherent monocytes measured by quantitative immunoassays. *Eur J Haematol* 1992;49:199–207.
14. Oster W, Lindemann A, Mertelsmann R, et al. Production of macrophage-, granulocyte-, granulocyte-macrophage- and multi-colony-stimulating factor by peripheral blood cells. *Eur J Immunol* 1989;19:543–547.
15. Oster W, Lindemann, A, Mertelsmann R, et al. Granulocyte-macrophage colony-stimulating factor (CSF) and multilineage CSF recruit human monocytes to express granulocyte CSF. *Blood* 1989;73:64–67.
16. Wieser M, Bonifer R, Oster W, et al. Interleukin-4 induces secretion of CSF for granulocytes and CSF for macrophages by peripheral blood monocytes. *Blood* 1989;73:1105–1108.
17. Ishizaka Y, Motoyoshi K, Hatake K, et al. Mode of action of human urinary colony-stimulating factor. *Exp Hematol* 1986;14:1–8.
18. Motoyoshi K, Yoshida K, Hatake K, et al. Recombinant and native human urinary colony-stimulating factor directly augments granulocytic and granulocyte-macrophage colony-stimulating factor production of human peripheral blood monocytes. *Exp Hematol* 1989;17:68–71.
19. Dokter WH, Dijkstra AJ, Koopmans SB, et al. G(AnH)MTetra, a naturally occurring 1,6-anhydro muramyl dipeptide, induces granulocyte colony-stimulating factor expression in human monocytes: a molecular analysis. *Infect Immun* 1994;62:2953–2957.
20. Lu L, Walker D, Graham CD, et al. Enhancement of release from MHC class II antigen-positive monocytes of hematopoietic colony stimulating factors CSF-1 and G-CSF by recombinant human tumor necrosis factor–alpha: synergism with recombinant human interferon-gamma. *Blood* 1988;72:34–41.
21. Hartung T, Wendel A. Immunomodulatory properties of filgrastim (r-met-HuG-CSF) in preclinical models. In: Morstyn G, et al., eds. *Filgrastim in clinical practice*. New York: Marcel Dekker, 1998:397–427.
22. Fattorini L, Xiao Y, Li B, et al. Induction of IL-1 beta, IL-6, TNF-alpha, GM-CSF and G-CSF in human macrophages by smooth transparent and smooth opaque colonial variants of *Mycobacterium avium*. *J Med Microbiol* 1994;40:129–133.
23. Ichinose Y, Hara N, Ohta M, et al. Recombinant granulocyte colony-stimulating factor and lipopolysaccharide maintain the phenotype of and superoxide anion generation by neutrophils. *Infect Immun* 1990;58:1647–1652.
24. Fibbe WE, van Damme J, Billiau A, et al. Interleukin 1 induces human marrow stromal cells in long-term culture to produce granulocyte colony-stimulating factor and macrophage colony-stimulating factor. *Blood* 1988;71:430–435.
25. Koeffler HP, Gasson J, Tobler A. Transcriptional and posttranscriptional modulation of myeloid colony-stimulating factor expression by tumor necrosis factor and other agents. *Mol Cell Biol* 1988;8:3432–3438.
26. Nelson S. Role of granulocyte colony-stimulating factor in the immune response to acute bacterial infection in the nonneutropenic host: an overview. *Clin Infect Dis* 1994;18(Suppl 2):S197–S204.
27. Demetri GD, Zenzie BW, Rheinwald JG, et al. Expression of colony-stimulating factor genes by normal human mesothelial cells and human malignant mesothelioma cells lines *in vitro*. *Blood* 1989;74:940–946.
28. Lai CF, Baumann H. Interleukin-1 beta induces production of granulocyte colony-stimulating factor in human hepatoma cells. *Blood* 1996;87:4143–4148.
29. Vellenga E, Dokter W, de Wolf JT, et al. Interleukin-4 prevents the induction of G-CSF mRNA in human adherent monocytes in response to endotoxin and IL-1 stimulation. *Br J Haematol* 1991;79:22–26.
30. Hamilton JA. Coordinate and noncoordinate colony stimulating factor formation by human monocytes. *J Leukoc Biol* 1994;55:355–361.
31. Lee MT, Kaushansky K, Ralph P, et al. Differential expression of M-CSF, G-CSF, and GM-CSF by human monocytes. *J Leukoc Biol* 1990;47:275–282.
32. Kruger M, Coorevits L, De Wit TP, et al. Granulocyte-macrophage colony-stimulating factor antagonizes the transforming growth factor-beta-induced expression of Fc gamma RIII (CD16) on human monocytes. *Immunology* 1996;87:162–167.
33. Cheers C, Haigh AM, Kelso A, et al. Production of colony-stimulating factors (CSFs) during infection: separate determinations of macrophage-, granulocyte-, granulocyte-macrophage-, and multi-CSFs. *Infect Immun* 1988;56:247–251.
34. Barsig J, Bundschuh DS, Hartung T, et al. Control of fecal peritoneal infection in mice by colony-stimulating factors. *J Infect Dis* 1996;174:790–799.

35. Dale DC, Lau S, Nash R, et al. Effect of endotoxin on serum granulocyte and granulocyte-macrophage colony-stimulating factor levels in dogs. *J Infect Dis* 1992;165:689–694.
36. Watari K, Asano S, Shirafuji N, et al. Serum granulocyte colony-stimulating factor levels in healthy volunteers and patients with various disorders as estimated by enzyme immunoassay. *Blood* 1989;73:117–122.
37. Kawakami M, Tsutsumi H, Kumakawa T, et al. Levels of serum granulocyte colony-stimulating factor in patients with infections. *Blood* 1990;76:1962–1976.
38. Metcalf D. The role of the colony-stimulating factors in resistance to acute infections. *Immunol Cell Biol* 1987;65:35–43.
39. Cebon J, Layton JE, Maher D, et al. Endogenous haematopoietic growth factors in neutropenia and infection. *Br J Haematol* 1994;86:265–274.
40. Robins HI, Kutz M, Wiedenmann GJ, et al. Cytokine induction by 41.8°C whole body hyperthermia. *Cancer Lett* 1995;97:195–201.
41. Omori F, Okamura S, Shimoda K, et al. Levels of human serum granulocyte colony-stimulating factor and granuloctye-macrophage colony-stimulating factor under pathological conditions. *Biotherapy* 1992;4:147–153.
42. Misago M, Kikuchi M, Tsukada J, et al. Serum levels of G-CSF, M-CSF and GM-CSF in a patient with cyclic neutropenia. *Eur J Haematol* 1991;46:312–313.
43. Tanaka H, Ishikawa K, Nishino M, et al. Changes in granulocyte colony-stimulating factor concentration in patients with trauma and sepsis. *J Trauma* 1996;40:718–726.
44. Lieschke GJ, Burgess AW. Granulocyte colony-stimulating factor and granulocyte-macrophage colony-stimulating factor (1). *N Engl J Med* 1992;327:28–35.
45. Freund M, Kleine HD. The role of GM-CSF in infection. *Infection* 1992;20 Suppl 2:S84–92
46. Gough NM, Gough J, Metcalf D, et al. Molecular cloning of cDNA encoding a murine haematopoietic growth regulator, granulocyte-macrophage colony stimulating factor. *Nature* 1984;309:763–767.
47. Wong GG, Witek JS, Temple PA, et al. Human GM-CSF: molecular cloning of the complementary DNA and purification of the natural and recombinant proteins. *Science* 1985;228:810–815.
48. Cantrell MA, Anderson D, Cerretti DP, et al. Cloning, sequence, and expression of a human granulocyte/macrophage colony-stimulating factor. *Proc Natl Acad Sci USA* 1985;82:6250–6254.
49. Huebner K, Isobe M, Croce CM, et al. The human gene encoding GM-CSF is at 5q21-q32, the chromosome region deleted in the 5q-anomaly. *Science* 1985;230:1282–1285.
50. Ruef C, Coleman DL. Granulocyte-macrophage colony-stimulating factor: pleiotropic cytokine with potential clinical usefulness. *Rev Infect Dis* 1990;12:41–62.
51. Collins HL, Bancroft GJ. Cytokine enhancement of complement-dependent phagocytosis by macrophages: synergy of tumor necrosis factor-alpha and granulocyte-macrophage colony-stimulating factor for phagocytosis of *Cryptococcus neoformans*. *Eur J Immunol* 1992;22:1447–1454.
52. Mayer P, Lam C, Obenaus H, et al. Recombinant human GM-CSF induces leukocytosis and activates peripheral blood polymorphonuclear neutrophils in nonhuman primates. *Blood* 1987;70:206–213.
53. Denzlinger C, Tetzloff W, Gerhartz HH, et al. Differential activation of the endogenous leukotriene biosynthesis by two different preparations of granulocyte-macrophage colony-stimulating factor in healthy volunteers. *Blood* 1993;81:2007–2013.
54. Metcalf D. The molecular biology and functions of the granulocyte-macrophage colony-stimulating factors. *Blood* 1986;67:257–267.
55. D'Alesandro MM, Gruber DF, O'Halloran KP, et al. *In vitro* modulation of canine polymorphonuclear leukocyte function by granulocyte-macrophage colony stimulating factor. *Biotherapy* 1991;3:233–239.
56. Munker R, Gasson J, Ogawa M, et al. Recombinant human TNF induces production of granulocyte-monocyte colony-stimulating factor. *Nature* 1986;323:79–82.
57. Bickel M, Cohen RB, Pluznik DH. Post-transcriptional regulation of granulocyte-macrophage colony-stimulating factor synthesis in murine T cells. *J Immunol* 1990;145:840–845.
58. Nimer SD, Gates MJ, Koeffler HP, et al. Multiple mechanisms control the expression of granulocyte-macrophage colony-stimulating factor by human fibroblasts. *J Immunol* 1989;143:2374–2377.
59. Wodnar-Filipowicz A, Heusser CH, Moroni C. Production of the haematopoietic growth factors GM-CSF and interleukin-3 by mast cells in response to IgE receptor–mediated activation. *Nature* 1989;339:150–152.
60. Sieff CA, Tsai S, Faller DV. Interleukin 1 induces cultured human endothelial cell production of granulocyte-macrophage colony-stimulating factor. *J Clin Invest* 1987;79:48–51.
61. Galy AH, Spits H. IL-1, IL-4, and IFN-gamma differentially regulate cytokine production and cell surface molecule expression in cultured human thymic epithelial cells. *J Immunol* 1991;147:3823–3830.
62. Churchill L, Friedman B, Schleimer RP, et al. Production of granulocyte-macrophage colony-stimulating factor by cultured human tracheal epithelial cells. *Immunology* 1992;75:189–195.
63. Akahane K, Pluznik DH. Interferon-gamma destabilizes interleukin-1–induced granulocyte-macrophage colony-stimulating factor mRNA in murine vascular endothelial cells. *Exp Hematol* 1993;21:878–884.
64. Cuturi MC, Anegon I, Sherman F, et al. Production of hematopoietic colony-stimulating factors by human natural killer cells. *J Exp Med* 1989;169:569–583.
65. Broudy VC, Kaushansky K, Segal GM, et al. Tumor necrosis factor type alpha stimulates human endothelial cells to produce granulocyte/macrophage colony-stimulating factor. *Proc Natl Acad Sci USA* 1986;83:7467–7471.

66. Munker R, Gasson J, Ogawa M, et al. Recombinant human TNF induces production of granulocyte-monocyte colony-stimulating factor. *Nature* 1986;323:79–82.
67. Demetri GD, Zenzie BW, Rheinwald JG, et al. Expression of colony-stimulating factor genes by normal human mesothelial cells and human malignant mesothelioma cells lines *in vitro*. *Blood* 1989;74:940–946.
68. Filonzi EL, Zoellner H, Stanton H, et al. Cytokine regulation of granulocyte-macrophage colony stimulating factor and macrophage colony-stimulating factor production in human arterial smooth muscle cells. *Atherosclerosis* 1993;99:241–252.
69. Omori F, Okamura S, Shimoda K, et al. Levels of human serum granulocyte colony-stimulating factor and granulocyte-macrophage colony-stimulating factor under pathological conditions. *Biotherapy* 1992;4:147–153.
70. Jung HC, Eckmann L, Yang SK, et al. A distinct array of proinflammatory cytokines is expressed in human colon epithelial cells in response to bacterial invasion. *J Clin Invest* 1995;95:55–65.
71. Gabrilove JL, Jakubowski A. Hematopoietic growth factors: biology and clinical application. *J Natl Cancer Inst Monogr* 1990;10:73–77.
72. Metcalf D, Nicola NA. Proliferative effects of purified granulocyte colony-stimulating factor (G-CSF) on normal mouse hemopoietic cells. *J Cell Physiol* 1983;116:198–206.
73. Tamura M, Hattori K, Nomura H, et al. Induction of neutrophilic granulocytosis in mice by administration of purified human native granulocyte colony-stimulating factor (G-CSF). *Biochem Biophys Res Commun* 1987; 142:454–460.
74. Ulich TR, del Castillo J, Guo K, et al. The hematologic effects of chronic administration of the monokines tumor necrosis factor, interleukin-1, and granulocyte-colony stimulating factor on bone marrow and circulation. *Am J Pathol* 1989;134:149–159.
75. Cairo MS, VandeVen C, Toy C, et al. Lymphokines: Enhancement by granulocyte-macrophage and granulocyte colony-stimulating factors of neonatal myeloid kinetics and functional activation of polymorphonuclear leukocytes. *Rev Infect Dis* 1990;12 :S492–S497.
76. Tkatch LS, Tweardy DJ. Human granulocyte colony-stimulating factor (G-CSF), the premier granulopoietin: biology, clinical utility, and receptor structure and function. *Lymphokine Cytokine Res* 1993;12:477–488.
77. Hartung T, Docke WD, Gantner F, et al. Effect of granulocyte colony-stimulating factor treatment on *ex vivo* blood cytokine response in human volunteers. *Blood* 1995;85:2482–2489.
78. Morstyn G, Campbell L, Souza LM, et al. Effect of granulocyte colony stimulating factor on neutropenia induced by cytotoxic chemotherapy. *Lancet* 1988;1:667–672.
79. Gabrilove JL, Jakubowski A, Fain K, et al. Phase I study of granulocyte colony-stimulating factor in patients with transitional cell carcinoma of the urothelium. *J Clin Invest* 1988;82:1454–1461.
80. van der Wouw PA, van Leeuwen R, van Oers RH, et al. Effects of recombinant human granulocyte colony-stimulating factor on leucopenia in zidovudine-treated patients with AIDS and AIDS related complex, a phase I/II study. *Br J Haematol* 1991;78:319–324.
81. Sica S, Rutella S, Di Mario A, et al. rhG-CSF in healthy donors: mobilization of peripheral hematopoietic progenitors and effect on peripheral blood leukocytes. *J Hematother* 1996;5:391–397.
82. Kerrigan DP, Castillo A, Foucar K, et al. Peripheral blood morphologic changes after high-dose antineoplastic chemotherapy and recombinant human granulocyte colony-stimulating factor administration. *Am J Clin Pathol* 1989;92:280–285.
83. Hartung T, Docke WD, Bundschuh DS, et al. Effect of filgrastim treatment on inflammatory cytokines and lymphocyte functions. *Clin Pharmacol Ther* 1999, 66:415–424.
84. Dexter TM, Heyworth CM. Growth factors and the molecular control of haemato. *Eur J Clin Microbiol Infect Dis* 1994;13(suppl 2):S3–S8.
85. Metcalf D. The granulocyte-macrophage colony-stimulating factors. *Science* 1985;229:16–22.
86. Rapoport AP, Abboud CN, Di Persio JF. Granulocyte-macrophage colony-stimulating factor (GM-CSF) and granulocyte colony-stimulating factor (G-CSF): receptor biology, signal transduction, and neutrophil activation. *Blood* Rev 1992;6:43–57.
87. Donahue RE, Emerson SG, Wang EA, et al. Demonstration of burst-promoting activity of recombinant human GM-CSF on circulating erythroid progenitors using an assay involving the delayed addition of erythropoietin. *Blood* 1985;66:1479–1481.
88. Sieff CA, Emerson SG, Donahue RE, et al. Human recombinant granulocyte-macrophage colony-stimulating factor: a multilineage hematopoietin. *Science* 1985;230:1171–1173.
89. Povolny BT, Lee MY. The role of recombinant human M-CSF, IL-3, GM-CSF and calcitriol in clonal development of osteoclast precursors in primate bone marrow. *Exp Hematol* 1993;21:532–537.
90. Inaba K, Steinman RM, Pack MW, et al Identification of proliferating dendritic cell precursors in mouse blood. *J Exp Med* 1992;175:1157–1167.
91. Donahue RE, Wang EA, Stone DK, et al Stimulation of haemato in primates by continuous infusion of recombinant human GM-CSF. *Nature* 1986;321:872–875.
92. Scarffe JH. Emerging clinical uses for GM-CSF. *Eur J Cancer* 1991;27:1493–1504.
93. Bokemeyer C, Schmoll H-J. Clinical results obtained with granulocyte-macrophage colony-stimulating factor (GM-CSF) in patients with testicular cancer. In: Nissen NI, Dexter TM, eds. *Granulocyte-macrophage colony-stimulating factor (GM-CSF). Current use and future applications. Proceedings from an international symposium, Lucerne, Switzerland, September 9–11 1993.* Cheshire, UK: Pennine Press, 1995:8–14.
94. Hast R, Bernell P, Kimby E, et al. rhGM-CSF in combination with standard induction chemotherapy for the

treatment of acute myeloid leukemia—an overview. In: Nissen NI, Dexter TM, eds. *Granulocyte-macrophage colony-stimulating factor (GM-CSF). Current use and future applications. Procceedings from an international symposium, Lucerne, Switzerland, September 9–11 1993.* Cheshire, UK: Pennine Press, 1995:24–26.

95. Kropec A, Lemmen SW, Grundmann HJ, et al. Synergy of simultaneous administration of ofloxacin and granulocyte colony-stimulating factor in killing of *Escherichia coli* by human neutrophils. *Infection* 1995;23: 298–300.
96. Daschner FD, Grundmann H, Anding K, et al. Combined effect of human neutrophils, ceftazidime and granulocyte colony-stimulating factor on killing of *Escherichia coli. Eur J Clin Microbiol Infect Dis* 1995;14: 536–539.
97. Roilides E, Walsh TJ, Pizzo PA, et al. Granulocyte colony-stimulating factor enhances the phagocytic and bactericidal activity of normal and defective human neutrophils. *J Infect Dis* 1991;163:579–583.
98. Kitagawa S, Yuo A, Souza LM, et al. Recombinant human granulocyte colony-stimulating factor enhances superoxide release in human granulocytes stimulated by the chemotactic peptide. *Biochem Biophys Res Commun* 1987;144:1143–1146.
99. Balazovich KJ, Almeida HI, Boxer LA. Recombinant human G-CSF and GM-CSF prime human neutrophils for superoxide production through different signal transduction mechanisms. *J Lab Clin Med* 1991;118: 576–584.
100. Khwaja A, Carver JE, Linch DC. Interactions of granulocyte-macrophage colony-stimulating factor (CSF), granulocyte CSF, and tumor necrosis factor alpha in the priming of the neutrophil respiratory burst. *Blood* 1992; 79:745–753.
101. Katsura Y, Tsuru S, Noritake M, et al. Granulocyte colony-stimulating factor enhances the extracellular emission of reactive oxygen from neutrophils stimulated with formylmethionylleucylphenylalanine. *Cell Immunol* 1993;148:10–17.
102. Valerius T, Repp R, de Wit TP, et al. Involvement of the high-affinity receptor for IgG (Fc gamma RI; CD64) in enhanced tumor cell cytotoxicity of neutrophils during granulocyte colony-stimulating factor therapy. *Blood* 1993;82:931–939.
103. Hartung T, Volk H-D, Wendel A. G-CSF—an anti-inflammatory cytokine. *J Endotox Res* 1995;2:195–201.
104. Shirafuji N, Matsuda S, Ogura H, et al. Granulocyte colony-stimulating factor stimulates human mature neutrophilic granulocytes to produce interferon-alpha. *Blood* 1990;75:17–19.
105. Görgen I, Hartung T, Leist M, et al. Granulocyte colony-stimulating factor treatment protects rodents against lipopolysaccharide-induced toxicity via suppression of systemic tumor necrosis factor-alpha. *J Immunol* 1992;149:918–924.
106. Kitabayashi A, Hirokawa M, Hatano Y, et al. Granulocyte colony-stimulating factor downregulates allogeneic immune responses by posttranscriptional inhibition of tumor necrosis factor-alpha production. *Blood* 1995;86:2220–2227.
107. Pan L, Delmonte Jr J, Jalonen CK, et al. Pretreatment of donor mice with granulocyte colony-stimulating factor polarizes donor T lymphocytes toward type-2 cytokine production and reduces severity of experimental graft-versus-host disease. *Blood* 1995;86:4422–4442.
108. Hartung T. Anti-flammatory effects of G-CSF. *Curr Opin Hematol* 1998;5:221–225.
109. Boneberg EM, Gantner F, Hareng L, et al. Human monocytes express functional receptors for granulocyte colony-stimulating factor. *Blood* 2000;95: 270–276.
110. Pajkrt D, Manten A, van der Poll T, et al. Modulation of cytokine release and neutrophil function by granulocyte colony-stimulating factor during endotoxemia in humans. *Blood* 1997;90:1415–1424.
111. DiPersio JF, Abboud CN. Activation of neutrophils by granulocyte-macrophage colony-stimulating factor. In: Coffey RG, ed. *Granulocyte responses to cytokines. Basic and clinical research.* New York: Marcel Dekker, 1992:457–484.
112. Weisbart RH, Gasson JC, Golde DW. Colony-stimulating factors and host defense. *Ann Intern Med* 1989;110: 297–303.
113. Cannistra SA, Vellenga E, Groshek P, et al. Human granulocyte-monocyte colony-stimulating factor and interleukin 3 stimulate monocyte cytotoxicity through a tumor necrosis factor–dependent mechanism. *Blood* 1988;71:672–676.
114. Sisson SD, Dinarello CA. Production of interleukin-1 alpha, interleukin-1 beta and tumor necrosis factor by human mononuclear cells stimulated with granulocyte-macrophage colony-stimulating factor. *Blood* 1988;72:1368–1374.
115. Randow F, Döcke W-D, Bundschuh DS, et al. *In vitro* prevention and reversal of lipopolysaccharide desensitization by IFN-γ, IL-12, and granulocyte-macrophage colony-stimulating factor. *J Immun* 1997;158:2911–2918.
116. Bundschuh DS, Barsig J, Hartung T, et al. Granulocyte-macrophage colony-stimulating factor and IFN-γ restore the systemic TNF-α response to endotoxin in lipopolysaccharide-desensitized mice. *J Immun* 1997; 158:2862–2871.
117. Tiegs G, Barsig J, Matiba B, et al. Potentiation by granulocyte macrophage colony-stimulating factor of lipopolysaccharide toxicity in mice. *J Clin Invest* 1994;93:2616–2622.
118. Hartung T, von Aulock S, Freitag M, et al. Blood cytokine response of low-dose molgramostim (rhGM-CSF)–treated patients. *Cytokine* 2000;12:1570–1574.
119. Nelson S, Daifuku R, Andresen J. Use of filgrastim (r-metHu-G-CSF) in infectious diseases. In: Morstyn G, Dexter G, eds. *Filgrastim in clinical practice.* New York: Marcel Dekker, 1994:253–266

120. Schwab G, Hecht T. Recombinant methionyl granulocyte colony-stimulating factor (filgrastim): a new dimension in immunotherapy. *Ann Hematol* 1994;69:1–9.
121. Nicola NA, Metcalf D. Binding of 125I-labeled granulocyte colony-stimulating factor to normal murine hemopoietic cells. *J Cell Physiol* 1985;124:313–321.
122. Shimoda K, Okamura S, Harada N, et al. Identification of a functional receptor for granulocyte colony-stimulating factor on platelets. *J Clin Invest* 1993;91:1310–1313.
123. Avalos BR. Molecular analysis of the granulocyte colony-stimulating factor receptor. *Blood* 1996;88:761–777.
124. Welte K, Bonilla MA, Gillio AP, et al. Recombinant human granulocyte colony-stimulating factor. Effects on hemato in normal and cyclophosphamide-treated primates. *J Exp Med* 1987;165:941–948.
125. Avalos BR, Gasson JC, Hedvat C, et al. Human granulocyte colony-stimulating factor: biologic activities and receptor characterization on hematopoietic cells and small cell lung cancer cell lines. *Blood* 1990;75:851–857.
126. Matsuda S, Shirafuji N, Asano S. Human granulocyte colony-stimulating factor specifically binds to murine myeloblastic NFS-60 cells and activates their guanosine triphosphate binding proteins/adenylate cyclase system. *Blood* 1989;74:2343–2348.
127. Di Persio J, Billing P, Kaufman S, et al. Characterization of the human granulocyte-macrophage colony-stimulating factor receptor. *J Biol Chem* 1988;263:1834–1841.
128. Gearing DP, King JA, Gough NM, et al. Expression cloning of a receptor for human granulocyte-macrophage colony-stimulating factor. *EMBO J* 1989;8:3667–3676.
129. Hayashida K, Kitamura T, Gorman DM, et al. Molecular cloning of a second subunit of the receptor for human granulocyte-macrophage colony-stimulating factor (GM-CSF): reconstitution of a high-affinity GM-CSF receptor. *Proc Natl Acad Sci USA* 1990;87:9655–9659.
130. Kitamura T, Sato N, Arai K, et al. Expression cloning of the human IL-3 receptor cDNA reveals a shared beta subunit for the human IL-3 and GM-CSF receptors. *Cell* 1991;66:1165–1174.
131. Lopez AF, Elliott MJ, Woodcock J, et al. GM-CSF, IL-3 and IL-5: cross-competition on human haemopoietic cells. *Immunol Today* 1992;13:495–500.
132. Sullivan R, Griffin JD, Simons ER, et al. Effects of recombinant human granulocyte and macrophage colony-stimulating factors on signal transduction pathways in human granulocytes. *J Immunol* 1987;139:3422–3430.
133. McColl SR, Di Persio JF, Caon AC, et al. Involvement of tyrosine kinases in the activation of human peripheral blood neutrophils by granulocyte-macrophage colony-stimulating factor. *Blood* 1991;78:1842–1852.
134. Okuda K, Sanghera JS, Pelech SL, et al. Granulocyte-macrophage colony-stimulating factor, interleukin-3, and steel factor induce rapid tyrosine phosphorylation of p42 and p44 MAP kinase. *Blood* 1992;79:2880–2887.
135. Coffey RG, Diaz S, Coffey CS. Effects of inhibition of lipoxygenase and guanylate cyclase on human neutrophil responses to formyl peptide and granulocyte-macrophage colony-stimulating factor. *J Leukoc Biol* 1993;54:89–96.
136. Lieschke GJ, Grail D, Hodgson G, et al. Mice lacking granulocyte colony-stimulating factor have chronic neutropenia, granulocyte and macrophage progenitor cell deficiency, and impaired neutrophil mobilization. *Blood* 1994;84:1737–1746.
137. Matsumoto M, Matsubara S, Matsuno T, et al. Protective effect of human granulocyte colony-stimulating factor on microbial infection in neutropenic mice. *Infect Immun* 1987;55:2715–2720.
138. Ono M, Matsumoto M, Matsubara S, et al. Protective effect of human granulocyte colony-stimulating factor on bacterial and fungal infections in neutropenic mice. *Behring Inst Mitt* 1988;83:216–221.
139. Mooney DP, Gamelli RL, O'Reilly M, et al. Recombinant human granulocyte colony-stimulating factor and Pseudomonas burn wound sepsis. *Arch Surg* 1988;123:1353–1357.
140. Silver GM, Gamelli RL, O'Reilly M. The beneficial effect of granulocyte colony-stimulating factor (G-CSF) in combination with gentamicin on survival after Pseudomonas burn wound infection. *Surgery* 1989;106: 452–456.
141. Sartorelli KH, Silver GM, Gamelli RL. The effect of granulocyte colony-stimulating factor (G-CSF) upon burn-induced defective neutrophil chemotaxis. *J Trauma* 1991;31:523–530.
142. Abraham E, Stevens P. Effects of granulocyte colony-stimulating factor in modifying mortality from *Pseudomonas aeruginosa* pneumonia after hemorrhage. *Crit Care Med* 1992;20:1127–1133.
143. Cairo MS, Plunkett JM, Mauss D, et al. Seven-day administration of recombinant human granulocyte colony-stimulating factor to newborn rats: modulation of neonatal neutrophilia, myelo, and group B Streptococcus sepsis. *Blood* 1990;76:1788–1794.
144. Cairo MS, Mauss D, Kommareddy S, et al. Prophylactic or simultaneous administration of recombinant human granulocyte colony stimulating factor in the treatment of group B streptococcal sepsis in neonatal rats. *Pediatr Res* 1990;27:612–616.
145. Cairo MS, Plunkett JM, Nguyen A, et al. Effect of stem cell factor with and without granulocyte colony-stimulating factor on neonatal hemato: *in vivo* induction of newborn myelo and reduction of mortality during experimental group B streptococcal sepsis. *Blood* 1992;80:96–101.
146. Novales JS, Salva AM, Modanlou HD, et al. Maternal administration of granulocyte colony-stimulating factor improves neonatal rat survival after a lethal group B streptococcal infection. *Blood* 1993;81:923–927.
147. Iguchi K, Inoue S, Kumar A. Effect of recombinant human granulocyte colony-stimulating factor administration in normal and experimentally infected newborn rats. *Exp Hematol* 1991;19:352–358.
148. Dale DC. Potential role of colony-stimulating factors in the prevention and treatment of infectious diseases. *Clin Infect Dis* 1994;18(suppl 2):S180–S188.

149. Root RK, Dale DC. Granulocyte colony-stimulating factor and granulocyte-macrophage colony-stimulating factor: comparisons and potential for use in the treatment of infections in nonneutropenic patients. *J Infect Dis* 1999;179 Suppl 2:S342–S352.
150. Kanazawa M, Ishizaka A, Hasegawa N, et al. Granulocyte colony-stimulating factor does not enhance endotoxin-induced acute lung injury in Guinea pigs. *Am Rev Respir Dis* 1988;148:1030–1035.
151. Fink MP, O'Sullivan BP, Menconi MJ, et al. Effect of granulocyte colony-stimulating factor on systemic and pulmonary responses to endotoxin in pigs. *J Trauma* 1993;34:571–578.
152. O'Reilly M, Silver GM, Greenhalgh DG, et al. Treatment of intra-abdominal infection with granulocyte colony-stimulating factor. *J Trauma* 1992;33:679–682.
153. Goya T, Torisu M, Doi F, et al. Effects of granulocyte colony stimulating factor and monobactam antibiotics (Aztreonam) on neutrophil functions in sepsis. *Clin Immunol Immunopathol* 1993;69:278–284.
154. Toda H, Murata A, Matsuura N, et al.Therapeutic efficacy of granulocyte colony stimulating factor against rat cecal ligation and puncture model. *Stem Cells (Dayt)*1993;11:228–234.
155. Lundblad R, Nesland JM, Giercksky KE. Granulocyte colony-stimulating factor improves survival rate and reduces concentrations of bacteria, endotoxin, tumor necrosis factor, and endothelin-1 in fulminant intra-abdominal sepsis in rats. *Crit Care Med* 1996;24:820–826.
156. Lorenz W, Reimund KP, Weitzel F, et al. Granulocyte colony-stimulating factor prophylaxis before operation protects against lethal consequences of postoperative peritonitis. *Surgery* 1994;116:925–934.
157. Dunne JR, Dunkin BJ, Nelson S, et al. Effects of granulocyte colony stimulating factor in an nonneutropenic rodent model of *Escherichia coli* peritonitis. *J Surg Res* 1996;61:348–354.
158. Eichacker PQ, Waisman Y, Natanson C, et al. Cardiopulmonary effects of granulocyte colony-stimulating factor in a canine model of bacterial sepsis. *J Appl Physiol* 1994;77:2366–2373.
159. Lister PD, Gentry MJ, Preheim LC. Granulocyte colony-stimulating factor protects control rats but not ethanol-fed rats from fatal pneumococcal pneumonia. *J Infect Dis* 1993;168:922–926.
160. Nelson S, Summer W, Bagby G, et al. Granulocyte colony-stimulating factor enhances pulmonary host defenses in normal and ethanol-treated rats. *J Infect Dis* 1991;164:901–906.
161. Smith WS, Sumnicht GE, Sharpe RW, et al. Granulocyte colony-stimulating factor versus placebo in addition to penicillin G in a randomized blinded study of gram-negative pneumonia sepsis: analysis of survival and multisystem organ failure. *Blood* 1995;86:1301–1309.
162. Freeman BD, Correa R, Karzai W, et al. Controlled trials of rG-CSF and CD11b-directed MAb during hyperoxia and *E. coli* pneumonia in rats. *J Appl Physiol* 1996;80:2066–2076.
163. Yasuda H, Ajiki Y, Shimozato T, et al. Therapeutic efficacy of granulocyte colony-stimulating factor alone and in combination with antibiotics against *Pseudomonas aeruginosa* infections in mice. *Infect Immun* 1990;58: 2502–2509.
164. Lazard T, Perronne C, Cohen Y, et al. Efficacy of granulocyte colony-stimulating factor and RU-40555 in combination with clarithromycin against *Mycobacterium avium* complex infection in C57BL/6 mice. *Antimicrob Agents Chemother* 1993;37:692–695.
165. Kayashima S, Tsuru S, Hata N, et al. Therapeutic effect of granulocyte colony-stimulating factor (G-CSF) on the protection against Listeria infection in SCID mice. *Immunology* 1993;80:471–476.
166. Azuma I, Ishihara C, Iida J, et al. Stimulation of host-defense mechanism with synthetic adjuvants and recombinant cytokines against viral infection in mice. *Adv Exp Med Biol* 1992;319:253–263.
167. Uchida K, Yamamoto Y, Klein TW, et al. Granulocyte-colony stimulating factor facilitates the restoration of resistance to opportunistic fungi in leukopenic mice. *J Med Vet Mycol* 1992;30:293–300.
168. Hamood M, Bluche PF, De Vroey C, et al. Effects of recombinant human granulocyte-colony stimulating factor on neutropenic mice infected with *Candida albicans*: acceleration of recovery from neutropenia and potentiation of anti–*C. albicans* resistance. *Mycoses* 1994;37:93–99.
169. Polak-Wyss A. Protective effect of human granulocyte colony-stimulating factor (hG-CSF) on Cryptococcus and Aspergillus infections in normal and immunosuppressed mice. *Mycoses* 1991;34:205–215.
170. Polak-Wyss A. Protective effect of human granulocyte colony stimulating factor (hG-CSF) on Candida infections in normal and immunosuppressed mice. *Mycoses* 1991;34:109–118.
171. Tanaka T, Okamura S, Okada K, et al. Protective effect of recombinant murine granulocyte-macrophage colony-stimulating factor against *Pseudomonas aeruginosa* infection in leukocytopenic mice. *Infect Immun* 1989;57: 1792–1799.
172. Liehl E, Hildebrandt J, Lam C, et al. Prediction of the role of granulocyte-macrophage colony-stimulating factor in animals and man from *in vitro* results. *Eur J Clin Microbiol Infect Dis* 1994;13(suppl 2):S9–S17.
173. Canturk NZ, Vural B, Esen N, et al. Effects of granulocyte-macrophage colony-stimulating factor on incisional wound healing in an experimental diabetic rat model. *Endocrinol Res* 1999;25:105–116.
174. Molloy RG, Holzheimer R, Nestor M, et al. Granulocyte-macrophage colony-stimulating factor modulates immune function and improves survival after experimental thermal injury. *Br J Surg* 1995;82:770–776.
175. Frenck RW, Sarman G, Harper TE, et al. The ability of recombinant murine granulocyte-macrophage colony-stimulating factor to protect neonatal rats from septic death due to *Staphylococcus aureus*. *J Infect Dis* 1990; 162:109–114.
176. Wheeler JG, Givner LB. Therapeutic use of recombinant human granulocyte-macrophage colony-stimulating factor in neonatal rats with type III group B streptococcal sepsis. *J Infect Dis* 1992;165:938–941.
177. Givner LB, Nagaraj SK. Hyperimmune human IgG or recombinant human granulocyte-macrophage colony-

stimulating factor as adjunctive therapy for group B streptococcal sepsis in newborn rats. *J Pediatr* 1993; 122:774–779.

178. Gennari R, Alexander JW, Gianotti L, et al. Granulocyte macrophage colony-stimulating factor improves survival in two models of gut-derived sepsis by improving gut barrier function and modulating bacterial clearance. *Ann Surg* 1994;220:68–76.
179. Toda H, Murata A, Oka Y, et al. Effect of granulocyte-macrophage colony-stimulating factor on sepsis-induced organ injury in rats. *Blood* 1994;83:2893–2898.
180. Collins HL, Bancroft GJ. Cytokine enhancement of complement-dependent phagocytosis by macrophages: synergy of tumor necrosis factor-alpha and granulocyte-macrophage colony-stimulating factor for phagocytosis of *Cryptococcus neoformans*. *Eur J Immunol* 1992;22:1447–1454.
181. Murray HW, Cervia JS, Hariprashed J, et al. Effect of granulocyte-macrophage colony-stimulating factor in experimental visceral Leishmaniasis. *J Clin Invest* 1995;95:1183–1192.
182. Grau GE, Kindler V, Piguet PF, et al. Prevention of experimental cerebral malaria by anticytokine antibodies. Interleukin 3 and granulocyte macrophage colony-stimulating factor are intermediates in increased tumor necrosis factor production and macrophage accumulation. *J Exp Med* 1988;168:1499–1504.
183. Reed SG, Grabstein KH, Pihl DL, et al. Recombinant granulocyte-macrophage colony-stimulating factor restores deficient immune responses in mice with chronic *Trypanosoma cruzi* infections. *J Immunol* 1990;145: 1564–1570.
184. Lejeune M, Sariban E, Cantinieaux B, et al. Granulocytes functions in children with cancer are differentially sensitive to the toxic effect of chemotherapy. *Pediatr Res* 1996;39:835–842.
185. Lejeune M, Ferster A, Cantinieaux B, et al. Prolonged but reversible neutrophil dysfunctions differentially sensitive to granulocyte colony-stimulating factor in children with acute lymphoblastic leukaemia. *Br J Haematol* 1998;102:1284–1291.
186. Iki S, You A, Yagisawa M, et al. Increased neutrophil respiratory burst in myeloproliferative disorders: selective enhancement of superoxide release triggered by receptor mediated agonists and low responsiveness to *in vitro* cytokine stimulation. *Exp Hematol* 1997;25:26–33.
187. Glaspy JA, Baldwin GC, Robertson PA, et al. Therapy for neutropenia in hairy cell leukemia with recombinant human granulocyte colony-stimulating factor. *Ann Intern Med* 1988;109:789–795.
188. Wiltschke C, Krainer M, Nanut M, et al. *In vivo* administration of granulocyte-macrophage colony-stimulating factor and granulocyte colony-stimulating factor increases neutrophil oxidative burst activity. *J Interferon Cytokine Res* 1995;15:249–253.
189. Harazmi A, Nielsen H, Hovgaard D, et al. Modulation of neutrophil and monocyte function by recombinant human granulocyte-macrophage colony-stimulating factor in patients with lymphoma. *Eur J Clin Invest* 1991;21:219–224.
190. Gaviria JM, Liles WC, Dale DC. The influence of colony-stimulating factors on neutrophil production, distribution and function. In: Wingard JR, Demetri GD, eds. *Clinical applications of cytokines and growth factors*, 1st ed. Norwell, MA: Kluwer Academic Publishers, 1999:118–136.
191. Ozer H, Armitage JO, Bennett CL, et al. 2000 update of recommendations for the use hematopoietic colony-stimulating factors: evidence-based, clinical practice guidelines. *J Clin Oncol* 2000;18:3558–3585.
192. Maher DW, Lieschke GJ, Green M, et al. Filgrastim in patients with chemotherapy-induced febrile neutropenia: a double-blind, placebo-controlled trial. *Ann Intern Med* 1994;121:492–501.
193. Aviles A, Guzman R, Garcia EL, et al. Results of a randomized trial of granulocyte colony-stimulating factor in patients with infection and severe granulocytopenia. *Anti-Cancer Drugs* 1996;7:392–397.
194. Yau JC, Neidhart JA, Triozzi P, et al. Randomized placebo-controlled trial of granulocyte-macrophage colony-stimulating factor support for dose-intensive cyclophosphamide, etoposide, and cisplatin. *Am J Hematol* 1996;51:289–303.
195. Mayordomo JI, Rivera F, Diaz-Puente MT, et al. Improving treatment of chemotherapy-induced neutropenic fever by administration of colony-stimulating factors. *J Natl Cancer Inst* 1995;87:803–808.
196. Lyman GH, Lyman CG, Sanderson RA, et al. Decision analysis of hematopoietic growth factors use in patients receiving cancer chemotherapy. *J Natl Cancer Inst* 1993;85:488–493.
197. Frumkin LR. Role of granulocyte colony-stimulating factor and granulocyte-macrophage colony-stimulating factor in the treatment of patients with HIV infection. *Curr Opin Hematol* 1997;4:200–206.
198. Coffey MJ, Phare SM, George S, et al. Granulocyte colony-stimulating factor administration to HIV-infected subjects augments reduced leukotriene synthesis and anticryptococcal activity in neutrophils. *J Clin Invest* 1998;102:663–670.
199. Esser R, Glienke W, Von Briesen H, et al. Differential regulation of proinflammatory and hematopoietic cytokines in human macrophages after infection with HIV. *Blood* 1996;88:3474–3481.
200. Pitrak DL, Tsai HC, Mullane KM, et al. Accelerated neutrophil apoptosis in the acquired immunodeficiency syndrome. *J Clin Invest* 1996;98:2714–2719.
201. Newman GW, Guarnaccia JR, Remold HG, et al. Cytokines enhance neutrophils from human immunodeficiency virus-negative donors and AIDS patients to inhibit the growth of *Mycobacterium avium in vitro*. *J Infect Dis* 1997;175:891–900.
202. Pitrak DL, Sutton SH, Tsai HC, et al. Reversal of accelerated neutrophil apoptosis and restoration of respiratory burst activity with r-metHuG-CSF (filgrastim) therapy in patients with AIDS. *AIDS* 1999;13:427–428.
203. Baldwin GC, Gasson JC, Quan SG, et al. Granulocyte-macrophage colony-stimulating factor enhances neu-

trophil function in acquired immunodeficiency syndrome patients. *Proc Natl Acad Sci USA* 1988;85: 2763–2766.

204. Moore RD, Keruly JC, Chaisson RE. Neutropenia and bacterial infection in acquired immunodeficiency syndrome. *Arch Intern Med* 1995;155:1965–1970.
205. Kuritzkes DR, Parenti D, Ward DJ, et al. Filgrastim prevents severe neutropenia and reduces infective morbidity in patients with advanced HIV infection: results of a randomized, multicenter, controlled trial. *AIDS* 1998;12:65–74.
206. Hermans P, Rozenbaum W, Jou A, et al. Filgrastim to treat neutropenia and support myelosuppressive medication dosing in HIV infection. *AIDS* 10:1627–1633.
207. Keiser P, Rademacher S, Smith J, et al. G-CSF association with prolonged survival in HIV-infected patients with disseminated *Mycobacterium avium* complex infection. *Int J STD AIDS* 1998;9:394–399.
208. Hartung T, Pitrak DL, Foote M, et al. Filgrastim (r-metHuG-CSF) restores IL-2 production of blood from advanced HIV patients. *J Infect Dis* 1998;178:686–692.
209. Hardy WD. Combined ganciclovir and recombinant granulocyte-macrophage colony-stimulating factor in the treatment of cytomegalovirus retinitis in AIDS patients. *J Acquir Immune Defic Syndr* 1991;4:S22–S28.
210. Kaplan LD, Kahn JO, Crowe S, et al. Clinical and virologic effects of recombinant human granulocyte-macrophage colony-stimulating factor in patients receiving chemotherapy for human immunodeficiency virus–associated non-Hodgkin's lymphoma: results of a randomized trial. *J Clin Oncol* 1991;9:929–940.
211. Angel JB, High K, Rhame F, et al. Phese III study of granulocyte-macrophage colony-stimulating factor in advance HIV disease: effect on infections, CD4 cell counts and HIV suppression. Leukine/HIV study group. *AIDS* 2000;14:387–395.
212. Kedzierska K, Mak J, Mijch A, et al. Granulocyte-macrophage colony-stimulating factor augments phagocytosis of *Mycobacterium avium* complex by human immunodeficiency virus type 1–infected monocytes/macrophages *in vitro* and *in vivo*. *J Infect Dis* 2000;181:390–394.
213. Crowe SM. Role of macrophages in the pathogenesis of human immunodeficiency virus (HIV) infection. *Aust N Z J Med* 1995;25:777–783.
214. Lieschke GJ, Burgess AW. Granulocyte colony-stimulating factor and granulocyte-macrophage colony-stimulating factor (2). *N Engl J Med* 1992;327:99–106.
215. Sato N, Kashima K, Tanaka Y et al. Effect of granulocyte colony-stimulating factor on generation of oxygen-derived free radicals and myeloperoxidase activity in neutrophils from poorly controlled NIDDM patients. *Diabetes* 1997;46:133–137.
216. Bagdade JD, Stewart M, Walters E. Impaired granulocyte adherence a reversible defect in host defense in patients with poorly controlled diabetes. *Diabetes* 1978;27:677–681.
217. Bagdade JD, Root RK, Bulger RJ. Impaired leukocyte function in patients with poorly controlled diabetes. *Diabetes* 1974;23:9–15.
218. Repine JE, Clawson CC, Goetz FC. Bactericidal function on neutrophils from patients with acute bacterial infections and from diabetics. *J Infect Dis* 1980;142:869–875.
219. Gough A, Clapperton M, Rolando N, et al. Randomized placebo-controlled trial of granulocyte colony-stimulating factor in diabetic foot infection. *Lancet* 1997;350:855–859.
220. Remes K, Ronnemaa T. Healing of chronic leg ulcers in diabetic necrobiosis lipoidica with local granulocyte-macrophage colony-stimulating factor treatment. *J Diabetes Complications* 1999;13:115–118.
221. Gaviria JM, Dale DC, Root RK. Neutrophils: function and role in sepsis syndrome. *Sepsis* 1998;2:107–117.
222. Gamelli RL, He LK, Liu H. Macrophage suppression of granulocyte and macrophage growth following burn wound infection. *J Trauma* 1994;37:888–892.
223. Natanson C, Hoffman WD, Suffredini AF, et al. Selected treatment strategies for septic shock based on proposed mechanisms of pathogenesis. *Ann Intern Med* 1994;120:771–783.
224. Fiorentino DF, Zlotnik A, Mosman TR, et al. IL-10 inhibits cytokine production by activated macrophages. *J Immunol* 1991;147:3815–3822.
225. Marchant A, Alegre ML, Hakim A, et al. Clinical and biological significance of interleukin-10 plasma levels in patients with septic shock. *J Clin Immunol* 1995;15:266–273.
226. Volk HD, Thieme M, Heym S, et al. Alterations in function and phenotype of monocytes from patients with septic disease: predictive value and new therapeutic strategies. *Behring Inst Mitt* 1991:208–215.
227. Pinsky MR, Vincent JL, Deviere J, et al. Serum cytokine levels in human septic shock: relation to multiple-system organ failure and mortality. *Chest* 1993;103:565–575.
228. Marty C, Misset B, Tamion F, et al. Circulating interleukine-8 concentrations in patients with multiple organ failure of septic and nonseptic origin. *Crit Care Med* 1994;22:673–679.
229. Kragsbjerg P, Holmberg H, Vikerfors T. Dynamics of blood cytokine concentrations in patients with bacteremic infections. *Scand J Infect Dis* 1996;28:391–398.
230. Patton JH, Lyden SP, Ragsdale DN, et al. Granulocyte colony-stimulating factor improves host defense to resuscitated shock and polymicrobial sepsis without provoking generalized neutrophil-mediated damage. *J Trauma* 1998;44:750–759.
231. Presneill JJ, Waring PM, Layton JE, et al. Plasma granulocyte colony-stimulating factor and granulocyte-macrophage colony-stimulating factor levels in critical illness including sepsis and septic shock: relation to disease severity, multiple organ dysfunction, and mortality. *Crit Care Med* 2000;28:2344–2354.

232. Arslan E, Yavuz M, Dalay C. The relationship between tumor necrosis factor (TNF)–alpha and survival following granulocyte colony-stimulating factor (G-CSF) administration in burn sepsis. *Burns* 2000;26:521–524.
233. Nishida T, Hasegawa J-I, Nakao K, et al. Granulocyte colony-stimulating factor for gastrointestinal perforation in patients with leukopenia. *J Trauma* 1996;40:727–732.
234. Ishikawa K, Tanaka H, Matsuoka T, et al. Recombinant human granulocyte colony-stimulating factor attenuates inflammatory responses in septic patients with neutropenia. *J Trauma* 1998;44:1047–1055.
235. Ishikawa K, Tanaka H, Takaoka M, et al. Granulocyte colony-stimulating factor ameliorates life-treatening infections after combined therapy with barbiturates and mild hypothermia in patients with severe head injuries. *J Trauma* 1999;46:999–1007.
236. Weiss M, Gross-Weege W, Harms B, et al. Filgrastim (RHG-CSF) related modulation of the inflammatory responses in patients at risk of sepsis or with sepsis. *Cytokine* 1996;8:260–265.
237. Flohe S, Borgermann J, Dominguez FE, et al. Influence of granulocyte-macrophage colony-stimulating factor (GM-CSF) on whole blood endotoxin responsiveness following trauma, cardiopulmonary bypass, and severe sepsis. *Shock* 1999;12:17–24.
238. Fanning NF, Kell MR, Shorten GD, et al. Circulating granulocyte-macrophage colony-stimulating factor in plasma of patients with the systemic inflammatory response syndrome delays neutrophil apoptosis through inhibition of spontaneous reactive oxygen species generation. *Shock* 1999;11:167–174.
239. Roilides E, Uhlig K, Venzon D, et al. Neutrophil oxidative burst in response to blastoconidia and pseudohyphae of *Candida albicans*: augmentation by granulocyte colony-stimulating factor and interferon-γ. *J Infect Dis* 1992;166:668–673.
240. Roilides E, Holmes A, Blake C, et al. Effects of granulocyte colony-stimulating factor and interferon-γ on antifungal activity of human polymorphonuclear neutrophils against pseudohyphae of different medically important candida species. *J Leukocyte Biol* 1995;57:651–656.
241. Roilides E, Uhlig K, Venzon D, et al. Enhancement of oxidative response and damage caused by human neutrophils to *Aspergillus fumigatus* hyphae by granulocyte colony-stimulating factor and gamma interferon. *Infect Immun* 1993;61:1185–1193.
242. Roilides E, Holmes A, Blake C, et al. Antifungal activity of elutriated human monocytes against *Aspergillus fumigatus* hyphae: enhancement by granulocyte-macrophage colony-stimulating factor and interferon-γ. *J Infect Dis* 1994;170:894–899.
243. Gaviria JM, van Burik J-A, Dale DC, et al. Comparison of interferon-γ, granulocyte colony-stimulating factor, and granulocyte-macrophage colony-stimulating factor for priming leukocyte-mediated hyphal damage of opportunistic fungal pathogens. *J Infect Dis* 1999;179:1038–1041.
244. Roilides E, Holmes A, Blake C, et al. Impairment of neutrophil antifungal activity against hyphae of *Aspergillus fumigatus* in children infected with human immunodeficiency virus. *J Infect Dis* 1993;167:905–911.
245. Roilides E, Uhlig K, Venzon D, et al. Prevention of corticosteroid-induced suppression of human polymorphonuclear leukocyte-induced damage of *Aspergillus fumigatus* hyphae by granulocyte colony-stimulating factor and gamma interferon. *Infect Immun* 1993;61:4870–4877.
246. Roilides E, Blake C, Holmes A, et al. Granulocyte-macrophage colony-stimulating factor and interferon-γ preven dexamethasone-induced immunosuppression of antifungal monocyte activity against *Aspergillus fumigatus* hyphae. *J Med Vet Mycol* 1996;34:63–69.
247. Gaviria JM, Grohskopf LA, Barnes R, et al. Successful treatment of rhinocerebral zygomycosis: a combined-strategy approach. *Clin Infect Dis* 1999;28:160–161.
248. Sahin B, Paydas S, Cosar E, et al. Role of granulocyte colony-stimulating factor in the treatment of mucormaycosis. *Eur J Microbiol Infect Dis* 1996;15:866–868.
249. Gonzalez CE, Couriel DR, Walsh TJ. Disseminated zygomycosis in a neutropenic patient: successful treatment with amphotericin B lipid complex and granulocyte colony-stimulating factor. *Clin Infect Dis* 1997;24: 192–196.
250. Leleu X, Sendid B, Fruit J, et al. Combined anti-fungal therapy and surgical resection as treatment of pulmonary zygomycosis in allogeneic bone marrow transplantation. *Bone Marrow Transplant* 1999;24:417–420.
251. Vecchiarelli A, Monari C, Baldelli F, et al. Beneficial effect of recombinant human granulocyte colony-stimulating factor on fungicidal activity of polymorphonuclear leukocytes from patients with AIDS. *J Infect Dis* 1995;171:1448–1454.
252. Kullberg BJ, Vandewoude K, Herbrecht R, et al. A double-blind, randomized, placebo-controlled phase II study of filgrastim (recombinant granulocyte colony-stimulating factor) in combination with fluconazole for treatment of invasive candidiasis and candidemia in nonneutropenic patients [Abstract]. In: *38th Interscience Conference on Antimicrobial Agents and Chemotherapy.* American Society of Microbiology, Washington, DC, 1998:479.
253. Smith JA. Neutrophils, host defense, and inflammation: a double-edged sword. *J Leukoc Biol* 1994;56: 672–686.
254. Dallaire F, Ouellet N, Simard M, et al. Efficacy of rhG-CSF in a murine model of pneumococcal pneumonia: effect of lung inflammation and precocity of treatment [Abstract]. In: *39th Interscience Conference on Antimicrobial Agents and Chemotherapy.* American Society of Microbiology, Washington, DC, 1999:386.
255. DeBoisblanc BP, Mason CM, Andresen J, et al. Phase I safety trial of filgrastim (r-metHuG-CSF) in non-neutropenic patients with severe community-acquired pneumonia. *Respir Med* 1997;91:387–394.
256. Nelson S, Belknap SM, Carlson RW, et al. A randomized controlled trial of filgrastim as an adjunct to antibi-

otics for treatment of hospitalized patients with community-acquired pneumonia. *J Infect Dis* 1998;178:1075–1080.
257. Wunderink RG, Leeper KV, Schein RMH, et al. Clinical response to filgrastim (rMetHuG-CSF) in pneumonia with severe sepsis [Abstract]. *Am J Respir Clin Med* 1996;153:123.
258. Nelson S, Heyder AM, Stone J, et al. A randomized controlled trial of filgrastim for treatment of hospitalized patients with multilobar pneumonia. *J Infect Dis* 2000;182:970–973.
259. Root RK, Nelson S, Dale DC, et al. Filgrastim (r-metHuG-CSF) As adjunctive therapy in the treatment of patients with pneumonia and severe sepsis. Results of a placebo-controlled trial. *Am J Respir Crit Care Med* 2000;161:A91.
260. Faist E, Schinkel C, Zimmer S. Update on the mechanisms of immune suppression of injury and immune modulation. *World J Surg* 1996;20:545–559.
261. Schafer H, Hubel K, Bohlen H, et al. Perioperative treatment with filgrastim stimulates granulocyte function and reduces infectious complications after esophagectomy. *Ann Hematol* 2000;79:143–151.
262. Wenisch C, Werkgartner T, Sailer H, et al. Effect of preoperative prophylaxis with filgrastim in cancer neck dissection. *Eur J Clin Invest* 2000;30:460–466.
263. Meropol NJ, Petrelli NJ, Lipman BJ, et al. Granulocyte-macrophage colony-stimulating factor as infection prophylaxis in high-risk oncologic surgery. *Am J Surg* 1996;172:299–302.
264. Neupogen (filgrastim). In: *Physicians' desk reference (PDR),* 54th ed. Montvale, NJ: Medical Economics Company, 2000:528–533.
265. Leukine (sargramostim). In: *Physician's desk reference (PDR),* 54th ed. Montvale, NJ: Medical Economics Company, 2000:1419–1423.
266. Kinstler OB, Brems DN, Lauren SL, et al. Characterization and stability of N-terminally PEGylated rhG-CSF. *Pharm Res* 1996;13:996–1002.
267. Johnston E, Crawford J, Blackwell S, et al. Randomized, dose-escalation study of SD/01 compared with daily filgrastim in patients receiving chemotherapy. *J Clin Oncol* 2000;18:2522–2528.
268. Decoster G, Rich W, Brown SL. Safety profile of filgrastim (r-metHuG-CSF). In: Morstyn G, Dexter TM, eds. *Filgrastim (r-metHuG-CSF) in clinical practice.* New York: Marcel Dekker, 1994:267–290.
269. Peters WP, Shogan JS, Shpall EJ, et al. Recombinant human granulocyte-macrophage colony-stimulating factor produces fever. *Lancet* 1988;1:950.
270. Lieschke GJ, Cebon J, Morstyn G. Characterization of the clinical effects after the first dose of bacterially synthesized recombinant granulocyte-macrophage colony-stimulating factor. *Blood* 1989;74:2634–2643.
271. Ibelgaufts H. *Lexikon der Zytokine.* Munich: Medikon Verlag, 1992.
272. Frumkin LR, Dale DC. The role of colony-stimulating factors in HIV disease. *AIDS Reader* 1996;6:185–193.

10

The Interferons

Steven M. Holland

Immunopathogenesis Unit, Laboratory of Host Defenses, National Institute of Allergy and Infectious Diseases, National Institutes of Health, Bethesda, Maryland

The interferons were first identified and named for their ability to interfere with viral infections of eukaryotic cells (1,2). They were early on broken into three categories, based on the predominant cells of origin: interferons predominantly produced by leukocytes (now known collectively as IFNα), an interferon produced predominantly by fibroblasts (now known as IFNβ), and an interferon produced mainly by T cells (immune or IFNγ). These properties were further refined biochemically, and it became apparent that there were important differences in acid stability, molecular size, and activity. IFNα and IFNβ, and the similar IFNω, share similar biochemical properties, gene proximity, induction, receptor, and signaling pathways, and are collectively referred to as "type I interferons." In contrast, IFNγ is quite distinct in many of these features and is referred to as a "type II interferon." However, all the interferons share certain parts of the signaling pathways in common, and they all interfere with viral replication *in vitro* and *in vivo*.

All the interferons share the same basic signal transduction approach: the IFN molecule binds to a heterodimeric receptor on the cell surface, the polypeptide chains of which are constitutively associated with protein tyrosine kinase molecules of the Janus kinase family (3). These signaling molecules transphosphorylate each other, leading to tyrosine phosphorylation of the respective ligand binding or α chains of the receptor. These phosphorylation steps in turn lead to phosphorylation of the latent signal transduction and activator of transcription molecules (STATs), which then combine in various arrangements and, with other molecules, translocate to the nucleus and upregulate DNA transcription.

Among the most important molecules involved in the further refinement of intracellular signaling are the interferon regulatory factors (IRFs). These are a growing family of related transcriptional regulators that have DNA-binding and protein–protein interacting domains, and can act as activators or inhibitors of downstream signaling. Although there is a certain degree of accident in the discovery and nomenclature of the type I and type II interferons, the sharing of several of these intracellular signal transduction pathways shows the functional overlap of these molecules and their effects (4).

Since their discovery in the 1950s, these cytokines have served as the basis for numerous studies of the biology of cancers, infections, and autoimmunity (5). They are now the standard of care in the treatment of malignancy [IFNα and chronic myeloid leukemia (CML)], autoimmune disorders [IFNβ and multiple sclerosis (MS)], and infectious diseases [IFNγ and chronic granulomatous disease (CGD)]. This chapter outlines the differences and the important similarities of these three related cytokines, their receptors and signaling pathways, and their clinical applications, both approved and investigational.

INTERFERON-α

IFNα is produced by fibroblasts and leukocytes, among others. It signals, through a heterodimeric transmembrane receptor, the activation of the tyrosine kinases Jak1 and Tyk2, which in turn lead to the assembly of the IFNα-stimulated gene factor 3 (ISGF3) complex, composed of STAT1, STAT2, and the associated protein p48 (6). IFNα also upregulates expression of the IL-12β2 receptor (7), thereby enhancing IL-12 responsiveness. There are several different forms of the IFNα receptor (IFNαR)that can be synthesized and expressed, each with slightly different *in vitro* and *in vivo* reactivity (8). For instance, the IFNαRα chain has only one, full-length form, whereas the IFNαRβ has both long (fully functional) and short (binding but not full biological activity) forms. These receptor molecules have some homology to each other, and IFNαRα has some homology to IFNγR1 as well.

There are at least 26 different type I interferon genes clustered around 9p22 (9), comprised predominantly of IFNα genes and pseudogenes, genes and pseudogenes for IFNω, and the single gene for IFNβ at the most distal end of the cluster. The type I IFN genes are all closely spaced and intronless (10,11). Recently, Siegal et al. (12) identified the critical peripheral blood progenitor responsible for high level IFNα production as a dendritic cell precursor. The IFNαRα and IFNαRβ chains are located at 21q22 and are responsible for signaling for IFNα, IFNβ, and IFNω.

Among the proteins activated by IFNα signaling is interferon consensus-sequence binding protein (ICSBP). Gabriele et al. (13) analyzed the function of ICSBP in the knockout mouse. They found a critical role for ICSBP in the control of myeloid apoptosis, since these animals developed a disease characterized by expansion of granulocytes and macrophages with progression to a fatal blast crisis similar to CML in humans. In contrast, human tumor cell lines overexpressing ICSBP had higher rates of spontaneous apoptosis. Schmidt et al. (14) examined the expression of ICSBP transcripts in human myeloid leukemias. Seventy-nine percent of cells from patients with CML, and 66% of cells from patients with acute myeloid leukemia showed little to no transcription of ICSBP, compared to only 6% of normals. However, this relative deficit of ICSBP expression could be overcome by *in vitro* exposure to IFNγ or *in vivo* treatment of CML patients with IFNα. However, with progression of CML, the relative level of ICSBP induction by IFNα waned. Cells from patients with acute lymphoblastic/lymphocytic leukemia and chronic monoblastic/monocytic leukemia did not show the same phenotype. This may in part explain the susceptibility reported in patients with CML to nontuberculous mycobacterial infections (15).

Another shared signaling molecule, Jak1, is more dramatically required for survival. Jak1 is needed for the IFN receptors, the receptors that use the common γ chain (IL-2, -4, -7, -9, -13, and 15), and the receptors that use the gp130 chain, IL-6, LIF, and CNTF. Rodig et al. (16) created a Jak1-deficient mouse, which was runted, unable to nurse, and died perinatally. They failed to develop a normal lymphocyte compartment and showed effects on B cells, T cells, myocytes, and neurons. Interestingly, there were no effects on erythroid, myeloid, or platelet development.

IFNα and IFNγ are differentially regulated and differentially regulate each other. McRae et al. (17) found that IFNα inhibited dendritic cell IL-12 p40 production and therefore served to reduce commitment to the Th1 pathway and IFNγ production. IFNα *in vitro* also reduced TNFα and LT production, but the effect on TNF and LT was not apparently mediated by reduction in IL-12. Fantuzzi et al. (18) showed that IFNα downregulated the IL-12Rβ1 chain and therefore IFNγ production through IL-12, whereas IL-

18 led to an increase in IL-12Rβ1, indicating that these two cytokines have somewhat opposite roles in modulating the pathways leading to IFNγ production. The type I interferons, but not IFNγ, are also modulated by nitric oxide (NO), which seems to repress IFNα and IFNβ expression, but does not affect IFNγ expression. This activity can be derepressed in the presence of nitric oxide synthase (NOS) inhibitors or scavengers (19). IFNα generally antagonizes IFNγ production through regulation of IL-12 and the IL-12Rβ1 chain. IFNα is downregulated by NO, which is potently induced by IFNγ and IL-12, through the agency of the IL-12R. Interestingly, studies on isolated neutrophils showed no effect of IFNα on the standardly tested activities such as superoxide production, phagocytosis, chemotaxis, or bactericidal activity (20).

Viruses have also shown great skill in regulating IFNα activity. Vaccinia and other poxviruses have adopted soluble type I IFN receptor genes as a method of host immune avoidance (21–23).

Animal Models

Muller et al. (24) explored the role for IFNα in mice through the creation of animals deficient in the IFNα or type 1 IFN receptor. These animals are highly susceptible to most viruses, including DNA and RNA types. For most viruses, having an intact IFNγ pathway does not compensate this defect, nor does deficiency of the IFNγR much influence outcomes. However, for some viruses, notably vaccinia virus and Theiler's virus, IFNγ and IFNα both play critical roles. Van den Broek et al. (25) have carefully reviewed the different effects of type 1 and type 2 IFNR knockouts. In general, the type 1 IFNs are needed for early and rapid responses, whereas the type 2 IFN, IFNγ, acts later, after immune induction.

Mice deficient in the receptor for IFNα/β are highly susceptible to a plethora of viral infections. Weck et al. (26) studied mice deficient in various IFN signaling pathways following infection by the murine γ herpesvirus 68 (γHV68). Mice without STAT1 or the IFNα/β receptor succumbed rapidly (within 4 days) to viral infection. Normal control animals had no mortality. In contrast, mice deficient in the IFNγR had an intermediate phenotype, with longer survival, depending on the age at which they were inoculated. They cleared infection from viscera, albeit slower than normal animals. However, IFNγR-deficient mice developed large vessel arteritis several weeks after inoculation, involving the entire thickness of the vessel. This is being explored as a model for arteritis.

Human Defects

Following on the identification of type 1 IFN as a major component of viral defense, several investigators reported cases of severe or recurrent viral infections associated with low or absent IFNα production *in vitro* (27–30). Biron et al. (31) identified a case of severe recurrent herpes virus infection with eventual development of non-Hodgkin's lymphoma in a young man with impaired IFNα production and absence of natural killer (NK) cells. However, none of these cases has had a genetic diagnosis indicating a lesion in any of the IFNα genes or in the IFNα signal transduction pathway. Neustock et al. (32) showed that newborn mononuclear cells were deficient in IFNα response to Newcastle disease virus but not to Sendai virus *in vitro* on the basis of diminished IFNα production, but not due to a diminished number of cells producing IFNα. Although this may explain in part the more severe neonatal susceptibility to viral infection, it is not a genetic defect.

Similar findings have been made with IFNγ responsiveness early in life. This lack of immune maturation with neonatal hyporesponsiveness to interferons and at least some of their inducers is not likely to be accidental, but presumably serves some benefit not yet recognized.

Schmidt et al. (14) showed defective production of ICSBP in CML as cited above. Olapade et al. (9) showed frequent deletions of the gene region, including 9p21 and the type 1 IFN gene cluster in a variety of human cancers, but this seems to be more critically related to deletions in the CDKN2 gene (cyclin-dependent kinase inhibitor 2A).

Hourihane et al. (33) described two siblings with a novel syndrome of CD4 lymphocytopenia and disseminated molluscum contagiosum who responded extremely well to IFNα therapy. However, they were unable to identify an underlying defect.

Despite the frequency and economic impact of viral infections, discrete defects involving IFNα, IFNβ, IFNω, or their receptors have not been reported as underlying human infection susceptibility. This stands in sharp contrast to the susceptibilities associated with the IFNγ receptor and associated pathways. This paucity of recognized genetic defects may reflect the large number of IFNα genes. However, the majority of cytokine defects identified to date have been among receptors, and the work in mice suggests that there is only one set of IFNα/β receptors. Therefore, either there is such low survival capacity in the IFNα-deficient/unresponsive children that they have not been identified, or the conditions in which these defects have been sought are not the right ones.

IFNα Therapy

Therapeutic use of various preparations of IFNα have been tried for the last several decades, most notably in the treatment of respiratory infections, warts (34), hepatitis (35), vascular malformations (36), and certain cancers. The role of IFNα in the treatment of CML is now widely accepted and is reviewed elsewhere (37).

Almost two decades ago, Hayden and Gwaltney (38) showed that IFNα administered intranasally was effective at prevention of rhinovirus infection at doses ranging from 11 to 43 million IU/dose given over 5 days. The highest dose could be administered daily and prevented 75% of symptomatic colds. However, that high dose caused mild leukopenia in a few participants. In a closer look at longer term prophylaxis, Hayden and Gwaltney showed that 28 days of 8 million IU of IFNα daily by spray led to development of nasal ulcerations or bloody mucus in about one-fourth of the patients, and extensive submucosal lymphocytic and mononuclear cell infiltrates in over half. These abnormalities resolved within 2 months. Subsequently, Hayden et al. (39) studied intrafamilial exposure to rhinovirus as modified by use of 7 days of IFNα 5 million units intranasally daily. There was a highly significant reduction in symptomatic colds among recipients of IFNα compared to placebo. Again, mild but transient nasal irritation was noted. Surprisingly, similar trials with IFNβ serine showed no benefit (40), suggesting that there may be important biologic differences between IFNα and IFNβ, despite their sharing of the same receptor pathway.

Schafer et al. (41) identified low levels of IFNα in mouse milk, and reported that IFNα imbibed in mother's milk by suckling mice protected against subsequent viral challenge. This observation initiated a persistent interest in oral administration of IFN for prophylaxis and treatment of viral infections. One principle underlying this application is that the physiologic exposure of the mucosa to IFNα in respiratory secretions is at quite modest levels, unlike the millions of units used in systemic therapy. Oral administration of natural human IFNα (nHuIFNα) has been tried in several animal studies (reviewed in

42). A recurrent finding is that oral administration of natural human IFNα is more effective at lower doses (200 IU and less) than higher doses. Moore et al. (43) showed a significant effect of low-dose (50 and 150 IU) oral nHuIFNα on lower respiratory inflammatory cytology in standard-bred racehorses. Neutrophils, macrophages, and lymphocytes were significantly reduced in animals receiving 50 and 150 IU, but not those receiving 450 IU, when compared to placebo recipients. These effects were seen 8 days after initiation and 3 days after cessation of nHuIFNα. Interestingly, the proportions of $CD4^+$, $CD5^+$, or $CD8^+$ lymphocytes in bronchoalveolar lavage fluid were not affected by administration of nHuIFNα. Subsequently, Moore et al. (44) showed similar significant reductions in other markers of lower airway inflammation, such as total protein, IgG, and IgA concentration 8 days after administration of 50 IU and 150 IU nHuIFNα. These differences persisted at a significant level even out to 15 days after administration of 50 IU nHuIFNα. In a study of calves infected by bovine respiratory disease complex, Cummins et al. (45) showed a therapeutic effect on mean daily weight gain of nHuIFNα 20 IU or 200 IU, but not 2,000 IU, administered orally daily over 3 days. A onetime prophylactic dose of 200 IU nHuIFNα showed a trend toward protection as well. Therefore, in these animal studies, oral nHuIFNα appears to be effective in modulation of inflammatory markers and treatment of viral infections at low more than high doses. In addition, it may have prophylactic value.

Papillomavirus infections have been a target of great interest and have been the occasion of some of the early successes in IFNα therapy. Although there have been many reports of small series showing significant benefit to IFNα in anogenital warts, randomized trials have, in general, not shown such impressive results (reviewed in 46). Avidano et al. (47) retrospectively reviewed the use of IFNα in addition to laser surgery as adjuvant treatment of recurrent respiratory papillomatosis in 34 patients. They found that 16/34 had complete and 12/34 partial responses to IFNα, with better rates of response among those with earlier onset disease. The toxicity profile was favorable.

Hepatitis

The use of IFNα in the treatment of hepatitis has been extensive and is now quite promising. Hoofnagle et al. (48) treated 10 patients with non-A non-B hepatitis in an open-label pilot study with varying doses of IFNα for varying periods of time up to 1 year. They found rapid reductions in transaminases and improvement in liver histology, but rebound liver function elevation was rapid in those treated for only a relatively short time (4 months). Subsequently, Davis et al. (49) randomized 166 patients with chronic HCV infection to receive either 3 MU IFNα subcutaneously three times weekly, 1 MU subcutaneously three times weekly, or no treatment for 6 months. The rates of normalization or near normalization of transaminases were 46%, 28%, and 8%, respectively. Complete normalization occurred in 85% of treatment responders in the 3 MU group, but only 56% of responders in the 1 MU group. Hepatic histologic improvement was seen at the higher dose level as well. However, relapse within the first 6 months after study completion was seen in over half in both low- and high-dose cohorts. DiBisceglie et al. (50) treated 21 patients with HCV in a smaller randomized prospective trial using IFNα 2 MU subcutaneously three times weekly as monotherapy in the treatment of HCV. IFNα recipients had improvements in histologic and liver function parameters. About half had complete responses in terms of normalization of transaminases. However, similar to previous studies, they still saw relapse of the great majority of cases within 6 to 12 months following discontinuation of IFNα.

The above studies suggested that dose and duration were important factors in clearing HCV. Therefore, Poynard et al. (51) randomized patients to receive 6 months of therapy with 3 MU IFNα subcutaneously three times weekly followed by 12 months of the same regimen, 12 months of 1 MU subcutaneously three times weekly, or no further treatment. Significantly more patients in the longer duration higher dose arm cleared their infections at 18 months of study (45%) than did either of the other two groups (around 30% in each). However, over the ensuing 2 years of follow-up, half of the responders in the high-dose group relapsed, as did about two-thirds of the patients in the low- or no-dose groups. Poynard et al. (52) went on to conduct a metaanalysis to examine the issues of dose and duration in the IFNα monotherapy of HCV. There were clear benefits in terms of improvement of transaminases and persistence of remission that accrued to higher dose regimens (6 versus 3 MU) given over longer periods (12 versus 6 months). However, even in the best case scenarios, the long-term clearance rate was still only in the 20% range.

The addition of ribavirin to IFNα therapy for HCV has greatly increased the rates of early and sustained clearance of HCV from blood as well as normalization of transaminases and improvement in histology. McHutchison et al. (53) randomized 912 patients to receive IFNα 3 MU subcutaneously three times weekly with or without ribavirin for 24 or 48 months with follow-up over 6 months. They found greater rates of clearance at 6 months in those patients receiving both agents compared to those receiving IFNα alone (53% versus 29%, respectively). During follow-up off drugs, the rate of sustained clearance in recipients of IFN alone fell to 6%, compared to 31% in the dual therapy arm. There were further benefits to longer duration of therapy, but there were also higher rates of drug-related toxicity and subject dropout. Poynard et al. (54) conducted a similar study among 832 subjects and found a 43% response rate for patients receiving both IFNα 3 MU subcutaneously three times weekly and ribavirin (RBV) for 12 months, compared to 19% for those receiving IFNα alone. They identified several factors that were important in successful IFNα therapy of HCV: genotype of HCV other than type 1, lower viral load, age less than 40 years, minimal hepatic fibrosis, and female sex. They found that patients who did not have as many of the favorable factors benefited more from prolonged (48 weeks) of therapy. Combination therapy was also effective in successful retreatment of those who had relapsed following IFNα alone (55). Therefore, IFNα therapy for chronic HCV is effective and tolerable, but has a low level of sustained virologic and biochemical clearance. This therapeutic effect is somewhat dependent on dose and duration and greatly augmented by coadministration of ribavirin.

These issues of dose and duration have been partially addressed by covalent attachment of polyethylene glycol (pegolation) to the IFNα itself to allow less frequent dosing but more sustained levels. The pegolated IFNα (PEG-interferon-α_{2a}) has a slower absorption and a much longer plasma half-life than its unmodified counterpart. Zeuzem et al. (56) compared PEG-interferon-α_{2a} 180 μg subcutaneously once weekly for 48 weeks to unmodified IFNα 6 MU subcutaneously three times weekly for 12 weeks followed by 3 MU subcutaneously three times weekly for 36 weeks. All patients were followed up at 24 weeks after treatment cessation (72 weeks total). PEG-interferon-α_{2a} was associated with excellent virologic response rates at 48 and 72 weeks compared to IFNα (69% and 39%, compared to 28% and 19%, respectively, $p = 0.001$). Biochemical response showed similar impressive trends. Similar benefits extended to the effect of PEG-interferon-α_{2a} on treatment of chronic HCV and cirrhosis (57). The toxicity profiles were similar for both the PEG-interferon-α_{2a} and IFNα groups, with 7% and 10% discontinuing therapy, respectively (56). Of note, about 20% of each group required dose modifications for signs or symptoms associated with IFN. Common toxicities in this non–placebo-controlled trial included headache, fatigue, fever, myalgia, rigors, nausea, insomnia, and anorexia. The fact that this study was done without added antivirals suggests that future regimens that include antivirals will be able to achieve much higher rates of early and sustained response.

Another approach to trying to enhance IFNα response in hepatitis C is the construction of an IFNα that contains the most common amino acids at polymorphic positions throughout the different available natural IFNα genes (58). Consensus interferon (CIFN) is a composite protein designed in the expectation of increased activity by combining the most active components of the various natural interferons. In fact, CIFN shows a 10-fold higher *in vitro* biological activity as compared to single recombinant IFNα2b or IFNα2a, possibly due to its greater binding affinity to interferon receptors. In addition, it is clinically more active, as shown by its use in patients who have failed or broken through on IFNα2b. CIFN 9 μg, three times weekly for 24 weeks, was similar to the standard 3 MU IFNα. However, in subjects who had responded but relapsed following 6 months of standard dose IFNα, 15 μg CIFN three times weekly for 48 weeks resulted in a sustained virologic response rate of 58%. Those who had not responded to standard IFN therapy had a 13% sustained response to the same higher dose, longer duration CIFN regimen. Higher dose CIFN was well tolerated. The ability of CIFN to achieve responses in relapsed or nonresponsive patients suggests that it may have greater biological activity without a significant change in toxicity. However, as pointed out by Heathcote et al. (59), close monitoring during therapy with standard regimens must be carried out to identify those patients who have transient responses followed by breakthrough and those that achieve no response to IFNα at all. CIFN may also be a target for enhancement, such as pegolation, in future studies if the increased activity can be reproduced.

Treatment of hepatitis B virus (HBV) infection is less straightforward. The efficacy of IFNα in HBV is very dependent on underlying host immune status relative to the virus. That is, elevated transaminases at the time of initiation of therapy and a short duration of disease are markers that are associated with better responses to therapy (60,61). A short burst of prednisolone, presumably allowing for an increase in viral replication and further opportunities for priming of an immune response, appears to be helpful for induction of IFNα clearance of HBeAg (62–64). Lin et al. (63) showed long-term benefits of IFNα therapy in a randomized study of Taiwanese men with chronic HBV infection. Seroconversion of HBeAg was seen in 42% of IFNα-treated patients compared to 24% of untreated patients. Importantly, in the years following IFNα therapy, 56% of the remaining patients who had not seroconverted in the IFNα group went on to clear their HBeAg, compared to only 19% of comparable patients in the control group. The cumulative incidence of sustained response was highest in the steroid-primed group. Development of hepatocellular carcinoma (HCC), a lethal consequence of chronic HBV infection, was only 1.5% in treated patients compared to 12% in untreated patients. Cumulative survival was significantly higher in the treated than the control group. IFN therapy, cirrhosis, and age at entry were independent factors for survival and HCC development. Maintenance of HBeAg seroconversion is sustained in the vast majority of individuals following therapy. Overall, success of IFNα therapy in HBV has been correlated with higher transaminases and lower levels of HBV DNA in the blood (reviewed in 65).

More recently, the development of the nucleoside analog lamivudine has been investigated in chronic HBV infection. Lamivudine is orally available, easily administered, has a favorable toxicity profile, and can be delivered over prolonged courses. Similar to IFNα, there is a benefit of preexisting elevation of transaminases, again suggesting an important role for underlying host response in viral clearance (66). However, there is not yet persuasive evidence for a benefit to combined therapy of IFNα and lamivudine (65).

Overall, these data in hepatitides suggest that host immune response is critical to viral control and clearance and that IFNα is a potent modulator of that activity. The mechanisms by which this occurs are not clear (i.e., mediated by acquired or innate immune responses), but their understanding will be critical to further development of rational therapeutics. The development of antivirals with moderate specificity, low toxicity, easy delivery, and low cost may eventually make efforts at immune augmentation redundant.

Tuberculosis

Giosue et al. (67) investigated the effects of different doses of IFNα aerosol on markers of immune activation in normals and patients with chronic bronchitis. Doses of 3 MU administered by aerosol for 5 consecutive days caused no significant toxicity and were associated with increased peripheral blood 2′-5′ oligoadenylate synthetase (OAS) levels and increased nitroblue tetrazolium reduction by phagocytes. Despite finding some IFNα-induced activities, IFNα levels in peripheral blood were not altered by aerosol administration. In contrast, the aerosol delivery of IFNγ reported by Jaffee et al. (68) did not lead to detected induction of IFNγ-inducible genes in peripheral blood mononuclear cells.

Having identified a biologically active dose and favorable toxicity profile, Giosue et al. (69) used aerosolized IFNα in the treatment of drug-sensitive pulmonary tuberculosis. They examined two groups of pulmonary tuberculosis patients: 10 received IFNα aerosol (3 MU three times weekly for 8 weeks) along with standard appropriate chemotherapy, and 10 received chemotherapy alone. The IFNα group had earlier resolution of clinical signs, radiographic signs (nodules of 2 to 10 mm, consolidation), and sputum smears than did the group on chemotherapy alone. These findings were accompanied in IFNα recipients by increased numbers of lymphocytes and HLA-DR expression in brancho alveolar lavage fluid (bALF) cells at 8 weeks, and significantly lower levels of previously elevated BALF IL-6 and TNFα. Levels of IFNαR were no different on BALF lymphocytes or monocytes in recipients or controls. Giosue et al. (70) have repeated this study of adjuvant aerosolized IFNα 3 MU three times weekly for 6 months in seven patients with clinically nonresponsive multidrug-resistant tuberculosis (MDRTB) following at least 6 months of failure to clear sputum of tuberculosis on antimycobacterial therapy alone. Five out of seven patients converted their sputum smears to negative during the initial 2 months of IFNα treatment, but no cultures converted. Sputum colony counts fell during therapy and rebounded following it. Chest computed tomography (CT) scans were slightly improved in all patients. These data suggest that IFNα by aerosol does have some effect on refractory MDRTB and that this effect is more profound during, rather than following, administration. Similar effects (transient reduction in smear positivity, but persistence of culture positivity) were reported for the use of aerosolized IFNγ for MDRTB by Condos et al. (71).

Palmero et al. (72) used systemic IFNα 3 MU subcutaneously three times weekly for 12 weeks in patients with MDRTB. Of five patients treated, two achieved long-term cures of their infections, one had a sputum smear conversion but remained culture positive, and two had no change. This difference between aerosolized IFNα (high-level clearance of sputum smears but not cultures) and systemic IFNα in resistant tuberculosis is mirrored in the experience with IFNγ. Whether this is a reproducible difference in these routes of administration remains unclear. The study sizes have been quite small, and there are no standardized treatment regimens for MDRTB, making baseline criteria, and therefore underlying host factors, heterogeneous. Clearly, larger randomized trials are needed.

Although IFNγ is often considered the critical cytokine for mycobacterial control, these therapeutic data suggest that IFNα may either directly augment mycobacterial killing or modulate host response in a way that makes mycobacterial killing more effective (e.g., regulation of IFNγ production or IL-12 response). Further experiments in animal models are imperative to understand the mechanisms involved. Since STAT1 is phosphorylated during both IFNα and IFNγ stimulation, there may be overlapping activation of specific antimycobacterial pathways. This may have important implications for treatment of patients with IFNγR defects, since stimulation of the IFNαR in patients with IFNγR deficiency still leads to normal STAT1 phosphorylation (G. Uzel and S. M. Holland, unpublished observations, 2000).

IFN-β

IFNβ has had its largest application in the treatment of MS, a disease of widely presumed, but not proven, infectious etiology. Although MS is more commonly discussed in the neurologic literature, brief mention will be made of it here because of the management of the toxicities and the likely increasing use of this cytokine for this and other "autoimmune" diseases over the years to come. MS has been recently reviewed by Noseworthy et al. (73).

There are currently three formulations of IFNβ in clinical use: IFNβ-1a (Avonex; Biogen) and IFNβ-1b (Betaseron; Berlex) are available in the United States; a higher dose formulation of IFNβ-1a (Rebif; Serono) is licensed for use in Europe and Canada.

Several reports have indicated a clinical benefit to the use of IFNβ in the early treatment of relapsing-remitting MS. Paty et al. (74) showed a marked effect of IFNβ-1b in the reduction of new lesions on magnetic resonance imaging (MRI) in a prospective, blinded, placebo-controlled trial. This effect was sustained over longer term therapy using 8 MIU of IFNβ-1b subcutaneously every other day (75). Miller et al. (76) showed a similar effect of IFNβ-1b on progression of secondary MS using the same 8 MIU dose every other day subcutaneously. However, although these studies showed a benefit for therapy on the rate of progression as measured by appearance and accumulation of new hyperintense inflammatory lesions on serial MRI scanning, there was not an overall retardation of brain atrophy, suggesting that IFNβ-1b therapy may slow but not stop the deleterious effects of MS on brain (77).

IFNβ-1a also shows activity against MS. Significant benefits accrue using 6 MIU (30 Mμg) of IFNβ-1a intramuscularly in patients with relapsing and remitting MS (78). In a multicenter, blinded, placebo-controlled trial of 22 μg (6 MΩng-remitting MS (79). Further exploration of dose interval and dependence was carried out by looking at the 22 μg and 44 μg doses delivered weekly (80). There was a clear effect of the 44 μg dose even at this lower, less frequent level, but it was less than that seen with the three times weekly dose regimen.

The rate of development of neutralizing antibody to IFNβ during the course of therapy is between 5% and 30%, and appears higher with IFNβ-1b than IFNβ-1a (81). These antibodies appear to be biologically significant insofar as they inhibit the elaboration of neopterin and β2 microglobulin, but their effect on the clinical effect of IFNβ in the treatment of MS is less clear. However, these antibodies are transient, and their long-term impact on clinical response is unclear (82).

Chofflon (83) reviewed the four major placebo-controlled trials of IFNβ in relapsing-remitting multiple sclerosis (RRMS), which confirmed the benefit of IFNβ therapy. He also reviewed the three IFN-β products currently available and licensed for use in RRMS, their relative indications, doses, and routes of administration. He suggests that optimal results are likely to be achieved with the highest tolerable dosage of IFNβ instituted early in the course of disease to delay progression.

Mechanisms of IFNβ action in MS are not yet proven. IFNβ has effects on HLA display as measured by β2 microglobulin, lymphocyte proliferation, antigen presentation, and cytokine production in the periphery and in the brain (84). Rothuizen et al. (85) explored effects of different IFNβ-1a (Rebif) doses administered *in vivo* on *in vitro* cytokine expression. They found no difference in serum or resting *in vitro*–produced cytokine levels. However, there was significant inhibition of mitogen-stimulated production of IL-1b, IL-6, IFN-γ, TNF-α, and TNF-β within 24 to 48 hours after injection. There was no evidence for either tolerance or augmentation over 1 month of administration at weekly or thrice-weekly intervals. Dose dependence was observed, with three times weekly dosing (22 μg) having more suppression of inflammatory cytokine production than weekly injections (66 μg > 22 μg). Importantly, IL-10 secretion remained unchanged. Whereas there was a clear effect of proximity of the dose of IFNβ on cytokine elaboration, the increases in serum β2-microglobulin, neopterin, and 2-5A-synthetase were more sustained over the dosing interval. The inhibition of IL-12 production by the type 1 interferons has been proposed by Karp et al. (86) as a unifying hypothesis for the mechanism of action in MS. In addition, IFNβ decreases synthesis of matrix metalloproteinases, which may act to reduce cellular migration into areas of inflammation (87,88).

The toxicities of IFNβ in the treatment of MS are similar to those encountered with IFNα (reviewed in 89). In general, these toxicities are more marked early in the course of administration, tend to ameliorate with continued therapy, and are somewhat dose dependent. The most common reactions are flu-like syndrome, transient liver enzyme elevations or leukopenias, menstrual irregularity, and increased spasticity. Injection site erythema, edema, and occasional necrosis can occur after subcutaneous application of IFNβ-1b and IFNβ-1a (90). Most of the acute symptomatic toxicities occur within the 6 to 24 hours immediately following the dose. More rare toxicities, some of which may not be related to IFNβ administration, include autoimmune reactions, capillary leak syndrome, anaphylactic shock, and thrombotic-thrombocytopenic purpura. Alopecia has been seen in about 4% of recipients. Depression has been reported with all the interferons (IFNα, IFNβ, IFNγ), but seems to be most clearly associated with IFNα, although whether this is due to dose or cytokine-specific issues, or is some interaction of the cytokine with the underlying diseases (hepatitis and CML) is not clear (Chapter 13).

IFN-γ

IFNγ is encoded by a single gene with three exons located on chromosome 12q14 in humans and chromosome 10 in mouse. IFNγ is produced by lymphocytes ($CD4^+$, $CD8^+$, NK cells) as well as macrophages and perhaps neutrophils (91). It is induced by a number of signals, including IL-12 and IL-18 (92,93) and in turn induces hundreds of genes, including its own inducers (94,95). IFNγ also induces enzymes important in the killing of intracellular organisms, including the ATP receptor P2X7 (96,97). IFNγ activates neutrophils and macrophages to produce superoxide and nitric oxide, increase surface display of MHC antigens and Fc receptors, decrease lysosomal pH, and increase the intracellular concentration of certain antibiotics (98,99). IFNγ potently upregulates MHC class 2 expression and has been implicated in the etiology of aplastic anemia (100). However, the effects of IFNγ and its inducer IL-12 on bone marrow transplantation and graft versus host disease (GVHD) are surprisingly salutary (101,102), and IFNγ is not needed for acute GVHD in animal models (103).

Aguet et al. (104) cloned the ligand binding chain of the IFNγR, initially referred to as IFNγRα, but now as IFNγR1. Bohni et al. (105) showed that this receptor was species-nonspecific in its intracellular signaling (i.e., human receptors could use the intracellular signaling molecules of murine cells), whereas the ligand–receptor interaction was fairly tightly conserved (i.e., human and mouse IFNγ do not activate each other's receptors). However, it was early on appreciated that there were other factors required for IFNγ signaling in addition to the IFNγR1 chain. Subsequently, Hemmi et al. (106) and Soh et al. (107) identified the accessory factor as the IFNγ signal transducing chain, or IFNγRβ, now referred to as IFNγR2. These two chains were shown to be necessary and sufficient for IFNγ activation of cells, although there has been some discussion of a possible third chain that more potently mediates antiviral activity (107). Bach et al. (108) showed that IFNγR2 is specifically downregulated in mature CD4 cells of either Th1 or Th2 phenotype, providing a means of desensitization of mature T cells to IFNγ through modulation of the signaling but the binding chain.

Dighe et al. (109) created an autosomal dominant form of the IFNγR1 by truncation of the intracellular domain of the molecule leading to unusual expression characteristics in murine cells. The mutant molecule was overabundant on the cell surface and retained its IFNγ-binding activity, although it had lost its signaling capacity and the receptor recycling motif. This led to a dominant negative inhibition of IFNγ signaling.

IFNγ signals through a membrane-bound receptor composed of two chains, IFNγR1 and IFNγR2, which are constitutively bound to their respective Janus kinases Jak1 and Jak2. On binding of homodimeric IFNγ, the Jaks reciprocally transphosphorylate, leading to phosphorylation of the intracellular domain of IFNγR1 at tyrosine 440 (Y440). This then serves as a binding site for the latent activator of signal transduction and transcription 1 (STAT1), which is in turn phosphorylated. Phosphorylated STAT1 (STAT1-P) homodimerizes, creating a complex that moves to the nucleus and binds nuclear DNA at sites that contain γ activation sequences (GAS) (6,99,110).

Animal Models

With the creation of IFNγ-deficient (111) and IFNγR-deficient (112) mice, the door was opened to a deeper understanding of the multiple roles of IFNγ in the regulation of both innate and acquired immunity. The demonstration of enhanced susceptibility to low-dose inocula of *M. bovis* presaged the discoveries of the critical roles of IFNγ in protection against mycobacteria. In addition, IFNγ was shown to have roles in the activity of NK cells and in the control of cellular proliferation. The remarkable similarities of IFNγ-deficient and IFNγR-deficient mice suggested that the IFNγR and its ligand appear to be relatively mutually monogamous and to control a large number of host innate and acquired immune responses. However, as shown in these early papers and many subsequent publications, the activities of IFNγ are not required for normal growth, development, or protection from normal flora under normal conditions. Therefore, IFNγ (as well as IFNα and IFNβ) are cytokines whose function is only apparently required during infection. In contrast, some of the signaling molecules that they activate, most notably Jak1, are absolutely required for normal development (16). Nguyen et al. (113) have shown that, during acute viral infection in mice, IFNα inhibits IFNγ production through a pathway that is dependent on the type 1 IFN receptor and is STAT1 mediated. In addition, IFNα inhibits IL-12–mediated IFNγ production.

Dighe et al. (114) showed that IFNγ responsiveness is necessary for tumor rejection. Expression of a dominant negative IFNγR1 (ADIFNγR1) mutant impaired immune rejection of a fibrosarcoma (Meth A) and overcame resistance in immune animals. Dighe et al. (115) also created mice transgenic for ADIFNγR1 mutants under specific promoters that targeted IFNγ unresponsiveness to specific compartments (mature macrophage or T cell) by placing the construct under the control of the human lysozyme or lck promoters, respectively. In animals with macrophages rendered unresponsive to IFNγ, susceptibility to listeriosis was enhanced, both in terms of mortality and microbial burden. This was not markedly augmented by wholesale neutralization of IFNγ, suggesting that the macrophage is the critical compartment for listeriacidal activity. In animals with the ADIFNγR1 construct under the lck promoter, the total numbers of T cells and B cells were normal, indicating that IFNγ responsiveness is not needed for lymphoid development. However, functional expression of the transgene was limited to the $CD3^+$ T cell compartment. When animals with T cells unresponsive to IFNγ were challenged with *Listeria*, there was no difference between transgenics and normals in terms of mortality or body burden of organisms. There was no skewing of Th phenotype in animals transgenic for $CD3^+$ ADIFNγR1, suggesting that Th1 phenotype development is not dependent on T cell IFNγ responsiveness. What appears to determine Th1 development is IFNγ enhancement of IL-12 production.

Muller et al. (116) and van den Broek et al. (25) used type 1 and type 2 IFNR knockout animals to demonstrate that for some viruses, such as vaccinia or Theiler's virus, both IFN systems are essential for antiviral defense and are functionally nonredundant. Whereas IFNα and IFNβ are essential for early response to viruses, IFNγ is typically produced later in the course of the immune response and is active against intracellular bacteria and parasites as well. Weck et al. (26) used γHV 68 to show that, in contrast to mice with defects affecting type 1 IFN or STAT1, which died very early after viral infection, IFNγR-deficient mice had longer survival, depending on the age at which they were inoculated. Although IFNγR-deficient mice eventually cleared virus from their viscera, they went on to develop large vessel arteritis several weeks after inoculation, involving the entire thickness of the vessel. Control animals had no mortality from virus and formed no arteritis.

Yap and Sher (117) examined the relative contributions of hematopoietic and parenchymal IFNγR expression by the creation of reciprocal bone marrow chimeric mice. They found that while resistance to *Listeria* required only hematopoietic IFNγR expression, resistance to toxoplasmosis required expression in both compartments. Since the IFNγR is expressed on all nucleated cells, this result suggests a critical role in host defense for nonhematopoietic cells. In addition, it provides a note of caution for the presumed curative effect of bone marrow transplantation for IFNγR deficiency. Although successfully transplanted patients will have normal leukocytes, they may still be at risk for specific infections.

Human Polymorphisms and Defects

Tanaka et al. (118) studied a polymorphism in the signal peptide of IFNγR1 (G88A) leading to the conversion of amino acid 14 from Val to Met ($Val_{14}Met$). They found significant overrepresentation of this polymorphism in Japanese patients with systemic lupus erythematosus (SLE) compared to normals. The presence of the polymorphism led to reduced HLA-DR expression in response to IFNγ stimulation. The amino acid change occurs at the end of the signal peptide and may therefore impede maturation of the receptor. However, subsequently, Nakashima et al. (119) followed up this work on the IFNγR1 by looking at another polymorphism seen in the IFNγR2, as reported in the initial paper by Soh et al. (107). The IFNγR2 polymorphism is an arginine to glutamine change at amino acid 64 (Arg64Gln). This polymorphism carried no independent risk of SLE, but when combined with the previously described polymorphism Val14Met in IFNγR1, it conferred an odds ratio for SLE of 9.6, compared to individuals bearing homozygous Val14 and homozygous Arg64. Retrospectively, Nakashima et al. (119) also recognized that the effects previously ascribed to the Val14Met polymorphism in IFNγR1 were only seen when that was associated with the homozygous Gln64 polymorphism in IFNγR2. Therefore, this is an example of a phenotype (increased risk of SLE) conferred only in the presence of a complex genotype (polymorphisms in both IFNγR1 and IFNγR2). Whether this genotype has an infection-related phenotype as well has not been determined.

Multiple defects have been identified in the IFNγR1 and IFNγR2 (reviewed in 110). These have, in general, been identified due to severe infections with intracellular organisms such as nontuberculous mycobacteria and salmonella, but have also been associated with severe viral infections as well (120). Defects in the extracellular domains of IFNγR1 and IFNγR2 have been associated predominantly with severe, IFNγ-unresponsive infections (120–124). However, partial phenotypes with some preserved IFNγ responsiveness have been identified in both receptors (125,126). A common intracellular deletion due to a mutational hotspot has been identified in IFNγR1 at bp 818 (127). This common mutation, 818del4, is similar in effect to the autosomal dominant mutation described by Dighe et al. (109). Because it retains the transmembrane domain but is lacking the intracellular STAT1 and Jak 1 binding domains, it leads to accumulation of the extracellular, IFNγ-binding domain of IFNγR1 on the cell surface (127). In addition to the lack of the signaling molecule binding domains for Jak1 and STAT1, the deleted protein is missing the receptor recycling domain, and therefore this particular mutant has impaired removal from the cell surface. Therefore, these mutant, incompetent receptors accumulate on the cell surface and combine with normal receptors in complexes (both IFNγR1 and IFNγR2), leading to dominant inhibition of signaling.

As would be expected from the complex interrelationships of IFNγ and IL-12 and the downstream signaling molecule STAT1, mutations in these genes or their receptors also lead to infection susceptibility to intracellular infections, most notably with nontuberculous mycobacteria and salmonella (128–130). In addition, there has been one report of IL-12p40 deficiency, leading to recurrent infection with nontuberculous mycobacteria and salmonella (131).

Why do these mutations in the IFNγ /IL-12 synthesis and use pathways recurrently present with nontuberculous mycobacterial infections and salmonella and not tuberculosis, leishmaniasis, or severe viral infections? Perhaps they do present as these other infections, but in regions outside Western Europe and North America where access to health care and complex molecular diagnosis may not be as readily available. Patients may die or be treated successfully and never be diagnosed. The search for these mutations in other disease populations is imperative, as it is likely that we have only touched the tip of the iceberg in regard to the population-based phenotype of these defects. On the other hand, perhaps these pathways are genuinely necessary only for dealing with these particularly ubiquitous environmental organisms (especially the nontuberculous mycobacteria), and there are other mechanisms adduced for dealing with rarer encounters with true pathogens, such as tuberculosis. At this point, no single answer can be given with certainty, but it is clear that these patients exist in larger numbers than have been identified so far, and that the spectrum of infection is much broader than initially thought, including the environmental mycobacteria, salmonella, several viruses, and histoplasmosis (reviewed in 110).

IFNγ THERAPY

In humans, IFNγ has been studied in various clinical trials for infectious and noninfectious diseases since the mid-1980s. Nathan et al. (132) first demonstrated the ability of IFNγ to upregulate the production of superoxide by macrophages *in vitro*. They went on to demonstrate how IFNγ had the same effect in patients with advanced malignancy, namely upregulation of hydrogen peroxide formation (133). These seminal papers suggested that IFNγ was likely to have a critical role in host defense that was dependent on the reduced nicotinamide adenine dinucleotide phosphate (NADPH) oxidase, the cellular mechanism that transfers an electron from NADPH to molecular oxygen, resulting in superoxide anion production and the downstream metabolites, hydrogen peroxide and bleach (reviewed in 134). This early recognition of the relationship between IFNγ exposure and macrophage and neutrophil superoxide production led to experiments in patients with CGD, in whom the NADPH oxidase is genetically deficient. Early experiments suggested that certain CGD patients could respond to IFNγ *in vitro* with increased superoxide production and bacterial killing (135–137). In addition, it was noted that IFNγ upregulated the expression of the major X-linked gene involved in CGD, $gp91_{phox}$ (138). Ezekowitz et al. (139) and Sechler et al. (136) showed partial correction of the superoxide production defect in CGD by *in vivo* administration of IFNγ.

Schiff et al. (140) administered IFNγ to normal volunteers and examined markers of cellular adhesion, cellular activation, and opsonic potential. They found a significant increase in neutrophil expression of the high-affinity Fcγ-receptor (FcγR1) that peaked 48 hours after IFNγ treatment. In addition, monocyte expression of FcγR1, FcγRII, FcγRIII, CD11a, CD11b, CD18, and HLA-DR all increased over the same time course. Neutrophil phagocytosis of opsonized killed bacteria was also enhanced due to upregulation of Fc-γRI. Lipopolysaccharide-binding protein in serum also increased. These data suggested that IFNγ has broad effects on cellular activation, trafficking, and opsonic activity that may underlie some of its benefits in terms of innate immunity.

Chronic Granulomatous Disease

The above observations in superoxide production led to an international, double-blinded, placebo-controlled trial of IFNγ therapy as prophylaxis in CGD. This trial was highly successful in terms of demonstrating that IFNγ reduced the number and severity of infections in CGD by about 70%, regardless of antibiotic prophylaxis or genetic subtype of CGD (141). However, this pivotal study did not show that the administration of IFNγ led to upregulation of superoxide formation in the recipients: although IFNγ was indeed effective in reducing infections in CGD, the mechanism was not through the induction of superoxide or changes in the *in vitro* killing of bacteria. However, there was augmentation of *in vitro* killing of *Aspergillus* hyphae by CGD cells from patients treated with IFNγ (142). Therefore, the salutary effects of IFNγ on infection susceptibility in CGD are likely independent of regulation of the NADPH oxidase. Despite the lack of clear mechanism, IFNγ was licensed in the United States in 1991 for the prophylactic treatment of CGD. Subsequently, long-term follow-up of these patients who have received over 10 years of IFNγ (50 $\mu g/m^2$ subcutaneously three times weekly) has shown no unexpected toxicity or impairment of growth or development (143,144). These long-term IFNγ safety data include pediatric populations and show that long-term therapy is safe and well tolerated.

Subsequent studies of IFNγ prophylaxis in CGD mice have confirmed the earlier human study and the absence of alteration in superoxide production through NADPH oxidase (145). However, this study has been no more successful than the human one in trying to identify the mechanisms of action that are working in the setting of CGD.

Osteopetrosis

Osteopetrosis is a genetic disease in which bone becomes sclerotic, compromising bone marrow space and cranial nerve foramina. Patients suffer from anemia, blindness, deafness, and recurrent pathologic fractures. In addition, patients with osteopetrosis have recurrent infections, and their neutrophils are partially defective in superoxide production, as evinced by granulocyte-macrophage colony-forming unit (GM-CFU) that are low reducers of nitroblue tetrozolium (NBT). Presumably, their osteoclasts are as well, and this may have something to do with their failure to correctly remodel bone. Key et al. (146) showed that IFNγ increased bone resorption and increased superoxide production were linked in humans with osteopetrosis. They showed that if one treats rat calvaria *in vitro* with parathyroid hermone (PTH), it leads to an increase in NBT staining and calcium release. This effect is inhibited by deferral manganese, suggesting that superoxide is important in bone resorption. However, it is presumably superoxide produced from an oxidase other than the NADPH oxidase, since CGD patients (NADPH oxidase deficient) do not get osteopetrosis, pathologic fractures, or severe anemia. Key et al. (147) used IFNγ in the treatment of osteopetrosis at the same dose as that used in patients with CGD (50 μg/m^2 subcutaneously three times weekly). They found increased bone resorption, markedly decreased incidence of infections, an increase in GM-CFU NBT reduction, decreased transfusion requirement, and increased growth. The drug was well tolerated. All patients experienced some fever, and two had fever of >40°C. These severe fevers disappeared with reduction of the dose by 50%, and all patients were tolerating the drug well after 6 months of therapy. Osteopetrosis has been accepted as a licensed indication for the use of IFNγ in the United States.

ROUTE AND DOSE CONSIDERATIONS

Aulitzky et al. (148) studied longitudinal administration of IFNγ to patients with renal cell carcinoma. They looked at the downstream markers of IFNγ activation β2 microglobulin and neopterin. Using these two markers, they showed robust activation by IFNγ following the first dose, but there was tachyphylaxis at high doses (500 μg) and daily administration. In contrast, alternate day administration and lower dose levels (100 μg) retained responsiveness. These data were used to determine the dosing regimens that were used in the CGD trial (50 μg/m^2 subcutaneously three times weekly). Subsequently, Ahlin et al. (149) examined the effects of 50 μg/m^2 and 100 μg/m^2 IFNγ on neutrophil responses in CGD. They examined two small, randomized groups of patients with CGD of several different genotypes. Doses were given on two successive days, and effects were monitored over 18 days. There was some induction of superoxide production in some patients in both groups, an increase in CD64 (FcγR1) expression that was somewhat dose dependent, and a modest increase in aspergillicidal activity that was slightly greater at the higher dose than the lower one. Unfortunately, the authors did not address the effect of long-term therapy. Therefore, the suggestion that there is a prophylactic or long-term therapeutic benefit to the higher dose is hard to confirm.

Jaffee et al. (68) administered IFNγ by aerosol to normal volunteers over a range of doses up to 1 mg for up to 2 weeks. The volunteers showed good tolerance of the drug and good local induction of macrophage activation. Jaffee et al. (68) looked at peripheral blood monocyte activation simultaneous with aerosol administration and found no induction of IP-10, an IFNγ-responsive chemokine. In contrast, using peripherally administered IFNγ, they found no induction of pulmonary macrophage IP-10. These data were taken to show immunologic selectivity of pulmonary and systemic administration regimens. However, whether these data can be extrapolated to patients with ongoing pulmonary inflammation or those receiving chronic therapy in either compartment (pulmonary or systemic) is still unknown.

Kunzmann et al. (150) showed the expansion of γ/δ T cells in patients receiving the aminobisphosphonates alendronate, ibandronate, and pamidronate. This in turn leads to a significant increase in IFNγ production *in vitro*, if not *in vivo*, and may have unanticipated clinical implications for those being treated with these drugs.

Trauma and Burns

Following the demonstration that IFNγ activates phagocytes to increased production of superoxide and general activation, there was great interest in the ability of IFNγ to reduce infection rates in several settings in which infection remains the major cause of morbidity and mortality. Hershman et al. (151) showed that cell surface HLA-DR, a marker of monocyte activation, is significantly reduced in patients with severe injury or trauma. They corrected this abnormality in HLA-DR display by incubation of blood from injured patients *in vitro* with IFNγ.

Polk et al. (152) conducted a study of 213 trauma patients at high risk for infection who received either placebo or IFNγ 100 μg subcutaneously daily for 10 days. IFNγ significantly increased monocyte HLA-DR antigen expression and outcome predictive score. Although there were fewer severe complications and fewer deaths in the IFNγ arm, these differences were not statistically significant. This tantalizing result suggested that IFNγ might be useful in patients with severe trauma, but required a larger and perhaps differently structured trial to be proven.

To address these issues, Dries et al. (153) conducted a large multicenter, double-blinded, randomized controlled trial in 416 patients with a longer treatment arm (21 days). In this study, there was a significant benefit conferred by IFNγ treatment in terms of the number of deaths due to infection and deaths overall, but this effect was dominated by the results of one center, leaving the overall utility of IFNγ in this setting not proven. Mock et al. (154) discussed the shortcoming of the major trials of IFNγ in trauma and opined that there were severe systematic flaws in the studies that precluded successful conclusions as to the efficacy of IFNγ.

Kox et al. (155) treated patients with sepsis or systemic inflammatory response syndrome (SIRS) with IFNγ 100 μg sc daily if they had <30% of monocytes expressing HLA-DR. They continued IFNγ until expression was >50% for 3 consecutive days. Eight patients responded within the first 24 hours, and the remainder took 2 to 3 days. IFNγ was associated with early rises in plasma TNF and IL-6 levels, but there was no clear effect on mortality or morbidity.

To explore the possible benefits of IFNγ prophylaxis in burns, Wasserman et al. (156) conducted a randomized, double-blind, placebo-controlled, phase III multicenter trial at 23 European burn centers. They enrolled 216 patients with severe burns to receive either IFNγ 100 μg subcutaneously daily for up to 90 days or placebo. They found no differences between the groups in terms of death, infection rate, duration of intensive care stay or overall hospitalization, or scar formation.

The ability of IFNγ to influence scar formation has been of great interest in view of the data regarding IFNγ's ability to downregulate collagen synthesis (157). There have been numerous small studies of IFNγ in the prevention of keloid formation (158–160). These studies for the most part have used intralesional IFNγ at doses of 10 to 100 μg three times weekly. Of note, in the study by Granstein et al. (159), the design called for simultaneous injection of keloids on patients at two sites—one to receive IFNγ, the other placebo. Only the IFNγ sites showed any significant alteration, indicating that there is not adequate systemic effect of IFNγ to affect distant lesions. This may in part explain the lack of effect of IFNγ on scarring in the study by Wasserman et al. (156) in severe burns. Similar effects of IFNα on collagen synthesis and keloid formation have been reported (160,161).

Collagen Vascular Diseases

Although the collagen vascular diseases are not clearly infections or are not currently clearly known to be so, they are diseases in which infections occur with a higher frequency than in the general population, due in large part to aggressive therapies, especially those that induce immunosuppression. The question of the suitability of IFNγ therapy in these diseases arises, and it is useful to review the literature here in brief to clarify the effects of this proinflammatory cytokine in these inflammatory diseases.

There have been numerous studies of IFNγ in rheumatoid arthritis. In general, they have shown a modest benefit, at doses ranging from 50 to 100 μg subcutaneously daily up to twice weekly (162–165). However, not all studies have shown benefit (166). In particular, there has been greater demonstration of benefit in Europe than in the United States. More importantly than the demonstration of benefit for our purpose is that there was no demonstration of exacerbation in any of these large studies. Cannon et al. (167) conducted a 5-year follow-up on 70 rheumatoid arthritis patients who completed a 12-week multicenter double-blind placebo-controlled trial of IFNγ and then entered a continuation protocol. Eight patients continued IFNγ for 5 years, 47 discontinued IFNγ for lack of efficacy, and three developed suspected adverse drug reactions.

Although the most common side effects in most studies were transient fever and transient flu-like symptoms, there have been more severe complications in patients initially thought to have rheumatoid arthritis. Machold and Smolen (168) reported a life-threatening flare of SLE in a patient who had been erroneously thought to have rheumatoid arthritis. Graninger et al. (169) noted the development of SLE in a patient with rheumatoid arthritis after over 3 years of IFNγ therapy. Therefore, IFNγ is safe to use in rheumatoid arthritis but may exacerbate SLE.

The ability of IFNγ to inhibit fibroblast collagen synthesis led to studies of the effect of IFNγ in progressive systemic sclerosis (scleroderma). Rosenbloom et al. (170) showed that IFNγ was able to reduce collagen production from fibroblasts derived from scleroderma patients. This led to a series of studies over the ensuing decade to evaluate the possible benefit of IFNγ in scleroderma. Kahan et al. (171) enrolled 10 scleroderma patients in a dose escalation study of IFNγ, going from 10 μg/day to 100 μg/day. After 6 months, they observed significant improvement in multiple parameters, including skin, oral opening, joint range of motion, dysphagia, and creatinine clearance. A significant decrease in peripheral blood leukocytes was noted. Hein et al. (172) enrolled 14 patients with scleroderma, nine of whom completed the study, at 50 μg IFNγ subcutaneously three times weekly for 12 months. They found a significant improvement in skin score and in pulmonary fibrosis, as measured by improved blood gasses on IFNγ. Dysphagia, Raynaud's phenomenon, and cardiac involvement were not affected, and there were no serious toxicities.

Freundlich et al. (173) enrolled 18 patients with rapidly progressive scleroderma in an 18-week open-label dose ranging trial; 14 patients completed at least 16 weeks of the study. Patients received intramuscular IFNγ three times weekly at either 100 or 500 μg/m^2. The mean skin thickness decreased significantly, and three patients experienced disease remission after discontinuation of drug. Of the five patients who withdrew, three developed renal crisis. However, in a randomized controlled multicenter trial, Grassegger et al. (174) found overall skin improvement in more severe patients as well as improvements in mouth opening without any renal crises. Interestingly, in their study, the quality-of-life measures increased in the control group but not the IFNγ group.

Narayanan et al. (175) showed an effect of IFNγ *in vitro* on lung fibroblast collagen synthesis and mRNA transcription from normals and those with pulmonary fibrosis. They found that most cell lines derived from lung responded to IFNγ, and the effect lasted for at least 48 hours after withdrawal of IFNγ from the media. This observation as well as those listed above led to a trial of IFNγ in patients with idiopathic pulmonary fibrosis. Ziesche et al. (176) conducted a 12-month trial of oral prednisolone alone compared to prednisolone plus IFNγ 200 μg subcutaneously three times weekly in patients with idiopathic pulmonary fibrosis unresponsive to steroids or other immunosuppressives. Pulmonary function, as measured by total lung capacity and arterial oxygenation, increased significantly in the IFNγ plus prednisolone group, and the same parameters decreased significantly in the prednisolone-alone group. IFNγ toxicities such as fever, chills, and myalgias were transient and resolved within the first 3 months.

In summary, IFNγ has marked effects on collagen synthesis *in vitro*, which make it attractive for diseases in which fibrosis is a major complication. For some of these syndromes, systemic therapy is adequate (e.g., pulmonary fibrosis, scleroderma), whereas for others (e.g., keloid formation), local injection may be needed. IFNγ does not appear to worsen rheumatoid arthritis but does exacerbate SLE. In this regard, it is interesting to note that IL-12 is thought to exacerbate rheumatoid arthritis, further illustrating that, although IL-12 potently induces IFNγ, it is also induces numerous other pathways that may have distinct toxicities.

Leishmaniasis

The critical role of active infection in the suppression of cytokine infection was clearly demonstrated by Carvalho et al. (177) in their classic experiments involving patients with active visceral leishmaniasis. Whereas mitogen-stimulated IFNγ production was normal in patients with active visceral leishmaniasis, IFNγ production in response to Leishmania antigen was absent during active disease, but normalized after successful chemotherapy. This observation suggested that restoration of IFNγ systemically during visceral leishmaniasis might be therapeutic. Subsequently, Murray et al. (178) demonstrated synergy of IFNγ and sodium stibogluconate (Pentostam) in *Leishmania donovani*–infected human macrophages *in vitro* and in mice *in vivo*.

These observations *in vitro* and in mice led to the critical trail Badaro et al. (179) of IFNγ plus pentostam in patients with visceral leishmaniasis who had been refractory to pentostam alone. Six of eight patients with refractory visceral leishmaniasis responded to treatment with IFNγ at doses of 100 to 400 μg/m^2/day in addition to pentostam 20 mg/kg/day for 10 to 40 days. This was expanded with nine treatment-naive patients with severe visceral leishmaniasis, eight of whom responded to treatment with IFNγ plus pentostam. Responders had marked improvement in symptoms, anemia, leukopenia, weight gain, decreased spleen size, and organisms in splenic aspirates. No relapse or recurrence was seen in up to 8 months. The major toxicity was fever. Badaro and Johnson (180) expanded this experience to include South American patients with diffuse cutaneous leishmaniasis.

Sundar et al. (181) treated 15 Indian patients with visceral leishmaniasis who were refractory to conventional therapy with 30 days of pentostam and IFNγ. In the remaining 13 patients, IFNγ plus antimony treatment was associated with daily fever but no other adverse reactions. Two patients withdrew for intolerance and subsequently died. The remaining 13 patients were cured, and this appeared to be durable. Sundar et al. (182) then went on to show that, in previously untreated patients with visceral leishmaniasis, IFNγ plus antimonials dramatically shortened the time to parasitologic cure compared to antimonials alone (63% versus 10%, respectively, at 10 days). Further, Sundar et al. (182) had 100% response in the combined therapy group, all of whom had durable cures. This was a level of response higher than in the conventional monotherapy arm. Sundar and Murray (183) tested the efficacy of IFNγ monotherapy in visceral leishmaniasis in nine patients. After 20 days of IFNγ therapy, four patients had no parasitologic change. In the other five patients, parasite loads in splenic aspirates declined about 75% but did not resolve completely. Therefore, although IFNγ was able to induce some degree of clearing, it was unable to execute a cure as monotherapy. Similar results have been seen in mycobacterial infections. Sundar et al. (184) went on to show equivalence of short-course (15 days) therapy with IFNγ plus stibogluconate to long-course combined therapy (30 days) and long-course conventional monotherapy with stibogluconate (30 days).

In summary, active visceral leishmaniasis is associated with antigen-specific immune suppression, but the cells are still IFNγ responsive. IFNγ has a potent synergistic effect on therapy with conventional antimonials, but is of relatively modest effect in the absence of concurrently administered antiparasitics. The mechanisms involved in this activity are unclear, but increased intracellular concentration of antiparasitics appears to be important.

Mycobacterial Infections

Although the mechanisms involved in IFNγ control of mycobacterial infection are unknown, its role in regulating mycobacterial growth is widely accepted. The recognition of hypersusceptibility to nontuberculous mycobacterial infections in patients with mutations affecting IFNγ synthesis or response serves as a final human proof of the central role of IFNγ in mycobacterial control.

Appelberg and Orme (185) demonstrated a mycobacteriostatic effect of IFNγ in mouse cells *in vitro* and suggested that its main effect was to enhance the acidification of mycobacteria-containing vesicles. Toxic oxygen radicals appeared unnecessary for control of *Mycobacterium bovis* infection in mouse bone marrow cells *in vitro* (186). Mice lacking the NADPH oxidase, and hence unable to produce phagocyte superoxide in response to infection, were no more susceptible to *Mycobacterium avium* infection than wild-type animals (187). For *Mycobacterium tuberculosis*, the NADPH oxidase appears to be more important for early but not late control of infection in the lung (188,189). However, nitric oxide (NO) is critically important for mycobacterial control in mice (188). Human cells have given inconsistent results in terms of IFNγ-activated mycobacterial killing *in vitro*: some studies show that IFNγ has mycobactericidal and mycobacteriostatic activities (190), but others do not (191). In one study, IFNγ enhanced the growth of *M. avium* complex (MAC) in macrophages (192).

IFNγ knockout mice develop widespread tuberculosis with very poor granulomatous response and die rapidly (193,194). The surprising inability of administered IFNγ to restore normal resistance to tuberculosis suggested that IFNγ might play a critical role in immune development or that systemically administered IFNγ does not activate critical local defenses as well as IFNγ supplied by adjacent or contiguous T or NK cells (193). Similar susceptibilities were seen in IFNγR-deficient mice (195) and in mice lacking the IFNγ-induced interferon regulatory factor–1 (IRF-1; 196). Similar hypersusceptibility to MAC infection was reported in IFNγ-deficient mice (187). In wild-type mice infected with MAC, elevated prostaglandin E_2 production (an inhibitor of macrophage function) was successfully downregulated by IFNγ leading to enhanced mycobacterial clearance (197).

Hussain et al. (198) found that soon after MAC infection of the mouse, macrophage levels of IFNγR1 and IFNγR2 begin to decline, followed by inhibition of the ability to activate STAT1. This in turn leads to the decrease of inducibility of many IFNγ-responsive genes (e.g., IRF-1) and a relative inability of the cell to be activated to the antimycobacterial state. Ting et al. (199) showed that *M. tuberculosis* infection of human macrophages blocks certain distal effects of IFNγ, including killing of *Toxoplasma gondii* and induction of FcγRI. *M. tuberculosis* inhibits the association of STAT1 with the transcriptional coactivators CREB binding protein and p300. Irradiated whole organisms, isolated cell walls, and, to a lesser degree, lipoarabinomannan (LAM) have effects similar to those of live organisms. Therefore, in this human macrophage system, *M. tuberculosis* inhibits distal aspects of IFNγ signaling while leaving proximal processes (Jak-STAT interaction) intact.

IFNγ has been used successfully as an adjuvant in the treatment of the three major human mycobacterial infections: *Mycobacterium leprae, M. avium* complex, and *M. tuberculosis*. Nathan et al. (200) first used short-course, low-dose, intradermal IFNγ in the treatment of lepromatous leprosy (1 to 10 μg daily for 3 days) in conjunction with antimycobacterials. Monocyte hydrogen peroxide production was enhanced, granuloma formation increased, local activation markers upregulated, and the cutaneous bacterial burden decreased.

When Sampaio et al. (201) used longer term IFNγ therapy (10 months) in conjunction with antimycobacterials, they noted a rate of erythema nodosum leprosum (ENL), a toxic inflammatory reaction in leprosy that can lead to neuropathy or death, in IFNγ recipients that was much higher than in those receiving antimycobacterials alone (60% versus 17%, respectively). ENL correlated with TNFα message and protein in peripheral blood mononuclear cells and peripheral blood. Thalidomide, long used in the treatment of ENL, decreased TNFα levels in cells and blood through what was thought to be destabilization of TNFα mRNA (202). In an effort to achieve rapid clearance of organisms and prevent ENL, IFNγ was given to patients with lepromatous leprosy in conjunction with thalidomide and antimycobacterial chemotherapy. In this setting, there was no increase in IFNγ-induced clearance of infection over that observed with antimycobacterials alone (203). This indicated that thalidomide modulates the factors that underlie the IFNγ effect on mycobacterial clearance. On the other hand, thalidomide successfully blocked the development of ENL. It remains to reconcile thalidomide's apparent blockade of IFNγ-induced killing of *M. leprae*, on the one hand, and its reported enhancement of IL-12 and IFNγ production in tuberculosis, on the other.

The fundamental causes of ENL are still unknown, but it is clear that ENL is a response to the presence of organisms and does not occur in IFNγ-treated leprosy patients who have previously received antimycobacterial therapy to the point that they are free of bacilli (203). ENL has not been seen in the therapy of other mycobacterial diseases for which long-term IFNγ has been used, suggesting that ENL is leprosy-specific. Haslett et al. (204) have now shown that thalidomide enhances $CD8^+$ T-lymphocyte proliferation as well as IL-12 and IFNγ production. Bekker et al. (205) used thalidomide in patients with tuberculosis and HIV, and showed enhancement of antigen-specific proliferative responses, preferentially through $CD8^+$ T-lymphocytes. The clinical trials in tuberculosis showed little, if any, effect of thalidomide on TNFα levels. These findings leave the mechanism by which thalidomide affects ENL somewhat unclear.

In all of the studies to date in leprosy, IFNγ reduced bacterial load only when combined with antimycobacterials: when used alone, it induced immunological changes but did not significantly affect clearing of the infection. This is similar to the effects seen with IFNγ monotherapy of leishmaniasis by Sundar and Murray (183). Both IFNγ and TNFα significantly increase the intracellular concentration of the macrolide antibiotic azithromycin, a mechanism that may be relevant for other antibiotics as well (206).

Squires et al. (207,208) were the first to use IFNγ in the treatment of MAC infection. They treated six MAC-bacteremic AIDS patients with IFNγ with or without concurrent antimycobacterials. The treatment trials lasted up to 6 weeks. In those patients who received IFNγ plus antimycobacterials, there was a clear decline in mycobacteremia, but when IFNγ was used without concurrent antimycobacterials, there was no change in bacterial counts. After discontinuation of IFNγ, bacterial counts rebounded. These results were independent of $CD4^+$ T-lymphocyte counts, indicating that IFNγ activity did not require normal numbers of $CD4^+$ T cells.

Patients in whom disseminated nontuberculous mycobacteria (NTM) infection occurs in the absence of HIV infection are a group with heterogeneous abnormalities in IFNγ generation associated with abnormal IL-12 production (209), idiopathic $CD4^+$ T-lymphocytopenia (210), and mutations in the IFNγ or IL-12 receptors (reviewed in 110). All of these patients share the *in vitro* phenotype of low mitogen-stimulated IFNγ production from peripheral blood mononuclear cells. In patients with refractory MAC or other NTM infections and intact IFNγ receptors, including the ADIFNγR1, IFNγ has produced very favorable results, with cure rates of up to 60% (210 and S.M. Holland, unpublished observations, 2001). Prolonged IFNγ therapy (>1 year) may be needed in some cases.

Numerous patients with autosomal recessive, complete defects in the IFNγR have been identified and reported, and there have been suggestions of IFNγ benefit in some of these cases (121,211). However, these benefits have not been demonstrable *in vitro*. In contrast, the patients with autosomal dominant (AD) IFNγR1 mutations respond well to IFNγ therapy (212). Patients with mutations in the IL-12 p40 gene (131) and the IL-12Rβ1 chain (129,130) are also highly responsive to IFNγ therapy, as would be expected. In these patients, the IFNγ receptor pathways are intact, but due to the lack of IL-12–driven IFNγ production, the IFNγ receptor is understimulated.

Chatte et al. (213) used aerosolized IFNγ, 500 μg by nebulizer 3 days/week in a 38-year-old man with silicosis and severe cavitary MAC disease who had failed medical therapy. Aerosolized IFNγ converted his smears to negative, although his cultures persisted positive. With the cessation of aerosolized IFNγ, his sputum smears reverted to their previous level and his disease progressed fatally. This was the first report of aerosolized IFNγ in the treatment of mycobacterial disease. The finding of rapid conversion of sputum to smear negative was remarkable in such a long-term refractory patient. Condos et al. (214) used IFNγ aerosol (500 μg three times weekly for 4 weeks) in five patients with longstanding MDRTB refractory to medical therapy. All five showed clearing of the sputum smears within that month. With this short course of therapy, no cultures converted, and all patients returned to smear positive after cessation of IFNγ. Importantly, no patient worsened during therapy, and there were no significant systemic or local complaints.

Placebo-controlled, randomized, multicenter prospective trials of aerosolized IFNγ are underway in both pulmonary MDRTB and in severe or refractory pulmonary MAC (Intermune Pharmaceuticals; http://www.intermune.com/trials/html/trials1.html). There is very little adverse event experience with aerosol IFNγ, but so far it appears relatively safe. Hemoptysis has been seen in one recipient each with invasive pulmonary fungal disease and severe cavitary mycobacterial disease (S.M. Holland, unpublished observations, 1997), but that cannot be directly attributed to IFNγ. There is very little systemic toxicity from aerosol administration, although we have had one patient with significant arthralgias on aerosol therapy (S.M. Holland, unpublished observations, 1998). We have used subcutaneous IFNγ in patients with refractory pulmonary MAC infections; the best results appeared in patients with noncavitary disease.

The overall experience with IFNγ and tuberculosis is limited. Raad et al. (215) reported a patient with acute lymphocytic leukemia in remission with biopsy-proven MDRTB involving the brain and spinal cord that was steroid dependent due to infection-related edema. Subcutaneous IFNγ allowed rapid reduction in steroid dose and led to cure without any exacerbation of CNS inflammation. The ability of IFNγ to induce a cure without an exacerbation of local inflammation is encouraging in terms of its safety in the treatment of inflammatory diseases. This result was somewhat presaged by the experience in CGD, in which there was no exacerbation of inflammatory conditions (141). Therefore, IFNγ appears well tolerated in both CNS and severe pulmonary MDRTB in these small series. Systemic IFNγ, in addition to antimycobacterials, can effect a cure of nontuberculous infections when used for prolonged courses, and aerosolized IFNγ can convert sputa in short periods.

For patients with known or suspected mutations in the IFNγ receptors, the advisability of IFNγ therapy depends on whether the specific mutation is complete, partial, or dominant. Patients with complete ARIFNγR1 or complete ARIFNγR2 deficiency demonstrate absolute refractoriness to IFNγ stimulation *in vitro* and *in vivo*. In contrast, patients with partial defects, whether in IFNγR1 or IFNγR2, show *in vitro* response to addition of IFNγ at levels 10- to 100-fold higher than normals. Patients with the dominant forms of IFNγR1 deficiency show attenuated IFNγ responsiveness *in vitro* at higher doses. IFNγ therapy *in vivo* is clearly effective in patients with ADIFNγR1 deficiency, even at the standard 50 $\mu g/m^2$ dose. In some cases of ADIFNγR1 deficiency that are slow to respond, higher doses may be effective (S. M. Holland, unpublished observations, 2001).

CONCLUSIONS

The mechanisms by which any of the interferons perform their desired effects are still shrouded and obscure, in large part as a reflection of our persistent ignorance of fundamental aspects of microbial susceptibility and host defense. Even though we now have incontrovertible proof that IFNγ is necessary for mycobacterial control, we still do not know why. This ignorance in turn leaves open numerous hypotheses about mechanism of action in certain disease states. However, our areas of ignorance notwithstanding, it is clear that the interferons are critical components of normal host response and that they can be therapeutically manipulated over a wide range of diseases, from cancers to MS to tuberculosis (Table 10.1). It makes the most sense to push forward simultaneously on the basic and the therapeutic fronts, with a vigilant eye on the convergence of information that will lead to deeper understanding of these critical components of host defense.

Table 10-1. *Licensed Therapeutic Interferons, United States*

Interferon	Manufacturer	Source	Size	Licensed indications[2]	Dose[1]
Interferon α preparations					
IFNα-2a	(Roferon-A; Roche)	*E. coli*	165 aa 19 kD	Hepatitis C Hairy cell leukemia AIDS related KS Early Ph+ CML	3 MIU TIW 3 MIU daily 36 MIU daily 9 MIU daily
IFNα-2b	(Intron A; Schering)	*E. coli*	19 kD	Chronic Hepatitis C Chronic Hepatitis B Hairy cell leukemia Malignant melanoma Follicular lymphoma Condyloma accuminata AIDS related KS	3 MIU TIW 5 MIU daily 2 MIU/m^2 TIW 20 MIU/m^2 IV/D 5 MIU TIW 1 MIU IL TIW 30 MIU/m^2 TIW
IFNα-2b+ Ribavirin	(Rebetron; Schering)	*E. coli*	19 kD	Chronic Hepatitis C	3 MIU TIW combined with ribavirin twice daily
IFN alfacon-1 (consensus IFN)	(Infergen; Amgen)	*E. coli*	166 aa 19 kD	Chronic Hepatitis C	9 μg TIW
IFNα-N3	(Alferon N; Interferon Sciences)	pooled human leuko-cytes	~166 aa 16–27 kD	Condyloma accuminata	250,000 IU BIW
Interferon β preparations					
IFNβ-1a	(Avonex; Biogen)	CHO cells	166 aa 22.5 kD	Relapsing MS	30 μg IM weekly
IFNβ-1b	(Betaseron; Berlex)	*E. coli* (cys17 ser)	165 aa 18.5 kD	Relapsing-remitting MS	250 μg alternate days
Interferon γ preparations					
IFNγ-1b	(Actimmune; InterMune)	*E. coli*	140 aa	Chronic granulomatous disease	50 μg/m^2 TIW*
			16.5 kD	Severe osteopetrosis	50 μg/m^2 TIW*

*equivalent to 1MIU/m^2

KS, Kaposi's sarcoma; MS, multiple sclerosis; QD, daily; BIW, twice weekly; TIW, three times weekly; MIU, million international units; aa, amino acids; kD, kilodalton; CHO, Chinese Hamster Ovary; IL, intralesional; IM, intramuscular; IV, intravenous.

[1]Dose reflects the initial (induction) doses used in various regimens and are often lower for maintainance. Note the extremely broad dose ranges for different applications. Certain preparations come in several different dose vials, so care must be taken in the writing of prescriptions and the drawing up of doses. All dosage is subcutaneous except where stated.

[2]As of January, 2001.

REFERENCES

1. Nagano Y, Kojima Y. Pouvoir immunisant du virus vaccinal inactive par des rayons ultraviolets. *C R Soc Biol (Paris)* 1954;148:1700–1702.
2. Isaacs A, Lindemann J. Virus interferone. I: The interferons. *Proc R Soc Lond (Biol)* 1957;147:258–267.
3. David M. Transcription factors in interferon signaling. *Pharmacol Ther* 1995;65:149–161.

4. Nguyen H, Hiscott J, Pitha PM. The growing family of interferon regulatory factors. *Cytokine Growth Factor Rev* 1997;8:293–312.
5. Baron S, Tyring SK, Fleischmann WR Jr, et al. The interferons. Mechanisms of action and clinical applications. *JAMA* 1991;266:1375–1383.
6. Schindler C, Darnell JE, Jr. Transcriptional responses to polypeptide ligands: The JAK-STAT pathway. *Annu Rev Biochem* 1995;64:621–651.
7. Rogge L, Barberis-Maino L, Biffi M, et al. Selective expression of an interleukin-12 receptor component by human T helper 1 cells. *J Exp Med* 1997;185:825–831.
8. Domanski P, Colamonici OR. The type-I interferon receptor. The long and short of it. *Cytokine Growth Factor Rev* 1996;7:143–151.
9. Olopade, OI, Bohlander SK, Pomykala H, et al. Mapping of the shortest region of overlap of deletions of the short arm of chromosome 9 associated with human neoplasia. *Genomics* 1992;14:437–443.
10. Diaz MO, Bohlander S, Allen G. Nomenclature of the human interferon genes. *J Interferon Cytokine Res* 1996; 16:179–180.
11. Fountain JW, Karayiorgou M, Taruscio D, et al. Genetic and physical map of the interferon region on chromosome 9p. *Genomics* 1992;14:105–112.
12. Siegal FP, Kadowaki N, Shodell M, et al. The nature of the principal type 1 interferon-producing cells in human blood. *Science* 1999;284:1835–1837.
13. Gabriele L, Phung J, Fukumoto J, et al. Regulation of apoptosis in myeloid cells by interferon consensus sequence-binding protein. *J Exp Med* 1999;190:411–421.
14. Schmidt M, Nagel S, Proba J, et al. Lack of interferon consensus sequence binding protein (ICSBP) transcripts in human myeloid leukemias. *Blood* 1998;91:22–29.
15. Akiyama H, Maruyama T, Uetake T, et al. Systemic infection due to atypical mycobacteria in patients with chronic myelogenous leukemia. *Rev Infect Dis* 1991;3:815–818.
16. Rodig SJ, Meraz MA, White JM, et al. Disruption of the Jak1 gene demonstrates obligatory and nonredundant roles of the Jaks in cytokine-induced biologic responses. *Cell* 1998;93:373–383.
17. McRae BL, Semnani RT, Hayes MP, et al. Type I IFNs inhibit human dendritic cell IL-12 production and Th1 cell development. *J Immunol* 1998;160:4298–4304.
18. Fantuzzi G, Reed DA, Dinavello CA. IL-12 induced IFN-gamma is dependent on easpase-l processing of the IL-18 precursor. *J Clin Invest* 1999;104:761–767.
19. Guillemard E, Varano B, Belardelli F, et al. Inhibitory activity of constitutive nitric oxide on the expression of alpha/beta interferon genes in murine peritoneal macrophages. *J Virol* 1999;73:7328–7333.
20. Farr B, Gwaltney JM Jr, Hayden FG, et al. Human polymorphonuclear neutrophil functions are unaffected by human interferon-alpha$_2$. *Infect Immun* 1983;42:1195–1197.
21. Symons JA, Alcami A, Smith GL. Vaccinia virus encodes a soluble type I interferon receptor of novel structure and broad species specificity. *Cell* 1995;81:551–560.
22. Liptakova H, Kontsekova E, Alcami A, et al. Analysis of an interaction between the soluble vaccinia virus-coded type I interferon (IFN)–receptor and human IFN-alpha$_1$ and IFN-alpha$_2$. *Virology* 1997;232:86–90.
23. Alcami A, Symons JA, Smith GL. The vaccinia virus soluble alpha/beta interferon (IFN) receptor binds to the cell surface and protects cells from the antiviral effects of IFN. *J Virol* 2000;74:11230–11239.
24. Muller U, Steinhoff U, Reis LF, et al. Functional role of type I and type II interferons in antiviral defense. *Science* 1994;264:1918–1921.
25. van den Broek MF, Muller U, Huang S, et al. Immune defence in mice lacking type I and/or type II interferon receptors. *Immunol Rev* 1995;148:5–18.
26. Weck KE, Dal Canto AJ, Gould JD, et al. Murine gamma-herpesvirus 68 causes severe large-vessel arteritis in mice lacking interferon-gamma responsiveness: a new model for virus-induced vascular disease. *Nat Med* 1997;3:1346–1353.
27. Virelizier JL, Lenoir G, Griscelli C. Persistent Epstein-Barr virus infection in a child with hypergammaglobulinaemia and immunoblastic proliferation associated with a selective defect in interferon secretion. *Lancet* 1978;II:231–234.
28. Lipinski M, Virelizier JL, Tursz T, et al. Natural killer and killer cell activities in patients with primary immunodeficiencies or defects in immune interferon production. *Eur J Immun* 1980;10:246–249.
29. Virelizier JL, Griscelli C. Defaut selectif de secretion d'interferon associe a un deficit d'activite cytotoxique naturelle. *Arch Franc Pediatr* 1981;38:77–81.
30. Isaacs D, Clarke JR, Tyrrell DAJ, et al. Deficient production of leucocyte interferon (interferon-alpha) *in vitro* and *in vivo* in children with recurrent respiratory tract infections. *Lancet* 1981;II:950–952.
31. Biron CA, Byron KS, Sullivan JL. Severe herpesvirus infections in an adolescent without natural killer cells. *N Engl J Med* 1989;320:1731–1735.
32. Neustock P, Kruse A, Bock S, et al. Deficient interferon-alpha response of newborns in comparison to adults. *Lymphokine Cytokine Res* 1993;12:109–114.
33. Hourihane J, Hodges E, Smith J, et al. Interferon alpha treatment of molluscum contagiosum in immunodeficiency. *Arch Dis Child* 1999;80:77–79.
34. Finter NB, Chapman S, Dowd P, et al. The use of interferon-alpha in virus infections. *Drugs* 1991;42:749–765.
35. Heathcote J. Antiviral therapy for patients with chronic hepatitis C. *Semin Liver Dis* 2000;20:185–199.
36. Powell J. Update on hemangiomas and vascular malformations. *Curr Opin Pediatr* 1999;11:457–463.

37. Sawyers CL. Chronic myeloid leukemia. *N Engl J Med* 1999;340:1330–1340.
38. Hayden FG, Gwaltney JM Jr. Intranasal interferon-alpha$_2$ for prevention of rhinovirus infection and illness. *J Infect Dis* 1983;148:543–550.
39. Hayden FG, Albrecht JK, Kaiser DL, et al. Prevention of natural colds by contact prophylaxis with intranasal alpha$_2$-interferon. *N Engl J Med* 1986;314:71–75.
40. Sperber SJ, Levine PA, Sorrentino JV, et al. Ineffectiveness of recombinant interferon-beta serine nasal drops for prophylaxis of natural colds. *J Infect Dis* 1989;160:700–705.
41. Schafer TW, Lieberman M, Cohen M, et al. Interferon administered orally: protection of neonatal mice from lethal virus challenge. *Science* 1972;176:1326–1327.
42. Cummins JM, Beilharz MW, Krakowka S. Oral use of interferon. *J Interferon Cytokine Res* 1999;19:853.
43. Moore BR, Krakowka S, Cummins JM, et al. Changes in airway inflammatory cell populations in standardbred racehorses after interferon-alpha administration. *Vet Immunol Immunopathol* 1996;49:347–358.
44. Moore BR, Krakowka S, Mcvey DS, et al. Inflammatory markers in bronchoalveolar lavage fluid of standardbred racehorses with inflammatory airway disease: response to interferon-alpha. *Equine Vet J* 1997;29: 142–147.
45. Cummins JM, Guthrie D, Hutcheson DP, et al. Natural human interferon-alpha administered orally as a treatment of bovine respiratory disease complex. *J Interferon Cytokine Res* 1999;19:907–910.
46. Rockley PF, Tyring SK. Interferons alpha, beta and gamma therapy of anogenital human papillomavirus infections. *Pharmacol Ther* 1995;65:265–287.
47. Avidano MA, Singleton GT. Adjuvant drug strategies in the treatment of recurrent respiratory papillomatosis. *Otolaryngol Head Neck Surg* 1995;112:197–202.
48. Hoofnagle JH, Mullen KD, Jones DB, et al. Treatment of chronic non-A, non-B hepatitis with recombinant human alpha interferon: a preliminary report. *N Engl J Med* 1986;315:1575–1578.
49. Davis GL, Balart LA, Schiff ER, et al. Treatment of chronic hepatitis C with recombinant interferon alpha. A multicenter randomized controlled study. *N Engl J Med* 1989;321:1501–1506.
50. DiBisceglie AM, Martin P, Kassianides C, et al. Recombinant interferon alpha therapy for chronic hepatitis C. A randomized, double-bind, placebo-controlled trial. *N Engl J Med* 1989;321:1506–1510.
51. Poynard T, Bedossa P, Chevallier M, et al. A comparison of three interferon-alpha$_{2b}$regimens for the long-term treatment of chronic non-A, non-B hepatitis. Multicenter Study Group. *N Engl J Med* 1995;332:1457–1462.
52. Poynard T, Leroy V, Cohard M, et al. Meta-analysis of interferon randomized trials in the treatment of viral hepatitis C: effects of dose and duration. *Hepatology* 1996;24:778–789.
53. McHutchison JG, Gordon S, Schiff ER, et al. Interferon-alpha$_{2b}$ monotherapy versus interferon-alpha$_{2b}$ plus ribavirin as initial treatment for chronic hepatitis C: Results of a U.S. multicenter randomized controlled study. *N Engl J Med* 1998;339:1485–1492.
54. Poynard T, Marcellin P, Lee S, et al. Randomised trial of interferon alpha$_{2b}$ plus ribavirin for 48 weeks or for 24 weeks versus interferon alpha$_{2b}$ plus placebo for 48 weeks for treatment of chronic infection with hepatitis C virus. *Lancet* 1998;352:1426–1432.
55. Davis GL, Esteban-Mur R, Rustgi V, et al. Recombinant interferon alpha$_{2b}$ (Intron A) alone or in combination with ribavirin (Rebetol) for retreatment of interferon relapse in chronic hepatitis C. *N Engl J Med* 1998;339: 1493–1499.
56. Zeuzem S, Feinman SV, Rasenack J, et al. PEG-interferon-alpha$_{2a}$ in patients with chronic hepatitis C. *N Engl J Med* 2000;343:1666–1672.
57. Heathcote EJ, Shiffman ML, Cooksley WG, et al. PEG-interferon-alpha$_{2a}$ in patients with chronic hepatitis C and cirrhosis. *N Engl J Med* 2000;343:1673–1680.
58. Heathcote J. Consensus interferon: a novel interferon for the treatment of hepatitis C. *J Viral Hepat* 1998; 5(suppl 1):13–18.
59. Heathcote EJ, James S, Mullen KD, et al. Chronic hepatitis C virus patients with breakthroughs during interferon treatment can successfully be retreated with consensus interferon. The Consensus Interferon Study Group. *Hepatology* 1999;30:562–566.
60. Perrillo RP. The management of chronic hepatitis B. *Am J Med* 1994;96:34S–39S.
61. Perrillo RP, Mason AL. Therapy for hepatitis B virus infection. *Gastroenterol Clin North Am* 1994;23:581–601.
62. Liaw YF, Lin SM, Chen TJ, et al. Beneficial effect of prednisolone withdrawal followed by human lymphoblastoid interferon on the treatment of chronic type B hepatitis in Asians: a randomized controlled trial. *J Hepatol* 1994;20:175–180.
63. Lin SM, Sheen IS, Chien RN, et al. Long-term beneficial effect of interferon therapy in patients with chronic hepatitis B virus infection. *Hepatology* 1999;29:971–975.
64. Liaw YF, Tsai SL, Chien RN, et al. Prednisolone priming enhances Th1 response and efficacy of subsequent lamivudine therapy in patients with chronic hepatitis B. *Hepatology* 2000;32:604–609.
65. Farrell G. Hepatitis B and antigen seroconversion: effects of lamivudine alone or in combination with interferon alpha. *J Med Virol* 2000;61:374–379.
66. Chien RN, Liaw YF, Atkins M. Pretherapy alanine transaminase level as a determinant for hepatitis B e antigen seroconversion during lamivudine therapy in patients with chronic hepatitis B. Asian Hepatitis Lamivudine Trial Group. *Hepatology* 1999;30:770–774.
67. Giosue S, Casarini M, Ameglio F, et al. Minimal dose of aerosolized interferon-alpha in human subjects: biological consequences and side effects. *Eur Respir J* 1996;9:42–46.

68. Jaffee HA, Buhl R, Mastrangeli A, et al. Organ specific cytokine therapy: local activation of mononuclear phagocytes by delivery of an aerosol of recombinant interferon-gamma to the human lung. *J Clin Invest* 1991; 88:297–302.
69. Giosue S, Casarini M, Alemanno L, et al. Effects of aerosolized interferon-alpha in patients with pulmonary tuberculosis. *Am J Respir Crit Care Med* 1998;158:1156–1162.
70. Giosue S, Casarini M, Ameglio F, et al. Aerosolized interferon-alpha treatment in patients with multi-drug-resistant pulmonary tuberculosis. *Eur Cytokine Netw* 2000;11:99–104.
71. Condos R, Rom WN, Schluger NW. Treatment of multidrug-resistant pulmonary tuberculosis with interferon-gamma via aerosol. *Lancet* 1997;349:1513–1515.
72. Palmero D, Eiguchi K, Rendo P, et al. Phase II trial of recombinant interferon-alpha$_{2b}$ in patients with advanced intractable multidrug-resistant pulmonary tuberculosis: long-term follow-up. *Int J Tuberc Lung Dis* 1999;3:214–218.
73. Noseworthy JH, Lucchinetti C, Rodriguez M, et al. Multiple sclerosis. *N Engl J Med* 2000;343:938–952.
74. Paty DW, Li DK, UBC MS/MRI Study Group, IFNB Multiple Sclerosis Study Group. Interferon-beta$_{1b}$ is effective in relapsing-remitting multiple sclerosis. II. MRI analysis results of a multicenter, randomized, double-blind, placebo-controlled trial. *Neurology* 1993;43:662–667.
75. The IFNB Multiple Sclerosis Study Group, University of British Columbia MS/MRI Analysis Group. Interferon-beta$_{1b}$ in the treatment of multiple sclerosis: final outcome of the randomized controlled trial. *Neurology* 1995;45:1277–1285.
76. Miller DH, Molyneux PD, Barker GJ, et al. Effect of interferon-beta$_{1b}$ on magnetic resonance imaging outcomes in secondary progressive multiple sclerosis: results of a European multicenter, randomized, double-blind, placebo-controlled trial. European Study Group on interferon-beta$_{1b}$ in secondary progressive multiple sclerosis. *Ann Neurol* 1999;46:850–859.
77. Molyneux PD, Kappos L, Polman C, et al. The effect of interferon-beta$_{1b}$ treatment on MRI measures of cerebral atrophy in secondary progressive multiple sclerosis. *Brain* 2000;123:2256–2263.
78. Jacobs LD, Cookfair DL, Rudick RA, et al. Intramuscular interferon-beta$_{1a}$ for disease progression in relapsing multiple sclerosis. The Multiple Sclerosis Collaborative Research Group. *Ann Neurol* 1996;39:285–294.
79. Li DK, Paty DW. Magnetic resonance imaging results of the PRISMS trial: a randomized, double-blind, placebo-controlled study of interferon-beta$_{1a}$ in relapsing-remitting multiple sclerosis. Prevention of relapses and disability by interferon-beta$_{1a}$subcutaneously in multiple sclerosis. *Ann Neurol* 1999;46:197–206.
80. The Once Weekly Interferon for MS Study Group. Evidence of interferon-beta$_{1a}$ dose response in relapsing-remitting MS. *Neurology* 1999;53:679–686.
81. Rudick RA, Simonian NA, Alam JA, et al. Incidence and significance of neutralizing antibodies to interferon-beta$_{1a}$ in multiple sclerosis. Multiple Sclerosis Collaborative Research Group. *Neurology* 1998;50:1266–1272.
82. Rice GPA, Paszner B, Oger J, et al. The evolution of neutralizing antibodies in multiple sclerosis patients treated with interferon-β_{1b}. *Neurology* 1999;52:1277–1279.
83. Chofflon M. Recombinant human interferon-beta in relapsing-remitting multiple sclerosis: a review of the major clinical trials. *Eur J Neurol* 2000;7:369–380.
84. Yong VW, SChabot S, Stuve O, et al. Interferon-beta in the treatment of multiple sclerosis: mechanisms of action. *Neurology* 1998;51:682–689.
85. Rothuizen LE, Buclin T, Spertini F, et al. Influence of interferon-beta$_{1a}$ dose frequency on PBMC cytokine secretion and biological effect markers. *J Neuroimmunol* 1999;99:131–141.
86. Karp CL, Biron CA, Irani DN. Interferon-beta in multiple sclerosis: is IL-12 suppression the keyγ *Immunol Today* 2000;21:24–28.
87. Trojano M, Avolio C, Liuzzi GM, et al. Changes of serum ICAM-1 and MMP-9 induced by rIFNb-1b treatment in relapsing-remitting MS. *Neurology* 1999;53:1402–1408.
88. Bever CT Jr, Rosenberg GA. Matrix metalloproteinases in multiple sclerosis: targets of therapy or markers of injuryγ *Neurology* 1999;53:1380–1381.
89. Walther EU, Hohlfeld R. Multiple sclerosis: side effects of interferon-beta therapy and their management. *Neurology* 1999;53:1622–1627.
90. Sasseville D, Ghamdi WA, Khenaizan SA. Interferon-induced cutaneous necrosis. *J Cutan Med Surg* 1999;3: 320–323.
91. Wang J, Wakeham J, Harkness R, et al. Macrophages are a significant source of type 1 cytokines during mycobacterial infection. *J Clin Invest* 1999;103:1023–1029.
92. Tomura M, Maruo S, Mu J, et al. Differential capacities of $CD4^+$, $CD8^+$, and $CD4^-$ $CD8^-$ T cell subsets to express IL-18 receptor and produce IFN-gamma in response to IL-18. *J Immunol* 1998;160:3759–3765.
93. Mountford AP, Coulson PS, Cheever AW, et al. Interleukin-12 can directly induce T-helper 1 responses in interferon-gamma (IFN-gamma) receptor–deficient mice, but requires IFN-gamma signalling to downregulate T-helper 2 responses. *Immunology* 1999;97:588–594.
94. Boehm U, Klamp T, Groot M, et al. Cellular responses to interferon-γ. *Annu Rev Immunol* 1997;15:749–795.
95. Pien GC, Satoskar AR, Takeda K, et al. Cutting edge: selective IL-18 requirements for induction of compartmental IFN-gamma responses during viral infection. *J Immunol* 2000;165:4787–4791.
96. Humphreys BD, Dubyak GR. Induction of the P2z/P2X7 nucleotide receptor and associated phospholipase D activity by lipopolysaccharide and IFN-gamma in the human THP-1 monocytic cell line. *J Immunol* 1996;157: 5627–5637.

97. Lammas DA, Stober C, Harvey CJ, et al. ATP-induced killing of mycobacteria by human macrophages is mediated by purinergic P2Z(P2X7) receptors. *Immunity* 1997;7:433–444.
98. Murray HW. Current and future clinical applications of interferon-gamma in host antimicrobial defense. *Intensive Care Med* 1996;22(suppl 4):S456–S461.
99. Darnell JE Jr. Studies of IFN-induced transcriptional activation uncover the Jak-Stat pathway. *J Interferon Cytokine Res* 1998;18:549–554.
100. Nistico A, Young NS. Gamma-interferon gene expression in the bone marrow of patients with aplastic anemia. *Ann Intern Med* 1994;120:463–469.
101. Murphy WJ, Welniak LA, Taub DD, et al. Differential effects of the absence of interferon-gamma and IL-4 in acute graft-versus-host disease after allogeneic bone marrow transplantation in mice. *J Clin Invest* 1998;102: 1742–1748.
102. Yang YG, Dey BR, Sergio JJ, et al. Donor-derived interferon-gamma is required for inhibition of acute graft-versus-host disease by interleukin 12. *J Clin Invest* 1998;102:2126–2135.
103. Saleem S, Konieczny BT, Lowry RP, et al. Acute rejection of vascularized heart allografts in the absence of IFN-gamma. *Transplantation* 1996;62:1908–1911.
104. Aguet M, Dembic Z, Merlin G. Molecular cloning and expression of the human interferon-gamma receptor. *Cell* 1988;55:273–280.
105. Bohni R, Hemmi S, Aguet M. Signaling steps involving the cytoplasmic domain of the interferon-gamma receptor alpha-subunit are not species-specific. *J Biol Chem* 1994;269:14541–14545.
106. Hemmi S, Bohni R, Stark G, et al. A novel member of the interferon receptor family complements functionality of the murine interferon-gamma receptor in human cells. *Cell* 1994;76:803–810.
107. Soh J, Donnelly RJ, Kotenko S, et al. Identification and sequence of an accessory factor required for activation of the human interferon-gamma receptor. *Cell* 1994;76:793–802.
108. Bach EA, Szabo SJ, Dighe AS, et al. Ligand-induced autoregulation of IFN-gamma receptor beta chain expression in T helper cell subsets. *Science* 1995;270:1215–1218.
109. Dighe AS, Farrar MA, Schreiber RD. Inhibition of cellular responsiveness to interferon-gamma (IFN-gamma) induced by overexpression of inactive forms of the IFN-gamma receptor. *J Biol Chem* 1993;268: 10645–10653.
110. Dorman SE, Holland SM. Interferon-gamma and interleukin-12 pathway defects and human disease. *Cytokine Growth Factor Rev* 2000;11:321–333.
111. Dalton DK, Pitts-Meek S, Keshav S, et al. Multiple defects of immune cell function in mice with disrupted interferon-gamma genes. *Science* 1993;259:1739–1742.
112. Huang S, Hendriks W, Althage A, et al. Immune response in mice that lack the interferon-gamma receptor. *Science* 1993;259:1742–1745.
113. Nguyen KB, Cousens LP, Doughty LA, et al. Interferon a/b-mediated inhibition and promotion of interferon g: STAT1 resolves a paradox. *Nat Immunol* 2000;1:70–76
114. Dighe AS, Richards E, Old LJ, et al. Enhanced *in vivo* growth and resistance to rejection of tumor cells expressing dominant negative IFN-gamma receptors. *Immunity* 1994;1:447–456.
115. Dighe AS, Campbell D, Hsieh CS, et al. Tissue-specific targeting of cytokine unresponsiveness in transgenic mice. *Immunity* 1995;3:657–666.
116. Muller U, Steinhoff U, Reis LF, et al. Functional role of type I and type II interferons in antiviral defense. *Science* 1994;264:1918–1921.
117. Yap GS, Sher A. Effector cells of both nonhemopoietic and hemopoietic origin are required for interferon (IFN)–gamma- and tumor necrosis factor (TNF)–alpha-dependent host resistance to the intracellular pathogen, Toxoplasma gondii. *J Exp Med* 1999;189:1083–1092.
118. Tanaka Y, Nakashima H, Hisano C, et al. Association of the interferon-gamma receptor variant (Val14Met) with systemic lupus erythematosus. *Immunogenetics* 1999;49:266–271.
119. Nakashima H, Inoue H, Akahoshi M, et al. The combination of polymorphisms within interferon-gamma receptor 1 and receptor 2 associated with the risk of systemic lupus erythematosus. *FEBS Lett* 1999;453:187–190.
120. Dorman SE, Holland SM. Mutation in the signal-transducing chain of the interferon-gamma receptor and susceptibility to mycobacterial infection. *J Clin Invest* 1998;101:2364–2369.
121. Levin M, Newport MJ, D'Souza S, et al. Familial disseminated atypical mycobacterial infection in childhood: a human mycobacterial susceptibility geneγ *Lancet* 1995;345:79–83.
122. Newport MJ, Huxley CM, Huston S, et al. A mutation in the interferon-gamma receptor gene and susceptibility to mycobacterial infection. *N Engl J Med* 1996;335:1941–1949.
123. Jouanguy E, Altare F, Lamhamedi S, et al. Interferon-gamma receptor deficiency in an infant with fatal bacille Calmette-Guerin infection. *N Engl J Med* 1996;335:1956–1961.
124. Holland SM, Dorman SE, Kwon A, et al. Abnormal regulation of interferon-gamma, interleukin-12, and tumor necrosis factor–alpha in human interferon-gamma receptor 1 deficiency. *J Infect Dis* 1998;178:1095–1104.
125. Jouanguy E, Lamhamedi-Cherradi S, Altare F, et al. Partial interferon-gamma receptor 1 deficiency in a child with tuberculoid bacillus Calmette-Guerin infection and a sibling with clinical tuberculosis. *J Clin Invest* 1997; 100:2658–2664.
126. Doffinger R, Jouanguy E, Dupuis S, et al. Partial interferon-gamma receptor signaling chain deficiency in a patient with bacille Calmette-Guerin and *Mycobacterium abscessus* infection. *J Infect Dis* 2000;181:379–384.

127. Jouanguy E, Lamhamedi-Cherradi S, Lammas D, et al. A human IFNGR1 small deletion hotspot associated with dominant susceptibility to mycobacterial infection. *Nat Genet* 1999;21:370–378.
128. Doffinger, et al. STAT1 2001 (submitted).
129. de Jong R, Altare F, Haagen IA, et al. Severe mycobacterial and Salmonella infections in interleukin-12 receptor-deficient patients. *Science* 1998;280:1435–1438.
130. Altare F, Durandy A, Lammas D, et al. Impairment of mycobacterial immunity in human interleukin-12 receptor deficiency. *Science* 1998a;280:1432–1435.
131. Altare F, Lammas D, Revy P, et al. Inherited interleukin 12 deficiency in a child with bacille Calmette-Guerin and Salmonella enteritidis disseminated infection. *J Clin Invest* 1998 Dec 15;102:2035–2040.
132. Nathan CF, Murray HW, Wiebe ME, et al. Identification of interferon-gamma as the lymphokine that activates human macrophage oxidative metabolism and antimicrobial activity. *J Exp Med* 1983;158:670–689.
133. Nathan CF, Horowitz CR, de la Harpe J, et al. Administration of recombinant interferon-gamma to cancer patients enhances monocyte secretion of hydrogen peroxide. *Proc Natl Acad Sci USA* 1985;82:8686–8690.
134. Segal BH, Leto TL, Gallin JI, et al. Genetic, biochemical, and clinical features of chronic granulomatous disease. *Medicine (Baltimore)* 2000;79:170–200.
135. Gallin JI, Sechler JM, Malech HL. Reconstitution of defective phagocyte function in chronic granulomatous disease of childhood with recombinant human interferon-gamma. *Trans Assoc Am Physicians* 1988;101: 12–17.
136. Sechler JM, Malech HL, White CJ, et al. Recombinant human interferon-gamma reconstitutes defective phagocyte function in patients with chronic granulomatous disease of childhood. *Proc Natl Acad Sci USA* 1988;85: 4874–4878.
137. Ezekowitz RA, Orkin SH, Newburger PE. Recombinant interferon-gamma augments phagocyte superoxide production and X-chronic granulomatous disease gene expression in X-linked variant chronic granulomatous disease. *J Clin Invest* 1987;80:1009–1016.
138. Newburger PE, Ezekowitz RA, Whitney C, et al. Induction of phagocyte cytochrome b heavy chain gene expression by interferon-gamma. *Proc Natl Acad Sci USA* 1988;85:5215–5219.
139. Ezekowitz RA, Dinauer MC, Jaffe HS, et al. Partial correction of the phagocyte defect in patients with X-linked chronic granulomatous disease by subcutaneous interferon-gamma. *N Engl J Med* 1988;319:146–151.
140. Schiff DE, Rae J, Martin TR, et al. Increased phagocyte Fc gamma RI expression and improved Fc gamma receptor–mediated phagocytosis after *in vivo* recombinant human interferon-gamma treatment of normal human subjects. *Blood* 1997;90:3187–3194.
141. The International Chronic Granulomatous Disease Cooperative Study Group. A controlled trial of interferon-gamma to prevent infection in chronic granulomatous disease. *N Engl J Med* 1991;324:509–516.
142. Rex JH, Bennett JE, Gallin JI, et al. *In vivo* interferon-gamma therapy augments the *in vitro* ability of chronic granulomatous disease neutrophils to damage *Aspergillus hyphae. J Infect Dis* 1991;163:849–852.
143. Bemiller LS, Roberts DH, Starko KM, et al. Safety and effectiveness of long-term interferon-gamma therapy in patients with chronic granulomatous disease. *Blood Cells Mol Dis* 1995;21:239–247.
144. Gallin JI, Farber JM, Holland SM, et al. Interferon-gamma in the management of infectious diseases. *Ann Intern Med* 1995;123:216–224.
145. Jackson SH, Segal BH, Domachowski J, et al. Interferon gamma is effective in reducing infections in the mouse model of chronic granulomatous disease. *J Interferon Cytokine Res*, (in press).
146. Key LL Jr, Oexmann MJ, Green L. Nutrition in patients with osteopetrosis on interferon-gamma. *Nutrition* 1997;13:988–990.
147. Key LL Jr, Rodriguiz RM, Willi SM, et al. Long-term treatment of osteopetrosis with recombinant human interferon-gamma. *N Engl J Med* 1995;332:1594–1599.
148. Aulitzky W, Gastl G, Aulitzky WE, et al. Interferon-gamma for the treatment of metastatic renal cancer: dose-dependent stimulation and downregulation of beta-2 microglobulin and neopterin responses. *Immunobiology* 1987;176:85–95.
149. Ahlin A, Elinder G, Palmblad J. Dose-dependent enhancements by interferon-gamma on functional responses of neutrophils from chronic granulomatous disease patients. *Blood* 1997;89:3396–3401.
150. Kunzmann V, Bauer E, Feurle J, et al. Stimulation of gamma/delta T cells by aminobisphosphonates and induction of antiplasma cell activity in multiple myeloma. *Blood* 2000;96:384–392.
151. Hershman MJ, Appel SH, Wellhausen SR, et al. Interferon-gamma treatment increases HLA-DR expression on monocytes in severely injured patients. *Clin Exp Immunol* 1989;77:67–70.
152. Polk HC Jr, Cheadle WG, Livingston DH, et al. A randomized prospective clinical trial to determine the efficacy of interferon-gamma in severely injured patients. *Am J Surg* 1992;163:191–196.
153. Dries DJ, Jurkovich GJ, Maier RV, et al. Effect of interferon-gamma on infection-related death in patients with severe injuries. A randomized, double-blind, placebo-controlled trial. *Arch Surg* 1994;129:1031–1041.
154. Mock CN, Dries DJ, Jurkovich GJ, et al. Assessment of two clinical trials: interferon-gamma therapy in severe injury. *Shock* 1996;5:235–240.
155. Kox WJ, Bone RC, Krausch D, et al. Interferon-gamma$_{1b}$ in the treatment of compensatory anti-inflammatory response syndrome. A new approach: proof of principle. *Arch Intern Med* 1997;157:389–393.
156. Wasserman D, Ioannovich JD, Hinzmann RD, et al. Interferon-gamma in the prevention of severe burn-related infections: a European phase III multicenter trial. The Severe Burns Study Group. *Crit Care Med* 1998;26: 434–439.

157. Jaffe HA, Gao Z, Mori Y, et al. Selective inhibition of collagen gene expression in fibroblasts by an interferon-gamma transgene. *Exp Lung Res* 1999;25:199–215.
158. Larrabe WF, East CA, Jaffe HS, et al. Intralesional interferon-gamma treatment for keloids and hypertrophic scars. *Arch Otolaryngol Head Neck Surg* 1990;116:1159–1162.
159. Granstein RD, Rook A, Flotte TJ, et al. A controlled trial of intralesional recombinant interferon-gamma in the treatment of keloidal scarring. *Arch Dermatol* 1990;126:1295–1301.
160. Berman B, Flores F. Recurrence rates of excised keloids treated with postoperative triamcinolone acetonide injections or interferon alpha-2b injections. *J Am Acad Dermatol* 1997;37:755–757.
161. Berman B, Duncan MR. Short-term keloid treatment *in vivo* with human interferon-alpha2a results in a selective and persistent normalization of keloid fibroblast collagen, glycosaminoglycan and collagenase production *in vitro*. *J Am Acad Dermatol* 1989;21:694–706.
162. Lemmel EM, Brackertz D, Franke M, et al. Results of a multicenter placebo-controlled double-blind randomized phase III clinical study of treatment of rheumatoid arthritis with recombinant interferon-gamma. *Rheumatol Int* 1988;8:87–93.
163. Veys EM, Mielants H, Verbruggen G, et al. Interferon-gamma in rheumatoid arthritis: a double-blind study comparing human recombinant interferon-gamma with placebo. *J Rheumatol* 1988;15:570–574.
164. German Lymphokine Study Group Double-blind controlled phase III multicenter clinical trial with interferon-gamma in rheumatoid arthritis. *Rheumatol Int* 1992;12:175–185.
165. Machold KP, Neumann K, Smolen JS. Recombinant human interferon-gamma in the treatment of rheumatoid arthritis: double-blind placebo-controlled study. *Ann Rheum Dis* 1992;51:1039–1043.
166. Cannon GW, Pincus SH, Emkey RD, et al. Double-blind trial of recombinant gamma-interferon versus placebo in the treatment of rheumatoid arthritis. *Arthritis Rheum* 1989;32:964–973.
167. Cannon GW, Emkey RD, Denes A, et al. Prospective 5-year followup of recombinant interferon-gamma in rheumatoid arthritis. *J Rheumatol* 1993;20:1867–1873.
168. Machold KP, Smolen JS. Interferon-gamma–induced exacerbation of systemic lupus erythematosus. *J Rheumatol* 1990;17:831–832.
169. Graninger WB, Hassfeld W, Pesau BB, et al. Induction of systemic lupus erythematosus by interferon-gamma in a patient with rheumatoid arthritis. *J Rheumatol* 1991;18:1621–1622.
170. Rosenbloom J, Feldman G, Freundlich B, et al. Inhibition of excessive scleroderma fibroblast collagen production by recombinant gamma-interferon. Association with a coordinate decrease in types I and III procollagen messenger RNA levels. *Arthritis Rheum* 1986;29:851–856.
171. Kahan A, Amor B, Menkes CJ, et al. Recombinant interferon-gamma in the treatment of systemic sclerosis. *J Med* 1989;87:273–277.
172. Hein R, Behr J, Hundgen M, et al. Treatment of systemic sclerosis with gamma-interferon. *Br J Dermatol* 1992; 126:496–501.
173. Freundlich B, Jimenez SA, Steen VD, et al. Treatment of systemic sclerosis with recombinant interferon-gamma. A phase I/II clinical trial. *Arthritis Rheum* 1992;35:1134–1142.
174. Grassegger A, Schuler G, Hessenberger G, et al. Interferon-gamma in the treatment of systemic sclerosis: a randomized controlled multicentre trial. *Br J Dermatol* 1998;139:639–648.
175. Narayanan AS, Whithey J, Souza A, etal. Effect of gamma-interferon on collagen synthesis by normal and fibrotic human lung fibroblasts. *Chest* 1992;101:1326–1331.
176. Ziesche R, Hofbauer E, Wittmann K, et al. A preliminary study of long-term treatment with interferon-gamma$_{1b}$ and low-dose prednisolone in patients with idiopathic pulmonary fibrosis. *N Engl J Med* 1999;341:1264–1269.
177. Carvalho EM, Badaro R, Reed SG, et al. Absence of gamma-interferon and interleukin-2 production during active visceral leishmaniasis. *J Clin Invest* 1985;76:2066–2069.
178. Murray HW, Berman JD, Wright SD. Immunochemotherapy for intracellular *Leishmania donovani* infection: gamma-interferon plus pentavalent antimony. *J Infect Dis* 1988;157:973–978.
179. Badaro R, Falcoff E, Badaro FS, et al. Treatment of visceral leishmaniasis with pentavalent antimony and interferon-gamma. *N Engl J Med* 1990;322:16–21.
180. Badaro R, Johnson WD Jr. The role of interferon-gamma in the treatment of visceral and diffuse cutaneous leishmaniasis. *J Infect Dis* 1993;167(suppl 1):S13–S17.
181. Sundar S, Rosenkaimer F, Murray HW. Successful treatment of refractory visceral leishmaniasis in India using antimony plus interferon-gamma. *J Infect Dis* 1994;170:659–662.
182. Sundar S, Rosenkaimer F, Lesser ML, et al. Immunochemotherapy for a systemic intracellular infection: accelerated response using interferon-gamma in visceral leishmaniasis. *J Infect Dis* 1995;171:992–996.
183. Sundar S, Murray HW. Effect of treatment with interferon-gamma alone in visceral leishmaniasis. *J Infect Dis* 1995;172:1627–1629.
184. Sundar S, Singh VP, Sharma S, et al. Response to interferon-gamma plus pentavalent antimony in Indian visceral leishmaniasis. *J Infect Dis* 1997;176:1117–1119.
185. Appelberg R, Orme IM. Effector mechanisms involved in cytokine-mediated bacteriostasis of *Mycobacterium avium* infections in murine macrophages. *Immunology* 1993;80:352–359.
186. Flesch IE, Kaufmann SH. Attempts to characterize the mechanisms involved in mycobacterial growth inhibition by gamma-interferon–activated bone marrow macrophages. *Infect Immun* 1988;56:1464–1469.
187. Doherty TM, Sher A. Defects in cell-mediated immunity affect chronic, but not innate, resistance of mice to *Mycobacterium avium* infection. *J Immunol* 1997;58:4822–4831.

188. Adams LB, Dinauer MC, Morgenstern DE, et al. Comparison of the roles of reactive oxygen and nitrogen intermediates in the host response to *Mycobacterium tuberculosis* using transgenic mice. *Tuber Lung Dis* 1997; 78:237–246.
189. Cooper AM, Segal BH, Frank AA, et al. Transient loss of resistance to pulmonary tuberculosis in p47(phox–/) mice. *Infect Immun* 2000;68:1231–1234.
190. Bermudez LE, Young LS. Oxidative and non-oxidative intracellular killing of *Mycobacterium avium* complex. *Microbiol Pathol* 1989;7:289–298.
191. Denis M, Gregg EO, Ghandirian E. Cytokine modulation of *Mycobacterium tuberculosis* growth in human macrophages. *Int J Immunopharmacol* 1990;12:721–727.
192. Douvas GS, Looker DL, Vatter AE, et al. Gamma-interferon activates human macrophages to become tumoricidal and leishmanicidal but enhances replication of macrophage-associated mycobacteria. *Infect Immun* 1985;50:1–8.
193. Flynn JL, Chan J, Triebold KJ, et al. An essential role for interferon-gamma in resistance to *Mycobacterium tuberculosis* infection. *J Exp Med* 1993;178:2249–2254.
194. Cooper AM, Dalton DK, Stewart TA, et al. Disseminated tuberculosis in interferon-gamma gene–disrupted mice. *J Exp Med* 1993;178:2243–2247.
195. Kamijo R, Le J, Shapiro D, et al. Mice that lack the interferon-gamma receptor have profoundly altered responses to infection with Bacillus Calmette-Guerin and subsequent challenge with lipopolysaccharide. *J Exp Med* 1993;178:1435–1440.
196. Kamijo R, Harada H, Matsuyama T, et al. Requirement for transcription factor IRF-1 in NO synthase induction in macrophages. *Science* 1994;263:1612–1615.
197. Edwards CKd, Hedegaard HB, Zlotnik A, et al. Chronic infection due to *Mycobacterium intracellulare* in mice: association with macrophage release of prostaglandin E_2 and reversal by injection of indomethacin, muramyl dipeptide, or interferon-gamma. *J Immunol* 1986;136:1820–1827.
198. Hussain S, Zwilling BS, Lafuse WP. *Mycobacterium avium* infection of mouse macrophages inhibits IFN-gamma Janus kinase-STAT signaling and gene induction by down-regulation of the IFN-gamma receptor. *J Immunol* 1999;163:2041–2048.
199. Ting LM, Kim AC, Cattamanchi A, et al. *Mycobacterium tuberculosis* inhibits IFN-gamma transcriptional responses without inhibiting activation of STAT1. *J Immunol* 1999;163:3898–3906.
200. Nathan CF, Kaplan G, Levis WR, et al. Local and systemic effects of intradermal recombinant interferon-gamma in patients with lepromatous leprosy. *N Engl J Med* 1986;315:6–15.
201. Sampaio EP, Moreira AL, Sarno EN, et al. Prolonged treatment with recombinant interferon-gamma induces erythema nodosum leprosum in lepromatous leprosy patients. *J Exp Med* 1992;175:1729–1737.
202. Sampaio EP, Kaplan G, Miranda A, et al. The influence of thalidomide on the clinical and immunologic manifestation of erythema nodosum leprosum. *J Infect Dis* 1993;168:408–414.
203. Sampaio EP, Malta AM, Sarno EN, et al. Effect of rhuIFN-gamma treatment in multibacillary leprosy patients. *Int J Lepr Other Mycobact Dis* 1996;64:268–273.
204. Haslett PA, Klausner JD, Makonkawkeyoon S, et al. Thalidomide stimulates T cell responses and interleukin 12 production in HIV-infected patients. *AIDS Res Hum Retroviruses* 1999;15:1169–1179.
205. Bekker LG, Haslett P, Maartens G, et al. Thalidomide-induced antigen-specific immune stimulation in patients with human immunodeficiency virus type 1 and tuberculosis. *J Infect Dis* 2000;81:954–965.
206. Bermudez LE, Inderlied C, Young LS. Stimulation with cytokines enhances penetration of azithromycin into human macrophages. *Antimicrob Agents Chemother* 1991;35:2625–2629.
207. Squires KE, Murphy WF, Madoff LC, et al. Interferon-gamma and *Mycobacterium avium*–intracellulare infection. *J Infect Dis* 1989;159:599–600.
208. Squires KE, Brown ST, Armstrong D, et al. Interferon-gamma treatment for *Mycobacterium avium*–intracellular complex bacillemia in patients with AIDS [Letter]. *J Infect Dis* 1992;166:686–687.
209. Frucht DM, Holland SM. Defective monocyte costimulation for IFN-gamma production in familial disseminated *Mycobacterium avium* complex infection: abnormal IL-12 regulation. *J Immunol* 1996;157:411–416.
210. Holland SM, Eisenstein EM, Kuhns DB, et al. Treatment of refractory disseminated nontuberculous mycobacterial infection with interferon-gamma. A preliminary report. *N Engl J Med* 1994;330:1348–1355.
211. Vesterhus P, Holland SM, Abrahamsen TG, et al. Familial disseminated infection due to atypical mycobacteria with childhood onset. *Clin Infect Dis* 1998;27:822–825.
212. Jouanguy E, Lamhamedi-Cherradi S, Lammas D, et al. A human IFNGR1 small deletion hotspot associated with dominant susceptibility to mycobacterial infection. *Nat Genet* 1999;21:370–378.
213. Chatte G, Panteix G, Perrin-Fayolle M, et al. Aerosolized interferon-gamma for *Mycobacterium avium*–complex lung disease. *Am J Respir Crit Care Med* 1995;152:1094–1096.
214. Condos R, Rom WN, Schluger NW. Treatment of multidrug-resistant pulmonary tuberculosis with interferon-gamma via aerosol. *Lancet* 1997;349:1513–1515.
215. Raad I, Hachem R, Leeds N, et al. Use of adjunctive treatment with interferon-gamma in an immunocompromised patient who had refractory multidrug-resistant tuberculosis of the brain. *Clin Infect Dis* 1996;22: 572–574.

11

Myeloid Growth Factors in Supportive Care of Cancer and Marrow Transplant Therapies

Thomas Lehrnbecher and *Stephen J. Chanock

*Immunocompromised Host Section, Pediatric Oncology Branch, Advanced Technology Center, National Cancer Institute, National Institutes of Health, Bethesda, Maryland; and *Senior Investigator, Pediatric Oncology Branch, National Cancer Institute, Bethesda, Maryland*

Infectious complications are a major cause of morbidity and mortality in patients receiving therapy for malignancy (1–5). Of the three major modalities used to treat cancer, the risk for infectious complications is substantially greater following myelotoxic chemotherapy than either surgery or radiation therapy (6). Over the past three decades, the success of managing infectious complications in the immunocompromised host has evolved mainly on the basis of applying the lessons of the past to current algorithms. In the process, a more refined appreciation of the relative importance of different risk factors has evolved (7). More potent antibiotics used judiciously, coupled with better diagnostic modalities, have contributed significantly to the successes of supportive care for the cancer patient. Consequently, advances in the supportive care of cancer patients have led directly to the improvements in survival for selected cancers, such as acute leukemia and lymphoma (8). At the same time, these improvements in supportive care have permitted the oncology community to consider more intensive, myelosuppressive therapies, which often include autologous stem cell rescue afterwards.

Over the past three decades, it has become apparent that the loss of neutrophils due to standard or intensive chemotherapy places the cancer patient at high risk for bacterial and fungal infections (9). Neutropenia is defined as an absolute circulating count of less than 500/μL, but when the circulating neutrophil count falls below 100/μL, the risk for dangerous bacterial and fungal infections increases substantially (10–12). In early studies, the incidence of documented bacteremia or fungemia in febrile and neutropenic cancer patients approached 100% in patients untreated for up to 3 weeks. In response to the poor outcome observed in the majority of these patients, early use of empirical antibiotic therapy has evolved and now nearly eliminated mortality, which is less than 2% to 3% (3,13,14). The presence of fever (greater than 38.00°C to 38.50°C) in the neutropenic cancer patient is to be considered a harbinger for potential, serious infection, even if no clinically apparent site is identified (3,15–17). The risk of waiting until a pathogen is identified by diagnostic studies, usually on the order of 24 to 48 hours, is too great. Accordingly, initiation of empirical antibiotics is indicated at the first sign of fever in the neutropenic host. For these reasons, it is not surprising that fever in the neutropenic patient is one of the most common reasons for admission to the hospital for cancer patients (9). Besides neutropenia, other therapy-induced alterations impact the likelihood of developing an infection. These include disruption of the integument (i.e., mucositis), long-term placement of central venous catheters, and impairment of humoral and cellular immunity, either due to underlying disease or therapeutic interventions with corticosteroids or other myelosuppressive agents (6). Though the relative contribution of these alterations varies between different combinations of chemotherapy and is also impacted by the underlying malignancy, the cumulative effect of cycles of therapy is most important. Nonetheless, of these contributing factors, neutropenia has emerged as the most important of the risk factors for infection.

One of the most notable and clinically useful byproducts of the revolution in recombinant DNA technology is the availability of a novel set of agents, poised to address a critical problem in the supportive care of cancer patients, the loss of neutrophils. The characterization and purification of granulocyte colony-stimulating factor (G-CSF) and granulocyte-monocyte colony-stimulating factor (GM-CSF) offers the promise of a new dimension for supportive care in the cancer patient (18–20). Both hematopoietic growth factors accelerate granulopoiesis and, thus, create the possibility of abbreviating and in some circumstances, eliminating the period of greatest risk, absolute neutropenia. These two naturally found hematopoietic growth factors, GM-CSF, have undergone commercial development and are now widely available for use in the form of recombinant proteins. However, their judicious use is not well defined and the source of ongoing controversy. During the investigation of the biology of G-CSF and GM-CSF, important similarities and critical differences have been uncovered, few of which influence clinical indications for use. In this regard, the two agents are more similar and thus can be used interchangeably in many, but not all clinical situations. This review will highlight some of the notable differences, but it is important to recognize that the clinical differences between using G- and GM-CSF are minimal.

THE BIOLOGY OF THE G-CSF AND GM-CSF

In the human genome, G-CSF and GM-CSF map to different chromosomes; the gene for G-CSF maps to 17q21-22, whereas the gene for GM-CSF maps to 5q21-31 (Table 11.1) (21–23). Both factors are produced by macrophages, fibroblasts, endothelial cells, and bone marrow stromal cells (24–28). GM-CSF, which acts on a wider range of target cells, is also produced by T- and B-lymphocytes, mast cells, and eosinophils (25,29,30). G- and GM-CSF interact with unique receptors that are highly expressed on neutrophils; in addition, the GM-CSF receptor is expressed on monocytes (31–33).

TABLE 11-1. *G-CSF and GM-CSF*

Factor	Generic name	Trade name	Chromosomal localization	Cellular source
G-CSF	Filgrastim (*E. coli* derived) Lenograstim (CHO cell derived)	Neupogen (Amgen) Neutrogin (Chugaï-Rhône Poulenc)	17q21-22	Macrophages, fibroblasts, endothelial cells, bone marrow stromal cells
GM-CSF	Sargramostim (yeast derived) Molgramostim (*E. coli* derived)	Leukine (Immunex) Leukomax (Sandoz, Schering-Plough)	5q21-31	Macrophages, endothelial cells, fibroblasts, bone marrow stromal cells, T and B lymphocytes, mast cells, eosinophils

CHO, Chinese hamster ovary.

The effects of G-CSF and GM-CSF are quite similar with respect to maturation of neutrophils; both expand circulating pools of neutrophils by stimulating proliferation and maturation of myeloid progenitor cells (34–36). GM-CSF also accelerates production of monocytes in bone marrow (37,38). The effects of G-CSF and GM-CSF on hematopoiesis appear to be late, in cells already committed to the white cell lineage, unlike another growth factor of current clinical interest, IL-3, which expands early hematopoietic progenitors (39–41). The observation that both G- and GM-CSF mobilize hematopoietic stem cells in the peripheral blood has had profound implications for harvesting stem cells for transplantation and stem cell rescue.

Both myeloid colony factors, G- and GM-CSF, can enhance phagocytic function in neutrophils *ex vivo*. GM-CSF also augments monocyte function in a manner comparable to neutrophils (42,43). In *ex vivo* studies, G- and GM-CSF enhance superoxide generation, phagocytosis, and fungicidal activity against *Candida albicans* and *Aspergillus fumigatus* (44–46). Also, GM-CSF has been reported to enhance uptake and destruction of bacterial and parasitic pathogens (47,48), augment antibody-dependent cellular cytotoxicity, and increase release of proinflammatory cytokines (51,52). One group has reported synergistic microbicidal activity between commonly used antibiotics and neutrophils treated with G-CSF (53).

Recently, G-CSF and GM-CSF have been shown to modulate apoptosis, by delaying programmed cell death in neutrophils *in vitro* (24,55). The effect appears to be independent of oxidative stress and is still not well characterized (56). Interestingly, these observations partly explain the observed persistence of high neutrophil counts in marrow recipients who received neutrophil transfusions from their original marrow donor (57).

CLINICAL INDICATIONS FOR THE USE OF G-CSF OR GM-CSF

Over the past decade, a large number of studies have been published reporting on the clinical usefulness of G-CSF and GM-CSF in supportive cancer therapy and marrow transplantation. In response to the widespread use of these growth factors in clinical oncology and transplantation, a series of reviews of the current literature (including information in abstracts and material only presented at meetings) has been conducted by a blue-ribbon panel of experts convened by the American Society of Clinical Oncology. The express purpose has been to formulate recommendations for the judicious use of myeloid growth factors, particularly since the cost of the factors is very high (58,59).

Use of G- and GM-CSF has been divided into three separate categories with respect to use in patients receiving myelotoxic chemotherapy and those undergoing bone marrow transplantation (BMT) (Table 11.2). At present, the strongest data support the use of growth factors shortly after receiving chemotherapy or marrow transplantation to prevent serious infection. The analysis of a wide spectrum of patients receiving different therapies underscores the importance of the specific recommendations for restricted use of

TABLE 11-2. *Recognized indications for hematopoietic growth factors in cancer patients*

Purpose	Timing of administration
Prevention of infectious events	Initiate 24–48 h postmyelosuppressive chemotherapy
Treatment of febrile, neutropenic episode	Initiate at admission
Augmentation of host defense	Initiate at diagnosis
Mobilization of stem cells	Short course and during recovery from therapy

these factors. In other words, not all patients receiving myelosuppressive chemotherapy should receive support with G- or GM-CSF following chemotherapy. Data do not support the use of myeloid growth factors at the onset of a febrile, neutropenic event, though many still employ this approach. Primarily on theoretical grounds and with only anecdotal reports of success in desperate cases, the use of myeloid growth factors to augment host defenses during a documented life-threatening infection has been advanced (3,58). Recently, a fourth application has emerged and has garnered significant interest in the transplant community: the use of myeloid growth factors for mobilization of granulocytes or hematopoietic stem cells.

PREVENTION OF INFECTIOUS COMPLICATIONS IN CANCER PATIENTS WHO ARE EXPECTED TO BE NEUTROPENIC

The ability to abrogate postchemotherapy neutropenia and reduce the risk for infection has been the underlying rationale for investigating G- and GM-CSF in cancer and marrow transplant patients. Interestingly, the most compelling data for use of either G-CSF and GM-CSF in preventing infections has been in patients receiving intensive chemotherapy (Tables 11.3 and 11.4). The burden of evidence has been accumulated in studies with G-CSF. In nearly all studies showing a positive benefit, the design has been to initiate G-CSF or GM-CSF shortly after completion of a cycle of chemotherapy, usually within 24 to 48 hours. In all but one study (60), it has been shown that G-CSF or GM-CSF significantly shortened the duration of neutropenia and frequently lessened the degree (i.e., depth) of neutropenia. However, the clinical implications of shortening neutropenia have not necessarily translated into a demonstrable reduction in infection. For the most part, the significant findings have been in indirect measurements of infection, such as days of fever, hospital days, duration of antibiotic therapy, and overall financial cost of hospitalization. Fewer studies have demonstrated a reduction in documented infections, and no study, as of yet, has shown that there is a statistically significant improvement in survival in cancer patients.

To date, no randomized studies have shown a difference between the different factors, G- and GM-CSF, following myelosuppressive chemotherapy. The initial licensing studies that lead to the approval of G-CSF were conducted in three separate cancer populations, all receiving different chemotherapy regimens (61,63). These studies showed that one could safely use G-CSF to reduce the duration of neutropenia and, in turn, reduce the number of febrile, neutropenic episodes as well as the use of antibiotics and hospitalization days. Additional studies have been published validating this approach in a variety of populations, which all have in common intensive therapy and high rates of documented or presumed infection, on the order of 30% or greater (Table 11.3) (64,65). However, other studies have not reached the same conclusions in different populations at lower risk, again underscoring the importance of the therapy given. Furthermore, negative studies have been reported in adults and children with a wide range of underlying malignancies and therapies (Table 11.3) (62,66–74). The specific use of G- or GM-CSF is not recommended in all patients. Instead, usage should be restricted to those patients with either a previous history of a serious infection during prior neutropenia or in patients in whom the expected likelihood of developing a febrile neutropenic event or documented infection is greater than 40% (58,59).

For prevention of possible infection during therapy-induced neutropenia, G- or GM-CSF must be given after a suitable interval, at least 24 to 48 hours after myelosuppressive chemotherapy, to prevent severe myeloablation and possible aplasia. Because G- and GM-CSF induce rapid mobilization and cell cycling of progenitors, the risk for enhanced marrow toxicity is greatest when high levels of chemotherapy are present (75–81). In an early study, concurrent administration of growth factors and etoposide led to more profound neutropenia and thrombocytopenia (82). In patients with lung cancer, the initiation of G-CSF on day 8 of a chemotherapy cycle instead of day 2 resulted in a lower incidence of intercycle neutropenia (80% versus 44%, $p<.05$) (79).

The use of G- and GM-CSF in patients with acute myelogenous leukemia (AML) is slightly more complicated than in other disease populations because of the theoretical risk that G- or GM-CSF could stimulate leukemogenesis directly. Leukemic blast cells express functional receptors (83). For example, it has been shown that G- and GM-CSF can induce proliferation of leukemic blasts in culture (84,87). In clinical studies, the burden of evidence suggests that it is safe to administer G- or GM-CSF to AML patients (Table 11.5) (88–90). Dombret et al. (91) reported a significantly higher remission rate in patients treated with G-CSF compared to controls (70% versus 47%, $p = 0.002$). Other studies have not correlated G- or GM-CSF use with higher rates of remission (88–90,92–94). Only one study has reported troubling findings that are not fully explained by G-CSF use alone (Table 11.5); administration of GM-CSF during the hypoplastic phase of an induction regimen with a daunorubicin/cytarabine combination for AML significantly decreased the rate of complete remission (95). Also, one published study supports the use of G- and GM-CSF after completion of induction chemotherapy for AML in patients ≥55 years of age (90).

In patients with acute lymphoblastic leukemia (ALL), the data for use of G- and GM-CSF is also controversial but not for the same reasons as AML. Most experts would agree that these agents have no role during support of maintenance chemotherapy, when the risk for infection is very low. If there is an indication in ALL therapy, it is during induction and intensification therapy. Currently, the data is slightly more persuasive in adults than in children. In a study of 53 adult patients, G-CSF markedly abbreviated neutropenia; time to recovery defined as an absolute neutrophil count >1,000/μL was shortened from 26 days in untreated controls to 16 days in the group that received G-CSF ($p < 0.001$) (96). The authors also observed a reduction in incidence in febrile neutropenic episodes as well as documented infections (12% versus 42% in controls, $p < 0.05$, and 40% versus 77%, $p < 0.05$, respectively) (96). In a prospective, randomized, open-label phase-III pediatric study, the G-CSF arm was associated with a significant reduction in febrile neutropenic events (17% in G-CSF patients versus 40% in the control group, $p = 0.007$), microbiologically defined infections (8% versus 15%, $p = 0.04$) and duration of intravenous antibiotic administration (18.2 days per patient versus 32.2 days, $p = 0.02$) (97). Furthermore, the authors reported that, in the G-CSF arm, better adherence to the treatment schedule was observed (97). On the other hand, Pui et al. (98) reported no advantage for G-CSF over placebo in a randomized study of pediatric ALL patients. Two earlier studies failed to demonstrate a significant advantage for growth factor in ALL therapy, one in children and one in adults (60,99).

There are fewer studies that have directly addressed the use of GM-CSF as a preventive measure during expected bouts of neutropenia (Table 11.4). Still, the reported data are comparable to the studies in G-CSF (60,67,68,70,71,100–104). GM-CSF accelerates neutrophil recovery and, in selected patients, reduces measurable indicators of infection or infectious risk. For example, in a cohort of non-Hodgkin's lymphoma patients, the use of GM-CSF significantly reduced the duration of neutropenia, days with fever (2.1 ver-

TABLE 11-3. *Summary of trials evaluating the effectiveness*

Dose, route, and preparation	Disease	Adult/ pediatric	*N*	Amelioration of depth and/or duration of neutropenia*	Decrease in neutropenic fever
5 μg/kg/d, s.c., filgrastim	ALL	Adult	198**	P < 0.001 20 vs 13 days (Note: ANC is defined < 1000/μL)	
5 μg/kg/d, s.c., added to induction, filgrastim	Neuroblastoma	Pediatric	59**	P < 0.001 26 vs 9 days	NS after first cycle P = 0.002, 0.008, 0.001 after cycle 2, 3, 4 resp.
5 μg/kg/d, s.c., filgrastim	Aggressive NHL	Adult	74**	NS (median neutrophil nadir)	NS
5 μg/kg/d, s.c., filgrastim	ALL	Adult	53**	P < 0.001 28 vs 16 days (Note: ANC is defined <1000/μL)	P = 0.035 42% vs 12%
5 μg/kg/d, s.c., lenograstim	Aggressive NHL	Adult	162**	P < 0.001 2–4 vs 0–1 days (dependent on cycle)	NS
5 μg/kg/d, s.c., filgrastim	Solid tumor, lymphoma	Adult	138**	P < 0.001 4 vs 2 days	
10 μg/kg/d, s.c., filgrastim	ALL	Pediatric	164**	P = 0.007 12.7 vs 5.3 days	NS
5 μg/kg/d, s.c., filgrastim	High-risk ALL	Pediatric	34**	P = 0.02 20.3 vs 6.2 days	P = 0.007 40% vs 17%
5 μg/kg/d, s.c., lenograstim	Breast cancer	Adult	120**	P < 0.001 5–6 vs 2 days (dependent on cycle)	
5 μg/kg/d, s.c., filgrastim	ALL	Adult	76**	P = 0.002 12.5 vs 6 days (Note: ANC is defined <1000/μL)	NS
5 μg/kg/d, s.c., filgrastim	Various	Pediatric	16	P < 0.0001 16.5 vs 4.8 days	P = 0.04 50% vs 10%
5 μg/kg/d, s.c., lenograstim	Small-cell lung cancer	Adult	65**	Median WBC nadir >1000/μL in each cycle for G-CSF group <1000/μL in cycle 2–6 for control group	NS
5 μg/kg/d, s.c., G-CSF (unspecified)	Aggressive NHL	Adult	67	P < 0.001 for incidence (56% vs 18%)	of neutropenia
230 μg/m²/d, s.c., filgrastim	Small-cell lung cancer	Adult	130**	P < 0.001 9–11 vs 1–3 days (dependent on cycle) (Note: ANC is defined <1000/μL)	P < 0.002 53% vs 26%
230 μg/m²/d, s.c., filgrastim	NHL	Adult	80**	P = 0.00001 for incidence of neutropenia 85% vs 37% (Note: ANC is defined <1000/μL)	NS
230 μg/m²/d, s.c., filgrastim	Small-cell lung cancer	Adult	199**	P < 0.001 6 vs 3 days	P < 0.001 57% vs 28%
200 μg/m²/d, i.v., filgrastim	ALL, AML, CML	Most adult	108**	P = 0.0002 28 vs 20 days	NS

*Neutropenia is defined as 500 neutrophils/mL except otherwise specified.
**The design of the study includes randomization with a control group.
***G-CSF was given to a febrile patients with severe neutropenia.

of G-CSF for prevention of infectious complications

Decrease in documented infections	Decrease in antibiotic usage	Decrease in hospitalization	Improvement in disease-free survival	Reduced cost	Reference
		P = 0.02 28 vs 22 days	NS		Larson et al., 1998 (65)
		NS	P = 0.072 2.4 vs 1.3 years		Michon et al., 1998(73)
NS	NS	NS	NS		Fridrik et al., 1997 (69)
P = 0.017 77% vs 40%			NS		Geissler et al., 1997 (96)
P < 0.05 34% vs 18.5% Severe infections: P = 0.001 61% vs 31%	P = 0.002 11.8 vs 6 days	P < 0.05 10 vs 5.3 days	NS		Gisselbrecht et al., 1997 (231)
NS	NS	NS			Hartmann et al., 1997 (74)***
P = 0.009 36% vs 16%	NS	P = 0.011 10 vs 6 days	NS	No	Pui et al., 1997 (98)
P = 0.04 15% vs 8%	P = 0.02 32.2 vs 18.2 days		NS		Welte et al., 1996 (97)
P = 0.042 22% vs 8.2%	P = 0.005 15.4 vs 8.7 days	P = 0.003 8.3 vs 3.7 days	NS		Chevallier et al., 1995 (64)
NS			NS		Ottmann et al., 1995 (99)
	P = 0.003 95 vs 13 days	P = 0.02 65 vs 13 days		$1,000 per cycle	Rilkonen et al., 1995 (105)
	NS	NS	NS		Woll et al., 1995 (72)
Trend			Trend		Bertini et al., 1994 (232)
NS	P < 0.02 58% vs 37%	P < 0.04 58% vs 39%	NS		Trillet-Lenoir et al., 1993 (63)
NS			NS		Pettengell et al., 1992 (62)
			NS		Crawford et al., 1991 (81)
P = 0.028 30% vs 10%			NS		Ohno et al., 1990 (66)

TABLE 11-4. *Summary of trials evaluating the effectiveness of*

Dose, route, and preparation	Disease	Adult/ pediatric	*N*	Amelioration of depth and/or duration of neutropenia*	Decrease in neutropenic fever
5 μg/kg/d, i.v., molgramostim	Advanced multiple myeloma	Adult	102**	P = 0.0468 29 vs 23.5 days	NS
250 μg/m²/d, s.c., sargramostim[1]	Breast cancer (II–III)	Adult	142**	P < 0.001 6.8 vs 2.8 days	
5–15 μg/kg/d, s.c., molgramostim	Sarcoma	Pediatric	37**	P < 0.0001 9 vs 7 days	NS
250 μg/m²/12 h, s.c., sargramostim	NHL, breast cancer	Adult	56**	P = 0.01 12 vs 10 days, only sign. in cycle 1	
10 μg/kg/d, s.c., molgramostim	Advanced/ relapsed germ cell tumors	Adult	104**	P = 0.02 for median neutrophil nadir, 96 vs 320/μL, only sign. in cycle 2	
250 μg/m²/12 h, s.c., sargramostim[2]	Small cell lung cancer	Adult	215**	P < 0.01 Incidence of grade 4 neutropenia 24% vs 18%	NS
250 μg/m²/d, i.v., molgramostim	Sarcoma	Pediatric	11 (82 cycles)**	P = 0.0001 5.7 vs 1.9 days	
5.5 μg/kg/d, s.c., regramostim	Poor prognosis ALL	Pediatric	40**	NS	NS
1,000 mg/m²/d, s.c., sargramostim	Solid tumor (recurrent)	Pediatric	20	P = 0.005 16.8 vs 10 days	NS
400 μg/d, s.c., molgramostim	NHL	Adult	125**	P between 0.04 and <0.01 for median leukocyte nadir, dependent on cycle (1,000–2,100 vs 1,600–2,600/mL)	NS

*Neutropenia is defined as 500 neutrophils/μL except otherwise specified.
**The design of the study includes randomization with a control group.
[1]Moderate-dose chemotherapy.
[2]Includes radiation.

GM-CSF as a preventive measure to decrease infectious complications

Decrease in documented infections	Decrease in antibiotic usage	Decrease in hospitalization	Improvement in disease-free survival	Decrease in cost	Reference
	NS	Trend	NS		Moreau et al., 1997 (71)
		NS	NS		Jones et al., 1996 (70)
NS	NS	NS	NS	NS	Wexler et al., 1996 (68)
		P = 0.035 8 vs 4 days only sign. in cycle 1			Yau et al., 1996 (104)
P = 0.01 for clinically relevant infections, 45% vs 24%, only sign. in cycle 1	P = 0.01 43% vs 20%, only sign. in cycle 1				Bajorin et al., 1995 (103)
	P = 0.04 (inverse) mean, 2.6 vs 3.3 days	P < 0.01 (inverse) mean, 5.2 vs 9.7 days	NS		Bunn et al., 1995 (100)
	NS				Burdach et al., 1995 (102)
NS	NS	NS	NS		Calderwood et al., 1994 (60)
NS		NS			Marina et al., 1994 (67)
P = 0.03 45% vs 27%	P = 0.02 8 vs 3.2 days	P = 0.01 8 vs 3.5 days	NS		Gerhartz et al., 1993 (101)

TABLE 11-5. *Growth factors*

CSF, dose, and route	Adult/ pediatric	*N*	Amelioration of depth and/or duration of neutropenia*	Decrease in neutropenic fever
Prophylaxis of infectious complications				
400 μg/m²/d, i.v., start day 11 of chemotherapy, filgrastim	Adult (>55 yrs)	234**	P = 0.014 24 vs 21 days	NS
5 μg/kg/d, unspecified route, start after 3rd cycle of chemotherapy filgrastim	Adult	249	P < 0.001 31.1 vs 20.5 days	
5 μg/kg/d, s.c., after induction therapy, filgrastim	Adult (median 54 yrs)	521**	P = 0.0001 25 vs 20 days	P = 0.009 8.5 vs 7 days
5 μg/kg/d, i.v., start day 9 of chemotherapy, lenograstim	Adult (>64 yrs)	173**	P < 0.001 27 vs 21 days (Note: ANC is defined <1000/μL)	
5 μg/kg/d, i.v., start day 2 of chemotherapy, molgramostim	Adult	240**	P = 0.0001 29 vs 24 days	NS
5 μg/kg/d, i.v., different arms: before/during and/or after chemotherapy molgramostim	Adult	102**	Trend (for GM-CSF after chemotherapy)	
250 μg/m²/d, i.v., start day 11 of chemotherapy, sagramostim	Adult (>55 to 70 yrs)	117**	P = 0.001 17 vs 13 days	
5 μg/kg/d, i.v., start day 2 of chemotherapy, molgramostim	Adult (>60 yrs)	388**	P = 0.02 17 vs 15 days	
Priming				
400 μg/m²/d, i.v., start 1 day before chemotherapy, G-CSF (unspecified)	Adult	123	P < 0.0001 34 vs 21 days (Note: ANC is defined <1000/μL)	
200 μg/m²/d, i.v., start 2 days before chemotherapy, filgrastim	Adult	58**	P < 0.001 29 vs 24 days	
250 μg/m²/d, s.c., 18 h before chemotherapy, molgramostim	Adult	80**	NS	NS
125 μg/m²/d (20 mg/m²/day for pts. >60 yrs.), s.c., up to 8 days before chemotherapy, molgramostim	Adult	58	NS	
250 μg/m²/d, i.v., start 48 or 24 hrs prior to chemotherapy, molgramostim	Adult	18	P < 0.05 25.2 vs 22.5 days	

*Neutropenia is defined as 500 neutrophils/mL except otherwise specified.
**The design of the study includes randomization with a control group.

in acute myelogenous leukemia

Decrease in documented infections	Decrease in antibiotic usage	Decrease in hospitalization	Improvement in rate of complete remission	Improvement in disease-free survival	Reference
NS	Trend	NS	NS	NS	Godwin et al., 1998 (93)
		P = 0.05 97% vs 85%	NS	NS	Moore et al., 1997 (94)
NS	P = 0.0001 18.5 vs 15 days	P = 0.0001 25 vs 20 days	NS	NS	Heli et al., 1997 (88)
NS			P = 0.002 47% vs 70%	NS	Dombret et al., 1995 (88)
NS	P = 0.018 25 vs 23 days	NS	NS	P = 0.003 21% vs 48%	Witz et al., 1998 (92)
NS			P = 0.008 (decreased with GM-CSF after chemotherapy, whether priming or not) 74% vs 47%		Zittoun et al., 1996 (95)
P = 0.002 36% vs 10% (grade-3/4 infections)		NS	NS	P = 0.048 4.8 vs 10.6 months	Rowe et al., 1995 (90)
NS		NS	NS	NS	Slone et al., 1995 (90)
NS			NS	NS	Estey et al., 1994 (260)
NS			NS	NS	Ohno et al., 1994 (263)
NS			NS	NS	Heli et al., 1995 (261)
			P = 0.011 (inverse) 65% vs 48%	Trend (inverse)	Estey et al., 1992 (264)
					Bettelheim et al., 1991 (262)

sus 4.0, $p = 0.04$), the frequency of clinically relevant infection (28 versus 69 infections, 16 versus 30 patients, $p = 0.2$), and days of hospitalization for presumed infection (3.5 versus 8.0 days, $p = 0.01$) (101).

Preliminary cost/benefit analysis studies looking at G- or GM-CSF have not generally shown a striking reduction in overall costs (68,98). While it has been shown that adjuvant growth factor support resulted in delivery of enhanced dose intensity of chemotherapy compared to controls who did not receive growth factor, no significant difference was apparent with respect to response or event free survival (63,68,98). In fact, one notable, prospective study showed that GM-CSF was associated with an increase in antibiotic usage and prolongation of hospitalization (100). Reports that G-CSF or GM-CSF retard recovery from thrombocytopenia and/or anemia are misleading; more likely the delivery of additional therapy accounts for some of the marrow toxicity (68,70,100). In conclusion, cost analyses have not demonstrated a substantial saving in real dollars associated with growth factor usage (68,98,105).

TABLE 11-6. *Trials evaluating myeloid growth factors*

CSF, dose, and route	Disease	Adult/ pediatric	*N*	Amelioration of depth and/or duration of neutropenia*	Decrease in fever
5 µg/kg/d, i.v filgrastim	Solid tumor, lymphoma, ALL, AML	Pediatric	112**	P = 0.02 5 vs 3 days	NS
5 µg/kg/d, i.v. filgrastim	Solid tumor, lymphoma	Adult	82**	P < 0.001 3 vs 2 days	NS
12 µg/kg/d, s.c. filgrastim	Solid tumor, lymphoma, ALL	Adult	218**	P = 0.005 4 vs 3 days	NS
5 µg/kg/d, s.c. molgramostim	Solid tumor, lymphoma	Adult	68**	Entire group: P = 0.024, 4 vs 3 days Low-risk chemotherapy: P = 0.011, 4 vs 2 days High-risk chemotherapy: NS	NS
3 µg/kg/d, i.v. molgramostim	Solid tumor, leukemia, lymphoma	Adult	107**	NS (Note: ANC is defined <1000/µL)	NS
5 µg/kg/d, s.c. molgramostim	Solid tumor, lymphoma, ALL	Adult	134**	NS	NS
5 µg/kg/d, i.v. molgramostim	Solid tumor, lymphoma	Adult	82**	P < 0.001 3 vs 2 days	NS
5 µg/kg/d, i.v. molgramostim	Solid tumor, ALL	Pediatric	40**	P < 0.05 6 vs 4.5 days	NS
2.8 µg/kg/d, i.v. GM-CSF (not specified)	Solid tumor, lymphoma, ALL	Adult	30**	NS	NS

*Neutropenia is defined as 500 neutrophils/µL except otherwise specified.
**The design of the study includes randomization with a control group.

ADMINISTRATION OF G-CSF AND GM-CSF AT THE TIME OF A FEBRILE, NEUTROPENIC EVENT

Withholding the use of G-CSF or GM-CSF until admission for fever and neutropenia has been studied extensively (Table 11.6). Despite the expected observation that neutropenia is abbreviated with use of either G-CSF or GM-CSF (106–114), the net effect is marginal. Most studies have shown no benefit whatsoever, while a handful have shown a modest reduction in indirect measurements, such as days in hospital and antibiotic use. Two randomized studies, one with G-CSF in children and one with GM-CSF in adults, resulted in a 1- or 2-day reduction in hospital stay (median, 5 versus 7 days, $p = 0.04$ in one, and by a day, $p = 0.018$, respectively) and a decrease in days of antibiotic therapy (median, 5 versus 6 days, $p = 0.02$, and a decrease by 1 day, $p = 0.01$, respectively) (106,111). In all studies published to date, neither documented infections nor overall survival were affected by use of these growth factors (113).

to support febrile, neutropenic events at the time of diagnosis

Decrease in documented infections	Decrease in antibiotic usage	Decrease in hospitalization	Improvement in disease-free survival	Decrease in cost	Reference
	P = 0.02 6 vs 5 days	P = 0.04 7 vs 5 days		P = 0.04 29% reduction	Mitchell et al, 1997 (111)
		P < 0.001 7 vs 5 days		NS	Mayordomo et al, 1995 (109)
	NS	NS			Maher et al, 1994 (114)
NS	Entire group: P = 0.01, 6 vs 5 days Low-risk chemotherapy: P < 0.001, 7 vs 3.5 days High-risk chemotherapy: NS	NS			Ravaud et al, 1998 (106)
NS	NS	NS	NS		Anaissie et al, 1996 (113)
	NS	NS	NS	P < 0.05 (inverse, GM-CSF more expensive)	Vellenga et al, 1996 (108)
		P < 0.001 7 vs 5 days		NS	Mayordomo et al, 1995 (109)
	P < 0.05 8.5 vs 7 days	P < 0.05 10 vs 9 days		Trend	Riikonen et al, 1994 (110)
	NS				Biesma et al, 1990 (107)

The financial impact for use of G- or GM-CSF at the time of fever and neutropenia is not clear at all. One group reported an analysis of 58 episodes of fever in children and found that GM-CSF saved more than $2,000 per febrile episode (110). Others calculated that the cost per hospital stay was $4,140 in the GM-CSF group versus $3,590 in the placebo group (108). Still, others have not reported significant differences in cost (109,111).

Although a modest reduction in hospital stay and use of antibiotic therapy has been demonstrated, the available data do not clearly support the routine initiation of growth factors as adjunctive therapy in all febrile, neutropenic cancer patients (58,59). In a study published by Ravaud et al. (106), the greatest benefit with GM-CSF was surprisingly in patients at low risk. The duration of hospitalization during the study was reduced from 7 to 4 days ($p = 0.003$), and the duration on antibiotics during hospitalization from 7 to 3.5 days ($p < 0.001$). In contrast, Maher et al. (111) found in an exploratory subset analysis of a randomized, double-blind, placebo-controlled trial of 218 adult cancer patients with fever and neutropenia, that the use of G-CSF appeared to provide the greatest benefit in patients with documented infection and in patients with neutrophil counts of less than 100/μL (114). On further analysis, G-CSF seemed to benefit three subgroups in particular: those with acute lymphoblastic leukemia, those with early onset (<10 days) of fever after chemotherapy, and those without documented septicemia or focal infection.

AUGMENTATION OF HOST DEFENSE IN DOCUMENTED INFECTIONS

As mentioned earlier, *in vitro* studies suggest that both G-CSF and GM-CSF augment phagocyte function, which has been confirmed *ex vivo* but not *in vivo* (42,43). Still, the potential for enhancing function, especially in critically ill, immunocompromised hosts has provided adequate rationale for directed use of these factors. The literature is limited to small uncontrolled studies or case reports detailing the administration of adjuvant G- or GM-CSF to critically ill patients with documented infection. Anecdotal reports suggest that growth factors can be useful in patients with life-threatening fungal infections. For example, together with amphotericin B, G-CSF or GM-CSF have been associated with successful outcome in patients with Candida spp. or Aspergillus spp. who otherwise had a poor prognosis (115). Closer examination of a subset of patients who received G-CSF did not show a significant improvement in the clinical course compared to those patients who did not receive growth factors (106,113).

Prospective studies, while clearly indicated, are difficult to perform because of the paucity of patients in one center with an invasive fungal infection on a comparable protocol. The current consensus is that the approach should be held in reserve for severe life-threatening infections in the neutropenic host.

In the past, there was considerable interest in another hematopoietic growth factor, macrophage colony-stimulating factor (M-CSF) partly because of its specificity for monocytes and partly because of antifungal activity observed in a phase I study (116,117). However, these studies have not been followed-up and this agent is not available for clinical use.

G-CSF AND GM-CSF IN HIGH-DOSE CYTOTOXIC TREATMENT AND PROGENITOR CELL TRANSPLANTATION

Recipients of autologous and allogeneic marrow transplantation are at especially high risk for infection during the period of recovery following marrow ablation, marked by neutropenia. Use of G- and GM-CSF have quickly assumed a central role in supportive care to accelerate recovery of marrow. In some ways, the depth and duration of neutropenia during induction therapy for a lymphoreticular malignancy (i.e., leukemia or lymphoma) does not differ significantly from risk for infection in the immediate post-transplant period. In the transplant setting, the severity of mucositis combined with lymphocyte depletion confer a greater risk that lasts for an extended period of time, depending upon the specific preparation and type of transplant.

THE USE OF G-CSF OR GM-CSF IN AUTOLOGOUS MARROW TRANSPLANTATION

The use of G- and GM-CSF in autologous BMT has been the focus of intensive clinical investigation. Already, the liberal use of these agents has been adopted as the standard of care until recovery of neutrophils. In a preliminary, observational study which compared outcomes to historical controls, Taylor et al. (118) showed that G-CSF given after autologous BMT significantly accelerated granulocyte recovery in 18 relapsed or refractory Hodgkin's disease patients (13 days versus 22 days, $p = 0.00189$). Subsequent studies have shown that both G- and GM-CSF can accelerate a recovery from ablative neutropenia (Table 11.7) and in some cases, can abbreviate the duration by as much as 50% (119–131). However, the promise of this intervention has not necessarily translated into a discernible reduction in risk for infection in all studies published thus far.

As expected, there is considerable variation in the impact on infection-related outcomes, with some studies reporting a clear reduction, while others reported only moderate changes in indirect measurements of infection. For example, G-CSF significantly reduced the duration of fever in early studies (120–122,132). Interestingly, reduction of febrile days posttransplant has not been well established in trials using GM-CSF. In three different trials, there is evidence to suggest that the use of growth factors could decrease documented infections overall but the evidence is not persuasive. In one prospective, randomized, placebo-controlled study of 245 patients, use of G-CSF at 5μg/kg/day resulted in a reduction of microbiologically documented infection (median, 12 versus 9 days, $p = 0.027$) (120). Similarly, the G-CSF arm was associated with less days of parenteral antibiotics (median days, 19 versus 15, $p < 0.001$) and hospitalization days (median days, 29 versus 25, $p = 0.02$). In a retrospective analysis of 141 patients undergoing BMT for treatment of lymphoid cancer, 40% of the patients not receiving GM-CSF developed a serious infection, whereas only 13% of patients given GM-CSF had serious infectious complications ($p = 0.001$) (133).

Different dosing schedules have been evaluated in small studies with no clear evidence that the higher dose, 10 μg/kg/day, confers an advantage (121–123,133). In a multicenter randomized study, the authors demonstrated that G-CSF (2 to 20 μg/kg/day) induced accelerated recovery in a dose-dependent manner (123). When doses were increased above 10 μg/kg/day, there was no appreciable advantage (121,122). In the context of marrow ablation, possible effects on other cells of hematopoietic lines were not predicted, one study reported accelerated platelet recovery in the group that received a growth factor (126). Another group reported that the use of GM-CSF reduced mucositis in patients who received total body irradiation (130).

Only one study has provided sufficient evidence to conclude that overall cost (including hospital days, antibiotics, etc.) can be reduced if hematopoietic growth factors are properly used (126). As observed in the studies of cancer patients receiving chemotherapy, not one study has demonstrated a significant improvement in survival. Unexpectedly,

TABLE 11-7. *Summary of trials using myeloid growth*

Dose, route, and preparation	Disease	Adult/ pediatric	*N*	Amelioration of depth and/or duration of neutropenia*	Decrease in fever
5 μg/kg/d, i.v. filgrastim	ALL, AML, CML, lymphoma, solid tumor	Pediatric	26	NS	P < 0.05 10 vs 6 days
10 μg/kg/d or 30 μg/kg/d, i.v. filgrastim	Lymphoma	Adult	54**	P = 0.0004 20 vs 12 days (10 μg/kg/d) 20 vs 14 days (30 μg/kg/d) (no sign. diff. between both groups)	P = 0.036 10 vs 5 days (10 μg/kg/d) 10 vs 6 days (30 μg/kg/d)
5 μg/kg/d, i.v. lenograstim	ALL, lymphoma, myeloma, solid tumor	2 to 70 years	245**	P < 0.001 20 vs 14 days	P = 0.014 5 vs 3 days***
10 μg/kg/d or 20 μg/kg/d, s.c. filgrastim	Lymphoma	Adult	43**	P < 0.0001 (whole CSF group) P < 0.00005 (10 μg/kg/d) 21.5 vs 10 days (no sign. diff. between both groups)	P = 0.0418 4 vs 1 days
2–20 μg/kg/d, G-CSF, unspecified	Non-myeloid malignancies	Adult	121**	P = 0.05 19 vs 13 days	
20 μg/kg/d, s.c. filgrastim	Leukemia, lymphoma	Adult	33	P < 0.0005 20 vs 11 days	NS
60 μg/kg/d, i.v. filgrastim	Relapsed Hodgkin's disease	Adult	18	P = 0.00189 22 vs 13 days	NS
15–250 μg/m²/d, i.v. GM-CSF, unspecified	ALL, lymphoma	Adult	141		
5.5 μg/kg/d, s.c. GM-CSF, unspecified	AML	Pediatric	22	NS	NS
125 μg/m²/d, i.v. GM-CSF, unspecified	Lymphomas, solid tumors	Pediatric	26	P < 0.007 23 vs 12 days	
250 μg/m²/d, i.v. molgramostim	NHL	Adult	91**	P < 0.0001 21 vs 14 days	NS
10 μg/kg/d, i.v. molgramostim	Relapsed Hodgkin's disease	Adult	24**	P = 0.02 27 vs 16 days (Note: ANC is defined <1000/μL)	
250 μg/m²/d, s.c. molgramostim	Lymphoma	Adult	58**	P = 0.0012 20 vs 14 days	NS
250 μg/m²/d, i.v. molgramostim	ALL, lymphoma	Adult	79**	P = 0.0001 28 vs 15 days	NS
5 μg/kg/d, s.c. or i.v. molgramostim	Solid tumor, ALL, Hodgkin's disease	Pediatric	16	P < 0.05 17 vs 14 days	NS
250 μg/m²/d, i.v. sargramostim	Leukemia, lymphoma	Adult	128**	P < 0.001 26 vs 19 days	NS

*Neutropenia is defined as 500 neutrophils/μL except otherwise specified.
**The design of the study includes randomization with a control group.
***Includes 20% of patients with allogeneic BMT.

factor support in autologous marrow transplantation

Decrease in documented infections	Decrease in antibiotic usage	Decrease in hospitalization	Improvement in disease-free survival	Decrease in cost	Reference
NS	NS	NS	NS		Dini et al, 1996 (132)
NS	NS	NS	NS		Schmitz et al, 1995 (121)
P = 0.027 12 vs 9 days***	P < 0.001 19 vs 15 days***	P = 0.02 29 vs 25 days***	NS***		Gisselbrecht et al, 1994 (120)
NS	NS	NS	NS		Stahel et al, 1994 (122)
	Trend	P = 0.01 15 vs 11 days			Linch et al, 1993 (123)
NS	P = 0.002 18 vs 11 days	Trend			Sheridan et al, 1989 (119)
NS					Taylor et al, 1989 (118)
P = 0.001 40% vs 13 %	Trend		NS (if matched)		Nemunaitis et al, 1998 (133)
NS	NS	NS	P = 0.05 80 vs 40% (inverse)		Calderwood et al, 1996 (134)
NS					Gordon et al, 1994 (130)
NS	NS	P < 0.05 28 vs 23 days	NS		Gorin et al, 1992 (129)
NS		P = 0.004 40.5 vs 32 days	NS	P = 0.005 $62,500 vs $39,800	Gulati et al, 1992 (126)
NS	NS	NS	NS		Khwaja et al, 1992 (131)
NS	NS	NS	NS		Link et al, 1992 (125)
	NS	NS			Saarinen et al, 1992 (128)
NS	P = 0.009 27 vs 24 days	P = 0.01 33 vs 27 days	NS		Nemunaitis et al, 1991 (124)

one study reported that in children with AML undergoing autologous BMT, the GM-CSF–treated group had a higher relapse and poorer overall survival rate after autologous BMT than the untreated group (134). In conclusion, G-CSF and GM-CSF can successfully shorten the period of neutropenia and potentially reduce infectious complications after autologous BMT. The routine use of growth factors requires further investigation, but in truth, it is already accepted in this clinical setting (58,59).

G-CSF OR GM-CSF IN ALLOGENEIC MARROW TRANSPLANTATION

The use of growth factors in support of allogeneic marrow transplantation has quickly been embraced but with little published data to demonstrate overall efficacy. While there is a strong rationale for giving G- or GM-CSF in the immediate transplant period, the issue has not been systematically studied but instead, adopted in nearly all centers. With two notable exceptions (132,135), the studies report abbreviation of neutropenia by as much as 50% (Table 11.8) (120,136–140). Like the data for autologous BMT, most published studies have shown a reduction in infection-related parameters but in some studies, the findings have not been replicated. Surprisingly, one placebo controlled study

TABLE 11-8. *Summary of trials using myeloid*

Dose, route, and preparation	Disease	Adult/ pediatric	*N*	Donors	Amelioration of depth and/or duration of neutropenia*	Decrease in fever
5 μg/kg/d, s.c. or i.v. G-CSF (unspecified)	Leukemia, lymphoma	Adult	196	HLA-identical	P < 0.0001 20 vs 12 days	
5 μg/kg/d, i.v. filgrastim	ALL, AML, CML, lymphoma, solid tumor	Pediatric	36	Matched sibling (N = 13) Unrelated donor (N = 5)	NS	NS
5 μg/kg/d, i.v. lenograstim	ALL, lymphoma, myeloma, solid tumor	2 to 70 years	70**	Unspecified	P < 0.01 20 vs. 14 days	
10 μg/kg/d, i.v. G-CSF (unspecified)	ALL, AML, CML, lymphoma	Adult	102	Matched sibling (N = 82) Unrelated donor (N = 20)	P < 0.01, 13 vs 10 days P < 0.05, 19 vs 16 days (depending on GVHD prophylaxis)	
250 μg/m²/d, i.v. sargramostim	Leukemia, lymphoma, myeloma	Adult	109**	HLA-identical	P = 0.0001 17 vs. 13 days	NS
10 μg/kg/d, i.v. molgramostim	Leukemia, lymphoma	Adult	53**	HLA-matched (N = 51) HLA-mismatched (N = 2)	P < 0.01 21 vs. 17 days	NS
5.5 μg/kg/d, i.v. GM-CSF (CHO-derived)	AML, ALL, CML, lymphoma	Adult	57**	HLA-identical	P < 0.05 15.6 vs 13.2 days	NS
5.5 μg/kg/d, i.v. GM-CSF (CHO-derived)	AML, ALL, CML	Adult	40**	HLA-matched siblings	NS	P < 0.005 (inverse)

*Neutropenia is defined as 500 neutrophils/μL except otherwise specified.
**The design of the study includes randomization with a control group.
***Reported for both autologous (*N* = 26) and allogeneic (*N* = 36).

showed that GM-CSF was associated with a greater likelihood of fever ($p = 0.005$) as well as a greater use of antibiotics (16 versus 13 days, $p = 0.019$) (135). Still, data from a randomized, double-blind placebo-controlled study in 109 patients showed a significant decrease in documented infections (64% versus 91%, $p = 0.001$) and a reduction in grade III or IV mucositis (8% of GM-CSF–patients versus 29% of placebo-treated patients, $p = 0.005$) (137). One trial concluded that pneumonia was less likely in the group of patients receiving a growth factor (139). Others have argued for use of G- or GM-CSF on the grounds that their use directly resulted in a shortening of hospitalization (136,137). Lastly, no study has shown an increase in graft-versus-host disease or graft rejection (120,135,138,139,141). Overall, survival is not changed but cost has been reported to be reduced (136,142).

GROWTH FACTORS AFTER FAILURE/DELAYED ENGRAFTMENT

In a minority of recipients, failure or delayed engraftment occurs, which, in turn, carries a substantially higher risk for infectious complications. The risk for graft failure is especially high in recipients who have received an allogeneic marrow purged of T cells

growth factors in allogeneic marrow transplantation

Decrease in documented infections	Decrease in antibiotic usage	Decrease in hospitalization	Improvement in disease-free survival	Decrease in cost	Reference
		P < 0.0001 23 vs 17 days	NS	P = 0.0373 $84,000 vs $80,600	Lee et al, 1998 (136)
NS***	NS***	NS***	NS***		Dini et al, 1996 (132)
					Gisselbrecht et al, 1994 (120)
			NS		Schriber et al, 1994 (140)
P = 0.001 91% vs 64 %	NS	P = 0.02 26 vs. 25 days	NS		Nemunaitis et al, 1995 (137)
NS			NS		Hiraoka et al, 1994 (138)
NS	NS	NS	Trend		De Witte et al, 1992 (139)
	P = 0.019 13 vs 16 days (inverse)	NS	NS		Powles et al, 1990 (135)

or treated *in vitro* with 4-hydroxycyclophosphamide (143,144). Consequently, these manipulations, which are intended to decrease the risk for graft-versus-host disease, come at a price. Therapeutic options for graft rejection or extended delayed engraftment are poor, as is the prognosis for a second transplant. In this context, therapy with G- or GM-CSF has been employed with moderate success (145,146). For example, GM-CSF was evaluated in 37 patients with marrow graft failure after allogeneic (n = 15), autologous (n = 21), or syngeneic (n = 1) BMT (144); GM-CSF was administered at doses between 60 and 1,000 μg/m^2/day for 14 or 21 days. Twenty-one patients achieved an absolute neutrophil count of more than 500/μL within 2 weeks of starting therapy, while no response was noted in the remaining 16 patients. While not conclusive, overall survival was better in the group who received GM-CSF compared to historical controls. Other studies have reported similar findings. Unfortunately, the effect is rarely sustained (147–150).

In this context, some investigators have pursued the use of these agents in combination, based upon subtle but important differences in the effect of the factors. It has been postulated that a response could be observed with G-CSF but not GM-CSF because theoretically G-CSF stimulates both early and late myeloid progenitor cells whereas GM-CSF mainly stimulates the intermediate myeloid progenitor cells (151). In fact, Boulad et al. (151) described one patient with graft failure following autologous BMT, who responded to GM-CSF only temporarily, but subsequently responded to G-CSF. However, no such advantage was observed in a prospective, randomized trial comparing GM-CSF versus sequential GM-CSF and G-CSF as treatment for primary or secondary graft failure in 47 BMT patients (152). Based on the available data, continuing growth factor therapy in patients with protracted posttransplantation neutropenia or reintroduction of growth factor therapy for those patients with recurrent myelosuppression may have potential benefit and is unlikely to cause harm (58,59).

G-CSF AND GM-CSF IN THE SUPPORT OF PERIPHERAL BLOOD PROGENITOR CELL INFUSIONS

Both G-CSF and GM-CSF stimulate the release of peripheral blood progenitor cells (PBPC) from the bone marrow into the peripheral blood (153–155). Thus, the ability to mobilize large quantities of stem cells offers an important advance in transplantation, namely, harvesting a greater number of progenitors, which, in turn, improves the likelihood of engraftment. In the past, insufficient number of cells for infusion was the primary cause of graft failure (156,157). Quantitatively, delayed or failed engraftment has been associated with infusion of less than 2.5 to 5.0 × 10^6 CD34$^+$ cells/kg (158–160). Efforts to harvest stem cells from peripheral blood had been hampered by two factors, the rarity of stem cells in the steady state in circulation, and the need to perform repetitive phereses to harvest adequate numbers (161,162). Now, infusion of growth factor mobilized PBPCs can lead to a more rapid hematologic recovery than harvested marrow (either allogeneic or autologous) (163–168). Furthermore, infusion of mobilized PBPCs has emerged as a new tool for support following intensive therapy. In particular, stem cell rescue can lessen toxicities, such as mucositis, antibiotic use, and hospitalization time (162,165,166,169–171).

For some time, it has been observed that nonablative chemotherapy can successfully mobilize progenitor cells for peripheral collection (172–176). Together with the use of G- or GM-CSF following cytotoxic chemotherapy, an effective mobilization regimen has been developed (177). In fact, several studies have shown that the combination of a myeloid growth factor and cytotoxic chemotherapy is superior to either alone (154,155, 157,161,162,165,175,177–181).

One of the major advantages of using growth factors with nonablative chemotherapy is that it is safe and feasible in infants and children as well as in adults (182–187). In the past, pheresis of children and infants has been associated with significant risk. Children have a greater volume of blood per kilogram of body weight and are therefore more susceptible to metabolic and hemodynamic disturbances. In this regard, use of growth factors further facilitates the harvest of an adequate number of stem cells. After mobilization with G-CSF, the CD34$^+$ cell yield of peripheral blood progenitor allografts in 41 normal donors exceeded that of bone marrow allografts by 3.7-fold (188). Peripheral stem cell harvest with G- or GM-CSF mobilization also eliminates the risk of anesthesia for allogeneic marrow donors.

The peak yield for stem cell harvest after mobilization with growth factors occurs after 4 to 8 days (57,189–191), whereas, if growth factors are given with chemotherapy, the best yield is shortly after recovery from neutropenia (175,192,193). In rare circumstances, escalating the dose has been effective in producing a better yield, even as late as three weeks afterwards (194). Existing data do not show any appreciable difference between G-CSF and GM-CSF for PBPC harvest following cytotoxic chemotherapy; they induce comparable yields of progenitors. The combination of G-CSF with GM-CSF has no significant clinical benefit over either factor alone (198).

Not only are growth factors useful for collection of PBPCs, but they are also indicated posttransplantation for the purpose of accelerating recovery of neutrophils (Table 11.9). Similar to the data reporting on G- and GM-CSF support of autologous or allogeneic marrow transplantation, growth factor support results in abbreviation of the period of neutrophil aplasia in patients who receive PBPCs (199–208). The efficacy of GM-CSF alone or in combination with PBPCs as support for patients receiving high-dose chemotherapy was compared in several trials that showed similar results (209–212). In a randomized study of 18 patients with advanced breast cancer undergoing high-dose chemotherapy, patients receiving GM-CSF–primed PBPCs and GM-CSF recovered neutrophil counts faster than patients receiving GM-CSF alone (12 versus 21 days, $p = 0.02$) (210).

Growth factor support after infusion of PBPCs has contributed to a decrease in the use of antibiotics and hospital days in multiple studies (199–206,213). A decrease in the duration of fever was reported in two nonrandomized studies using G-CSF (199,206), whereas in a double-blind randomized study, the administration of GM-CSF after the transfusion of mobilized PBPCs resulted in a significantly higher number of febrile days (6 versus 2 days, $p = 0.01$) (214). No single trial reported a better event-free or overall survival for patients receiving growth factors in this setting. It should be added that one study suggested a role for combination support with G- and GM-CSF (213).

In two separate, nonrandomized studies, growth factor support of PBPC transplantation had no beneficial effect on clinical endpoints (215,216). In one study, G-CSF approximately doubled the average cost of PBPC transplantation (215). Conversely, others have provided analyses that indicate that overall cost could be reduced, particularly in utilization of supportive care for infections (i.e., antibiotic usage and less hospitalization) (199,203,205,206). Since cost is a major issue in transplantation, several authors have investigated delaying administration of growth factors until well after infusion of autologous PBPCs; a delay of 6 days was not found to be detrimental to hematological recovery (217,218).

TABLE 11-9. *Summary of several recent trials of growth-factor*

Dose, route, and preparation	Disease	Adult/ pediatric	*N*	Amelioration of depth and/or duration of neutropenia*	Decrease in fever
300 μg/m²/d, i.v. filgrastim	ALL, NHL, solid tumor	Pediatric	58**	P = 0.046 12 vs 11 days	NS
5 μg/kg/d, i.v. filgrastim	NHL, Hodgkin's disease, myeloma	Adult	40	P < 0.0001 14 vs 10 days	P = 0.028 5 vs 2.5 days
5 μg/kg/d, s.c. filgrastim	High-grade NHL	Adult (<60 yrs)	23**	P < 0.0001 13.2 vs 9.7 days	NS
263 μg/kg/d, s.c. lenograstim	Lymphoma	Adult	62**	P = 0.0001 12.5 vs 9 days	
50 μg/m²/d, s.c. filgrastim	Myeloma, lymphoma	Adult	36**	P < 0.0001 14 vs 10 days	NS
5 μg/kg/d, s.c. filgrastim	NHL	Adult	40	NS	NS
5 μg/kg/d, i.v. G-CSF (unspecified)	NHL, Hodgkin's disease, solid tumor	Adult	41**	P = 0.0001 16 vs 10.5 days	NS
5 μg/kg/d, s.c. filgrastim***	NHL, Hodgkin's disease	Adult	60	P < 0.05 17 vs 10 days	
10 μg/kg/d, s.c. or i.v. filgrastim	NHL, Hodgkin's disease, myeloma, solid tumor	Adult	19	NS	NS
50 μg/m²/d, s.c. filgrastim	Lymphoma, leukemia, solid tumor	Adult	20	P < 0.01 14 vs 10 days	NS
5 μg/kg/d, s.c. molgramostim	NHL, Hodgkin's disease, myeloma, solid tumor	Adult	50**	NS	P = 0.01 4 vs 7 days (inverse)
10 μg/kg/d, i.v. molgramostim****	Lymphoma, leukemia, solid tumor	Adult	60**	P < 0.01 15 vs 12 days	NS*****
5 μg/kg/d, s.c. filgrastim (+ EPO – 150 U/kg/d)	Breast cancer, ovarian cancer	Adult	25	P < 0.0001 11 vs 8 days	P < 0.0001 4 vs 0 days
5 μg/kg/d, s.c. GM-CSF (unspecified) (+ EPO – 150 U/kg/d)	Breast cancer, ovarian cancer	Adult	25	NS	NS
Combination of G-CSF and GM-CSF, 7.5 μg/kg/d and 2.5 μg/kg/d, resp., i.v.	NHL, Hodgkin's disease, solid tumor	Adult	37**	P = 0.0004 16 vs 10 days	NS

*Neutropenia is defined as 500 neutrophils/μL, except otherwise specified.
**The design of the study includes randomization with a control group.
***Historical control group did not receive G-CSF at collection or after cell infusion.
****Autologous PBSC with or without bone marrow.
*****Includes patients with autologous BMT.

therapy after autologous peripheral blood stem–cell transplantation

Decrease in documented infections	Decrease in antibiotic usage	Decrease in hospitalization	Improvement in disease-free survival	Decrease in cost	Reference
					Kawano et al, 1998 (207)
NS	P = 0.019 11 vs 8 days	P = 0.0028 16 vs 13 days		Trend	Tarella et al, 1998 (206)
NS	NS	P = 0.001 15 vs 12 days		Trend	Lee et al, 1998 (205)
NS	NS	P = 0.0002 15.5 vs 13 days			Linch et al, 1997 (204)
	NS	P = 0.0003 16 vs 13 days		Trend	McQuaker et al, 1997 (203)
NS	NS	NS			Cortelazzo et al, 1995 (216)
	P = 0.03 15 vs 11 days	P = 0.002 24 vs 18 days	NS		Klumpp et al, 1995 (202)
P < 0.05 7 vs 0 cases		P < 0.05 30 vs 22 days			Brice et al, 1994 (201)
	NS	NS		Trend (inverse)	Dunlop et al, 1994 (215)
	P < 0.01 8.5 vs 2.2 days				Shimazaki et al, 1994 (200)
NS	NS	NS			Legros et al, 1997 (214)
NS****		NS	NS****		Greenberg et al, 1996 (208)
NS	P < 0.0001 7.5 vs 0 days	P = 0.0357 20 vs 18 days		Trend	Benedetti Panici et al, 1997 (199)
NS	P < 0.0001 7.5 vs 0 days	P = 0.0069 20 vs 16 days		Trend	Benedetti Panici et al, 1997 (199)
NS		P = 0.0112 21 vs 19 days			Spitzer et al, 1994 (213)

NEW HORIZONS FOR THE USE OF G- AND GM-CSF

The Use of G-CSF and GM-CSF to Enhance Dose Intensity

Retrospective analyses have correlated chemotherapy activity with dose intensity (219–221). Cheung et al. (222) have shown in a retrospective analysis of 44 clinical trials that maximal dose intensification of drugs over a short duration can improve outcome in patients with poor-risk neuroblastoma. Similar results have been reported for Ewing's sarcoma, osteogenic sarcoma and advanced-stage intermediate-grade lymphoma (219,223). These data suggest that patients who receive higher and more frequent doses of chemotherapy are more likely to benefit from more aggressive treatment. In light of the widespread use of G- and GM-CSF, oncologists have employed these agents to pursue dose-escalation of single or multiple agent chemotherapies. So far, several preliminary studies have shown that G-CSF or GM-CSF allow better adherence to dose intensification schedules of single agents, such as cyclophosphamide (224), paclitaxel (225), or mitoxantrone (226). In one study, 41 patients with locally advanced breast cancer who received epirubicin and cyclophosphamide plus G-CSF every 2 weeks were compared with patients who received the same regimen given every 3 weeks without G-CSF in a previous study (227). The authors suggested that the administration of G-CSF facilitated dose intensification of both drugs (a 59.5% increase of the actual dose intensity) with acceptable clinical side effects. Similar results were obtained in studies using different chemotherapy regimens for small cell lung cancer (72,228), metastatic or high-risk breast cancer (229,230), and aggressive non-Hodgkin's lymphoma (62,231,232).

So far, randomized studies have not provided a clear and persuasive answer. In advanced high-grade non-Hodgkin's lymphoma treated with a combination of cyclophosphamide, mitoxantrone, vincristine, etoposide, bleomycin, and prednisone, the delivery of dose intensity in patients who received G-CSF was no better than in those who did not receive the growth factor (233). It is not surprising that the administration of G-CSF or GM-CSF has little or no impact on dose-escalation, since other dose-limiting toxicities are unaffected by growth factors, such as thrombocytopenia, mucositis or neuropathy (234). Therefore, combinations of drugs that induce thrombocytopenia (e.g., carboplatin, thiotepa) or extramedullary toxicities (e.g., 5-fluouracil, paclitaxel) may be difficult to escalate with growth factor support (235–238). Loss of T lymphocytes is also a limiting factor in dose intensification. This is especially important for children, because age as well as specific agents are critical parameters in T cell loss and regeneration (6,239–241). In a pediatric study using high-dose cyclophosphamide and G-CSF for brain tumors, cycles of therapy were administered approximately every 14 days. Fifty-six percent of patients in this study developed opportunistic complications, such as pneumocystic pneumonia, severe adenoviral pneumonia, and herpes zoster (240).

On the other hand, two randomized trials in patients with small cell lung cancer report improved survival in patients who have received adjuvant growth factor. In one study with 64 patients, the median survival was 59 weeks in the G-CSF group compared to 32 weeks in controls ($p = 0.004$) (242). Similar results were observed in a trial of 65 patients in which the G-CSF group received a significantly higher dose-intensity. In this group, the overall 2-year survival rate was 32% compared to 15% in controls (72). In contrast, others, who have studied the same patient populations with small cell lung cancer and aggressive non-Hodgkin's lymphoma, have not reported similar results (63,231,243). In summary, the use of growth factors for intensification of chemotherapy outside of clinical trials is neither warranted nor recommended (58,59).

Hematopoietic Growth Factors in Cord Blood Transplantation

Successful transplantation of hematopoietic stem cells harvested from umbilical cord blood (i.e., placental blood) of human donors represents a major advance in transplantation biology. In addition, transplantation from both HLA-matched and HLA-mismatched unrelated donors have resulted in permanent engraftment with no greater risk for graft-versus-host disease (244–249). Not only does this approach increase the number of potential donors, but it also eliminates the risk to the donor. The small likelihood of transmitting clinically important infections is coupled with a low risk for severe graft-versus-host disease (245,247,249,250). A review of 562 recipients of cord blood transplants from unrelated donors illustrated the success of this approach (244); myeloid engraftment occurred at a median of 28 days and the cumulative rate of engraftment among the recipients by day 42 was 81% for a neutrophil count above 500/μL. Severe acute graft-versus-host disease occurred in 23% of the patients. In the majority of patients, either G-CSF or GM-CSF was used to accelerate neutrophil recovery following infusion of umbilical cord blood with no untoward complications (247–249). As this approach evolves, the judicious use of myelopoietic growth factors will be better defined by ongoing studies.

Granulocyte Transfusions

In the 1970s, there was intense interest in using granulocyte transfusions in the support of profoundly neutropenic patients with life-threatening infection. Among the many problems that plagued this approach was the difficulty in harvesting an adequate number of neutrophils from prospective donors. Other complications, such as a high rate of alloimmunization, poor leukocyte matching techniques, transmission of viral pathogens (i.e., first CMV, then HIV) further dampened enthusiasm. When it became clear that growth factors could easily and safely mobilize large numbers of neutrophils, attention turned back to the issue of granulocyte transfusions (251,252). G-CSF or GM-CSF given to normal volunteers can safely increase mobilization for collection by almost an order of magnitude (57,253,254). Close analysis of the primary description of the feasibility of G-CSF supported granulocyte transfusions also suggested that G-CSF–stimulated donor neutrophils might persist longer in circulation (57). Thus, with growth factor mobilization of healthy donors, a greater number of neutrophils can be harvested, infused and are expected to persist longer in circulation.

It is still not clear whether G-CSF–stimulated granulocyte transfusions will significantly improve survival. For the moment, granulocyte transfusions are generally reserved for patients with severe life-threatening infections. There have been anecdotal reports detailing successful use of G-CSF– or GM-CSF–stimulated granulocyte transfusions in patients with life-threatening fungal infections (255–257). However, a recent retrospective review of this modality in transplantation did not find an advantage for patients with fungal infection (258).

Growth factors can also influence the qualitative functions of neutrophils. G-CSF– or GM-CSF–treated granulocytes maintain functional capabilities and appear to survive longer (253,259). Preliminary data suggests that these agents may enhance microbicidal activity both in *ex vivo* and *in vivo* (45,46,113). In the future, it may be possible to use *ex vivo* manipulation of neutrophils to enhance microbicidal activity or to enable delivery of higher concentrations of a drug.

Priming With G-CSF and GM-CSF

What has been previously reported as a major contraindication, coadministration of growth factor support and myelotoxic chemotherapy has been used in selected circumstances to take advantage of the stimulatory effect of growth factors on leukemic cell cycle kinetics to move more leukemic cells out of the nonproliferative stage (G0 phase) and through G to S phase (84,87). Specifically, this approach has been investigated in AML. The rationale is based upon the observation that in transition from G to S phase, when active DNA synthesis is greatest, the largest number of leukemic blasts could be susceptible to cytotoxic chemotherapy. However, the possibility that "priming" could have a detrimental effect is considerable and led many to shy away from this approach. Clinical trials in AML patients have examined the feasibility of priming leukemic cells with G-CSF or GM-CSF for periods ranging from 18 hours to 8 days (Table 11.9) (260–264). In a preliminary study, 56 patients with newly diagnosed AML receiving GM-CSF (up to 8 days) were compared to 176 matched historical controls, all of whom also received ara-C and daunorubicin chemotherapy (264). The complete response rate in primed patients was 48%, whereas in control patients it was 65% ($p = 0.011$); survival data showed the same trend ($p = 0.035$). Other studies have reported similar findings. Since the overall results from the clinical trials with priming are not encouraging, ASCO guidelines do not recommend administration of growth factors either before and/or concurrent with chemotherapy (58,59).

PRACTICAL ISSUES OF USING G-CSF AND GM-CSF

Dosing and Route of Administration of G-CSF and GM-CSF

While there is widespread use of G- and GM-CSF in cancer patients, there has been little investigation of the proper dosage of G- and GM-CSF in the cancer therapy or transplant setting. To date, most published studies have employed G-CSF at 5 to 10 μg/kg/day subcutaneously, based upon the phase III licensing studies (61–63). However, it is not clear that 5 to 10 μg/kg/day is required, particularly as we gain a more refined understanding of the judicious use of these expensive agents. Similarly, the recommended dose for GM-CSF is between 5 and 10 μg/kg/day is based upon studies in cancer patients and autologous BMT patients who received a comparable dose of 250 μg/m^2/day. For the latter indication, several studies have shown a decrease in the time to neutrophil recovery, shortening of the duration of hospitalization, and received antibiotic use following autologous BMT (124,265). The data on GM-CSF dose is more complicated to evaluate because the studies are generally small and relatively few are prospective or randomized (67,80,266,267).

Dose-escalation studies have been conducted to investigate potential side effects unrelated to efficacy. In some phase I studies, G-CSF doses of 20 to 60 μg/kg/day accelerated recovery of neutrophils (268,269), whereas others have not replicated the effect (270–272). In several randomized trials comparing 5 and 10 μg/kg/day of G-CSF after intensive chemotherapy, no advantage was observed for the higher dose (273,274). On the other hand, some authors have argued that even lower doses could provide comparable effects in most clinical situations while saving considerable expense and avoiding potential toxicity (275–277). In some circumstances, low dose G-CSF, such as 1.5 to 2.0 μg/kg/day, is adequate and provides adequate acceleration of myelopoiesis (275–279). One of the challenges of the future will be to determine effective dosing based upon prospective studies.

For mobilization of PBPCs, a comparable controversy concerning the proper dose exists. One study has argued that there is no incremental benefit above 3 μg/kg of G-CSF per day, whereas other studies found little added benefit of 10 over 5 μg/kg/day (135). Moreover, more toxicity has been reported with the higher doses, especially in healthy volunteers (280). At this time, the current approach embraced by most centers is to use 3 to 5 μg/kg/day of G- or GM-CSF for mobilization of stem cells.

It is possible to administer G- and GM-CSF by subcutaneous or intravenous route; both achieve therapeutic levels that sustain neutrophil recovery. However, early reports of severe systemic manifestations related to intravenous administration have dampened interest in this route. Consequently, current use is generally by subcutaneous administration of both G- and GM-CSF. It is unlikely that this will change because of the ease of administration as an outpatient and the desire to minimize risk for systemic reactions. The pharmacokinetics permit administering the full dose once a day. While there are theoretical reasons to consider split dosing, such as to accelerate recovery in a patient with a life-threatening infection, there is little evidence to justify this schedule. There is no apparent difference in the pharmacokinetics between children and adults (281,282).

Discontinuing G- or GM-CSF support for the cancer patient or marrow recipient is recommended when an adequate number of circulating neutrophils is observed. There are no good data indicating the optimal threshold for stopping therapy. Most experts would agree that the circulating neutrophil count should exceed 5,000/μL and some advocate 10,000/μL. If G- or GM-CSF is discontinued as soon as the peripheral neutrophil count exceeds 500/μL, then there is substantial risk for the count to fall, even if transiently for a day or two. Since no studies have addressed this particular issue, one has to balance the cost against the relative risk for infection based upon a target level for circulating neutrophils.

Side Effects of Administration of G-CSF and GM-CSF

The toxicity profiles of G- and GM-CSF strongly resemble each other, but there are important subtle differences that have emerged from extensive clinical experience. In healthy volunteers, either factor can produce complaints which include fevers, bone pain, nausea and headache. These effects are accentuated by higher doses, which also can cause sleeplessness. For example, medullary bone pain is reported by 15% to 39% of patients receiving 5μg/kg/day, compared to 0% to 21% of control patients (61–63,68,110, 114). This side effect occurs especially when marrow activity is highest (283). Some have argued, but not necessarily demonstrated, that use shortly after high-dose chemotherapy can lead to accentuation of toxicities. Since the side effects of chemotherapy overlap with administration of growth factors, it is hard to differentiate the relative contribution of each. However, in several published reports in patients receiving high-dose chemotherapy followed by 250 μg/m^2/day of GM-CSF, there were no excessive systemic side effects when compared to placebo-treated controls (90,124,284).

Less common, but nonetheless significant complications of G- and GM-CSF have been described. For example, pulmonary reactions consisting of transient hypoxia and dyspnea have been reported (268,285). In selected patients, the first dose of GM-CSF can result in a systemic reaction that is characterized not only by dyspnea and hypoxia but also by transient flushing, tachycardia, hypotension, and rigor. In particular, the nonglycosylated form of GM-CSF has been associated with this rare, systemic effect (286,287). During phase I and II trials, pericarditis, atrial fibrillation, pleural effusion, capillary leak, and thrombosis have been reported after high doses or continuous administration of GM-CSF (288,295).

In some patients, splenomegaly is noted and, perhaps is the consequence of extramedullary hematopoiesis. Generally it is asymptomatic, but on occasion can result in left upper quadrant abdominal pain (296,297). Dermatological reactions associated with G-CSF or GM-CSF have been described, such as acute febrile neutrophilic dermatosis (Sweet syndrome) (298), transient leukemia cutis in a patient with CML (299), injection site inflammation (80,267,300–302), swipe rashes (283,296), and rare allergic reactions (283,303,304). Mild alopecia has been observed in patients receiving a growth factor chronically (296).

Some authors have suggested that GM-CSF could be associated with more toxicity because of the broader range of target cells (305–307). Sequential open-label trials comparing GM-CSF (molgramostim) and G-CSF (filgrastim) prophylaxis have provided preliminary evidence that GM-CSF may be associated with more toxicity than G-CSF (308–311). Others have not reported this difference, and argue that if it exists, the difference is relatively small. Nonetheless, head-to-head prospective studies have not been conducted but are needed to resolve this important issue.

Other components of peripheral blood are affected by the use of G- and GM-CSF. For example, some patients on G-CSF will experience an unexplained increase in monocytes and lymphocytes (312). Some investigators have noted an increase in eosinophil counts in patients receiving GM-CSF. On occasion, eosinophilia can reach 30% to 50% of the total white count before quickly dropping after cessation of GM-CSF. Elevated serum levels of enzymes classically associated with granulocyte production or function are frequently seen. These include elevations of lactate dehydrogenase, uric acid and alkaline phosphatase; the latter is frequently observed when there is rapid myeloid cell turnover (155,283,313–317).

So far, antibodies to recombinant preparations of G- and GM-CSF have not been a clinical problem. Anti–G-CSF antibodies have not been reported to date (61–63,318, 319), whereas 4% of patients have neutralizing antibodies to GM-CSF (284).

OTHER CYTOKINES

Interleukin-3

In the past, there has been intense interest in the clinical use of interleukin-3 (IL-3), a cytokine that has a broad range of effects on hematopoiesis. IL-3 acts directly on early progenitor cells, accelerating myelopoiesis and thrombopoiesis; IL-3 is also critical for lymphoid development and will increase circulating levels of peripheral lymphocytes (40,41). In clinical studies evaluating the use of IL-3 as adjuvant therapy for support of neutropenia following cytotoxic chemotherapy, the results have not conclusively demonstrated an overall benefit of IL-3. Furthermore, IL-3 is not as effective as G- or GM-CSF in accelerating recovery of neutrophils (320–325). Comparison of IL-3 supported autologous marrow recipients to historical controls receiving GM-CSF failed to show an advantage for IL-3. In a large, randomized, placebo controlled multicenter study in patients with ovarian cancer, the use of IL-3 did not significantly reduce indications for platelet transfusions nor result in a higher rate of compliance for scheduled chemotherapy (327).

Because IL-3 acts on early progenitors, studies have addressed the sequential use of IL-3 followed by GM-CSF, which acts at a later stage in granulopoiesis. A phase I study in patients with advanced tumors but normal hematopoiesis indicated that sequential treatment with IL-3 and GM-CSF could possibly accelerate neutrophil recovery and mobilize a larger pool of circulating progenitor cells but had no effect on platelet recovery

(328). However, follow-up studies have not confirmed the promise of these observations (329–332). Comparable data has been reported for patients undergoing autologous BMT. Unfortunately, a randomized study has not validated the conclusions of the previous study (333,334).

Preliminary data indicate that IL-3 could be an effective agent for mobilization of PBPCs but further studies are needed to confirm this observation. For example, the sequential administration of IL-3 followed by G-CSF permitted successful collection of PBSCs in 11 of 19 extensively pretreated patients, in whom prior PBSC mobilization with G-CSF had not been adequate (335).

Significant side effects associated with IL-3 use include fever and flu-like symptoms. Other side effects have been reported, such as facial flushing, headache, conjunctival inflammation, bone pain, local injection reactions, and rashes (320,323).

PIXY321

On the basis of preclinical data suggesting that IL-3 and GM-CSF together could accelerate marrow recovery, a recombinant molecule was generated that fused the active domains of GM-CSF and IL-3, designated PIXY321, to interact with both IL-3 and the GM-CSF receptors (336,337). In small, nonrandomized clinical trials, the effect of PIXY321 on neutrophil recovery appeared to be comparable to either G-CSF or GM-CSF (338–341). The salutary effect on platelet recovery was also observed (342,343). In two randomized studies, no benefit for PIXY321 over either G-CSF or GM-CSF was observed for neutrophil or platelet recovery (344,345). In a study of 39 pediatric patients, there was no demonstrable clinical benefit from PIXY321 (346). It is possible that the lack of clinical efficacy associated with PIXY321 could be partly explained by pharmacokinetic studies. In particular, low plasma concentrations correlated with increased clearance following prolonged administration (346).

The toxicity profile of PIXY321 is not unique. It approximates that of IL-3 and GM-CSF. Reactions at the site of injection and flu-like symptoms are the most commonly reported side effects of subcutaneous administration.

PERSPECTIVES

Hematopoietic colony-stimulating factors have been introduced into clinical practice as additional supportive measures that can reduce, but not eliminate infectious complications associated with therapy-induced neutropenia. Over the past decade, we have begun to appreciate the subtler aspects of the proper use of G-CSF and GM-CSF, identifying appropriate indications and contraindications. In the course of evaluating the corpus of studies, a set of formal recommendations have been propagated for the judicious use of these expensive growth factors (58,59). To prevent serious infection, the use of G- or GM-CSF is recommended in a subset of patients shortly after having received chemotherapy, a marrow transplant or stem cell rescue (58,59). In febrile neutropenic patients, current data do not support the use of growth factors as standard therapy. The use of G- or GM-CSF to augment host defense in neutropenic patients with a documented infection is reserved for extreme cases and the data is speculative, based upon *in vitro* and *ex vivo* observations. An exciting development is the use of G-CSF and GM-CSF to mobilize peripheral-blood progenitor cells. Current controversies include use of hematopoietic growth factors in AML and as adjuvant therapy for dose intensification treatment plans. Efforts must be directed at better defining the endpoints and in particular assigning value to reduction in treatment of possible infectious complications, such as days in hospital, antibiotic usage and costs.

Future studies are clearly warranted to address several issues. Prospective clinical trials are still needed to define specific treatment groups that can benefit from growth factor support. In addition, randomized studies are required to evaluate the proper dosage and duration of therapy, which most likely will vary between groups, depending upon underlying malignancy and therapy given. In addition, combinations of different growth factors have to be tested, particularly if *ex vivo* expansion and the storage of hematopoietic stem cells are to be utilized in a wider spectrum of patients.

ACKNOWLEDGMENTS

We would like to thank María Laura Lanzeni for her help in preparing the manuscript. Dr. Lehrnbecher was supported by a Dr. Mildred Scheel Stipendium, Deutsche Krebshilfe e.V.

REFERENCES

1. Freifeld A, Hathorn J, Pizzo P. Infectious complications in the pediatric cancer patient. In: Pizzo P, Poplack D, eds. *Principles and practice of pediatric oncology*. Philadelphia: Lippincott Co., 1993:987–1020.
2. Sculier JP, Weerts D, Klastersky J. Causes of death in febrile granulocytopenic cancer patients receiving empiric antibiotic therapy. *Eur J Cancer Clin Oncol* 1984;20:55–60.
3. Chanock SJ, Pizzo PA. Fever in the neutropenic host. *Infect Dis Clin North Am* 1996;10:777–796.
4. Bearman SI, Appelbaum FR, Back A, et al. Regimen-related toxicity and early posttransplant survival in patients undergoing marrow transplantation for lymphoma. *J Clin Oncol* 1989;7:1288–1294.
5. Kirk JL Jr, Greenfield RA, Slease RB, et al. Analysis of early infectious complications after autologous bone marrow transplantation. *Cancer* 1988;62:2445–2450.
6. Lehrnbecher T, Foster C, Vazquez N, et al. Therapy-induced alterations in host defense in children receiving chemotherapy. *J Pediatr Hematol Oncol* 1997;19:399–417.
7. Chanock SJ. Evolving risk factors for infectious complications of cancer therapy. In: Pizzo PA, ed. *Infectious complications in the immunocompromised host.* Philadelphia: W.B. Saunders Company, 1993:771–794.
8. Margolin JF, Poplack DG. Acute lymphoblastic leukemia. In: Pizzo PA, Poplack DG, eds. *Principles and practice of pediatric oncology*. Philadelphia: Lippincott–Raven Publishers, 1997:409–462.
9. Pizzo PA. Management of fever in patients with cancer and treatment-induced neutropenia. *N Engl J Med* 1993; 328:1323–1332.
10. Schimpff S, Satterlee W, Young V, et al. Empiric therapy with carbenicillin and gentamicin for febrile, patients with cancer and granulocytopenia. *N Engl J Med* 1971;284:1061–1065.
11. Schimpff SC, Young VM, Greene WH, et al. Origin of infection in acute nonlymphocytic leukemia: significance of hospital acquisition of potential pathogens. *Ann Intern Med* 1972;77:707–714.
12. Bodey GP, Buckley M, Sathe YS, et al. Quantitative relationships between circulating leukocytes and infections in patients with acute leukemia. *Ann Intern Med* 1966;64:328–340.
13. Freifeld AG, Walsh TJ, Marshall D, et al. Monotherapy for fever and neutropenia in cancer patients: a randomized comparison of ceftazadime versus imipenem. *J Clin Oncol* 1995;13:165–176.
14. De Pauw B, Deresinski S, Feld R, et al. Ceftazidime compared with piperacillin and tobramycin for the empiric treatment of fever in neutropenic patients with cancer. *Am J Med* 1994;120:834–844.
15. Talcott J, Finberg R, Mayer R, et al. The medical course of cancer patients with fever and neutropenia: clinical identification of a low-risk subgroup at presentation. *Arch Intern Med* 1988;148:2561–2568.
16. Talcott JA, Siegel RD, Finberg R, et al. Risk assessment in cancer patients with fever and neutropenia: a prospective, two-center validation of a prediction rule. *J Clin Oncol* 1992;10:316–322.
17. Freifeld AG, Pizzo PA. The outpatient management of febrile neutropenia in cancer. *Oncology* 1996;10: 599–606.
18. Wong GG, Witek JS, Temple PA, et al. Human GM-CSF: molecular cloning of the complementary DNA and purification of the natural and recombinant proteins. *Science*1985;228:810–815.
19. Welte K, Platzer E, Lu L, et al. Purification and biochemical characterization of human pluripotent hematopoietic colony-stimulating factor. *Proc Natl Acad Sci USA* 1985;82:1526–1530.
20. Souza LM, Boone TC, Gabrilove J, et al. Recombinant human granulocyte colony-stimulating factor: effects on normal and leukemic myeloid cells. *Science* 1986;232:61–65.
21. Huebner K, Isobe M, Croce CM, et al. The human gene encoding GM-CSF is at 5q21-q32, the chromosome region deleted in the 5q- anomaly. *Science* 1985;230:1282–1285.

22. Le Beau MM, Lemons RS, Carrino JJ, et al. Chromosomal localization of the human G-CSF gene to 17q11 proximal to the breakpoint of the t(15;17) in acute promyelocytic leukemia. *Leukemia* 1987;1:795–799.
23. Simmers RN, Webber LM, Shannon MF, et al. Localization of the G-CSF gene on chromosome 17 proximal to the breakpoint in the t(15;17) in acute promyelocytic leukemia. *Blood*1987;70:330–332.
24. Thorens B, Mermod JJ, Vassalli P. Phagocytosis and inflammatory stimuli induce GM-CSF mRNA in macrophages through posttranscriptional regulation. *Cell* 1987;48:671–679.
25. Munker R, Gasson J, Ogawa M, et al. Recombinant human TNF induces production of granulocyte-monocyte colony-stimulating factor. *Nature* 1986;323:79–82.
26. Bagby GC, Jr., Dinarello CA, Wallace P, et al. Interleukin 1 stimulates granulocyte macrophage colony-stimulating activity release by vascular endothelial cells. *J Clin Invest* 1986;78:1316–1323.
27. Zsebo KM, Yuschenkoff VN, Schiffer S, et al. Vascular endothelial cells and granulopoiesis: interleukin-1 stimulates release of G-CSF and GM-CSF. *Blood* 1988;71:99–103.
28. Koeffler HP, Gasson J, Ranyard J, et al. Recombinant human TNF alpha stimulates production of granulocyte colony-stimulating factor. *Blood* 1987;70:55–59.
29. Wimperis JZ, Niemeyer CM, Sieff CA, et al. Granulocyte-macrophage colony-stimulating factor and interleukin-3 mRNAs are produced by a small fraction of blood mononuclear cells. *Blood* 1989;74:1525–1530.
30. Pluznik DH, Bickel M, Mergenhagen SE. B lymphocyte derived hematopoietic growth factors. *Immunol Invest* 1989;18:103–116.
31. Gasson JC, Kaufman SE, Weisbart RH, et al. High-affinity binding of granulocyte-macrophage colony-stimulating factor to normal and leukemic human myeloid cells. *Proc Natl Acad Sci USA* 1986;83:669–673.
32. Nicola NA, Metcalf D. Binding of the differentiation-inducer, granulocyte-colony-stimulating factor, to responsive but not unresponsive leukemic cell lines. *Proc Natl Acad Sci USA* 1984;81:3765–3769.
33. Nicola NA, Metcalf D. Binding of ^{125}I-labeled granulocyte colony-stimulating factor to normal murine hemopoietic cells. *J Cell Physiol* 1985;124:313–321.
34. Gasson JC. Molecular physiology of granulocyte-macrophage colony-stimulating factor. *Blood* 1991;77: 1131–1145.
35. Welte K, Gabrilove J, Bronchud MH, et al. Filgrastim (r-metHuG-CSF): the first 10 years. *Blood* 1996;88: 1907–1929.
36. Strife A, Lambek C, Wisniewski D, et al. Activities of four purified growth factors on highly enriched human hematopoietic progenitor cells. *Blood* 1987;69:1508–1523.
37. Chen BD, Clark CR, Chou TH. Granulocyte/macrophage colony-stimulating factor stimulates monocyte and tissue macrophage proliferation and enhances their responsiveness to macrophage colony-stimulating factor. *Blood* 1988;71:997–1002.
38. Chen BD, Mueller M, Chou TH. Role of granulocyte/macrophage colony-stimulating factor in the regulation of murine alveolar macrophage proliferation and differentiation. *J Immunol* 1988;141:139–144.
39. Metcalf D. The molecular biology and functions of the granulocyte-macrophage colony-stimulating factors. *Blood* 1986;67:257–267.
40. Ganser A, Lindemann A, Seipelt G, et al. Effects of recombinant human interleukin-3 in patients with normal hematopoiesis and in patients with bone marrow failure. *Blood* 1990;76:666–676.
41. Ganser A, Lindemann A, Seipelt G, et al. Recombinant human interleukin-3 in patients with hematopoietic failure. *Recent Results Cancer Res* 1991;121:162–172.
42. Gadish M, Kletter Y, Flidel O, et al. Effects of recombinant human granulocyte and granulocyte-macrophage colony-stimulating factors on neutrophil function following autologous bone marrow transplantation. *Leuk Res* 1991;15:1175–1182.
43. Fabian I, Kletter Y, Bleiberg I, et al. Effect of exogenous recombinant human granulocyte and granulocyte-macrophage colony-stimulating factor on neutrophil function following allogeneic bone marrow transplantation. *Exp Hematol* 1991;19:868–873.
44. Cohen DM, Bhalla SC, Anaissie EJ, et al. Effects of *in vitro* and *in vivo* cytokine treatment, leukapheresis and irradiation on the function of human neutrophils. *Clin Lab Haematol* 1997;19:39–47.
45. Roilides E, Uhlig K, Venzon D, et al. Neutrophil oxidative burst in response to blastoconidia and pseudohyphae of candida albicans: augmentation by granulocyte colony-stimulating factor and interferon-gamma. *J Infect Dis* 1992;166:668–673.
46. Roilides E, Walsh TJ, Pizzo PA, et al. Granulocyte colony-stimulating factor enhances the phagocytic and bactericidal activity of normal and defective human neutrophils. *J Infect Dis* 1991;163:579–583.
47. Fleischmann J, Golde DW, Weisbart RH, et al. Granulocyte-macrophage colony-stimulating factor enhances phagocytosis of bacteria by human neutrophils. *Blood* 1986;68:708–711.
48. Villalta F, Kierszenbaum F. Effects of human colony-stimulating factor on the uptake and destruction of a pathogenic parasite *(Trypanosoma cruzi)* by human neutrophils. *J Immunol* 1986;137:1703–1707.
49. Baldwin GC, Gasson JC, Quan SG, et al. Granulocyte-macrophage colony-stimulating factor enhances neutrophil function in acquired immunodeficiency syndrome. *Proc Natl Acad Sci USA* 1988;85:2763–2766.
50. Baldwin GC, Fuller ND, Roberts RL, et al. Granulocyte- and granulocyte-macrophage colony-stimulating factors enhance neutrophil cytotoxicity toward HIV-infected cells. *Blood* 1989;74:1673–1677.
51. Lindemann A, Riedel D, Oster W, et al. Granulocyte/macrophage colony-stimulating factor induces interleukin 1 production by human polymorphonuclear neutrophils. *J Immunol* 1988;140:837–839.
52. Lindemann A, Riedel D, Oster W, et al. Granulocyte-macrophage colony-stimulating factor induces cytokine secretion by human polymorphonuclear leukocytes. *J Clin Invest* 1989;83:1308–1312.

53. Kropec A, Lemmen SW, Grundmann HJ, et al. Synergy of simultaneous administration of ofloxacin and granulocyte colony-stimulating factor in killing *Escherichia coli* by human neutrophils. *Infection* 1995;23:298–300.
54. Colotta F, Re F, Polentarutti N, et al. Modulation of granulocyte survival and programmed cell death by cytokines and bacterial products. *Blood* 1992;80:2012–2020.
55. Gottlieb RA, Giesing HA, Zhu JY, et al. Cell acidification in apoptosis: granulocyte colony-stimulating factor delays programmed cell death in neutrophils by up-regulating the vacuolar $H(^{+})$-ATPase. *Proc Natl Acad Sci USA* 1995;92:5965–5968.
56. Kasahara Y, Iwai K, Yachie A, et al. Involvement of reactive oxygen intermediates in spontaneous and CD95 (Fas/APO-1)–mediated apoptosis of neutrophils. *Blood* 1997;89:1748–1753.
57. Bensinger WI, Price TH, Dale DC, et al. The effects of daily recombinant human granulocyte colony-stimulating factor administration on normal granulocyte donors undergoing leukapheresis. *Blood* 1993;81:1883–1888.
58. American Society of Clinical Oncology. American Society of Clinical Oncology recommendations for the use of hematopoietic colony-stimulating factors: evidence-based clinical practice guidelines. *J Clin Oncol* 1994;12: 2471–2508.
59. American Society of Clinical Oncology. Update of recommendations for the use of hematopoietic colony-stimulating factors: evidence-based clinical practice guidelines. *J Clin Oncol* 1996;14:1957–1960.
60. Calderwood S, Romeyer F, Blanchette V, et al. Concurrent rhGM-CSF does not offset myelosuppression from intensive chemotherapy: randomized placebo-controlled study in childhood acute lymphoblastic leukemia. *Am J Hematol* 1994;47:27–32.
61. Crawford J, Ozer H, Stoller R, et al. Reduction by granulocyte colony-stimulating factor of fever and neutropenia induced by chemotherapy in patients with small-cell lung cancer. *N Engl J Med* 1991;325:164–170.
62. Pettengell R, Gurney H, Radford JA, et al. Granulocyte colony-stimulating factor to prevent dose-limiting neutropenia in non-Hodgkin's lymphoma: a randomized controlled trial. *Blood* 1992;80:1430–1436.
63. Trillet-Lenoir V, Green J, Manegold C, et al. Recombinant granulocyte colony stimulating factor reduces the infectious complications of cytotoxic therapy. *Eur J Cancer* 1993;29A:319–324.
64. Chevallier B, Chollet P, Merrouche Y, et al. Lenograstim prevents morbidity from intensive induction chemotherapy in the treatment of inflammatory breast cancer. *J Clin Oncol* 1995;13:1564–1571.
65. Larson RA, Dodge RK, Linker CA, et al. A randomized controlled trial of filgrastim during remission induction and consolidation chemotherapy for adults with acute lymphoblastic leukemia: CALGB study 9111. *Blood* 1998;92:1556–1564.
66. Ohno R, Tomonaga M, Kobayashi T, et al. Effect of granulocyte colony-stimulating factor after intensive induction therapy in relapsed or refractory acute leukemia. *N Engl J Med* 1990;323:871–877.
67. Marina NM, Shema SJ, Bowman LC, et al. Failure of granulocyte-macrophage colony-stimulating factor to reduce febrile neutropenia in children with recurrent solid tumors treated with ifosfamide, carboplatin, and etoposide chemotherapy. *Med Pediatr Oncol* 1994;23:328–334.
68. Wexler LH, Weaver-McClure L, Steinberg SM, et al. Randomized trial of recombinant human granulocyte-macrophage colony-stimulating factor in pediatric patients receiving intensive myelosuppressive chemotherapy. *J Clin Oncol* 1996;14:901–910.
69. Fridrik MA, Greil R, Hausmaninger H, et al. Randomized open label phase III trial of CEOP/IMVP-Dexa alternating chemotherapy and filgrastim versus CEOP/IMVP-Dexa alternating chemotherapy for aggressive non-Hodgkin's lymphoma (NHL). A multicenter trial by the Austrian Working Group for Medical Tumor Therapy. *Ann Hematol* 1997;75:135–140.
70. Jones SE, Schottstaedt MW, Duncan LA, et al. Randomized double-blind prospective trial to evaluate the effects of sargramostim versus placebo in a moderate-dose fluorouracil, doxorubicin, and cyclophosphamide adjuvant chemotherapy program for stage II and III breast cancer. *J Clin Oncol* 1996;14:2976–2983.
71. Moreau P, Fiere D, Bezwoda WR, et al. Prospective randomized placebo-controlled study of granulocyte-macrophage colony-stimulating factor without stem-cell transplantation after high-dose melphalan in patients with multiple myeloma. *J Clin Oncol* 1997;15:660–666.
72. Woll PJ, Hodgetts J, Lomax L, et al. Can cytotoxic dose-intensity be increased by using granulocyte colony-stimulating factor? A randomized controlled trial of lenograstim in small-cell lung cancer. *J Clin Oncol* 1995; 13:652–659.
73. Michon JM, Hartmann O, Bouffet E, et al. An open-label, multicentre, randomised phase 2 study of recombinant human granulocyte colony-stimulating factor (filgrastim) as an adjunct to combination chemotherapy in paediatric patients with metastatic neuroblastoma. *Eur J Cancer* 1998;34:1063–1069.
74. Hartmann LC, Tschetter LK, Habermann TM, et al. Granulocyte colony-stimulating factor in severe chemotherapy-induced afebrile neutropenia. *N Engl J Med* 1997;336:1776–1780.
75. Broxmeyer HE, Benninger L, Patel SR, et al. Kinetic response of human marrow myeloid progenitor cells to *in vivo* treatment of patients with granulocyte colony-stimulating factor is different from the response to treatment with granulocyte-macrophage colony-stimulating factor. *Exp Hematol* 1994;22:100–102.
76. Meropol NJ, Miller LL, Korn EL, et al. Severe myelosuppression resulting from concurrent administration of granulocyte colony-stimulating factor and cytotoxic chemotherapy. *J Natl Cancer Inst* 1992;84:1201–1203.
77. Grem JL, McAtee N, Murphy RF, et al. Phase I and pharmacokinetic study of recombinant human granulocyte-macrophage colony-stimulating factor given in combination with fluorouracil plus calcium leucovorin in metastatic gastrointestinal adenocarcinoma. *J Clin Oncol* 1994;12:560–568.
78. Rowinsky EK, Grochow LB, Sartorius SE, et al. Phase I and pharmacologic study of high doses of the topoi-

somerase I inhibitor topotecan with granulocyte colony-stimulating factor in patients with solid tumors. *J Clin Oncol* 1996;14:1224–1235.
79. Soda H, Oka M, Fukuda M, et al. Optimal schedule for administering granulocyte colony-stimulating factor in chemotherapy-induced neutropenia in non–small-cell lung cancer. *Cancer Chemother Pharmacol* 1996;38: 9–12.
80. Neidhart JA, Mangalik A, Stidley CA, et al. Dosing regimen of granulocyte-macrophage colony-stimulating factor to support dose-intensive chemotherapy. *J Clin Oncol* 1992;10:1460–1469.
81. Kaplan LD, Kahn JO, Crowe S, et al. Clinical and virologic effect of recombinant human granulocyte-macrophage colony-stimulating factor in patients receiving chemotherapy for human immunodeficiency virus-associated non-Hodgkin's lymphoma: results of a randomized trial. *J Clin Oncol* 1991;9:929–940.
82. Shaffer DW, Smith LS, Burris HA, et al. A randomized phase I trial of chronic oral etoposide with or without granulocyte-macrophage colony-stimulating factor in patients with advanced malignancies. *Cancer Res* 1993; 53:5929–5933.
83. Lowenberg B, Touw IP. Hematopoietic growth factors and their receptors in acute leukemia. *Blood* 1993;81: 281–292.
84. Griffin J, Young D, Hermann F, et al. Effects of recombinant human GM-CSF on proliferation of clonogenic cells in acute myeloblastic leukemia. *Blood* 1986;67:1448–1453.
85. Motoji T, Watanabe M, Uzumaki H, et al. Granulocyte colony-stimulating factor (G-CSF) receptors on acute myeloblastic leukaemia cells and their relationship with the proliferative response to G-CSF in clonogenic assay. *Br J Haematol* 1991;77:54–59.
86. Tafuri A, Andreeff M. Kinetic rationale for cytokine-induced recruitment of myeloblastic leukemia followed by cycle-specific chemotherapy *in vitro*. *Leukemia* 1990;4:826–834.
87. Aglietta M, Piacibello W, Sanavio F, et al. Kinetics of human hemopoietic cells after *in vivo* administration of granulocyte-macrophage colony-stimulating factor. *J Clin Invest* 1989;83:551–557.
88. Heil G, Hoelzer D, Sanz MA, et al. A randomized, double-blind, placebo-controlled, phase III study of filgrastim in remission induction and consolidation therapy for adults with de novo acute myeloid leukemia. The International Acute Myeloid Leukemia Study Group. *Blood* 1997;90:4710–4718.
89. Stone RM, Berg DT, George SL, et al. Granulocyte-macrophage colony-stimulating factor after initial chemotherapy for elderly patients with primary acute myelogenous leukemia. *N Engl J Med* 1995;332: 1671–1677.
90. Rowe JM, Andersen JW, Mazza JJ, et al. A randomized placebo-controlled phase III study of granulocyte-macrophage colony-stimulating factor in adult patients (>55 to 70 years of age) with acute myelogenous leukemia: a study of the Eastern Cooperative Oncology Group (E 1490). *Blood* 1995;86:457–462.
91. Dombret H, Chastang C, Fenaux P, et al. A controlled study of recombinant human granulocyte colony-stimulating factor in elderly patients after treatment for acute myelogenous leukemia. AML Cooperative Study Group. *N Engl J Med* 1995;332:1678–1683.
92. Witz F, Sadoun A, Perrin MC, et al. A placebo-controlled study of recombinant human granulocyte-macrophage colony-stimulating factor administered during and after induction treatment for de novo acute myelogenous leukemia in elderly patients. Groupe Ouest Est Leucemies Aigues Myeloblastiques (GOELAM). *Blood* 1998; 91:2722–2730.
93. Godwin JE, Kopecky KJ, Head DR, et al. A double-blind placebo-controlled trial of granulocyte colony-stimulating factor in elderly patients with previously untreated acute myeloid leukemia: a Southwest oncology group study (9031). *Blood* 1998;91:3607–3615.
94. Moore JO, Dodge RK, Amrein PC, et al. Granulocyte-colony stimulating factor (filgrastim) accelerates granulocyte recovery after intensive postremission chemotherapy for acute myeloid leukemia with aziridinyl benzoquinone and mitoxantrone: cancer and leukemia group B study 9022. *Blood* 1997;89:780–788.
95. Zittoun R, Suciu S, Mandelli F, et al. Granulocyte-macrophage colony-stimulating factor associated with induction treatment of acute myelogenous leukemia: a randomized trial by the European Organization for Research and Treatment of Cancer Leukemia Cooperative Group. *J Clin Oncol* 1996;14:2150–2159.
96. Geissler K, Koller E, Hubmann E, et al. Granulocyte colony-stimulating factor as an adjunct to induction chemotherapy for adult acute lymphoblastic leukemia-a randomized phase III study. *Blood* 1997;90:590–596.
97. Welte K, Reiter A, Mempel K, et al. A randomized phase-III study of the efficacy of granulocyte colony-stimulating factor in children with high-risk acute lymphoblastic leukemia. Berlin-Frankfurt-Munster Study Group. *Blood* 1996;87:3143–3150.
98. Pui CH, Boyett JM, Hughes WT, et al. Human granulocyte colony-stimulating factor after induction chemotherapy in children with acute lymphoblastic leukemia. *N Engl J Med* 1997;336:1781–1787.
99. Ottmann OG, Hoelzer D, Gracien E, et al. Concomitant granulocyte colony-stimulating factor and induction chemoradiotherapy in adult acute lymphoblastic leukemia: a randomized phase III trial. *Blood* 1995;86: 444–450.
100. Bunn PA Jr, Crowley J, Kelly K, et al. Chemoradiotherapy with or without granulocyte-macrophage colony-stimulating factor in the treatment of limited-stage small-cell lung cancer: a prospective phase III randomized study of the Southwest Oncology Group. *J Clin Oncol* 1995;13:1632–1641.
101. Gerhartz HH, Engelhard M, Meusers P, et al. Randomized, double-blind, placebo-controlled, phase III study of recombinant human granulocyte-macrophage colony-stimulating factor as adjunct to induction treatment of high-grade malignant non-Hodgkin's lymphomas [Abstract]. *Blood* 1993;82:2329–2339.

102. Burdach SE, Muschenich M, Josephs W, et al. Granulocyte-macrophage-colony stimulating factor for prevention of neutropenia and infections in children and adolescents with solid tumors. Results of a prospective randomized study. *Cancer 1995*;76:510–516.
103. Bajorin DF, Nichols CR, Schmoll HJ, et al. Recombinant human granulocyte-macrophage colony-stimulating factor as an adjunct to conventional-dose ifosfamide-based chemotherapy for patients with advanced or relapsed germ cell tumors: a randomized trial. *J Clin Oncol* 1995;13:79–86.
104. Yau JC, Neidhart JA, Triozzi P, et al. Randomized placebo-controlled trial of granulocyte-macrophage colony-stimulating-factor support for dose-intensive cyclophosphamide, etoposide, and cisplatin. *Am J Hematol* 1996; 51:289–295.
105. Riikonen P, Rahiala J, Salonvaara M, et al. Prophylactic administration of granulocyte colony-stimulating factor (filgrastim) after conventional chemotherapy in children with cancer. *Stem Cells (Dayt)* 1995;13:289–294.
106. Ravaud A, Chevreau C, Cany L, et al. Granulocyte-macrophage colony-stimulating factor in patients with neutropenic fever is potent after low-risk but not after high-risk neutropenic chemotherapy regimens: results of a randomized phase III trial. *J Clin Oncol* 1998;16:2930–2936.
107. Biesma B, de Vries EG, Willemse PH, et al. Efficacy and tolerability of recombinant human granulocyte-macrophage colony-stimulating factor in patients with chemotherapy-related leukopenia and fever. *Eur J Cancer* 1990;26:932–936.
108. Vellenga E, Uyl-de Groot CA, de Wit R, et al. Randomized placebo-controlled trial of granulocyte-macrophage colony-stimulating factor in patients with chemotherapy-related febrile neutropenia. *J Clin Oncol* 1996;14: 619–627.
109. Mayordomo JI, Rivera F, Diaz-Puente MT, et al. Improving treatment of chemotherapy-induced neutropenic fever by administration of colony-stimulating factors. *J Natl Cancer Inst* 1995;87:803–808.
110. Riikonen P, Saarinen UM, Mäkipernaa A, et al. Recombinant human granulocyte-macrophage colony-stimulating factor in the treatment of febrile neutropenia: a double-blind placebo-controlled study in children. *Pediatr Infect Dis J* 1994;13:197–202.
111. Mitchell PLR, Morland B, Stevens MCG, et al. Granulocyte colony-stimulating factor in established febrile neutropenia: a randomized study of pediatric patients. *J Clin Oncol* 1997;15:1163–1170.
112. Gerhartz HH, Stern AC, Wolf-Hornung B, et al. Intervention treatment of established neutropenia with human recombinant granulocyte-macrophage colony-stimulating factor (rhGM-CSF) in patients undergoing cancer chemotherapy. *Leuk Res* 1993;17:175–185.
113. Anaissie EJ, Vartivarian S, Bodey GP, et al. Randomized comparison between antibiotics alone and antibiotics plus granulocyte-macrophage colony-stimulating factor (*Escherichia coli*–derived) in cancer patients with fever and neutropenia. *Am J Med* 1996;100:17–23.
114. Maher DW, Lieschke GJ, Green M, et al. Filgrastim in patients with chemotherapy-induced febrile neutropenia. *Ann Intern Med* 1994;121:492–501.
115. Bodey GP, Anaissie E, Gutterman J, et al. Role of granulocyte macrophage colony-stimulating factor as adjuvant therapy for fungal infection in patients with cancer. *Clin Infect Dis* 1993;17:705–707.
116. Nemunaitis J, Meyers JD, Buckner CD, et al. Phase I trial of recombinant human macrophage colony-stimulating factor in patients with invasive fungal infections. *Blood* 1991;78:907–913.
117. Nemunaitis J, Shannon-Dorcy K, Appelbaum FR, et al. Long-term follow-up of patients with invasive fungal disease who received adjunctive therapy with recombinant human macrophage colony-stimulating factor. *Blood* 1993;82:1422–1427.
118. Taylor KM, Jagannath S, Spitzer G, et al. Recombinant human granulocyte colony-stimulating factor hastens granulocyte recovery after high-dose chemotherapy and autologous bone marrow transplantation in Hodgkin's disease. *J Clin Oncol* 1989;7:1791–1799.
119. Sheridan WP, Morstyn G, Wolf M, et al. Granulocyte colony-stimulating factor and neutrophil recovery after high-dose chemotherapy and autologous bone marrow transplantation. *Lancet* 1989;2:891–895.
120. Gisselbrecht C, Prentice HG, Bacigalupo A, et al. Placebo-controlled phase III trial of lenograstim in bone-marrow transplantation. *Lancet* 1994;343:696–700.
121. Schmitz N, Dreger P, Zander AR, et al. Results of a randomised, controlled, multicentre study of recombinant human granulocyte colony-stimulating factor (filgrastim) in patients with Hodgkin's disease and non-Hodgkin's lymphoma undergoing autologous bone marrow transplantation. *Bone Marrow Transplant* 1995;15: 261–266.
122. Stahel RA, Jost LM, Cerny T, et al. Randomized study of recombinant human granulocyte colony-stimulating factor after high-dose chemotherapy and autologous bone marrow transplantation for high-risk lymphoid malignancies. *J Clin Oncol* 1994;12:1931–1938.
123. Linch DC, Scarffe H, Proctor S, et al. Randomised vehicle-controlled dose-finding study of glycosylated recombinant human granulocyte colony-stimulating factor after bone marrow transplantation. *Bone Marrow Transplant* 1993;11:307–311.
124. Nemunaitis J, Rabinowe SN, Singer JW, et al. Recombinant granulocyte-macrophage colony-stimulating factor after autologous bone marrow transplantation for lymphoid cancer. *N Engl J Med* 1991;324:1773–1778.
125. Link H, Boogaerts MA, Carella AM, et al. A controlled trial of recombinant human granulocyte-macrophage colony-stimulating factor after total body irradiation, high-dose chemotherapy, and autologous bone marrow transplantation for acute lymphoblastic leukemia or malignant lymphoma. *Blood* 1992;80:2188–2195.

126. Gulati SC, Bennett CL. Granulocyte-macrophage colony-stimulating factor (GM-CSF) as adjunct therapy in relapsed Hodgkin disease. *Ann Intern Med* 1992;116:177–182.
127. Advani R, Chao NJ, Horning SJ, et al. Granulocyte-macrophage colony-stimulating factor (GM-CSF) as an adjunct to autologous hemopoietic stem cell transplantation for lymphoma. *Ann Intern Med* 1992;116:183–189.
128. Saarinen UM, Hovi L, Riikonen P, et al. Recombinant human granulocyte-macrophage colony-stimulating factor in children with chemotherapy-induced neutropenia. *Med Pediatr Oncol* 1992;20:489–496.
129. Gorin NC, Coiffier B, Hayat M, et al. Recombinant human granulocyte-macrophage colony-stimulating factor after high-dose chemotherapy and autologous bone marrow transplantation with unpurged and purged marrow in non-Hodgkin's lymphoma: a double-blind placebo-controlled trial. *Blood* 1992;80:1149–1157.
130. Gordon B, Spadinger A, Hodges E, et al. Effect of granulocyte-macrophage colony-stimulating factor on oral mucositis after hematopoietic stem-cell transplantation. *J Clin Oncol* 1994;12:1917–1922.
131. Khwaja A, Linch DC, Goldstone AH, et al. Recombinant human granulocyte-macrophage colony-stimulating factor after autologous bone marrow transplantation for malignant lymphoma: a British National Lymphoma Investigation double-blind, placebo-controlled trial. *Br J Haematol* 1992;82:317–323.
132. Dini G, Floris R, Pession A, et al. Phase II study of recombinant human granulocyte colony-stimulating factor in children undergoing bone marrow transplantation. *Bone Marrow Transplant* 1996;18(suppl 2):121–128.
133. Nemunaitis J, Buckner CD, Dorsey KS, et al. Retrospective analysis of infectious disease in patients who received recombinant human granulocyte-macrophage colony-stimulating factor versus patients not receiving a cytokine who underwent autologous bone marrow transplantation for treatment of lymphoid cancer. *Am J Clin Oncol* 1998;21:341–346.
134. Calderwood S, Doyle JJ, Hitzler JK, et al. Administration of recombinant human granulocyte-macrophage colony-stimulating factor after autologous bone marrow transplantation in children with acute myelogenous leukemia: a note of caution. *Bone Marrow Transplant* 1996;18:87–91.
135. Powles R, Smith C, Milan S, et al. Human recombinant GM-CSF in allogeneic bone-marrow transplantation for leukemia: double-blind, placebo-controlled trial. *Lancet* 1990;336:1417–1420.
136. Lee SJ, Weller E, Alyea EP, et al. Efficacy and costs of granulocyte colony-stimulating factor in allogeneic T-cell depleted bone marrow transplantation. *Blood* 1998;92:2725–2729.
137. Nemunaitis J, Rosenfeld CS, Ash R, et al. Phase III randomized, double-blind placebo-controlled trial of rhGM-CSF following allogeneic bone marrow transplantation. *Bone Marrow Transplant* 1995;15:949–954.
138. Hiraoka A, Masaoka T, Mizoguchi H, et al. Recombinant human non-glycosylated granulocyte-macrophage colony-stimulating factor in allogeneic bone marrow transplantation: double-blind placebo-controlled phase III clinical trial. *Jpn J Clin Oncol* 1994;24:205–211.
139. De Witte T, Gratwohl A, Van Der Lely N, et al. Recombinant human granulocyte-macrophage colony-stimulating factor accelerates neutrophil and monocyte recovery after allogeneic T-cell–depleted bone marrow transplantation. *Blood* 1992;79:1359–1365.
140. Schriber JR, Chao NJ, Long GD, et al. Granulocyte colony-stimulating factor after allogeneic bone marrow transplantation. *Blood* 1994;84:1680–1684.
141. De Witte T, Vreugdenhil G, Schattenberg A. Prolonged administration of recombinant granulocyte-macrophage colony-stimulating factor (GM-CSF) after T-cell–depleted allogeneic bone marrow transplantation. *Transplant Proc* 1993;25:57–60.
142. Lyman GH, Lyman CG, Sanderson RA, et al. Decision analysis of hematopoietic growth factor use in patients receiving cancer chemotherapy. *J Natl Cancer Inst* 1993;85:488–493.
143. Shpall EJ, Jones RB, Bast RC Jr, et al. 4-Hydroperoxycyclophosphamide purging of breast cancer from the mononuclear cell fraction of bone marrow in patients receiving high-dose chemotherapy and autologous marrow support: a phase I trial. *J Clin Oncol* 1991;9:85–93.
144. Nemunaitis J, Singer JW, Buckner CD, et al. Use of recombinant human granulocyte-macrophage colony-stimulating factor in graft failure after bone marrow transplantation. *Blood* 1990;76:245–253.
145. Bolger GB, Sullivan KM, Storb R, et al. Second marrow infusion for poor graft function after allogeneic marrow transplantation. *Bone Marrow Transplant* 1986;1:21–30.
146. Champlin RE, Horowitz MM, van Bekkum DW, et al. Graft failure following bone marrow transplantation for severe aplastic anemia: risk factors and treatment results. *Blood* 1989;73:606–613.
147. Ippoliti C, Przepiorka D, Giralt S, et al. Low-dose non-glycosylated rhGM-CSF is effective for the treatment of delayed hematopoietic recovery after autologous marrow or peripheral blood stem cell transplantation. *Bone Marrow Transplant* 1993;11:55–59.
148. Vose JM, Bierman PJ, Kessinger A, et al. The use of recombinant human granulocyte-macrophage colony stimulating factor for the treatment of delayed engraftment following high dose therapy and autologous hematopoietic stem cell transplantation for lymphoid malignancies. *Bone Marrow Transplant* 1991;7:139–143.
149. Brandwein JM, Nayar R, Baker MA, et al. GM-CSF therapy for delayed engraftment after autologous bone marrow transplantation. *Exp Hematol* 1991;19:191–195.
150. Klingemann HG, Eaves AC, Barnett MJ, et al. Recombinant GM-CSF in patients with poor graft function after bone marrow transplantation. *Clin Invest Med 1990*;13:77–81.
151. Boulad F, Gillio A, Small TN, et al. Correction of neutropenia with rHuG-CSF after loss of response to rHuGM-CSF following autologous bone marrow transplant. *Bone Marrow Transplant* 1994;13:661–663.
152. Weisdorf DJ, Verfaillie CM, Davies SM, et al. Hematopoietic growth factors for graft failure after bone mar-

row transplantation: a randomized trial of granulocyte-macrophage colony-stimulating factor (GM-CSF) versus sequential GM-CSF plus granulocyte-CSF. *Blood* 1995;85:3452–3456.
153. Duehrsen U, Villeval JL, Boyd J, et al. Effects of recombinant human granulocyte colony-stimulating factor on hematopoietic progenitor cells in cancer patients. *Blood* 1988;72:2074–2081.
154. Socinski M, Cannistra S, Elias A. Granulocyte-macrophage colony stimulating factor expands the circulating hematopoietic progenitor cell compartment in man. *Lancet* 1988;1:1194–1198.
155. Mangan K, Mullaney M, Klumpp T, et al. Mobilization of peripheral blood stem cells by subcutaneous injections of yeast-derived granulocyte macrophage colony stimulating factor: a phase I–II study. *Stem Cells (Dayt)* 1993;11:445–454.
156. Bensinger WI, Longin K, Appelbaum F, et al. Peripheral blood stem cells (PBSCs) collected after recombinant granulocyte colony stimulating factor (rhG-CSF): an analysis of factors correlating with the tempo of engraftment after transplantation. *Br J Haematol* 1994;87:825–831.
157. Nademanee A, Sniecinski I, Schmidt GM, et al. High-dose therapy followed by autologous peripheral-blood stem-cell transplantation for patients with Hodgkin's disease and non-Hodgkin's lymphoma using unprimed and granulocyte colony-stimulating factor-mobilized peripheral-blood stem cells. *J Clin Oncol* 1994;12: 2176–2186.
158. Bensinger W, Appelbaum F, Rowley S, et al. Factors that influence collection and engraftment of autologous peripheral-blood stem cells. *J Clin Oncol* 1995;13:2547–2555.
159. Schwartzberg L, Birch R, Blanco R, et al. Rapid and sustained hematopoietic reconstitution by peripheral blood stem cell infusion alone following high-dose chemotherapy. *Bone Marrow Transplant* 1993;11:369–374.
160. Weaver CH, Hazelton B, Birch R, et al. An analysis of engraftment kinetics as a function of the CD34 content of peripheral blood progenitor cell collections in 692 patients after the administration of myeloablative chemotherapy. *Blood* 1995;86:3961–3969.
161. Kessinger A, Armitage JO. The evolving role of autologous peripheral stem cell transplantation following high-dose therapy for malignancies [Editorial]. *Blood* 1991;77:211–213.
162. Chao NJ, Schriber JR, Grimes K, et al. Granulocyte colony-stimulating factor "mobilized" peripheral blood progenitor cells accelerate granulocyte and platelet recovery after high-dose chemotherapy. *Blood* 1993;81: 2031–2035.
163. Bensinger W, Singer J, Appelbaum F, et al. Autologous transplantation with peripheral blood mononuclear cells collected after administration of recombinant granulocyte stimulating factor. *Blood* 1993;81:3158–3163.
164. Shpall EJ, Jones RB, Bearman SI, et al. Transplantation of enriched CD34-positive autologous marrow into breast cancer patients following high-dose chemotherapy: influence of CD34-positive peripheral-blood progenitors and growth factors on engraftment. *J Clin Oncol* 1994;12:28–36.
165. Sheridan WP, Begley CG, Juttner CA, et al. Effect of peripheral-blood progenitor cells mobilised by filgrastim (G-CSF) on platelet recovery after high-dose chemotherapy. *Lancet* 1992;339:640–644.
166. Elias AD, Ayash L, Anderson KC, et al. Mobilization of peripheral blood progenitor cells by chemotherapy and granulocyte-macrophage colony-stimulating factor for hematologic support after high-dose intensification for breast cancer. *Blood* 1992;79:3036–3044.
167. Peters WP, Rosner G, Ross M, et al. Comparative effects of granulocyte-macrophage colony-stimulating factor (GM-CSF) and granulocyte colony-stimulating factor (G-CSF) on priming peripheral blood progenitor cells for use with autologous bone marrow after high-dose chemotherapy. *Blood* 1993;81:1709–1719.
168. Pettengell R, Morgenstern GR, Woll PJ, et al. Peripheral blood progenitor cell transplantation in lymphoma and leukemia using a single apheresis. *Blood* 1993;82:3770–3777.
169. Uyl-de Groot CA, Richel DJ, Rutten FF. Peripheral blood progenitor cell transplantation mobilised by r-metHuG-CSF (filgrastim): a less costly alternative to autologous bone marrow transplantation. *Eur J Cancer* 1994;11:1631–1635.
170. Gilbert C, Meisenberg B, Vredenburgh J. Sequential prophylactic oral and empiric once-daily parenteral antibiotics for neutropenia and fever after high-dose chemotherapy and autologous bone marrow support. *J Clin Oncol* 1994;12:1005–1011.
171. Gianni AM, Siena S, Bregni M, et al. Granulocyte-macrophage colony-stimulating factor to harvest circulating haemopoietic stem cells for autotransplantation. *Lancet* 1989;2:580–585.
172. To LB, Shepperd KM, Haylock DN, et al. Single high doses of cyclophosphamide enable the collection of high numbers of hemopoietic stem cells from the peripheral blood. *Exp Hematol* 1990;18:442–447.
173. Rowlings PA, Bayly JL, Rawling CM, et al. A comparison of peripheral blood stem cell mobilisation after chemotherapy with cyclophosphamide as a single agent in doses of 4 g/m^{2}or 7 g/m^2 in patients with advanced cancer. *Aust N Z J Med* 1992;22:660–604.
174. Weaver CH, Schwartzberg LS, Birch R, et al. Collection of peripheral blood progenitor cells after the administration of cyclophosphamide, etoposide, and granulocyte-colony-stimulating factor: an analysis of 497 patients. *Transfusion* 1997;37:896–903.
175. Schwartzberg LS, Birch R, Hazelton B, et al. Peripheral blood stem cell mobilization by chemotherapy with and without recombinant human granulocyte colony-stimulating factor. *J Hematother* 1992;1:317–327.
176. Takaue Y, Watanabe T, Abe T, et al. Experience with peripheral blood stem cell collection for autografts in children with active cancer. *Bone Marrow Transplant* 1992;10:241–248.
177. Haas R, Hohaus S, Egerer G, et al. Recombinant human granulocyte-macrophage colony-stimulating factor

(rhGM-CSF) subsequent to chemotherapy improves collection of blood stem cells for autografting in patients not eligible for bone marrow harvest. *Bone Marrow Transplantation* 1992;9:459–465.
178. Teshima T, Harada M, Takamatsu Y, et al. Granulocyte colony-stimulating factor (G-CSF)-induced mobilization of circulating haemopoietic stem cells. *Br J Haematol* 1993;84:570–573.
179. Bishop MR, Anderson JR, Jackson JD, et al. High-dose therapy and peripheral blood progenitor cell transplantation: effects of recombinant human granulocyte-macrophage colony-stimulating factor on the autograft. *Blood* 1994;83:610–616.
180. Bellido M, Sureda A, Martino R, et al. Collection of peripheral blood progenitor cells for autografting with low-dose cyclophosphamide plus granulocyte colony-stimulating factor. *Haematologica* 1998;83:428–431.
181. Charrier S, Chassagne J, Cure H, et al. Mobilization of peripheral blood progenitor cells after induction chemotherapy (THP-doxorubicin-vinorelbine-cyclophosphamide-fluorouracil) and granulocyte colony-stimulating factor in breast cancer. *Bone Marrow Transplant* 1998;22:845–851.
182. Leibundgut K, Hirt A, Luthy AR, et al. Single institution experience with mobilization, harvesting, and reinfusion of peripheral blood stem cells in children with a solid tumor or leukemia. *Pediatr Hematol Oncol* 1994; 11:215–221.
183. Leibundgut K, Hauser SP, Ridolfi-Luthy A, et al. Peripheral blood progenitor cell collections in children with low platelet counts are safe [Letter]. *Bone Marrow Transplant* 1997;20:345–346.
184. Kanold J, Rapatel C, Berger M, et al. Use of G-CSF alone to mobilize peripheral blood stem cells for collection from children. *Br J Haematol* 1994;88:633–635.
185. Demeocq F, Kanold J, Chassagne J, et al. Successful blood stem cell collection and transplant in children weighing less than 25 kg. *Bone Marrow Transplant* 1994;13:43–50.
186. Eguchi H, Takaue Y, Kawano Y, et al. Peripheral blood stem cell autografts for the treatment of children over 1 year old with stage IV neuroblastoma: a long-term follow-up. *Bone Marrow Transplant* 1998;21:1011–1014.
187. Kanold J, Halle P, Berger M, et al. Large-volume leukapheresis procedure for peripheral blood progenitor cell collection in children weighing 15 kg or less: efficacy and safety evaluation. *Med Pediatr Oncol* 1999;32:7–10.
188. Korbling M, Huh YO, Durett A, et al. Allogeneic blood stem cell transplantation: peripheralization and yield of donor-derived primitive hematopoietic progenitor cells ($CD34^{+}$Thy-1dim) and lymphoid subsets, and possible predictors of engraftment and graft-versus-host disease. *Blood* 1995;86:2842–2848.
189. Sato N, Sawada K, Takahashi TA, et al. A time course study for optimal harvest of peripheral blood progenitor cells by granulocyte colony-stimulating factor in healthy volunteers. *Exp Hematol* 1994;22:973–978.
190. Bishop MR, Tarantolo SR, Jackson JD, et al. Allogeneic-blood stem-cell collection following mobilization with low-dose granulocyte colony-stimulating factor. *J Clin Oncol* 1997;15:1601–1607.
191. Korbling M, Przepiorka D, Huh YO, et al. Allogeneic blood stem cell transplantation for refractory leukemia and lymphoma: potential advantage of blood over marrow allografts. *Blood* 1995;85:1659–1665.
192. Tarella C, Ferrero D, Bregni M, et al. Peripheral blood expansion of early progenitor cells after high-dose cyclophosphamide and rhGM-CSF. *Eur J Cancer* 1991;27:22–27.
193. Chao NJ, Long GD, Negrin RS, et al. G-CSF and peripheral blood progenitor cells [Letter]. *Lancet* 1992;339: 1410.
194. Lie AK, Hui CH, Rawling T, et al. Granulocyte colony-stimulating factor (G-CSF) dose-dependent efficacy in peripheral blood stem cell mobilization in patients who had failed initial mobilization with chemotherapy and G-CSF. *Bone Marrow Transplant* 1998;22:853–857.
195. Hohaus S, Martin H, Wassmann B, et al. Recombinant human granulocyte and granulocyte-macrophage colony-stimulating factor (G-CSF and GM-CSF) administered following cytotoxic chemotherapy have a similar ability to mobilize peripheral blood stem cells. *Bone Marrow Transplant* 1998;22:625–630.
196. Abboud C, Reykdal S, Liesveld J, et al. Prospective randomized trial (NCI/T92-0010), comparing the efficacy of hematopoietic growth factors for mobilizing peripheral blood stem cells (PBSC) in autologous bone marrow transplantation: II. Progenitor mobilization kinetics [Abstract]. *Blood* 1995;86:463a.
197. Meisenberg B, Brehm T, Schmeckel A, et al. A combination of low-dose cyclophosphamide and colony-stimulating factors is more cost-effective than granulocyte-colony-stimulating factors alone in mobilizing peripheral blood stem and progenitor cells. *Transfusion*1998;38:209–215.
198. Spitzer G, Adkins D, Mathews M, et al. Randomized comparison of G-CSF + GM-CSF vs. G-CSF alone for mobilization of peripheral blood stem cells: effects on hematopoietic recovery after high-dose chemotherapy. *Bone Marrow Transplant* 1997;20:921–930.
199. Benedetti Panici P, Pierelli L, Scambia G, et al. High-dose carboplatin, etoposide and melphalan (CEM) with peripheral blood progenitor cell support as late intensification for high-risk cancer: non-haematological, haematological toxicities and role of growth factor administration. *Br J Cancer* 1997;75:1205–1212.
200. Shimazaki C, Oku N, Uchiyama H, et al. Effect of granulocyte colony-stimulating factor on hematopoietic recovery after peripheral blood progenitor cell transplantation. *Bone Marrow Transplant* 1994;13:271–275.
201. Brice P, Divine M, Marolleau JP, et al. Comparison of autografting using mobilized peripheral blood stem cells with and without granulocyte colony-stimulating factor in malignant lymphomas. *Bone Marrow Transplant* 1994;14:51–55.
202. Klumpp TR, Mangan KF, Goldberg SL, et al. Granulocyte colony-stimulating factor accelerates neutrophil engraftment following peripheral-blood stem-cell transplantation: a prospective, randomized trial. *J Clin Oncol* 1995;13:1323–1327.

203. McQuaker IG, Hunter AE, Pacey S, et al. Low-dose filgrastim significantly enhances neutrophil recovery following autologous peripheral-blood stem-cell transplantation in patients with lymphoproliferative disorders: evidence for clinical and economic benefit. *J Clin Oncol* 1997;15:451–457.
204. Linch DC, Milligan DW, Winfield DA, et al. G-CSF after peripheral blood stem cell transplantation in lymphoma patients significantly accelerated neutrophil recovery and shortened time in hospital: results of a randomized BNLI trial. *Br J Haematol* 1997;99:933–938.
205. Lee SM, Radford JA, Dobson L, et al. Recombinant human granulocyte colony-stimulating factor (filgrastim) following high-dose chemotherapy and peripheral blood progenitor cell rescue in high-grade non-Hodgkin's lymphoma: clinical benefits at no extra cost. *Br J Cancer* 1998;77:1294–1299.
206. Tarella C, Castellino C, Locatelli F, et al. G-CSF administration following peripheral blood progenitor cell (PBPC) autograft in lymphoid malignancies: evidence for clinical benefits and reduction of treatment costs. *Bone Marrow Transplant* 1998;21:401–407.
207. Kawano Y, Takaue Y, Mimaya J, et al. Marginal benefit/disadvantage of granulocyte colony-stimulating factor therapy after autologous blood stem cell transplantation in children: results of a prospective randomized trial. The Japanese Cooperative Study Group of PBSCT. *Blood* 1998;92:4040–4046.
208. Greenberg P, Advani R, Keating A, et al. GM-CSF accelerates neutrophil recovery after autologous hematopoietic stem cell transplantation. *Bone Marrow Transplant* 1996;18:1057–1064.
209. Shea TC, Mason JR, Storniolo AM, et al. Sequential cycles of high-dose carboplatin administered with recombinant human granulocyte-macrophage colony-stimulating factor and repeated infusions of autologous peripheral-blood progenitor cells: a novel and effective method for delivering multiple courses of dose-intensive therapy. *J Clin Oncol* 1992;10:464–473.
210. Kritz A, Crown JP, Motzer RJ, et al. Beneficial impact of peripheral blood progenitor cells in patients with metastatic breast cancer treated with high-dose chemotherapy plus granulocyte-macrophage colony-stimulating factor. A randomized trial. *Cancer*1993;71:2515–2521.
211. Tepler I, Cannistra SA, Frei Ed, et al. Use of peripheral-blood progenitor cells abrogates the myelotoxicity of repetitive outpatient high-dose carboplatin and cyclophosphamide chemotherapy. *J Clin Oncol* 1993;11: 1583–1591.
212. Brugger W, Birken R, Bertz H, et al. Peripheral blood progenitor cells mobilized by chemotherapy plus granulocyte-colony stimulating factor accelerate both neutrophil and platelet recovery after high-dose VP16, ifosfamide and cisplatin. *Br J Haematol* 1993;84:402–407.
213. Spitzer G, Adkins DR, Spencer V, et al. Randomized study of growth factors post-peripheral-blood-stem-cell transplant: neutrophil recovery is improved with modest clinical benefit. *J Clin Oncol* 1994;12:661–670.
214. Legros M, Fleury J, Bay JO, et al. rhGM-CSF vs placebo following rhGM-CSF–mobilized PBPC transplantation: a phase III double-blind randomized trial. *Bone Marrow Transplant* 1997;19:209–213.
215. Dunlop DJ, Fitzsimons EJ, McMurray A, et al. Filgrastim fails to improve haemopoietic reconstitution following myeloablative chemotherapy and peripheral blood stem cell rescue. *Br J Cancer* 1994;70:943–945.
216. Cortelazzo S, Viero P, Bellavita P, et al. Granulocyte colony-stimulating factor following peripheral-blood progenitor-cell transplant in non-Hodgkin's lymphoma. *J Clin Oncol* 1995;13:935–941.
217. Faucher C, Le Corroller AG, Chabannon C, et al. Administration of G-CSF can be delayed after transplantation of autologous G-CSF-primed blood stem cells: a randomized study. *Bone Marrow Transplant* 1996;17: 533–536.
218. Bence-Bruckler I, Bredeson C, Atkins H, et al. A randomized trial of granulocyte colony-stimulating factor (Neupogen) starting day 1 vs day 7 post-autologous stem cell transplantation. *Bone Marrow Transplant* 1998; 22:965–969.
219. Meyer RM, Hryniuk WM, Goodyear MD. The role of dose intensity in determining outcome in intermediate-grade non-Hodgkin's lymphoma. *J Clin Oncol* 1991;9:339–347.
220. Hryniuk W, Bush H. The importance of dose intensity in chemotherapy of metastatic breast cancer. *J Clin Oncol* 1984;2:1281—128-8.
221. Kwak L, Halpern J, Olshen R, et al. Prognostic significance of actual dose intensity in diffuse large-cell lymphoma: results of a tree-structured survival analysis. *J Clin Oncol* 1990;8:963–977.
222. Cheung NV, Heller G. Chemotherapy dose intensity correlates strongly with response, median survival, and median progression-free survival in metastatic neuroblastoma. *J Clin Oncol* 1991;9:1050–1058.
223. Smith MA, Ungerleider RS, Horowitz ME, et al. Influence of doxorubicin dose intensity on response and outcome for patients with osteogenic sarcoma and Ewing's sarcoma. *J Natl Cancer Inst* 1991;83:1460–1470.
224. Lichtman SM, Ratain MJ, Van Echo DA, et al. Phase I trial of granulocyte-macrophage colony-stimulating factor plus high-dose cyclophosphamide given every 2 weeks: a Cancer and Leukemia Group B study. *J Natl Cancer Inst* 1993;85:1319–1326.
225. Sarosy G, Kohn E, Stone DA, et al. Phase I study of taxol and granulocyte colony-stimulating factor in patients with refractory ovarian cancer. *J Clin Oncol* 1992;10:1165–1170.
226. Demetri G, Hayes D, Shapiro C. Dose-intensification of mitoxantrone with adjunctive G-CSF (filgrastim) in patients with advanced breast cancer: a phase I trial [Abstract]. *Blood* 1992;80:292a.
227. Scinto AF, Ferraresi V, Campioni N, et al. Accelerated chemotherapy with high-dose epirubicin and cyclophosphamide plus r-met-HuG-CSF in locally advanced and metastatic breast cancer. *Ann Oncol* 1995;6:665–671.
228. Ardizzoni A, Sertoli MR, Corcione A, et al. Accelerated chemotherapy with or without GM-CSF for small cell lung cancer: a non-randomised pilot study. *Eur J Cancer* 1990;26:937–941.

229. Mamounas EP, Anderson S, Wickerham DL, et al. The efficacy of recombinant human granulocyte colony-stimulating factor and recombinant human granulocyte macrophage colony-stimulating factor in permitting the administration of higher doses of cyclophosphamide in a doxorubicin-cyclophosphamide combination. An NS-ABP pilot study in patients with metastatic or high-risk primary breast cancer. National Surgical Adjuvant Breast and Bowel Project. *Am J Clin Oncol* 1994;17:374–381.
230. Ardizzoni A, Venturini M, Sertoli MR, et al. Granulocyte-macrophage colony-stimulating factor (GM-CSF) allows acceleration and dose intensity increase of CEF chemotherapy: a randomised study in patients with advanced breast cancer. *Br J Cancer* 1994;69:385–391.
231. Gisselbrecht C, Haioun C, Lepage E, et al. Placebo-controlled phase III study of lenograstim (glycosylated recombinant human granulocyte colony-stimulating factor) in aggressive non-Hodgkin's lymphoma: factors influencing chemotherapy administration. Groupe d'Etude des Lymphomes de l'Adulte. *Leuk Lymphoma* 1997; 25:289–300.
232. Bertini M, Freilone R, Vitolo U, et al. P-VEBEC: a new 8-weekly schedule with or without rG-CSF for elderly patients with aggressive non-Hodgkin's lymphoma (NHL). *Ann Oncol* 1994;5:895–900.
233. Zinzani PL, Pavone E, Storti S, et al. Randomized trial with or without granulocyte colony-stimulating factor as adjunct to induction VNCOP-B treatment of elderly high-grade non-Hodgkin's lymphoma. *Blood* 1997;89: 3974–3979.
234. Miles DW, Fogarty O, Ash CM, et al. Received dose-intensity: a randomized trial of weekly chemotherapy with and without granulocyte colony-stimulating factor in small-cell lung cancer. *J Clin Oncol* 1994;12:77–82.
235. Rusthoven J, Levin L, Eisenhauer E, et al. Two phase I studies of carboplatin dose escalation in chemotherapy-naive ovarian cancer patients supported with granulocyte-macrophage colony-stimulating factor. *J Natl Cancer Inst* 1991;83:1748–1753.
236. O'Dwyer PJ, LaCreta FP, Schilder R, et al. Phase I trial of thiotepa in combination with recombinant human granulocyte-macrophage colony-stimulating factor. *J Clin Oncol* 1992;10:1352–1358.
237. Moore DF Jr, Pazdur R. Phase I study of 5-fluorouracil with folinic acid combined with recombinant human granulocyte-macrophage colony-stimulating factor. *Am J Clin Oncol* 1992;15:464–466.
238. Schiller JH, Storer B, Tutsch K, et al. Phase I trial of 3-hour infusion of paclitaxel with or without granulocyte colony-stimulating factor in patients with advanced cancer. *J Clin Oncol* 1994;12:241–248.
239. Petrini B, Wasserman J, Blomgren H, et al. T helper/suppressor ratios in chemotherapy and radiotherapy. *Clin Exp Immunol* 1983;53:255–256.
240. Mackall C, Fleisher T, Brown M, et al. Lymphocyte depletion during treatment with intensive chemotherapy for cancer. *Blood* 1994;84:2221–2228.
241. Mackall C, Fleisher T, Brown M, et al. Age, thymopoiesis, and CD 4^+ T-lymphocyte regeneration after intensive chemotherapy. *N Engl J Med* 1995;332:143–149.
242. Negoro S, Masuda N, Furuse K, et al. Dose-intensive chemotherapy in extensive-stage small-cell lung cancer. *Cancer Chemother Pharmacol* 1997;40:S70–S73.
243. Trillet-Lenoir V, Soler P, Arpin D, et al. The limits of chemotherapy dose intensification using granulocyte colony stimulating factor alone in extensive small cell lung cancer. *Lung Cancer* 1996;14:331–341.
244. Rubinstein P, Carrier C, Scaradavou A, et al. Outcomes among 562 recipients of placental-blood transplants from unrelated donors. *N Engl J Med* 1998;339:1565–1577.
245. Kurtzberg J, Laughlin M, Graham ML, et al. Placental blood as a source of hematopoietic stem cells for transplantation into unrelated recipients. *N Engl J Med* 1996;335:157–166.
246. Gluckman E, Broxmeyer HA, Auerbach AD, et al. Hematopoietic reconstitution in a patient with Fanconi's anemia by means of umbilical-cord blood from an HLA-identical sibling. *N Engl J Med* 1989;321:1174–1178.
247. Gluckman E, Rocha V, Boyer-Chammard A, et al. Outcome of cord-blood transplantation from related and unrelated donors. Eurocord Transplant Group and the European Blood and Marrow Transplantation Group. *N Engl J Med* 1997;337:373–381.
248. Wagner JE, Kernan NA, Steinbuch M, et al. Allogeneic sibling umbilical-cord-blood transplantation in children with malignant and non-malignant disease. *Lancet* 1995;346:214–219.
249. Wagner JE, Rosenthal J, Sweetman R, et al. Successful transplantation of HLA-matched and HLA-mismatched umbilical cord blood from unrelated donors: analysis of engraftment and acute graft-versus-host disease. *Blood* 1996;88:795–802.
250. Rubinstein P, Rosenfield RE, Adamson JW, et al. Stored placental blood for unrelated bone marrow reconstitution. *Blood* 1993;81:1679–1690.
251. Strauss RG. Clinical perspectives of granulocyte transfusions: efficacy to date. *J Clin Apheresis* 1995;10: 114–118.
252. Chanock SJ, Gorlin J. Granulocyte transfusions: time for a second look. *Infect Dis Clin North Am* 1996;10: 327–343.
253. Caspar CB, Seger RA, Burger J, et al. Effective stimulation of donors for granulocyte transfusions with recombinant methionyl granulocyte-colony stimulating factor. *Blood* 1993;81:2866–2871.
254. Jendiroba DB, Lichtiger B, Anaissie E, et al. Evaluation and comparison of three mobilization methods for the collection of granulocytes. *Transfusion* 1998;38:722–728.
255. Grigg A, Vecchi L, Bardy P, et al. G-CSF–stimulated donor granulocyte collections for prophylaxis and therapy of neutropenic sepsis. *Aust NZ J Med* 1996;26:813–818.
256. Hester JP, Dignani MC, Anaissie EJ, et al. Collection and transfusion of granulocyte concentrates from donors

primed with granulocyte stimulating factor and response of myelosuppressed patients with established infection. *J Clin Apheresis* 1995;10:188–193.
257. Catalano L, Fontana R, Scarpato N, et al. Combined treatment with amphotericin-B and granulocyte transfusion from G-CSF–stimulated donors in an aplastic patient with invasive aspergillosis undergoing bone marrow transplantation. *Haematologica* 1997;82:71–72.
258. Bhatia S, McCullough JJ, Perry EH, et al. Granulocyte transfusions: efficacy in fungal infections in neutropenic patients following bone marrow transplantation. *Transfusion* 1994;34:226–232.
259. Katoh M, Takada M, Nakatani N, et al. Chemotaxis and phagocytosis of the neutrophils mobilized by granulocyte colony-stimulating factor in healthy donors for granulocyte transfusions. *Am J Hematol* 1995;49:96–97.
260. Estey E, Thall P, Andreeff M, et al. Use of granulocyte colony-stimulating factor before, during, and after fludarabine plus cytarabine induction therapy of newly diagnosed acute myelogenous leukemia or myelodysplastic syndromes: comparison with fludarabine plus cytarabine without granulocyte colony-stimulating factor. *J Clin Oncol* 1994;12:671–678.
261. Heil G, Chadid L, Hoelzer D, et al. GM-CSF in a double-blind randomized, placebo controlled trial in therapy of adult patients with de novo acute myeloid leukemia (AML). *Leukemia* 1995;9:3–9.
262. Bettelheim P, Valent P, Andreeff M, et al. Recombinant human granulocyte-macrophage colony-stimulating factor in combination with standard induction chemotherapy in de novo acute myeloid leukemia. *Blood* 1991;77: 700–711.
263. Ohno R, Naoe T, Kanamaru A, et al. A double-blind controlled study of granulocyte colony-stimulating factor started two days before induction chemotherapy in refractory acute myeloid leukemia. Kohseisho Leukemia Study Group. *Blood* 1994;83:2086–2092.
264. Estey E, Thall PF, Kantarjian H, et al. Treatment of newly diagnosed acute myelogenous leukemia with granulocyte-macrophage colony-stimulating factor (GM-CSF) before and during continuous-infusion high-dose ara-C + daunorubicin: comparison to patients treated without GM-CSF. *Blood* 1992;79:2246–2255.
265. Hamm J, Schiller JH, Cuffie C, et al. Dose-ranging study of recombinant human granulocyte-macrophage colony-stimulating factor in small-cell lung carcinoma. *J Clin Oncol* 1994;12:2667–2676.
266. O'Reilly SE, Gelmon KA, Onetto N, et al. Phase I trial of recombinant human granulocyte-macrophage colony-stimulating factor derived from yeast in patients with breast cancer receiving cyclophosphamide, doxorubicin, and fluorouracil. *J Clin Oncol* 1993;11:2411–2416.
267. Furman WL, Fairclough DL, Huhn RD, et al. Therapeutic effects and pharmacokinetics of recombinant human granulocyte-macrophage colony-stimulating factor in childhood cancer patients receiving myelosuppressive chemotherapy. *J Clin Oncol* 1991;9:1022–1028.
268. Neidhart J, Mangalik A, Kohler W, et al. Granulocyte colony-stimulating factor stimulates recovery of granulocytes in patients receiving dose-intensive chemotherapy without bone marrow transplantation. *J Clin Oncol* 1989;7:1685–1692.
269. Link CJ, Jr., Bicher A, Kohn EC, et al. Flexible granulocyte colony-stimulating factor dosing in ovarian cancer patients who receive dose-intense taxol therapy. *Blood* 1994;83:1188–1192.
270. Morstyn G, Campbell L, Lieschke G, et al. Treatment of chemotherapy-induced neutropenia by subcutaneously administered granulocyte colony-stimulating factor with optimization of dose and duration of therapy. *J Clin Oncol* 1989;7:1554–1562.
271. Sheridan W, Maher D, Wolf M. Assessment of three different dosages of r-methuG-CSF (filgrastim) as support for marrow engraftment after autologous bone marrow transplantation [Abstract]. *Blood* 1992;80:331a.
272. Gabrilove JL, Jakubowski A, Scher H, et al. Effect of granulocyte colony-stimulating factor on neutropenia and associated morbidity due to chemotherapy for transitional-cell carcinoma of the urothelium. *N Engl J Med* 1988;318:1414–1422.
273. Cairo M, Shen W, Miser J, et al. A randomized trial of two doses of G-CSF (5.0 vs 10.0 mcg/kg/d) following ifosfamide, carboplatin, and etoposide (ICE) chemotherapy in children with recurrent solid tumors (RST): significant clinical activity but no improvement in hematopoietic recovery (HR) with increased dose of G-CSF [Abstract]. *Proc Am Soc Clin Oncol* 1995;14:255.
274. Demetri G, Berry D, Younger J. Dose-intensified cyclophosphamide/doxorubicin (CD) followed by taxol (T) as adjuvant systemic chemotherapy for node-positive breast cancer (CALGB 9141): randomized comparison of two dose levels of G-CSF [Abstract]. *Proc Am Soc Clin Oncol* 1994;13:65.
275. Kaneko T, Takaku F, Ogawa M. Outline of clinical studies on recombinant human granulocyte colony stimulating factor (KRN 8601) in Japan. *Tokai J Exp Clin Med* 1991;16:51.
276. Toner G, Wollett A, Laidlaw C. Low versus standard dose G-CSF prophylaxis after chemotherapy: a randomized, crossover comparison [Abstract]. *Proc Am Soc Clin Oncol* 1994;13:429.
277. Calabresi F, Papaldo P, Marolla P. Different schedules of G-CSF in adjuvant breast cancer therapy with higher dose epirubicin + cyclophosphamide +/– ionidamine [Abstract]. *Proc Am Soc Clin Oncol* 1995;14:257.
278. Eguchi K, Sasaki S, Tamura T, et al. Dose escalation study of recombinant human granulocyte-colony-stimulating factor (KRN8601) in patients with advanced malignancy. *Cancer Res* 1989;49:5221–5224.
279. Eguchi K, Shinkai T, Sasaki Y, et al. Subcutaneous administration of recombinant human granulocyte colony-stimulating factor (KRN8601) in intensive chemotherapy for patients with advanced lung cancer. *Jpn J Cancer Res* 1990;81:1168–1174.
280. Schmitz N, Dreger P, Suttorp M, et al. Primary transplantation of allogeneic peripheral blood progenitor cells mobilized by filgrastim (granulocyte colony-stimulating factor). *Blood* 1995;85:1666–1672.

281. Furman W, Crist W. Biology and clinical applications of hemopoietins in pediatric practice. *Pediatrics* 1992;90: 716–728.
282. Stute N, Santana VM, Rodman JH, et al. Pharmacokinetics of subcutaneous recombinant human granulocyte colony-stimulating factor in children. *Blood* 1992;79:2849–2854.
283. McLeish S, Decoster G, Rich W. Clinical trial and post-marketing safety profile of filgrastim in oncology patients (NeupogenR) [Abstract]. *Proc Am Soc Clin Oncol* 1994;13:189.
284. Immunex-Corporation Leukine (sargramostim). Package insert, 1991.
285. White K, Cebon J. Transient hypoxaemia during neutrophil recovery in febrile patients. *Lancet* 1995;345: 1022–1024.
286. Lieschke GJ, Cebon J, Morstyn G. Characterization of the clinical effects after the first dose of bacterially synthesized recombinant human granulocyte-macrophage colony-stimulating factor. *Blood* 1989;74: 2634–2643.
287. Shepherd FA, Goss PE, Rusthoven J, et al. Phase I trial of granulocyte-macrophage colony-stimulating factor with high-dose cisplatin and etoposide for treatment of small-cell lung cancer: a study of the National Cancer Institute of Canada Clinical Trials Group [Letter]. *J Natl Cancer Inst* 1992;84:59–60.
288. Edmonson JH, Hartmann LC, Long HJ, et al. Granulocyte-macrophage colony-stimulating factor. Preliminary observations on the influences of dose, schedule, and route of administration in patients receiving cyclophosphamide and carboplatin. *Cancer* 1992;70:2529–2539.
289. Ho AD, Del Valle F, Haas R, et al. Sequential studies on the role of mitoxantrone, high-dose cytarabine, and recombinant human granulocyte-macrophage colony-stimulating factor in the treatment of refractory non-Hodgkin's lymphoma. *Semin Oncol* 1990;17:14–19.
290. Lieschke GJ, Maher D, O'Connor M, et al. Phase I study of intravenously administered bacterially synthesized granulocyte-macrophage colony-stimulating factor and comparison with subcutaneous administration. *Cancer Res* 1990;50:606–614.
291. Logothetis CJ, Dexeus FH, Sella A, et al. Escalated therapy for refractory urothelial tumors: methotrexate-vinblastine-doxorubicin-cisplatin plus unglycosylated recombinant human granulocyte-macrophage colony-stimulating factor. *J Natl Cancer Inst* 1990;82:667–672.
292. Lieschke GJ, Maher D, Cebon J, et al. Effects of bacterially synthesized recombinant human granulocyte-macrophage colony-stimulating factor in patients with advanced malignancy. *Ann Intern Med* 1989;110: 357–364.
293. Steward WP, Scarffe JH, Austin R, et al. Recombinant human granulocyte macrophage colony stimulating factor (rhGM-CSF) given as daily short infusions—a phase I dose-toxicity study. *Br J Cancer* 1989;59:142–145.
294. Brandt SJ, Peters WP, Atwater SK, et al. Effect of recombinant granulocyte-macrophage colony-stimulating factor on hematopoietic reconstitution after high-dose chemotherapy and autologous bone marrow transplant. *N Engl J Med* 1988;318:869–876.
295. Antman KS, Griffin JD, Elias A, et al. Effect of recombinant human granulocyte-macrophage colony-stimulating factor on chemotherapy-induced myelosuppression. *N Engl J Med* 1988;319:593–598.
296. Bonilla M. The Severe Chronic Neutropenia Study Group in conjunction with Amgen I. Clinical efficacy of recombinant human granulocyte colony-stimulating factor (r-metHuG-CSF) in patients with severe chronic neutropenia [Abstract]. *Blood* 1990;76:133a.
297. Negrin RS, Stein R, Vardiman J, et al. Treatment of the anemia of myelodysplastic syndromes using recombinant human granulocyte colony-stimulating factor in combination with erythropoietin. *Blood* 1993;82: 737–743.
298. Park JW, Mehrotra B, Barnett BO, et al. The Sweet syndrome during therapy with granulocyte colony-stimulating factor. *Ann Intern Med* 1992;116:996–998.
299. Joyce R, Goldstein J, Baker R. Reversible G-CSF associated leukemia cutis in blast crisis of chronic myelocytic leukemia [Abstract]. *Blood* 1992;80:450a.
300. Mueller BU, Jacobsen F, Butler KM, et al. Combination treatment with azidothymidine and granulocyte colony-stimulating factor in children with human immunodeficiency virus infection. *J Pediatr* 1992;121:797–802.
301. Beveridge R, Kales A, Binder A, et al. Comparison of toxicities of G-CSF and yeast-derived GM-CSF [Abstract]. *Blood* 1993;82:495a.
302. Jones S, Schottstaedt M, Duncan L. A randomized prospective trial to evaluate the effects of rHuGM-CSF versus placebo in a high-dose chemotherapy program for stage II and stage III breast cancer [Abstract]. *Proc Am Soc Clin Oncol* 1995;14:106.
303. Hudis C, Lebwohl D, Crown J. Feasibility of adjuvant dose-intensive cyclophosphamide (C) with G-CSF after doxorubicin (A) in women with high-risk stage II/III resectable breast cancer [Abstract]. *Proc Am Soc Clin Oncol* 1992;11:55.
304. Platzer E, A. S, Gramatzki M, et al. Clinical and biological effects of rHuG-CSF in chemotherapy for advanced head and neck cancer. In: *Cytokines in hemopoiesis, oncology, and AIDS (Conference Proceedings).* Hannover, Germany, 1991:22.
305. Stehle B, Weiss C, Ho AD, et al. Serum levels of tumor necrosis factor alpha in patients treated with granulocyte-macrophage colony-stimulating factor [Letter]. *Blood* 1990;75:1895–1896.
306. Sisson SD, Dinarello CA. Production of interleukin-1 alpha, interleukin-1 beta and tumor necrosis factor by human mononuclear cells stimulated with granulocyte-macrophage colony-stimulating factor. *Blood* 1988;72: 1368–1374.

307. Smith M, Horowitz M, Balis F. Pediatric experience with granulocyte-macrophage colony-stimulating factor (GM-CSF): pharmacokinetics and cytokine induction [Abstract]. *Proc Amer Assoc Cancer Res* 1991;32:196.
308. Dimitrov N, Stoller R, Hamm J. An NSABP pilot study evaluating GM-CSF and G-CSF used with high-dose chemotherapy [Abstract]. *Proc Am Soc Clin Oncol* 1993;12:138.
309. Lu D, Guo N, Zhang J. Use of hemopoietic growth factors G-CSF, GM-CSF in allogeneic bone marrow transplantation: a single center study [Abstract]. *Blood* 1993;82:285a.
310. Buonadonna A, Frustaci S, Galligioni E, et al. Comparison between G-CSF and GM-CSF for prophylaxis of severe leukopenia after intensive chemotherapy [Abstract]. *Proc Am Soc Clin Oncol* 1994;13:462.
311. DePlacido S, Perrone F, Carlomagno C. Toxicity and activity comparison of GM-CSF and G-CSF: ancillary results from two parallel phase I studies of high-dose chemotherapy for metastatic breast cancer [Abstract]. *Proc Am Soc Clin Oncol* 1995;14:257.
312. Kerrigan DP, Castillo A, Foucar K, et al. Peripheral blood morphologic changes after high-dose antineoplastic chemotherapy and recombinant human granulocyte colony-stimulating factor administration. *Am J Clin Pathol* 1989;92:280–285.
313. Gabrilove JL, Jakubowski A, Fain K, et al. Phase I study of granulocyte colony-stimulating factor in patients with transitional cell carcinoma of the urothelium. *J Clin Invest* 1988;82:1454–1461.
314. De Haas M, Kerst JM, van der Schoot CE, et al. Granulocyte colony-stimulating factor administration to healthy volunteers: analysis of the immediate activating effects on circulating neutrophils. *Blood* 1994;84:3885–3894.
315. Majlis A, Sarris A, Younes A. Rising serum LDH during chemotherapy treatment of patients with lymphoma or myeloma is often caused by G-CSF or GM-CSF support and not always by tumor progression [Abstract]. *Proc Am Soc Clin Oncol* 1994;13:388.
316. Herrmann F, Schulz G, Lindemann A, et al. Hematopoietic responses in patients with advanced malignancy treated with recombinant human granulocyte-macrophage colony-stimulating factor. *J Clin Oncol* 1989;7:159–167.
317. Phillips N, Jacobs S, Stoller R, et al. Effect of recombinant human granulocyte-macrophage colony-stimulating factor on myelopoiesis in patients with refractory metastatic carcinoma. *Blood* 1989;74:26–34.
318. Dale DC, Bonilla MA, Davis MW, et al. A randomized controlled phase III trial of recombinant human granulocyte colony-stimulating factor (Filgrastim) for treatment of severe chronic neutropenia. *Blood* 1993;81:2496–2502.
319. Amgen Neupogen (filgrastim). Package insert, 1994.
320. Rusthoven JJ, Eisenhauer E, Mazurka J, et al. Phase I clinical trial of recombinant human interleukin-3 combined with carboplatin in the treatment of patients with recurrent ovarian carcinoma. *J Natl Cancer Inst* 1993;85:823–825.
321. Biesma B, Willemse PH, Mulder NH, et al. Effects of interleukin-3 after chemotherapy for advanced ovarian cancer. *Blood* 1992;80:1141–1148.
322. Tepler I, Elias A, Kalish L, et al. Effect of recombinant human interleukin-3 on haematological recovery from chemotherapy-induced myelosuppression. *Br J Haematol* 1994;87:678–686.
323. D'Hondt V, Weynants P, Humblet Y, et al. Dose-dependent interleukin-3 stimulation of thrombopoiesis and neutropoiesis in patients with small-cell lung carcinoma before and following chemotherapy: a placebo-controlled randomized phase Ib study. *J Clin Oncol* 1993;11:2063–2071.
324. Dercksen MW, Hoekman K, ten Bokkel Huinink WW, et al. Effects of interleukin-3 on myelosuppression induced by chemotherapy for ovarian cancer and small cell undifferentiated tumours. *Br J Cancer* 1993;68:996–1003.
325. Kudoh S, Sawa T, Kurihara N, et al. Phase II study of recombinant human interleukin 3 administration following carboplatin and etoposide chemotherapy in small-cell lung cancer patients. SDZ ILE 964 (IL-3) Study. *Cancer Chemother Pharmacol* 1996;38:S89–S95.
326. Nemunaitis J, Appelbaum FR, Singer JW, et al. Phase I trial with recombinant human interleukin-3 in patients with lymphoma undergoing autologous bone marrow transplantation. *Blood* 1993;82:3273–3278.
327. Hofstra LS, Kristensen GB, Willemse PH, et al. Randomized trial of recombinant human interleukin-3 versus placebo in prevention of bone marrow depression during first-line chemotherapy for ovarian carcinoma. *J Clin Oncol* 1998;16:3335–3344.
328. Ganser A, Lindemann A, Ottmann OG, et al. Sequential *in vivo* treatment with two recombinant human hematopoietic growth factors (interleukin-3 and granulocyte-macrophage colony-stimulating factor) as a new therapeutic modality to stimulate hematopoiesis: results of a phase I study. *Blood* 1992;79:2583–2591.
329. Brugger W, Bross K, Frisch J, et al. Mobilization of peripheral blood progenitor cells by sequential administration of interleukin-3 and granulocyte-macrophage colony-stimulating factor following polychemotherapy with etoposide, ifosfamide, and cisplatin. *Blood* 1992;79:1193–1200.
330. O'Shaughnessy JA, Venzon DJ, Gossard M, et al. A phase I study of sequential versus concurrent interleukin-3 and granulocyte-macrophage colony-stimulating factor in advanced breast cancer patients treated with FLAC (5-fluorouracil, leucovorin, doxorubicin, cyclophosphamide) chemotherapy. *Blood* 1995;86:2913–2921.
331. Brugger W, Frisch J, Schulz G, et al. Sequential administration of interleukin-3 and granulocyte-macrophage colony-stimulating factor following standard-dose combination chemotherapy with etoposide, ifosfamide, and cisplatin. *J Clin Oncol* 1992;10:1452–1459.

332. Frisch J, Ganser A, Hoelzer D, et al. Interleukin-3 and granulocyte-macrophage colony-stimulating factor in combination: clinical implication. *Med Pediatr Oncol Suppl* 1992;2:34–37.
333. Fay JW, Lazarus H, Herzig R, et al. Sequential administration of recombinant human interleukin-3 and granulocyte-macrophage colony-stimulating factor after autologous bone marrow transplantation for malignant lymphoma: a phase I/II multicenter study. *Blood* 1994;84:2151–2157.
334. Fay J, Felser J, Abboud C. Sequential administration of recombinant human interleukin-3 (IL-3) and granulocyte-macrophage-stimulating factor (GM-CSF) after autologous bone marrow transplantation (ABMT) therapy for lymphoma: results of a phase III multicenter study [Abstract]. *Blood* 1995;86:222a.
335. Kolbe K, Peschel C, Rupilius B, et al. Peripheral blood stem cell (PBSC) mobilization with chemotherapy followed by sequential IL-3 and G-CSF administration in extensively pretreated patients. *Bone Marrow Transplant* 1997;20:1027–1032.
336. Curtis BM, Williams DE, Broxmeyer HE, et al. Enhanced hematopoietic activity of a human granulocyte/macrophage colony-stimulating factor-interleukin 3 fusion protein. *Proc Natl Acad Sci USA* 1991; 88:5809–5813.
337. Williams DE, Park LS. Hematopoietic effects of a granulocyte-macrophage colony-stimulating factor/interleukin-3 fusion protein. *Cancer* 1991;67:2705–2707.
338. Vadhan-Raj S, Broxmeyer HE, Andreeff M, et al. *In vivo* biologic effects of PIXY321, a synthetic hybrid protein of recombinant human granulocyte-macrophage colony-stimulating factor and interleukin-3 in cancer patients with normal hematopoiesis: a phase I study. *Blood* 1995;86:2098–2105.
339. Vadhan-Raj S, Papadopoulos NE, Burgess MA, et al. Effects of PIXY321, a granulocyte-macrophage colony-stimulating factor/interleukin-3 fusion protein, on chemotherapy-induced multilineage myelosuppression in patients with sarcoma. *J Clin Oncol* 1994;12:715–724.
340. Runowicz CD, Mandeli J, Speyer JL, et al. Phase I/II study of PIXY321 in combination with cyclophosphamide and carboplatin in the treatment of ovarian cancer. *Am J Obstet Gynecol*1996;174:1151–1160.
341. Collins C, Livingston R, Ellis G, et al. Effect of PIXY321 on hematologic recovery after high-dose cyclophosphamide (CTX), etoposide (VP-16), and cisplatin (CDDP) (CEP) in women with breast carcinoma [Abstract]. *Blood* 1993;82(suppl 1):366a.
342. Raptis G, Gilewski T, Gabrilove J. Evaluation of PIXY321 (PIXY) as a myeloprotective agent in patients with metastatic breast cancer receiving doxorubicin and thiotepa [Abstract]. *Proc Am Soc Clin Oncol* 1993;12:108.
343. Taylor C, Modiano M, Garrison L, et al. PIXY321 plus carboplatin (C) and adriamycin (A) in patients with advanced gastrointestinal malignancy [Abstract]. *Proc Am Soc Clin Oncol* 1993;12:195.
344. O'Shaughnessy JA, Tolcher A, Riseberg D, et al. Prospective, randomized trial of 5-fluorouracil, leucovorin, doxorubicin, and cyclophosphamide chemotherapy in combination with the interleukin-3/granulocyte-macrophage colony-stimulating factor (GM-CSF) fusion protein (PIXY321) versus GM-CSF in patients with advanced breast cancer. *Blood* 1996;87:2205–2211.
345. Schuster M, Beveridge R, Sosman J. Randomized phase II study of PIXY321 or Neupogen (rHuG-CSF) in combination with DHAP as salvage therapy for lymphoma [Abstract]. *Blood* 1995;86:54a.
346. Furman WL, Rodman JH, Tonda ME, et al. Clinical effects and pharmacokinetics of the fusion protein PIXY321 in children receiving myelosuppressive chemotherapy. *Cancer Chemother Pharmacol* 1998;41: 229–236.

12

Cytokine Signal Transduction

*David M. Frucht, †Samuel Fan, ‡Richard M. Siegel, *Roberta Visconti, and *John J. O'Shea

**Arthritis and Rheumatism Branch, National Institute of Arthritis and Musculoskeletal and Skin Diseases, Bethesda, Maryland; †Associate Professor, Department of Biology, Bradley University, Peoria, Illinois; and ‡Laboratory of Immunology, National Institutes of Allergy and Infectious Disease, Bethesda, Maryland*

Understanding the molecular basis of cytokine action is an important goal in cytokine research. However, because cytokines are an extremely diverse group of secreted factors, it is a challenge to provide a logical framework for discussing the different modes of signaling. Moreover, while cytokines are often grouped functionally (e.g., inflammatory, hematopoietic, or immunoregulatory cytokines), this classification is not necessarily informative if the goal is to understand intracellular signaling. This is because ligands that bind to entirely distinct families of receptors and utilize very different signaling pathways may, nevertheless, have similarities in their biological actions. Therefore, for the purposes of this chapter, it is simplest to group the cytokines according to the type of receptor that they bind. These receptors include the following family members: the so-called type I (hematopoietin family) and type II (interferon receptor family) cytokine receptors, receptor tyrosine kinases, receptor serine kinases, tumor necrosis factor (TNF) family receptors, interleukin-1 (IL-1) and closely related Toll-like receptors (TLRs), and G-protein coupled receptors (1) (Color Fig. 12.1). A great deal has been learned about how these various receptors signal, and this wealth of new information will be briefly reviewed.

TYPE I AND II CYTOKINE RECEPTORS

Type I receptors bind a family of cytokines that structurally have, as a central feature, a similar arrangement of four α-helical bundles (2). These proteins include hormones such as erythropoietin (EPO), thrombopoietin, prolactin (PRL), growth hormone (GH), and leptin; colony-stimulating factors (CSF) such as granulocyte colony-stimulating factors (G-CSF), macrophage colony-stimulating factors (M-CSF), and granulocyte-macrophage colony-stimulating factors (GM-CSF); and interleukins (IL-2 through IL-7, IL-9 through IL-13). Also included in this family are the cytokines ciliary neurotrophic factor (CNTF), leukemia inhibitory factor (LIF), oncostatin M (OSM), and cardiotropin 1 (CT-1) (1). Structurally, receptors in the type I family have conserved cysteine residues and a conserved Trp-Ser-X-Trp-Ser motif (where X indicates any amino acid) in their extracellular domains (Color Fig. 12.2). One interesting feature of this family of receptors is that subfamilies exist that use a shared receptor subunit in conjunction with a ligand-specific subunit (3). For instance, IL-2, IL-4, IL-7, IL-9, and IL-15 all use the common cytokine gamma chain, γc, as part of the receptors along with a ligand-specific chain. Similarly, gp130 is a shared subunit for IL-6 family cytokines (IL-6, IL-11, CNTF, LIF, OSM, and CT-1). The common beta subunit, βc, is shared by IL-3, IL-5, and GM-CSF. The use of common receptor subunits helps explain shared biological activities of some of these cytokines, while their distinct actions can be attributed in part to their ligand specific subunits. Unlike type I receptors, no shared receptor subunits have been identified in the type II cytokine receptor family, which includes interferon and IL-10 receptors. Both type I and II receptors have no intrinsic enzymatic activity. However, the membrane proximal segment of these receptors is conserved and is the region through which these receptors bind Janus kinases (Jaks). They have a single transmembrane domain and divergent cytoplasmic domains. Indeed, it has become clear through a variety of studies that Jaks play a pivotal role in signaling via this family of cytokine receptors (Color Fig. 12.2).

Janus Kinases

Presently, only four vertebrate Jaks have been identified (Jak1, Jak2, Jak3, and Tyk2) (4–6), making this is an exceedingly small family of protein tyrosine kinases. The essential functions of the Jaks in signaling by interferons and cytokines were first established using a panel of mutagenized cell lines made resistant to the effects of interferons (7,8). Through reconstitution experiments, it was first shown that Jaks are required for interferon signaling (9). Subsequently, cytokines using type I receptors were analyzed, and it is now known that all of the type I and II cytokine receptors activate various Jaks in some combination (Table 12.1). A few general concepts are clear from these studies (6). First, some Jaks (Jak1 and Jak2) are used by a variety of cytokine receptors. Second, Jak3, in

TABLE 12-1. *Signaling pathways utilized by Jaks and Stats*

Jak/Stat	Signaling pathway	Murine knockout phenotype
Jak1	**γc- and gp130-using cytokines, IL10, IFN-α, IFN-β, IFN-γ,** IL13	Neurological defect, mice die perinatally
Jak2	**EPO, βc-using cytokines,** TPO, IFN-γ, gp130-using cytokines, IL12, IL13, GH, Prolactin	Embryonically lethal, failure of red blood cell development
Jak3	**IL2, IL7, IL15,** other **gc**-using cytokines	Severe combined immunodeficiency
Tyk2	gp130-using cytokines, IL13, **IL12**, IFN-α, IFN-β, IL10	Reduced IFN and IL-12 responses
Stat1	**IFN-α, IFN-β, IFN-γ, FGF,** IL2, IL6, IL10	Susceptibility to viral and bacterial infections, Defective IFN signaling
Stat2	**IFN-α, IFN-β**	Defective IFN signaling
Stat3	**LIF, IL10, IL6,** other gp130-using cytokines, γc cytokines, GH	Embryonically lethal, conditional knockout showed defective IL-6 and IL-10 signaling
Stat4	**IL12,** IFN-α (human)	Defective Th1 development
Stat5a	**Prolactin, IL2, EPO,** γc- and βc-**sing** cytokines, GH, TPO	Defective lobul-alveolar development of the breast
Stat5b	**GH, GM-CSF, IL2, EPO,** γc/βc cytokines, prolactin, TPO	Required for sexual dimorphism, defective GM-CSF and IL-2 signaling
Stat5a/b	**GH, IL2, EPO**	Infertile, mammary gland defects, growth defect (GH signaling)
Stat6	**IL-4, IL-13**	Defective Th2 development

The γc-using cytokines include IL-2, IL-4, IL-7, IL-9, and IL-15; gp130-utilizing cytokines include IL-6, IL-11, OSM, CNTF, LIF, CT-1, and Leptin; and βc-using cytokines include IL-3, IL-5, and GM-CSF. Cytokines for which these signaling molecules have been shown to be essential in knockouts are in boldfaced type.

contrast, is used only by cytokines whose receptors contain the common cytokine γ chain, γc. Finally, as indicated above, the Jaks are physically associated with cytokine receptors.

The critical function of the Jaks is best illustrated in mice or humans deficient in these kinases. The first deficiency of a mammalian Jak was identified as the basis of one form of the human disease, severe combined immunodeficiency (SCID) (10,11), a heterogeneous group of disorders manifested by abnormalities in T and B lymphocyte function associated with severe infections early in life. The most common form of SCID, X-SCID, is due to mutations of γc. Accordingly, these patients have impaired signaling via all the cytokines that utilize this receptor subunit (IL-2, IL-4, IL-7, IL-9, and IL-15). Since Jak3 associates with γc, the possibility of Jak3 mutations was investigated in selected SCID patients. Indeed, it is now clear that mutation of either γc or Jak3 leads to the same functional defects. Shortly thereafter, Jak3 knockout mice were generated, and they, too, have defects of T, B and NK cells (12–14). The explanation for the T and B lymphocyte abnormalities in γc and Jak3-deficient mice and humans appears to be due to the failure of IL-7 signaling. Mice and humans with IL-7R mutations also have SCID (15). On the other hand, defective NK development in these SCID patients is likely the result of defective IL-15 signaling (16,17). Occasionally in Jak3-SCID patients, and more consistently in Jak3 –/– mice, the few T cells that are produced have an activated phenotype (18). This may be attributable to a lack of IL-2 signaling, as IL-2–, IL-2Rα– and IL-2Rβ–deficient mice have lymphoproliferative disease thought to be the result of inefficient apoptosis (19–21).

In contrast to Jak3-deficient mice and humans, gene targeting of Jak1 and Jak2 resulted in more diverse abnormalities (22–24). Jak1 –/– mice die perinatally, apparently due to an ill-characterized neurological defect (22). Similar to Jak3 –/– mice, these mice also have SCID, which is explained by the fact that γc-using cytokines utilize Jak1 in association with their ligand-specific receptor subunit. Other cytokine receptors that are dependent upon Jak1 include gp130 cytokine receptors (for IL-6, LIF, OSM, CNTF, and IL-11) and type II cytokines receptors (for IL-10, IFN-α, IFN-β, and IFN-γ).

Gene targeting of Jak2 was embryonically lethal, principally because Jak2 is essential for the function of the cytokine, erythropoietin (23,24). Thus Jak2 –/– mice do not form blood. This phenotype is entirely consistent with that of EPO and EPOR –/– mice, though more severe, as Jak2 is also necessary for signaling of other cytokines, including IL-3. On the other hand, chromosomal translocations involving the 3′ region of Jak2 and the 5′ region of the Tel transcription factor have been found to be present in leukemic cells, indicating that uncontrolled Jak2 signaling can be transforming (25–27).

Some questions regarding the Jak family remain to be answered. For example, the crystal structure for the Jaks is unknown, so our understanding of Jak structure is quite limited. We can, however, make some predictions based on their primary structure. Jaks are characterized by regions of homology termed Janus homology (JH) domains. The Jaks have a C-terminal tyrosine kinase or JH1 domain that has extensive homology to other tyrosine kinases. Amino-terminal to the kinase domain is a segment that has homology to tyrosine kinase domains but has no catalytic activity; hence, this putative domain is termed the pseudo kinase or JH2 domain. It is notable that this feature is unique to the Jaks; no other mammalian tyrosine kinase has such a domain. While it lacks catalytic activity, mutation of this domain has significant effects on the function of the Jaks as kinases, thus appearing to be a regulatory domain. A number of patients with Jak3-SCID have been identified with mutations in the JH2 domain (18,28). The kinases encoded by the mutant alleles have poor *in vitro* kinase activity and are unable to transmit cytokine-dependent signals, suggesting a critical role of the JH2 domain in regulating Jak kinase activity.

A key feature of the Jaks is their association with cytokine receptors. This appears to be mediated by the N-terminus. For Jak3, a relatively small portion of the molecule confers most of its ability to bind γc (29,30). Other Jak/receptor interactions have been studied, and the amino terminus is clearly involved, but the segments that mediate this interaction may be more extended than those of Jak3 (31,32).

One proposed mechanism by which type I and II receptors signal involves the following scenario. First, ligand binding effects aggregation of receptor subunits, bringing Jaks in close proximity. Alternatively, an allosteric mechanism has been proposed, but in either case, ligand binding allows Jaks to phosphorylate one another on residues in the activation loop, enhancing catalytic activity. After activation, the Jaks phosphorylate receptor subunits on tyrosine residues allowing recruitment of proteins with SH2 or phosphotyrosine binding (PTB) domains. These proteins, too, are then phosphorylated by Jaks. This allows a number of pathways to become activated, including the Ras/Raf/MAPK pathway and the PI3′ kinase pathway. Most importantly, phosphorylation of cytokine receptors also generates docking sites for a class of SH2-containing transcription factors termed the Stats.

Signal Transducers and Activators of Transcription (Stats)

Signal transducers and activators of transcription (Stats), as the name implies, serve essential functions in transducing signals from cytokine receptors to the nucleus, where they bind DNA and regulate gene transcription (4,5,33–35). These functions can be explained by Stat structure; Stat molecules consist of a central DNA binding domain flanked by a coiled-coiled domain that binds other transcription factors and coactivators (36,37). They also have N-terminal domain involvement in dimer-dimer interactions. C-terminal of the DNA binding domain is a linker domain followed by the SH2 domain and a conserved site of tyrosine phosphorylation. The C-terminus of the Stats is variable and contains the transcriptional activation domain. Thus the cytokine signaling appears to occur as follows; Stats are latent, cytosolic transcription factors that are recruited via their SH2 domains to cytokine receptors, which have been phosphorylated on specific tyrosine residues. Different Stats bind to specific cytokine receptors (Table 12.1). Stats, in turn, are phosphorylated, enabling their dimerization via reciprocal SH2-phosphotyrosine interactions. This leads to their nuclear translocation where they regulate gene transcription. Stats bind two types of DNA motifs, ISREs (IFN-stimulated response elements, consensus AGTTTNCNTTTCC) and GAS (gamma-activated sequence) elements (consensus TTCNNNGAA). Some Stats are also phosphorylated on a conserved serine residue in the transcriptional activation domain; this appears to be mediated by a MAPK family member.

There are seven mammalian Stats: Stat1, Stat2, Stat3, Stat4, Stat5a, Stat5b, and Stat6. As previously mentioned, the critical functions of Stat1 and Stat2 in transmitting cytokine-dependent signals were established through the use of mutagenized cell lines defective in IFN responses; reconstitution of these cell lines with the missing Stat was shown to restore signaling. Stat1 –/– mice were found to develop normally, but had extreme susceptibility to both viral and bacterial infections (38,39). This is entirely consistent with the defects seen in IFNαR and IFNγR –/– mice and IFNγR-deficient humans. Stat1 also appears to be important in regulating apoptosis, and its absence is associated with tumorigenesis. Stat2 knockout mice also have extreme viral susceptibility consistent with its regulation by IFNα/β (C. Schindler, personal communication, 2000).

In contrast, gene targeting of Stat3 leads to early embryonic lethality (40). The lethality is related in part to interference with LIF function, as LIF –/– knockout mice also display embryonic lethality due to failure of implantation (41). Using conditional knockouts, it has been demonstrated that targeting of Stat3 in myeloid cells has a dramatic effect. These mice have an exaggerated inflammatory response, which appears to be due to the failure of IL-10 signaling (42). Stat4 –/– mice develop completely normally but have defective cell-mediated immune responses and T helper (Th)1 differentiation and augmented Th2 development, a phenotype consistent with the abnormalities seen in IL-12 –/–, IL-12R –/– mice, and IL-12R–deficient humans (43–47).

Stat6 was originally purified as factor induced by IL-4. In contrast to Stat4 knockouts, Stat6 –/– mice have defective Th2 development (48–50). They also have defective IgE response following infection with parasites. Lack of Stat6 dramatically attenuates allergic and asthmatic disease in animal models. The cytokine IL-13 shares a receptor subunit with IL-4, and consequently IL-13 also activates Stat6. IL-13–induced responses are also abrogated in Stat6 –/– mice (51).

Stat5a and Stat5b are about 91% identical at the amino acid level and are both activated by a variety of cytokines, including prolactin (PRL), growth hormone, erythropoietin, thrombopoietin, and IL-2. Nonetheless, they have very specific functions. Stat5a knockout mice have impaired mammary gland development and failure of lactation (52). Stat5b knockout mice, by contrast, have defective sexually dimorphic growth and growth hormone-dependent regulation of liver gene expression (53). Doubly deficient Stat5a/5b –/– mice suffer perinatal lethality, though the reason for this is not clear presently (54). The surviving mice are small and the dwarfism is reminiscent of Laron-type dwarfism. The females are infertile, likely due to the interruption of PRL signaling in the corpus luteum. T cells do develop in Stat5a/5b –/– mice, though they are very abnormal. While the cells fail to proliferate *in vitro*, the mice develop lymphoproliferative disease, suggesting a defect in apoptosis (55,56).

Attenuation of Type I and Type II Cytokine Signaling

Perhaps as important as the triggers that initiate signal transduction are the mechanisms involved in extinguishing the response. We will discuss several families of proteins that are involved in downregulating cytokine signaling including the following: phosphatases, cytokine-inducible inhibitor molecules, and transcriptional repressors (57).

Since activation of the Jaks and Stats requires phosphorylation, and phosphorylation of these substrates is transient, dephosphorylation of Jaks and Stats is likely one point of regulation of cytokine signaling. SHP-1 is an example of a phosphatase that has been proposed to interact with cytokine receptors and downregulate signaling. Both the motheaten and the viable motheaten mice strains have mutations in this gene. Motheaten mice die at an early age and have signs of uncontrolled immune responses, including severe pneumonitis characterized by activated macrophages, neutrophilic skin lesions, elevated immunoglobulin levels, and anti-dsDNA antibody production (58,59).

The suppressor of cytokine signaling (SOCS) family proteins (alternatively termed Jab, SSI, and CIS) act at a different points along the cascade, some at the level of the Jaks (60–63). There are at least eight members of this family, which is characterized by a central SH2 domain and a C-terminal region of homology, or "SOCS box." Several SOCS can bind the phosphorylated activation loop of Jaks, inhibiting Jak kinase activity. For example, after its induction, SOCS-1 binds the phosphorylated activation loop tyrosine residue (Y1007) in Jak2 via its SH2 domain (64). SOCS-1 –/– mice have been generated and the animals die within a few weeks of birth due almost entirely to systemic hyperresponsiveness to IFN-γ; anti–IFN-γ reverses much of the pathology observed in these mice (65). SOCS-3 –/– mice, on the other hand, demonstrate its essential role in down-regulating fetal hematopoiesis. This suggests that SOCS-3 has a specific role in attenuating Jak2 function, which transduces signals for the erythropoietin receptor (66,67). CIS-1, another member of the SOCS family, has been proposed to act using a somewhat different mechanism, directly binding to the IL-2 receptor β chain to inhibit signaling.

Other inhibitors of cytokine signaling act at the level of Stat function. One such family is the protein inhibitor of activated Stat (PIAS) family; their exact function is less clear than the SOCS family (68). They have been shown to negatively regulate the transcriptional activation of Stats, but do not inhibit Stat phosphorylation. At present the mechanism of this action is unknown. Similarly, the zinc-finger protein, Bcl-6, has been shown to inhibit Stat function. Bcl-6–deficient mice develop systemic inflammation characterized by Th-2 predominance, possibly due to the ability of Bcl-6 to compete for Stat6 DNA binding sites (69). Thus much has been learned about the signal transduction pathways underlying cytokine signaling through type I and type II receptors. Through a series of elegant experiments, a relatively simple mechanism has emerged. Membrane-associated receptors are coupled via Jaks and Stats to the nucleus where target genes are activated. Knockout mouse models have demonstrated the critical functional roles of this signaling in immune responses.

TNF RECEPTOR FAMILY

The TNF receptor (TNFR) superfamily encompasses a large number of cell surface receptors that bind ligands structurally related to TNF (Table 12.2). While TNF can exist as a soluble ligand, many of these ligands are transmembrane molecules. The receptors for these ligands are type-I transmembrane glycoproteins characterized by cysteine-rich repeats of about 40 amino acids in their N-terminal extracellular domains. Each extracellular domain consists of three or four of these regions containing four to six cysteines involved in intrachain disulfide bonds. Like type I and type II cytokine receptors, the intracellular domains of the TNFR family members lack intrinsic enzymatic activity. Rather, signaling is initiated by the recruitment of various adapter and signaling molecules by signaling domains in the intracellular portion of TNFR family members. Recruitment of adaptor molecules activates a number of characteristic signaling pathways that can lead to a remarkably diverse set of cellular responses including differentiation, activation, release of inflammatory mediators, and apoptosis. TNF family receptors can be divided into two subfamilies by the types of intracellular signaling molecules recruited. Fas, TNFR1, death receptor (DR) 3, DR4, and DR5 share a conserved intracellular domain termed the death domain (DD). This domain is required for recruitment of DD-containing adaptor molecules that are involved in the initiation of apoptotic programmed cell death, though other signaling pathways can be activated by certain adaptor molecules as well. For this reason, these receptors have been termed "death receptors" (Table 12.2A). The function of a number of death receptors may be regulated by decoy receptors, cell surface molecules that bind ligand but lack functional intracellular domains (70) (Table 12.2B). TNF family receptors without death domains [CD27, CD30, CD40, herpes virus entry mediator (HVEM), TNFR2, lymphotoxin-β receptor (LTβR), OX-40, and 4-1 BB] associate with different types of adapter molecules, most importantly members of the TRAF (TNFR-associated factor) family (Table 12.2C). Recruitment of adaptor molecules to these receptors activates a broad range of signaling cascades, including the sphingomyelinase, NF-κB, JNK, and ERK pathways, leading to gene induction and downstream events. TNFR family members can be viewed as mediating a spectrum of responses, from purely apoptotic (Fas and other death receptors) to mixed (TNFR1), to nonapoptotic (CD27, CD30, CD40, HVEM, TNFR2, LTβR, OX-40, and 4-1 BB). However, there is crosstalk between these two subfamilies, as signaling through nonapoptotic receptors has been found to regulate apoptosis initiated by death receptors. For simplicity, the focus of this section will be on signaling by the two best understood members of this family: Fas and the two TNF receptors (Color Fig. 12.3).

Fas and Related Death Receptors

Fas, also known as CD95 or APO-1, is the prototypical member of the TNFR death receptor subfamily. The Fas antigen was originally cloned based on the apoptosis-inducing properties of anti-Fas antibodies (71). The *in vivo* role of Fas signaling in regulation of the immune system was confirmed when the naturally arising lpr and gld mouse strains were found to harbor homozygous mutations of Fas and Fas-ligand, respectively (72,73). Both of these mouse strains are characterized by lymphadenopathy and splenomegaly due to accumulation of unusual CD4-CD8- T cells, as well as the production of autoantibodies similar to those found in humans with systemic lupus erythematosus (SLE). Subsequently, humans with heterozygous mutations in the Fas receptor were identified with similar symptoms and autoantibodies (74,75). In this disease, the autoimmune lymphoproliferative syndrome (ALPS), the Fas mutations act as dominant negative inhibitors of intracellular signaling, causing defective apoptosis in all carriers of Fas mutations and overt disease in a variable percentage of family members (76).

Fas signaling is mediated by recruitment of proteins that directly and indirectly trigger the activation of caspases, a specific family of intracellular cysteine proteases involved in apoptosis (77). The initiation of signaling by Fas and other members of the TNF receptor family has been thought to be mediated by ligand-induced trimerization of receptors. This notion is largely based on the crystal structures of TNFR1 bound to LTβ (78) and TRAIL/DR5 (79,80), in which three receptors lie at the apices of a triangle, with the chains of trimeric ligand interdigitating between them. However, there is recent evidence that Fas and other members of the TNFR family are noncovalently preassociated before ligand binding, with the ligand causing a conformational change that brings the intracellular domains of the receptor closer together (81,82). This is reminiscent of the rearrangement of dimers of the erythropoietin receptor that occurs after binding of erythropoietin or agonistic ligand mimetics (83,84).

Intracellularly, the key event in Fas signaling is the stable recruitment of the adaptor molecule, Fas-associated death domain protein (FADD), and subsequently caspase-8 to the death domain of Fas to form a signaling complex termed the death inducing signal complex (DISC) (85). The death domain of Fas consists of six alpha helices arranged in a characteristic fold, which binds to a similar death domain in the C-terminus of FADD through charge–charge interactions (86). The N-terminus of FADD contains a structurally similar domain, termed the death-effector domain (DED), because overexpression of the DED can by itself trigger apoptosis. The structure of the FADD DED contains two hydrophobic patches not present in the DDs, which are critical for binding to caspase-8/FLICE/MACH and for apoptotic activity (87). This latter protein has two N-terminal

TABLE 12-2. TNF superfamily receptors and their signaling pathways

A) Death-Domain Containing Receptors (Death Receptors)

Molecule	Other names	Ligand	Interacting molecules	Comments	References
Fas	DR1, APO-1, CD95	FasL	FADD, Caspase-8	Most consistently proapoptotic	Itoh et al., 1991; Oehm et al., 1992; Trauth et al., 1989
TNFR1	DR2, CD120a, p55, p60	TNF, LTβ	TRADD, RIP (indirect) FADD (indirect) TRAF2 (indirect)	Cytotoxicity can be modulated by NFκB	Loetscher et al., 1990; Schall et al., 1990
DR3	TRAMP/WSL/APO2/LARD	TWEAK (APO-3)	TRADD, FADD (indirect), TNFR1 Caspase-10	Expression thought to be restricted to lymphocytes; induced after DNA damage via p53-dependent mechanism	Chinnaiyan et al., 1996; Kitson et al., 1996; Screaton et al., 1997
DR4	TRAIL-R1	TRAIL	?	May bind FADD but no requirement for FADD in DR4-induced death found in FADD knockout mice.	Schneider et al., 1997; Schneider et al., 1997; Yeh et al., 1998
DR5	TRAIL-R2	TRAIL	?	Can heterodimerize with DR4, induced by DNA damage	Pan et al., 1997; Walczak et al., 1997; Wu et al., 1997

B) Decoy receptors

Molecule	Other names	Ligand	Comments	References
TRID	TRAIL-R3, DcR1	TRAIL	GPI-linked extracellular receptor; blocks TRAIL-induced apoptosis	Degli-Esposti et al., 1997; Pan et al., 1997; Sheridan et al., 1997
TRAIL-R4	DcR2	TRAIL	Incomplete death domain; blocks TRAIL-induced apoptosis	Degli-Esposti et al., 1997; Marsters et al., 1997
Dc-R3	DcR3	FasL	Soluble molecule that binds FasL with higher affinity than Fas; amplified in some lung and colon carcinomas	Pitti et al., 1998

C) Other Receptors in the TNF-R Superfamily

Molecule	Other names	Ligand	Interacting intracellular molecules	Signaling pathways activated	Comments	References
TNFR2	CD120b	TNF, LTα	TRAF-1, 2	NF-κB, JNK	In mature CD8 T cells, this receptor is required for antigen-receptor induced apoptosis	Speiser et al., 1997; Zheng et al., 1995
LTbR	Lymphotoxin receptor	LTβ, LT$\alpha\beta$ LIGHT	TRAF1, 2, 3, 5	NF-κB	Lymphotoxin can also bind to TNF receptors	Crowe et al., 1994; VanArsdale et al., 1997
CD27		CD70	TRAF1, 2, 3 Siva (for apoptosis)	NF-κB, JNK, apoptosis	Early activation marker on B and T cells, mediates costimulation and also apoptosis under some circumstances	Prasad et al., 1997
CD30		CD30L (CD153)	TRAF1, 2	NF-κB, JNK	Found to be involved in thymic negative selection	Amakawa et al., 1996; Lee et al., 1996
CD40		CD40L (CD154)	TRAF2	NF-κB	Expressed on B cells and other APC's—can protect from cell death during antigen presentation	Klaus et al., 1997; Rathmell et al., 1996
OX-40	CD134	OX-40L	TRAF2	NF-κB	Expression is enriched on autoreactive cells; potent costimulator of activated T cells	Godfrey et al., 1994; Gramaglia et al., 1998; Kaleeba et al., 1998
4-1BB	CD137, ILA	4-1 BBL	TRAF-1, 2	NF-κB	May be particularly important in stimulating CD8 T cell mediated antiviral and antitumor immunity	Arch and Thompson, 1998; DeBenedette et al., 1999; Jang et al., 1998; Melero et al., 1998
HVEM	TR2	LIGHT	TRAF-1, 2, 3, 5	?	Can enhance proliferation of resting T cells but also induce apoptosis in tumor lines; lymphoid-specific viral entry mediator	Harrop et al., 1998; Zhai et al., 1998

death effector domains and a C-terminal caspase domain. Once bound to FADD, the proteolytic activity of caspase-8 is activated, resulting in the cleavage of downstream substrates and the initiation of apoptotic events (88,89).

Signaling through Fas appears to differ substantially in different cell types (90). In some cells, termed type I cells, there is sufficient activation of caspase-8 to trigger cleavage of the effector caspases-3, -6, and -7. These effector caspases cleave key cellular substrates, resulting in apoptosis without the need for *de novo* transcription of new proteins. In other cell types, termed type II, the amount of caspase-8 activated in the Fas signaling complex does not seem to be enough to activate apoptosis. In these cells, amplification of the apoptotic signal occurs in mitochondria, probably mediated by the cleavage of proapoptotic molecules, such as Bid, by caspase-8. This results in the release of cytochrome c from mitochondria, which complexes with apoptotic protease activating factor 1 (Apaf1) and procaspase-9, leading to caspase-9 activation (91–93). In type II cells, but not type I cells, overexpression of antiapoptotic Bcl-2 family members can block cell death at the mitochondrial stage. Activated mature T cells appear to be type I, in that Fas-induced apoptosis is not blocked by Bcl-2 overexpression (94). A requirement for FADD has been shown in other death receptors, as demonstrated by defective apoptosis signaling through TNF and DR3 receptors in FADD –/– mice (95,96). However, how caspases are activated by other death receptors is not clear.

The recruitment and activation of caspase-8 may be an important regulatory step in Fas signaling. A cellular inhibitory protein, Flice-like Inhibitory Protein (c-FLIP/I-Flice/Usurpin/CASH) with homology to caspase-8 but containing a functionally inactive caspase domain, can be recruited to the Fas signaling complex, but blocks activation of caspase-8 when overexpressed (97–100). Overexpression of c-FLIP by retroviral transduction blocks B-cell apoptosis *in vivo* and leads to autoantibody production (101). However, endogenous levels of c-FLIP do not readily correlate with sensitivity to Fas-induced apoptosis, so the physiological role of this protein awaits mouse knockout studies. The TRAIL receptors DR4 and DR5 may preferentially recruit caspase-10, rather than caspase-8 in humans, as illustrated by experiments with transfection studies with dominant negative versions caspases-8 and -10 (102). Moreover, patients with a variant form of ALPS have been shown to have deleterious caspase-10 mutations, and these patients show a selective defect in TRAIL vs. Fas signaling (103).

Death receptor signaling may also be regulated extracellularly and at the cell surface by splice variants, proteolytic extracellular receptor fragments, and decoy receptors. The Fas gene is alternatively spliced to yield secreted versions that inhibit normal receptor signaling in transfection systems (104). In addition, separate gene products encoding truncated receptors with defective signaling domains have been described for both Fas and TRAIL. These molecules, termed decoy receptors, are potent blockers of signaling by their cognate ligands, and are overexpressed in various tumor lines, possibly accounting for resistance of these tumors to apoptotic stimuli (Table 12.2B).

In addition to apoptosis, the signaling molecules in the Fas pathway may have other functions. Cells from FADD-deficient mice or mice expressing a dominant-negative version of FADD are resistant to apoptosis induced by FasL and TRAIL. However, they also have cardiac developmental defects and a profound blockade of lymphocyte activation at the level of cell cycle entry, suggesting other functions of the FADD molecule (95,96,105). Caspase-8–deficient mice also have defective Fas and TRAIL-induced apoptosis, but effects on lymphocyte activation have not yet been studied.

TNF Receptors

TNF binding to its receptors, TNFR1(p60, p55, CD120a) and TNFR2 (p80, p75, CD120b) results in both proapoptotic and antiapoptotic signals (Color Fig. 12.3). Intracellularly, TNFR1 can be divided into three domains that contribute to these events: 1) a C-terminal death domain; 2) an adjacent neutral sphingomyelinase (N-Smase); and 3) an acidic (A)-Smase activating domains. The TNFR1 death domain recruits the adapter molecule TNF-R1 associated death domain protein (TRADD) (106). This adapter protein also links the TNFR to both pro and antiapoptotic events. It does so by binding at least three additional proteins. Ligand binding causes recruitment of FADD to TRADD. TRADD also associates with a death domain containing a serine/threonine kinase, receptor interacting protein (RIP), again via the C-terminal death domain. RIP interacts with another protein, RIP-associated Ich-1/CED3 homologous protein with death domain (RAIDD) causing the recruitment of Caspase 2 (107). In contrast to these proteins, a molecule designated SODD (silencer of death domains) is found in the TNFR1 complex before receptor activation that dissociates from the receptor after ligand binding (108). SODD can also associate with the death receptor DR3. It is thought that SODD preassociation with TNFR1 may prevent spontaneous signaling by death domain-containing receptors.

In contrast to TNFR1, TNFR2 lacks a DD and associates with another family of adapter molecules, the TRAFs (TNFR-associated factors). TRAFs form a family of cytoplasmic adapter proteins that mediate signal transduction from many members of the TNF-receptor superfamily (109). TRAFs are also involved in signaling through the interleukin-1 and Toll-like receptor (TLR) family. TNFR2 was found to associate with heterodimeric complexes of TRAF1 and TRAF2 with direct association between the cytoplasmic tail of TNFR2 and TRAF2 (110). All TRAF proteins contain a C-terminal TRAF domain that is required for self-association and interaction with receptors. It contains a predicted coiled-coil region that is followed by a highly conserved TRAF-C domain. The crystal structure of the TRAF domain is a trimer with each TRAF-C domain forming an eight-stranded antiparallel beta-sandwich structure. TNF receptors bind to a conserved shallow surface depression of one TRAF-C domain (111). A major TRAF2-binding consensus sequence, (P/S/A/T)X(Q/E)E, and a minor consensus motif, PXQXXD are present in all known TRAF2-binding regions (112). TRAF-2 was found to bind more efficiently to the intracellular domain of CD40 when both proteins were trimerized (113), suggesting that the appropriate alignment of intracellular domains is the principal function of ligand in triggering intracellular signaling.

Cells from TRAF2-deficient mice are hypersensitive to apoptosis induced by TNF, implicating this protein in the antiapoptotic effect of TNF (114,115). One pathway for this protective effect may be through the activation of the DNA binding protein nuclear factor kappa B (NF-κB), suggested by the fact that TRAF-2 overexpression can induce NF-κB activity (116). Cells with a blocked NF-κB pathway are also hypersensitive to the apoptotic effect of TNF (117). However, TRAF2-independent mechanisms of protection must also exist, since TRAF2-deficient mice have a normal NF-κB response to TNF despite their hypersensitivity to apoptosis (115,118).

Although it is known that signaling through TNF receptors can rapidly activate NF-κB, the precise steps involved in NF-κB activation and the mechanism of protection from apoptosis have not been entirely elucidated (119). However, some points are clear. NF-κB transcription factors are sequestered in the cytoplasm of cells by a protein called Iκb (inhibitor of kappa B). Phosphorylation of Iκb results in its degradation via ubiquitination (Color Fig. 12.3). Free NF-κB subunits then translocate to the nucleus where they regulate expression of a wide variety of genes involved in inflammatory responses (120). A complex of two kinases and a regulatory protein are responsible for IkB phosphorylation. The kinases are termed IκB kinases α (IKKα) and β (IKKβ), and are constitutively associated with the regulatory protein IKKγ or NEMO (121). IKKβ, but not IKKα, is the target for proinflammatory stimuli (122). Mice homozygous for a disrupted IKKβ gene have extensive liver damage from apoptosis and die as embryos, but this phenotype can be suppressed by the inactivation of the TNFR1 gene. Cells from IKKβ –/– embryos have marked reduction of TNF and IL-1–induced NF-κB activity and enhanced apoptosis in response to TNF (123–126). In contrast, IKKα-deficient mice show that this kinase subunit is not required for activation of IKK and degradation of IκB by proinflammatory stimuli. Instead, loss of IKKα interfered with multiple morphogenetic events, including limb and skeletal patterning and proliferation and differentiation of epidermal keratinocytes (127). Taken together, these results illustrate the dual nature of TNF signaling: without NF-κB activation, TNF-induced cell death is unmasked or enhanced.

The activation of the IKK complex is less well understood. The kinase NIK (NF-κB inducing kinase) has been suggested to be responsible for IKK phosphorylation. However, this remains controversial. A naturally occurring mouse mutation termed alymphoplasia (aly) is the result of a point mutation of NIK (128). This disorder is characterized by the absence of lymph nodes (LN) and Peyer's patches (PP) and disorganized splenic and thymic structures, and the abnormal immune response in aly/aly mice. These defects initially implicated NIK as potentially important in CD40, CD30, and LTβR signaling, but not in TNFR action.

TNF also activates other signaling pathways, but the physiological significance of these responses is not clear. C-Jun N-terminal kinase (JNK) is activated by TNF in a TRAF2-dependent manner. A TRAF-interacting protein termed TANK (TRAF-associated NF-κB activator) along with the germinal center kinase–related kinase (GCKR) appear to be involved in this process (129). More recently another TNFR1 binding DD protein named MADD was found; overexpression of this protein leads to MAPK activation, including ERK and JNK activation (130). N-Smase activation is thought to mediate some of the inflammatory and proliferative response to TNF through the activation of ERK and phospholipase A2. The protein factor associated with N-Smase activation (FAN) may couple the TNFR to activation of this enzyme activity (131). N-Smase activation results in the production of ceramide, which activates MAPK. N-Smase activation is thought to play a role in TNF-mediated apoptosis and NF-κB activation, but this pathway has not been clearly elucidated.

Despite the fact that TNFR2 lacks a DD and is only known to associate with the TRAF proteins, T cells from TNFR2-deficient mice are more defective in apoptotic responses to TNF than are cells from TNFR1-deficient mice, suggesting that this receptor plays an indirect role in apoptosis signaling (132). The relationship between signaling by these two receptors for the same ligand is complex. It was originally suggested that TNFR2 functions by capturing soluble TNF and delivering it to TNFR1—the "ligand passing" model (133). However, it has recently become clear that TNFR2 independently signals to enhance apoptotic signals through TNFR1, though the mechanism of this effect is not clear at present (134,135).

Interestingly, the extracellular domains of TNFR1, TNFR2, and possibly other members of the TNFR superfamily can be cleaved from the cell surface by unidentified proteases. This process may serve to downregulate signaling by removing cell surface receptors as well as producing soluble inhibitors (136). Defective TNFR1 cleavage may underlie the autoinflammatory syndromes seen in patients with dominant mutations in the extracellular domain of this receptor (137). Other members of the TNFR family play diverse roles in the development and function of the immune system (Table 12.2). CD40, OX-40, CD27, CD30, and 4-BB1 can mediate costimulation of T-cell activation, but through different mechanisms. CD40L on T cells triggers APC activation including upregulation of the CD28 ligands B7-1 and B7-2, indirectly boosting costimulation of the T cell responses. OX-40, CD27, CD30, and 4-BB1 more likely act as direct costimulators of T cell activation. CD30 may have a distinct role in the thymus as part of the machinery that governs negative selection of autoreactive thymocytes, as thymocytes from CD30-deficient mice have defective apoptosis induced by TCR cross-linking (138). The Lymphotoxin β receptor appears to play a unique role in development of secondary lymph nodes, as LTα mice lack lymph nodes and Peyer's patches, an effect mediated through the LTβ receptor (139,140).

With large numbers of different TNF-R family members coexisting on cells, and sharing common signaling pathways, it is not clear how specificity of signaling is maintained. Much of the data on binding of adaptor and other putative signaling molecules to TNF-Rs was obtained in overexpression systems, and it has become clear that these systems identify candidate proteins which are later found not to interact with the receptor under physiological conditions. Subtle changes in receptor levels and differential regulation by intracellular and extracellular regulatory molecules may further refine the specificity of signaling by these receptors *in vivo*. These mechanisms work in concert to allow signaling by TNF-R family members to integrate diverse stimuli and produce coordinated inflammatory and specific immune responses.

INTERLEUKIN-1/TOLL-LIKE RECEPTOR FAMILY

The IL-1R (IL1R)/Toll-like receptor family comprises the IL-1 receptors, the IL-18 receptor, and the newly discovered human homologs to the Drosophila protein, the Toll-like receptors (TLR 1-5). Even some molecules associated with resistance to plant pathogens, including the tobacco mosaic virus, have been shown to be related to this family of receptors (141,142). Their roles are broad, but they have prominent roles in innate immune responses and inflammation. Members of this family allow responses to bacterial proteins (TLR) and mediate fever (IL-1). In contrast, IL-18 promotes Th-1 differentiation (IL-18) in the adaptive immune response. In this manner, this family of receptors has evolved to perform a variety of new functions in higher organisms. The ligands for the IL-1R/TLR family are as varied as the physiological changes that they induce. The IL-1 receptors, IL-1RI and IL-1RII bind IL-1α, IL-1β, and IL-1 receptor antagonist (IL-1Ra) (143,144). All three appear to have been derived from a common ancestral gene and are characterized by a 12 β-pleated sheet tertiary structure and by the lack of a signal peptide. The ligand for IL-18R, IL-18, also shares a 12 β-pleated sheet structure with the IL-1 family (145). The TLR family ligands, on the other hand, are entirely different from those of IL-1R or IL-18R, which is consistent with the fact that the TLRs do not have the same three immunoglobulin-like domains in their extracellular regions as do IL-1R and IL-18R (146). Although the extent of the ligands for the TLRs is not fully known at present, it is clear that some of the TLRs are activated by the cell wall components of microbial pathogens. TLR4 enables cellular response to bacterial LPS, whereas TLR2 appears to transduce signal after interacting with other bacterial products such as lipoproteins (147,148,149). The major regions of homology, which are common to the IL-1R/TLR family, are located in the intracytoplasmic region, resulting in the utilization of common signaling intermediates. Since IL-1 signaling has been studied in more detail, this chapter will concentrate on this receptor complex and signaling components. Many of the signaling intermediates for IL-18R and TLRs appear to be the same, but important data are still lacking. Stimulation by either IL-1α or IL-1β leads to the formation of the initial IL-1/IL-1RI complex, resulting in association of the complex with another member of the IL-1R/TLR family, IL-1RI accessory protein (IL-1RacP). IL-1RacP is also a component of the IL-18R (145,150,151). This interaction stabilizes the initial complex (152,153). IL-1Ra binding to IL-1RI does not enable interaction with IL-1RacP, and therefore does not initiate signal transduction. In this manner, IL-1Ra can act as a competitive antagonist for the potent action of IL-1.

The cytoplasmic domain of IL-1RII is extremely short and does not interact with and activate intracellular effectors (154). Its function seems to be to compete with IL-1RI for binding IL-1, perhaps acting as another buffer for the extremely high efficiency of IL-1RI to transduce the IL-1 signal, so that signaling is not inadvertently triggered. Additionally, both IL-1RI and IL-1RII are susceptible to proteolytic cleavage near the membrane surface, and can therefore act as soluble IL1-binding proteins, revealing another mechanism to down-modulate IL-1 signaling (155).

Formation of the initial IL-1/IL-1RI complex allows recruitment of the adapter protein myeloid differentiation factor 88 (Color Fig. 12.4). IL-1 receptor–associated kinase (IRAK), related to the Drosophila protein kinase, Pelle, then associates with the IL-1RI complex via a death domain (DD) on MyD88 (156,157). IRAK rapidly autophosphorylates, dissociates from the complex, and associates with TNFR-associated factor–6 (TRAF6) (158). TRAF6 activation leads to activation of IκB kinase-α (IKK-α) and IKK-β, which leads to IκB phosphorylation and its degradation within proteosomes, thus freeing bound NF-κB for nuclear translocation. Initially, this was thought to occur via NF-κB–inducing kinase (NIK), but this may not be the case. Recent data suggests that the adaptor protein ECSIT (evolutionarily conserved signaling intermediate in Toll pathways) regulates IL-1–dependent NF-κB activation, by regulating processing of MEK kinase–1 (MEKK-1) (159).

In addition, the cytoplasmic domains of IL-1RI have been reported to bind the small G-proteins, RhoA and Rac-1 (160). With the observed early GTP hydrolysis after cellular stimulation with IL-1, this suggests that induction of G-protein activity may also be involved in the cellular response to IL-1 stimulation. Small G-proteins may directly or indirectly activate MAP kinases, causing serine/threonine phosphorylation, altering their substrates' activities. During IL-1R activation, these kinases phosphorylate some transcription factors specifically, including p42/44 (Erk-1, 2), which phosphorylates c-Myc; p38 (SAPK-2, 3), which phosphorylates CHOP and Max; and p54 (SAPK-1/JNK), which phosphorylates c-Jun. Other factors, including Elk-1, can be activated by multiple MAPK pathways following IL-1 stimulation. This is also consistent with the observation that signaling by IL-1α, and IL-1β culminates in nuclear translocation of the AP-1 complex, which consists of the transcription factors c-jun and c-fos. Another possible pathway for IL-1 to effect NF-κB activation is through IL-1RI–dependent activation of phosphatidylinositol 3 kinase (PI3K), which acts at a level different than the degradation of IκB (161). While the complete molecular mechanism is not yet elucidated, evidence now suggests that a PI3K-dependent pathway may be responsible for a substantial fraction of NFκB and AP-1 activation in response to IL-1.

IL-18R and Toll-like receptor family members share many of the same signaling intermediates as IL-1R, as would be expected given their high degree of homology. As mentioned previously, IL-18R shares IL-1Racp with IL-1RI. Additionally MyD88,

IRAK, and TRAF6 signaling intermediates are activated in response to IL-18R and TLR activation. Although much investigation is still required, the body of evidence from overexpression systems and knockout models indicates important roles for MyD88, IRAK, and TRAF6 in IL-18R and TLR signaling (162–166). Also, as with IL-1R, activation of MAP kinase signaling cascades may play a role as well.

The use of common signaling pathways by IL-1R–related proteins allows redundancy in the immune response. In this regard, IL-1RI–deficient mice were unresponsive to stimulation by IL-1, but had no overtly deleterious phenotype (167). Similarly, IRAK-deficient mice appear to develop DTH normally, and were able to clear Listeria monocytogenes, a process requiring normal phagocytic function and responsiveness to IFNγ, although cellular responsiveness to IL-1β and IL-18 stimulation was muted (164,165).

However, some signaling intermediates for the IL-1R–related family of receptors undoubtedly serve nonredundant functions. MyD88-deficient mice had T lymphocytes that were defective in proliferative response and cytokine production in response to IL-1, with a defective Th1 response as well (162). IL-18 was not effective in inducing IFNγ production and NK activation in these mice. In addition, TRAF6-deficient mice had decreased survival *in utero* (163). Of those born, few survived as much as 2 weeks. As one would predict, the cells from these mice were unable to transmit signals from IL-1, CD40, and LPS. Their phenotype was grossly abnormal, as animals exhibited splenomegaly, osteopetrosis, and defective bone remodeling and tooth eruption. Taken together these knockout mouse models highlight the importance of the IL-1R/Toll-like signaling cascade in promoting both innate and acquired immunity.

The IL-1R/TLR family is essential for functions in both the innate and acquired immune responses. It is clear that while the receptors in this family share common signaling intermediates, they serve to facilitate a variety of functions. The challenge for future research will be to determine the basis of this specificity. Undoubtedly these signaling intermediates are excellent targets for the development of novel antiinflammatory drugs.

RECEPTOR TYROSINE KINASES

Classic growth factors like epidermal growth factor (EGF), platelet-derived growth factor (PDGF), nerve growth factor (NGF), and insulin bind and activate surface receptors, which have intrinsic tyrosine kinase activity; thus they are termed receptor tyrosine kinases (RTKs) (168,169). This contrasts with type I and II cytokine receptors that lack kinase activity but instead associate with Jaks. Factors that bind the RTK class of receptors and are often discussed in the context of cytokines include CSF-1 (colony-stimulating factor–1), stem cell factor (SCF, c-kit ligand or steel factor), and Flt3 ligand (fms-like tyrosine kinase 3 ligand) (170). The receptors for CSF-1, SCF, and Flt3 ligand belong to the same subfamily of RTKs as the PDGF receptor. Some of these receptors were discovered as viral oncogenes (v-fms and v-kit for the CSF-1R and SCFR, respectively) (171–173). The receptors in this subfamily typically have 5 immunoglobulin-like loops involved in ligand binding in their extracellular domains. The cytoplasmic domain contains a tyrosine kinase catalytic domain interrupted by an "insert region" that is not homologous to other tyrosine kinases. This segment is used to recruit various signaling molecules (168).

The first step in signaling by the RTKs is ligand-induced receptor dimerization (Color Fig. 12.5). In the case of the PDGFR, the ligand itself is a dimer; thus, it is easy to envision how ligand binding can effect receptor dimerization. Receptor dimerization brings the two intrinsic kinase domains into proximity with one another. Typically, this results in transphosphorylation of tyrosine residues in the so-called activation loop of the kinase domain, which results in increased phosphotransferase activity. The increased catalytic activity results in autophosphorylation of the receptor subunits on tyrosine residues. These phosphorylated tyrosine residues are then bound by a variety of signaling molecules that initiate signal transduction (174). During this important step, the signaling and adapter molecules recognize phosphotyrosine residues on the RTKs by virtue of their SH2 (src homology 2) domains or phosphotyrosine binding (PTB) domains (175).

A major pathway activated by RTKs is the Ras/Raf/ERK pathway. CSF-1R and SCFR for instance, have been documented to activate this pathway (176–178). Ras, is a small G-protein with intrinsic low GDP/GTP exchange activity. Guanine nucleotide exchange factors (GEFs) promote formation of the active GTP-bound Ras, while GTPase activating proteins (GAPs) promote formation of the inactive GDP-bound Ras (179). For the RTKs, two adapter proteins, Grb2 and Shc, have important functions in Ras activation. For some receptors, Grb2 binds directly to phosphotyrosine residues on the cytoplasmic tail of the receptor via its SH2 domain. In the CSF-1R, for example, Y697 is essential for Grb2 recruitment (180). For other receptors, Shc can bind first and then recruit Grb2. In addition to an SH2 domain, Grb2 has two SH3 domains that are stably associated with a proline-rich segment of the GEF, son of sevenless protein (SOS). The adapter Grb2 thereby recruits SOS to the membrane, allowing it to activate Ras (179–182). Active Ras binds the serine/threonine kinase Raf, activating the latter. Activated Raf in turn phosphorylates a dual specificity kinase, MEK, which phosphorylates and activates ERK (extracellular-signal regulated kinase) (179,183,184). RTKs-dependent ERK activation appears to be regulated also by SH2-containing tyrosine phosphatase-2 (SHP-2) (185). In hematopoietic cells, a major SHP-2-binding protein is the adapter protein Grb-2–associated binder–2 (Gab2). Gab2 binds SHP-2 and Shc in response to stimulation with several growth factors, including CSF-1, and it is constitutively associated with Grb2 (186). The SHP-2–related phosphatase SHP-1 is tyrosine phosphorylated in response to CSF-1 but it may have both negative and positive effects on cytokine signaling (187,188). Activated ERK translocates to the nucleus where it phosphorylates and modulates the activity of various transcription factors, including Elk-1 (189). By regulating the transcription of several genes, the Ras/Raf/ERK pathway controls cellular differentiation and proliferation. Accordingly, mutations of Ras, leading to the constitutive activation of the ERK pathway, have been found in a wide variety of human cancers (190).

Another important pathway activated by RTKs is the phosphoinositide 3-kinase (PI3K) pathway (190). Y721 of the CSF-1R, for example, is important for recruiting PI3K (191). PI3K catalyzes the formation of phosphatidylinositol-3,4,5-trisphosphate [PtdIns(3,4,5)P3] and PtdIns(3,4)P2 (192). These phospholipids are recognized by proteins with pleckstrin homology (PH) domains. One such protein is protein kinase B (PKB or Akt). Akt activity is also regulated by another protein, 3-phosphoinositide-dependent protein kinase-1 (PDK1), which also has a PH domain (193). PDK1 also activates another important kinase, p70 S6 kinase (194). The PI3K pathway appears to be critical for protecting cells from apoptosis. Recently, it has been shown that activated Akt phosphorylates BAD, which functions as an antiapoptotic protein, promoting cell survival (195,196). Another mechanism by which the PI3K/Akt pathway appears to regulate apoptosis is by phosphorylating and thereby inhibiting members of the Forkhead family of transcription factors. These proteins trigger apoptosis by enhancing the transcription of the Fas ligand gene (197–201). It has been demonstrated that one of the Akt-phosphorylated Forkhead transcription factors is inhibited, because it is sequestered in the cytoplasm by anchoring to 14-3-3 proteins (197). Since BAD also has been shown to interact with 14-3-3 proteins (202), 14-3-3 may serve as a chaperone for Akt substrates. Akt can also regulate cell survival by both inhibiting the activity of the cell-death protease caspase-9 and by promoting the degradation of IκB and increasing the activity of NF-κB, thus leading to the transcription of antiapoptotic genes (203–205).

The PI3K pathway is inhibited by the lipid phosphatase PTEN (phosphatase and tensin homolog deleted on chromosome ten), which dephosphorylates PI3K-generated phosphatidylinositides (206). Cells with deletion or inactivation of PTEN show elevated levels of 3′-phosphorylated phospholipids, constitutive Akt activation and resistance to multiple proapoptotic signals. Accordingly, deletions of PTEN have been found in numerous tumor types, demonstrating a role for this protein as tumor suppressor (193,206). Another phosphatase that regulates RTK -initiated signaling pathways is the SH2-containing inositol phosphatase, SHIP. It associates with Shc in response to several growth factors like CSF-1, thereby modulating both Ras and inositol signaling pathways (207,208).

In addition, a large number of other molecules are activated in response to ligand binding to RTKs. These include Src family kinases, the proto-oncogene Vav, and Cbl (209–211). Some data also indicate that signals originated from the RTKs can activate the Jak/Stat pathway (212–215). However, at the moment, the only evidence supporting a nonredundant and obligatory role of the Jaks or the Stats in RTKs-originated signaling pathways comes from the analysis of the Stat1 –/– mice. Using this system it has, in fact, been shown that Stat1 is required to guarantee a homeostatic control of the growth of chondrocytes upon stimulation of the RTK for the fibroblast growth factor (FGF) (216).

In conclusion, therefore, it is now generally appreciated that RTKs activate multiple different signaling pathways, which regulate several cellular functions including development, differentiation, proliferation and apoptosis. The mechanism for recruitment of signaling molecules is direct, as the receptor itself is a kinase.

TGF-β AND OTHER RECEPTOR SERINE/THREONINE KINASES

The transforming growth factor–beta (TGF-β) family comprises a large number of structurally related polypeptide growth factors involved in numerous processes including cell growth and cell fate determination, as well as immunoregulation. Mutations of the elements in this pathway also contribute to malignant transformation. The mammalian ligands that belong to this family include the following: TGF-β1, -β2, and -β3, bone morphogenic proteins, activins and cartilage-derived morphogenic proteins (217–219). The monomeric forms of these ligands contain intrachain disulfide bonds that result in a structure termed a cystine knot. The bioactive forms of the factors are typically dimers held together by both hydrophobic interactions and intersubunit disulfide bonds. For the purposes of this chapter, we will focus only on signaling by TGF-βs (Color Fig. 12.6) (220).

TGF-β Family Receptors Are Transmembrane Serine Kinases

Like receptor tyrosine kinases (RTKs), the receptors of the TGF-β family encode kinase domains. In contrast, however, the latter family encodes serine/threonine kinases (217,219). The extracellular domains of these molecules are relatively small, but rich in cysteine residues (10 or more). They have a single transmembrane domain and an intracellular kinase domain. There are substantial differences in how these receptors signal compared to RTKs.

First, this family of receptors is subdivided into type I and type II receptors, which participate in signaling in rather distinct ways. For TGF-β receptors, the ligand binds to the type II receptor, allowing the recruitment of the type I receptor. The receptor subunits have some affinity for one another, and the complex of the receptor subunits bound to ligand is rather stable.

Secondly, the type II receptor is thought to be a constitutively active kinase. Upon ligand binding, the type II receptor phosphorylates the type I receptor. The type I receptor is structurally distinct from the type II receptor, having a juxtamembrane domain that precedes the kinase domain, referred to as the GS domain. It is this site that is phosphorylated by the type II receptor. The type I receptor, in turn, is responsible for phosphorylating key signaling intermediates. It is not clear however whether the activation of the type I receptor is due to enhancement of its kinase activity, the appearance of substrate binding sites, or a combination of the two mechanisms.

Smads-Latent Cytosolic Transcription Factors Phosphorylated By Type I Receptors

The next important intermediates in TGF-β signaling are the Smads (217,219,221). The genes encoding these proteins were first isolated from *Drosophila* and *C. elegans* (222). Based on the phenotype of mutant flies, the genes were termed Mad (mothers against decapentaplegic). The *C. elegans* genes were termed Sma genes because of the small size of the mutant worms. The vertebrate homologs were subsequently termed Smads; there are eight known mammalian Smads. These proteins do not contain any previously known structural or enzymatic motifs. However, they have two homology domains termed the MH1 and MH2 domains at the N- and C-termini, respectively, which are separated by a central linker domain. The extreme C-terminus of some Smads is a critical site of phosphorylation.

Smads are subdivided into three classes. The receptor-regulated Smads (R-Smads) directly interact with, and are phosphorylated by the type I receptor. These include Smad1, -2, -3, -5, and -8, with Smad2 and Smad3 being phosphorylated in response to TGF-β. R-Smads bind to the GS domain of type I receptors. The interaction of R-Smads with TGF-β receptors may also be regulated by another molecule termed SARA (Smad anchor for receptor activation). SARA binds unphosphorylated Smad2 and Smad3. By virtue of its FYVE domain, it may bind phospholipids and localize Smads to the plasma membrane, facilitating receptor binding.

Next, R-Smads are phosphorylated on C-terminal serine residues triggering homodimerization of R-Smads or heterodimerization with another class of Smads, the common Smad or C-Smad (223). Smad4 is the only known C-Smad in vertebrates; it is thought to function as the central and essential downstream mediator of other Smads. The Smad MH2 domain is important for both receptor interaction and Smad dimerization. Phosphorylation of Smads also permits dissociation from SARA (221).

The third subfamily of Smads is the inhibitory Smads or I-Smads. In mammals, Smad6 and Smad7 are the I-Smads (224,225). Smad7 is induced by TGF-β and binds to TGF-β receptors inhibiting the phosphorylation of R-Smads. Thus, it serves as a classic feedback inhibitor. Smad6 works slightly differently. It competes with Smad4 for binding to an R-Smad.

Consistent with their key functions in development, gene targeting of most Smad molecules produces rather severe phenotypes (226). Smad2 knockout mice lack anterior/posterior specification and fail to develop mesoderm. Smad3 knockout mice have limb malformations, defective immune function and develop colon carcinomas at 4-6 months (227,228). Smad3 –/– also showed defective TGF-β responses. However, these mice also displayed accelerated wound healing compared to normal mice, which seems to contradict its role as a positive regulator of TGF-β role in enhancing wound healing (229). Smad4 knockout mice have growth retardation and gastrulation defects. Notably, Smad4 (also known as DPC4 or deleted in pancreatic carcinoma locus 4) is deleted in half of all human pancreatic carcinomas. In addition, mutations of Smad4 are found in other cancers and mutations of TGF-β receptors are found in both sporadic and inherited gastrointestinal cancers. Smad6 knockout mice have cardiovascular defects (230).

Smads and Gene Regulation

Once phosphorylated, R-Smads dissociate from the receptor, bind Smad4 in the cytoplasm, translocate to the nucleus, and regulate gene expression. Nuclear translocation of R-Smads may not require Smad4, but the reverse is not the case; Smad4 requires binding to an R-Smad to permit nuclear transit. A Smad DNA binding element (SBE) has been described (AGAC) and, as one would predict, TGF-β target genes may have multiple SBEs. The Smad MH1 domain is the DNA binding domain, whereas the MH2 domain is the transcriptional activation domain. Smads are regulated by the ubiquitin-proteasome pathway, and this may be an important means by which TGF-β signaling is terminated.

Smads also interact with a variety of other transcription factors. For instance, FAST-1 (forkhead activin signal transducer), a winged helix forkhead transcription factor, associates with the Smad2/Smad4 complex (231–233). It is a nuclear protein, so it likely binds to the Smad complex after nuclear translocation. The ternary complex of FAST/Smad2/Smad4 strongly activates transcription. Smads also bind to c-Jun/c-Fos, and AP-1 sites can overlap with SBE sites. Smads can also bind ATF2, the vitamin D receptor and other transcription factors and can recruit the coactivators Creb binding protein/p300. The Ski and SnoN corepressors can interact with Smads and antagonize TGF-β signaling (234,235).

Other TGF-β–Activated Pathways

The kinase TGF-β–associated kinase–1 (TAK1), a member of the mitogen-activated protein kinase family, also appears to be involved in TGF-β signaling. It is activated in response to ligand binding (236). TAK1 coimmunoprecipitates with another molecule, Tak-1 binding protein (TAB1), which activates TAK1 kinase activity (237). Together they activate the MAPK pathways, leading to activation of p38/SAPK2 and c-Jun N-terminal kinase (JNK); this may occur via MKK6 and MKK4, respectively (238,239). The activation of JNK in response to TGF-β is rather slow and it may not be directly involved in TGF-β signaling. Overexpression of TAK1 has also been reported to activate NF-κB (240).

In summary, there are features of TGF-β receptor–mediated signaling that are reminiscent of other receptors discussed in this chapter. Like receptor tyrosine kinases, they are themselves kinases, but the TGF-β family members are serine/threonine kinases, not tyrosine kinases. In an analogous fashion to type I and II cytokine receptors that recruit Stat family transcription factors, TGF-β family receptors recruit and phosphorylate latent, cytosolic transcription factors known as Smads. Phosphorylated Smads dissociate from the receptor, homo- and heterodimerize, and translocate to the nucleus where they regulate gene expression in conjunction with other transcription factors. Thus, the TGF-β signal transduction pathway is a rapid and direct means to convey signals from the membrane to the nucleus. Not surprisingly, this pathway is conserved throughout evolution. It is important for development and regulation of many cell types whereas dysregulation of the pathway contributes to the pathogenesis of cancer.

CHEMOKINE RECEPTORS

The interaction of chemokines with their receptors represents a critical step in the inflammatory process, regulating both activation and migration of leukocytes during the immune response. Several recent reviews detail the significant advances that have been made in this field recently, particularly with regard to their roles in trafficking of specific leukocyte subsets and their essential role in the pathogenesis of HIV infection (241–243). For the purposes of this chapter, we will simply describe the general mechanism for chemokine receptor function and highlight several of these receptors whose functions have been defined (Color Fig. 12.7).

Chemokines are small proteins, of approximately 70 to 100 amino acids, which have been classified on the basis of conserved cysteine residues into the following 4 subclasses: C, CC, CXC, and CX3C. CC, CXC, and CX3C chemokines have 4 conserved cysteines, the first two of which adjacent (CC) or separated by one (CXC) or three (CX3C) intervening amino acid residues. The one known C chemokine, lymphotactin, has only the first and third conserved cysteine residues. Chemokine receptors have seven hydrophobic membrane spanning domains and are G protein–coupled receptors; that is, they are members of the receptor superfamily that includes β-adrenergic receptors, odorant receptors, histamine receptors, dopamine receptors, the fMLP receptor, and the C5a receptor. In general, receptors for chemokines may have more than one chemokine ligand, but subclass specificity is maintained.

IL-8 is one of the better-characterized chemokines in this family and is especially important in homing of neutrophils to sites of inflammation (242). It binds two distinct receptors, CXCR1 and CXCR2, which share 78% amino acid identity. While only IL-8 binds CXCR1 with high affinity, CXCR2 binds multiple CXC chemokines with high affinity; this specificity has been shown to be determined by the NH2-terminal domain through studies with chimerae. At present we are limited in our ability to ascertain the specific biological roles of each of the IL-8 receptors in humans, since there are no murine homologues to IL-8 or CXCR1.

Like other heptahelical receptors, chemokine receptors are G-protein coupled receptors (GPCR). That is, the receptors couple to trimeric guanine nucleotide binding proteins. G-proteins can activate or inhibit adenylate cyclase and thus regulate cyclic AMP (cAMP). cAMP binds to the regulatory subunit of kinase A, activating it. Kinase A has a variety of substrates, an important one being the transcription factor, CREBP. More relevant to chemokine receptor signaling, though, is that some GPCR can also activate phospholipase C. Phospholipase C acts to hydrolyze membrane phospholipids into diacylglycerol and inositol triphosphate, second messengers that active protein kinase C and promote intracellular calcium flux via IP3 receptors, respectively. The G protein Gi2α is thought to be essential for the IL-8 signal cascade, ultimately leading to protein kinase C activation, release of intracellular calcium stores, and chemotaxis and activation of neutrophils.

Chemokine receptors have recently attracted scientific attention due to their role in the pathogenesis in certain infectious diseases, including HIV (241). Two chemokine receptors, CXCR4 and CCR5, have been shown to be coreceptors for T cell line-tropic and macrophage cell line–tropic HIV strains, respectively. Also, studies with knockout mice are beginning to elucidate the roles of other chemokine/chemokine receptor interactions in orchestrating immune responses (243). For example, CXCR5 has an essential role in homing B cells to splenic B cell follicles, and CCR7 is needed for normal migration of mature DC to lymph nodes. The importance of chemokine receptors in normal immune function, as well as disease pathogenesis is becoming increasingly clear with time. Whether therapeutic targeting of chemokine signal transduction pathways is possible is yet to be determined.

CONCLUSION

Numerous essential processes that occur in humans require the production and recognition of soluble cytokines and growth factors. Understanding the cellular machinery underlying these processes allows us to classify these factors on the basis of the intracellular signal transduction pathways that they utilize. In this manner, we can identify not only their evolutionary origins, but can predict, for example, why particular cytokines have specific functions or share functions with other cytokines. As this knowledge base grows, it will be especially useful in designing therapeutic strategies that target the cytokine signaling network in a specific manner.

REFERENCES

1. Vilček J. *The cytokines: an overview*. In: Thompson A, ed. San Diego: Academic Press, 1998:1.
2. Davies DR, Wlodawer A. Cytokines and their receptor complexes. *FASEB J* 1995;9:50.
3. Leonard WJ. Type I cytokines and interferons and their receptors. In: Paul WE, ed. *Fundamental immunology*, 4th ed. New York: Lippincott-Raven, 1999, 741–774.
4. Leonard WJ, O'Shea JJ. Jaks and STATs: biological implications. *Annu Rev Immunol* 1998;16:293.
5. Ihle JN, Witthuhn BA, Quelle FW, et al. Signaling through the hematopoietic cytokine receptors. *Annu Rev Immunol* 1995;13:369.
6. Ihle JN. Cytokine receptor signalling. *Nature* 1995;377:591.
7. Muller M, Briscoe J, Laxton C, et al. The protein tyrosine kinase JAK1 complements defects in interferon-alpha/beta and -gamma signal transduction. *Nature* 1993;366:129.
8. Watling D, Guschin D, Muller M, et al. Complementation by the protein tyrosine kinase JAK2 of a mutant cell line defective in the interferon-gamma signal transduction pathway. *Nature* 1993;366:166.
9. Velazquez L, Fellous M, Stark GR, et al. A protein tyrosine kinase in the interferon alpha/beta signaling pathway. *Cell* 1992;70:313.
10. Macchi P, Villa A, Gillani S, et al. Mutations of Jak-3 gene in patients with autosomal severe combined immune deficiency (SCID). *Nature* 1995;377:65.
11. Russell SM, Tayebi N, Nakajima H, et al. Mutation of Jak3 in a patient with SCID: essential role of Jak3 in lymphoid development. *Science* 1995;270:797.
12. Nosaka T, van Deursen JM, Tripp RA, et al. Defective lymphoid development in mice lacking Jak3. *Science* 1995;270:800.
13. Thomis DC, Gurniak CB, Tivol E, et al. Defects in B lymphocyte maturation and T lymphocyte activation in mice lacking Jak3. *Science* 1995;270:794.
14. Park SY, Saijo K, Takahashi T, et al. Developmental defects of lymphoid cells in Jak3 kinase-deficient mice. *Immunity* 1995;3:771.
15. Puel A, Ziegler SF, Buckley RH, et al. Defective IL7R expression in T(–)B(+)NK(+) severe combined immunodeficiency. *Nat Genet* 1998;20:394.
16. Lodolce JP, Boone DL, Chai S, et al. IL-15 receptor maintains lymphoid homeostasis by supporting lymphocyte homing and proliferation. *Immunity* 1998;9:669.
17. Kennedy MK, Glaccum M, Brown SN, et al. Reversible defects in natural killer and memory CD8 T cell lineages in interleukin 15-deficient mice. *J Exp Med* 2000;191:771.
18. Candotti F, Oakes SA, Johnston JA, et al. Structural and functional basis for JAK3-deficient severe combined immunodeficiency. *Blood* 1997;90:3996.
19. Willerford DM, Chen J, Ferry JA, et al. Interleukin-2 receptor alpha chain regulates the size and content of the peripheral lymphoid compartment. *Immunity* 1995;3:521.
20. Sadlack B, Merz H, Schorle H, et al. Ulcerative colitis–like disease in mice with a disrupted interleukin-2 gene. *Cell* 1993;75:253.
21. Suzuki H, Kundig TM, Furlonger C, et al. Deregulated T cell activation and autoimmunity in mice lacking interleukin-2 receptor beta. *Science* 1995;268:1472.

22. Rodig SJ, Meraz MA, White JM, et al. Disruption of the Jak1 gene demonstrates obligatory and nonredundant roles of the Jaks in cytokine-induced biologic responses. *Cell* 1998;93:373.
23. Neubauer H, Cumano A, Muller M, et al. Jak2 deficiency defines an essential developmental checkpoint in definitive hematopoiesis. *Cell* 1998;93:397.
24. Parganas E, Wang D, Stravopodis D, et al. Jak2 is essential for signaling through a variety of cytokine receptors. *Cell* 1998;93:385.
25. Peeters P, Raynaud SD, Cools J, et al. Fusion of TEL, the ETS-variant gene 6 (ETV6), to the receptor-associated kinase JAK2 as a result of t(9;12) in a lymphoid and t(9;15;12) in a myeloid leukemia. *Blood* 1997;90: 2535.
26. Lacronique V, Boureux A, Valle VD, et al. A TEL-JAK2 fusion protein with constitutive kinase activity in human leukemia. *Science* 1997;278:1309.
27. Ho JM, Beattie BK, Squire JA, et al. Fusion of the ets transcription factor TEL to Jak2 results in constitutive Jak-Stat signaling. *Blood* 1999;93:4354.
28. Chen M, Cheng A, Candotti F, et al. Complex effects of naturally occurring mutations in the JAK3 pseudokinase domains: evidence for interactions between the kinase and pseudokinase domains. *Mol Cell Biol* 2000;20: 947.
29. Chen M, Cheng A, Chen YQ, et al. The amino terminus of JAK3 is necessary and sufficient for binding to the common gamma chain and confers the ability to transmit interleukin 2–mediated signals. *Proc Natl Acad Sci USA* 1997;94:6910.
30. Cacalano NA, Migone TS, Bazan F, et al. Autosomal SCID caused by a point mutation in the N-terminus of Jak3: mapping of the Jak3-receptor interaction domain. *EMBO J* 1999;18:1549.
31. Yan H, Piazza F, Krishnan K, et al. Definition of the interferon-alpha receptor-binding domain on the TYK2 kinase. *J Biol Chem* 1998;273:4046.
32. Richter MF, Dumenil G, Uze G, et al. Specific contribution of tyk2 JH regions to the binding and the expression of the interferon alpha/beta receptor component IFNAR1. *J Biol Chem* 1998;273:24723.
33. Darnell JEJ, Kerr IM, Stark GR. Jak-STAT pathways and transcriptional activation in response to IFNs and other extracellular signaling proteins. *Science* 1994;264:1415.
34. Schindler C, Darnell JEJ. Transcriptional responses to polypeptide ligands: the JAK-STAT pathway. *Annu Rev Biochem* 1995;64:621.
35. Hoey T, Grusby MJ. STATs as mediators of cytokine-induced responses. *Adv Immunol* 1999;71:145.
36. Chen X, Vinkemeier U, Zhao Y, et al. Crystal structure of a tyrosine phosphorylated STAT-1 dimer bound to DNA. *Cell* 1998;93:827.
37. Becker S, Groner B, Muller CW. Three-dimensional structure of the Stat3beta homodimer bound to DNA. *Nature* 1998;394:145.
38. Meraz MA, White JM, Sheehan KC, et al. Targeted disruption of the Stat1 gene in mice reveals unexpected physiologic specificity in the JAK-STAT signaling pathway. *Cell* 1996;84:431.
39. Durbin JE, Hackenmiller R, Simon MC, et al. Targeted disruption of the mouse Stat1 gene results in compromised innate immunity to viral disease. *Cell* 1996;84:443.
40. Takeda K, Noguchi K, Shi W, et al. Targeted disruption of the mouse Stat3 gene leads to early embryonic lethality. *Proc Natl Acad Sci USA* 1997;94:3801.
41. Escary JL, Perreau J, Dumenil D, et al. Leukaemia inhibitory factor is necessary for maintenance of haematopoietic stem cells and thymocyte stimulation. *Nature* 1993;363:361.
42. Takeda K, Clausen BE, Kaisho T, et al. Enhanced Th1 activity and development of chronic enterocolitis in mice devoid of Stat3 in macrophages and neutrophils. *Immunity* 1999;10:39.
43. Thierfelder WE, van Deursen JM, Yamamoto K, et al. Requirement for Stat4 in interleukin-12–mediated responses of natural killer and T cells. *Nature* 1996;382:171.
44. Kaplan MH, Sun YL, Hoey T, et al. Impaired IL-12 responses and enhanced development of Th2 cells in Stat4-deficient mice. *Nature* 1996;382:174.
45. Kaplan MH, Grusby MJ. Regulation of T helper cell differentiation by STAT molecules. *J Leukoc Biol* 1998; 64:2.
46. de Jong R, Altare F, Haagen IA, et al. Severe mycobacterial and Salmonella infections in interleukin-12 receptor–deficient patients. *Science* 1998;280:1435.
47. Altare F, Durandy A, Lammas D, et al. Impairment of mycobacterial immunity in human interleukin-12 receptor deficiency. *Science* 1998;280:1432.
48. Shimoda K, van Deursen J, Sangster MY, et al. Lack of IL-4–induced Th2 response and IgE class switching in mice with disrupted Stat6 gene. *Nature* 1996;380:630.
49. Kaplan MH, Schindler U, Smiley ST, et al. Stat6 is required for mediating responses to IL-4 and for development of Th2 cells. *Immunity* 1996;4:313.
50. Takeda K, Tanaka T, Shi W, et al. Essential role of Stat6 in IL-4 signalling. *Nature* 1996;380:627.
51. Takeda K, Kamanaka M, Tanaka T, et al. Impaired IL-13–mediated functions of macrophages in STAT6-deficient mice. *J Immunol* 1996;157:3220.
52. Liu X, Robinson GW, Wagner KU, et al. Stat5a is mandatory for adult mammary gland development and lactogenesis. *Genes Dev* 1997;11:179.
53. Udy GB, Towers RP, Snell RG, et al. Requirement of STAT5b for sexual dimorphism of body growth rates and liver gene expression. *Proc Natl Acad Sci USA*1997;94:7239.
54. Teglund S, McKay C, Schuetz E, et al. STAT5a and STAT5b proteins have essential and nonessential, or redundant, roles in cytokine responses. *Cell* 1998;93:841.

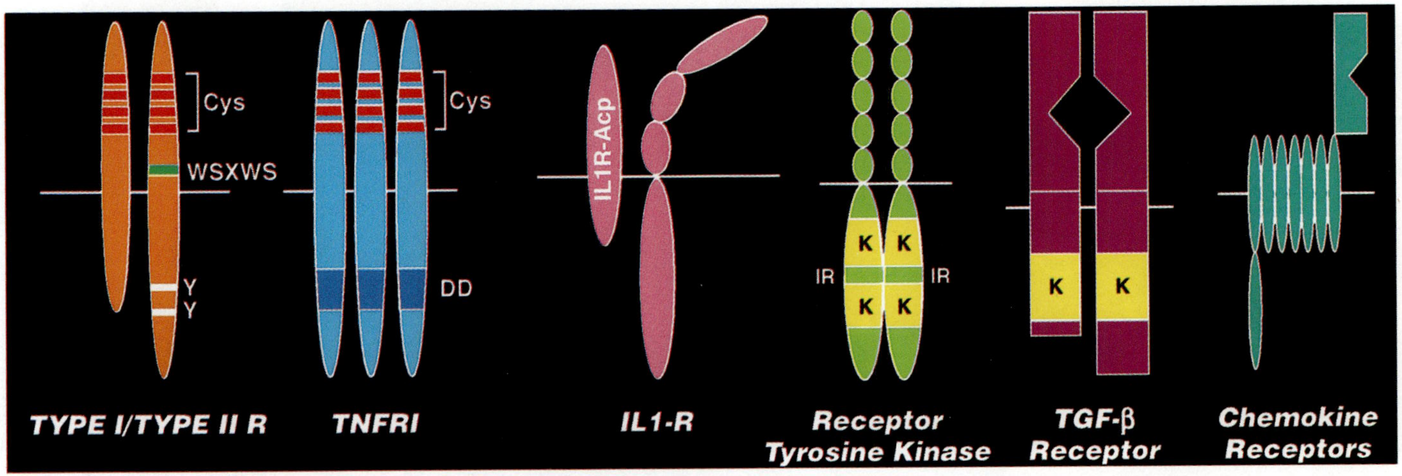

FIG. 12.1. Schematic representation of the different receptor families. Cys, cysteine-rich domain; Y, tyrosine; DD, death domain; K, kinase domain; IR, insert region.

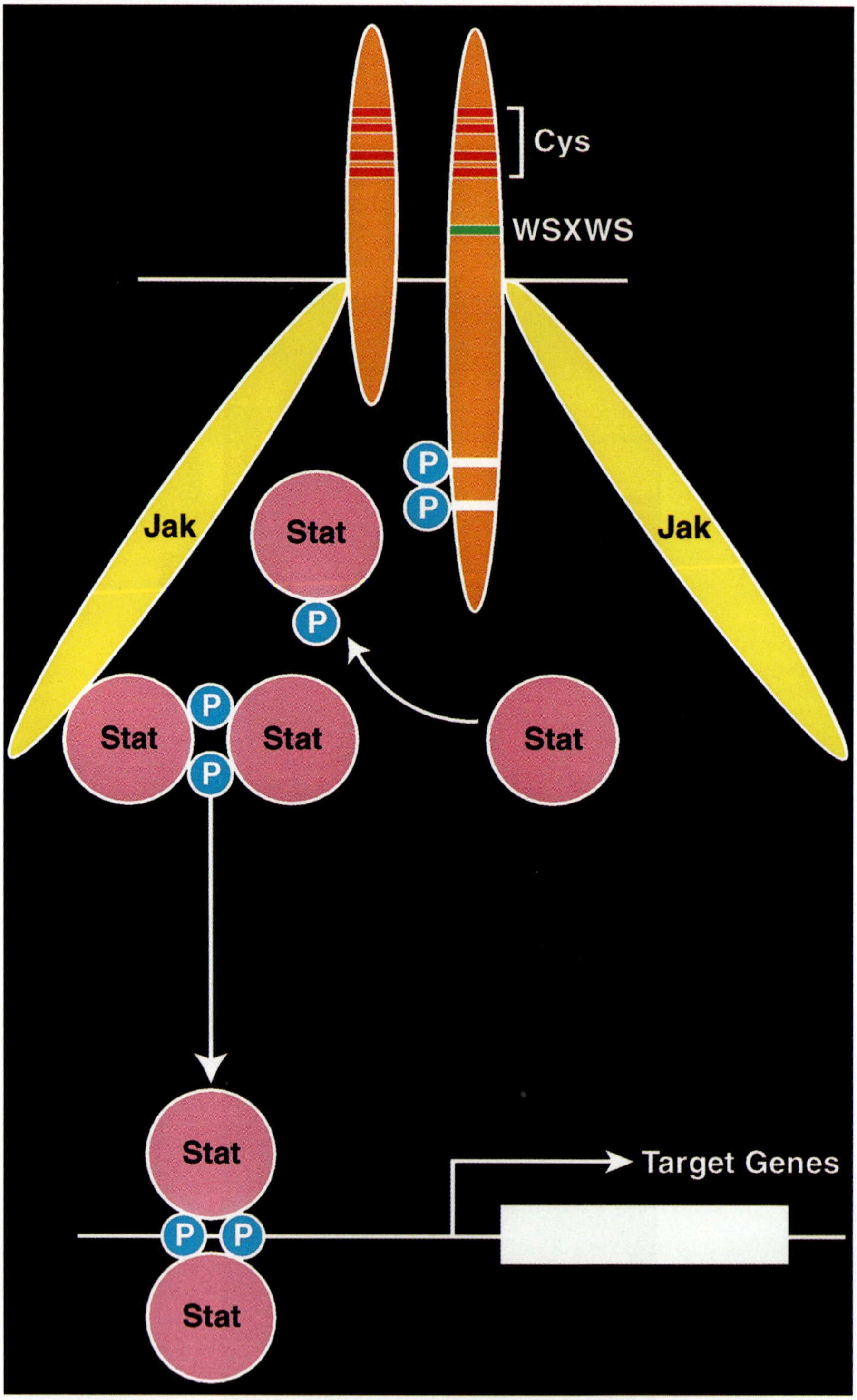

FIG. 12.2. Schematic representation of type 1 and type 2 cytokine signaling. Interaction of the receptor with its ligand causes activation of Jak kinase activity. The Jaks then phosphorylate receptor docking sites for the Stats, which are phosphorylated, leading to their dimerization and translocation to the nucleus, where they regulate gene transcription.

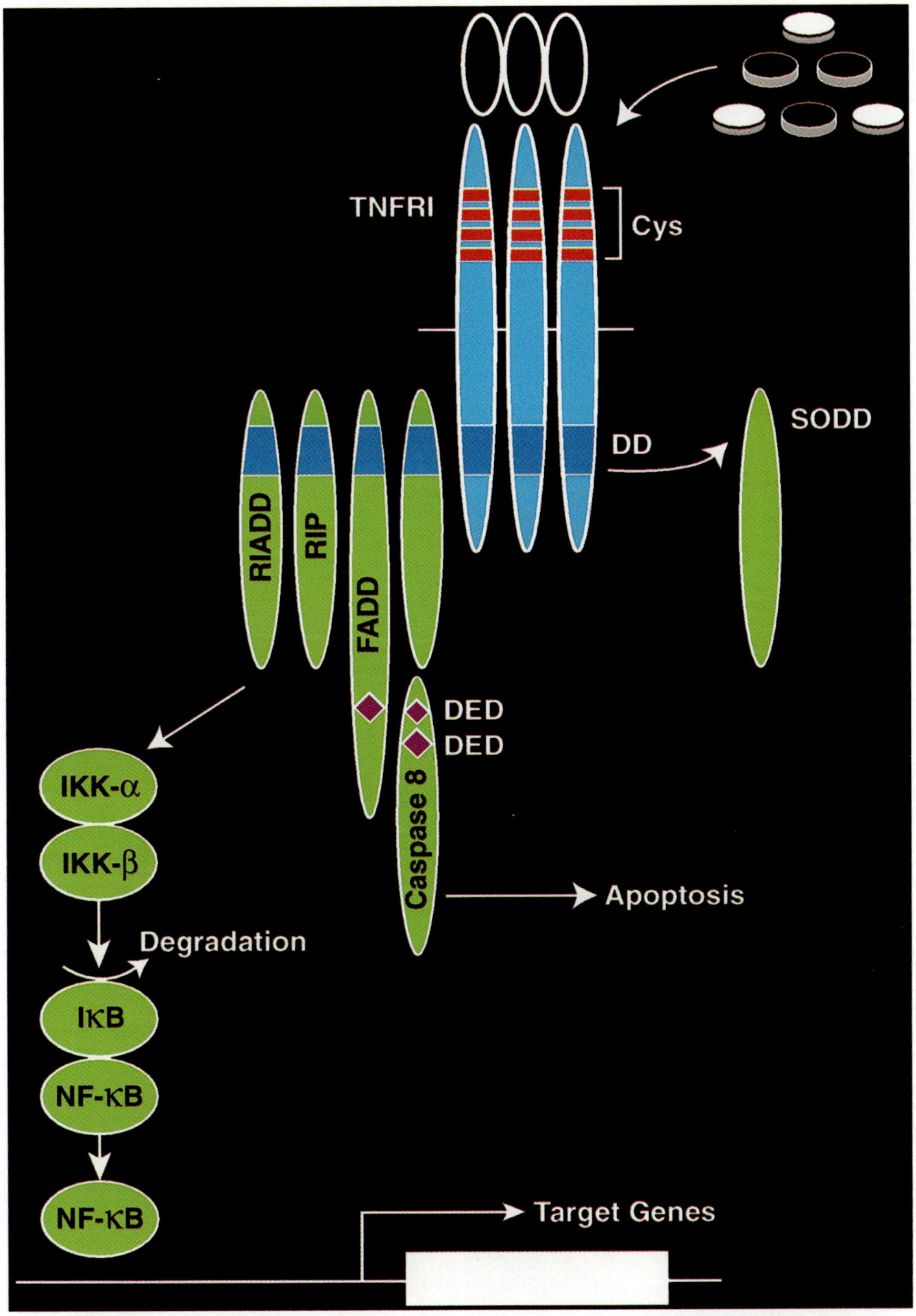

FIG. 12.3. Schematic representation of tumor necrosis factor receptor (TNFR) signaling. The TNF-α trimer binds trimeric TNFR1, dislodging SODD from its death domain (DD) association with the receptor. This allows TNFR-associated death domain protein (TRADD) to associate with the receptor via DD interaction. TRADD, in turn, can recruit Fas-associated death domain protein (FADD), receptor interacting protein (RIP), and RIP-associated Ich-1/CED3 homologous protein with death domain (RAIDD) to the complex via DD interactions, ultimately leading to NF-κB activation and to apoptosis via caspase-8.

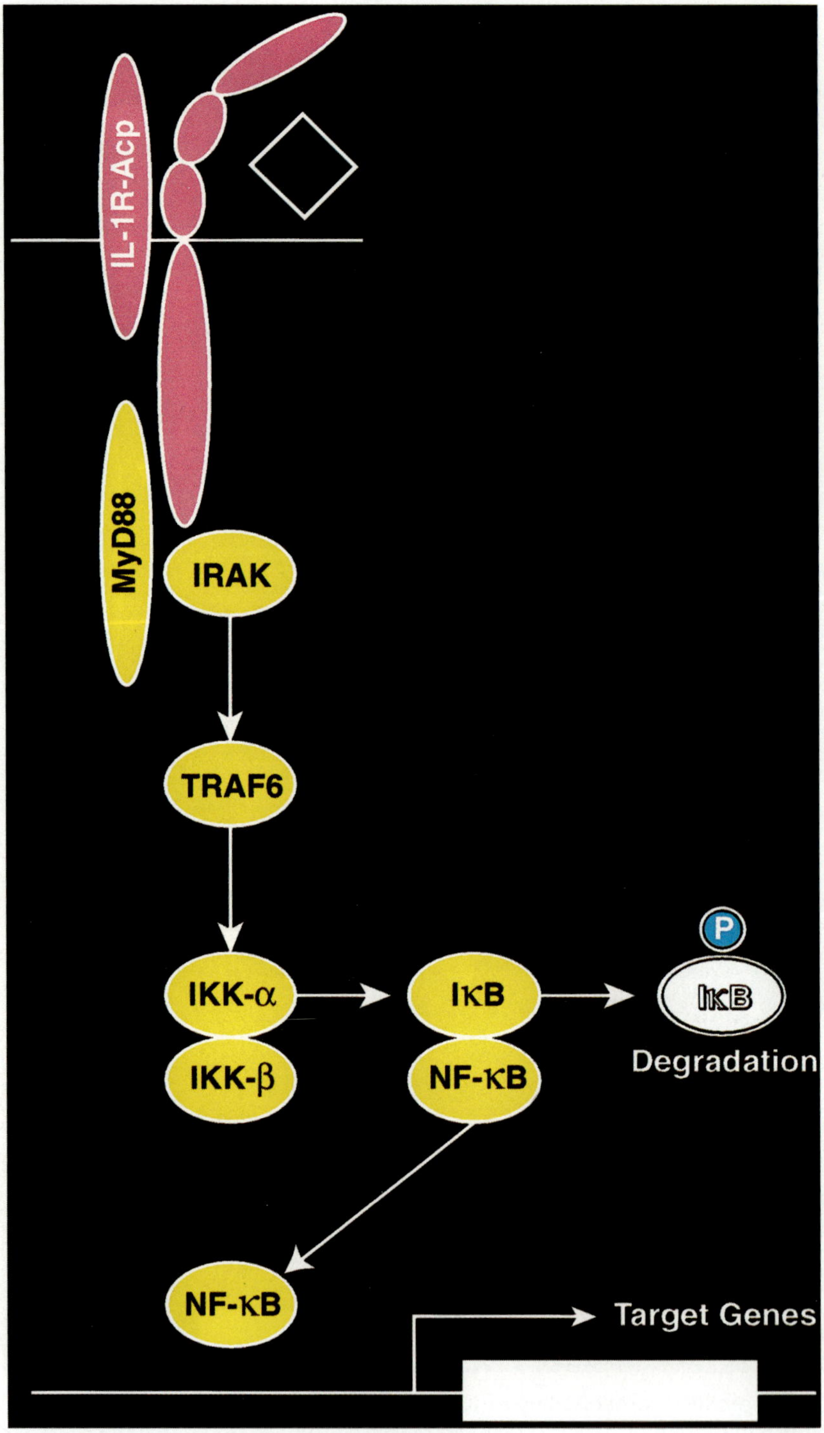

FIG. 12.4. Schematic representation of IL-1R signaling. IL-1 interaction with the IL-1R/IL-1R-Acp recruits MyD88 and IL-1 receptor–associated kinase (IRAK) to the receptor complex. IRAK then dissociates and activates TRAF6, leading to activation of NF-κB and target genes.

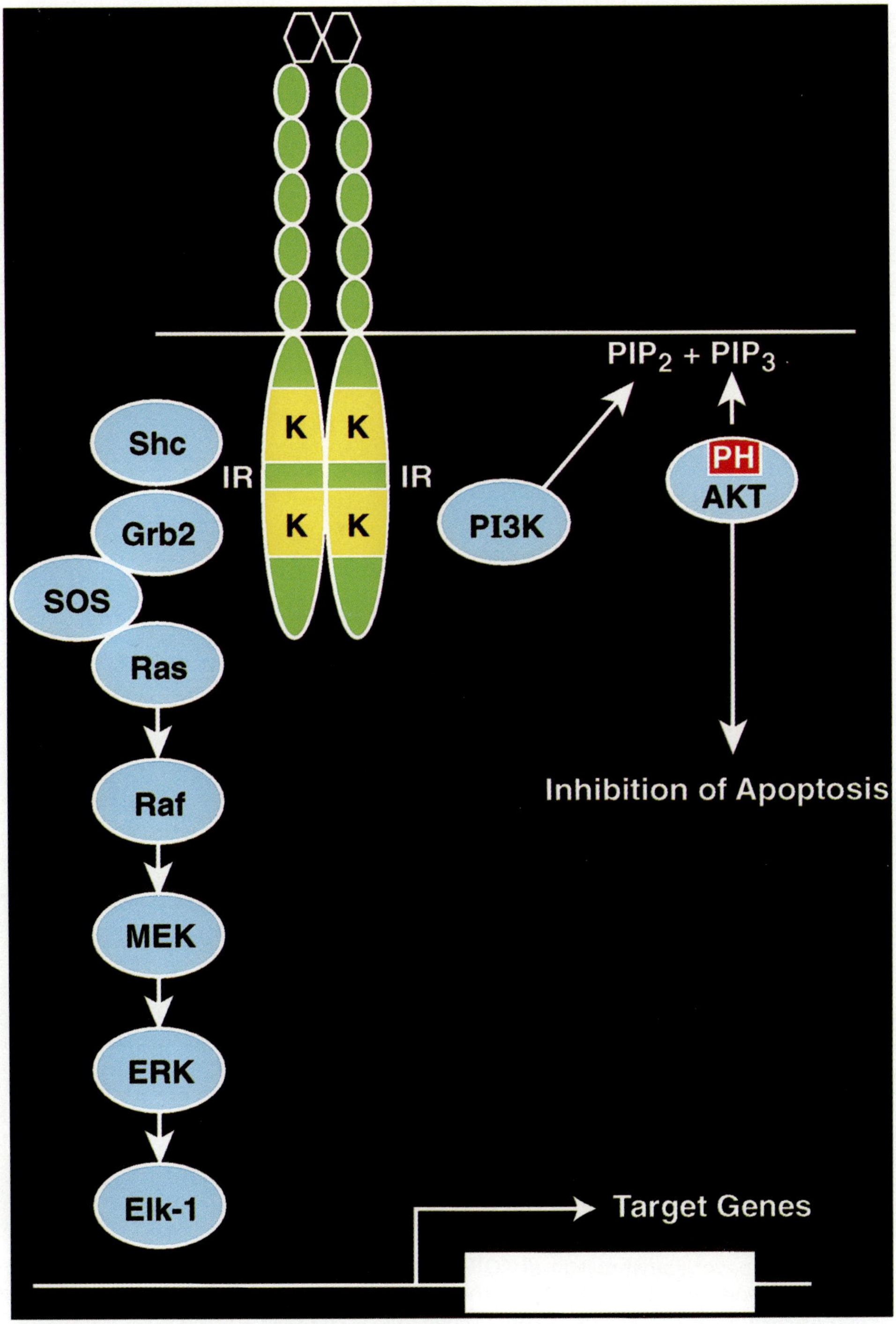

FIG. 12.5. Schematic representation of receptor tyrosine kinase (RTK) signaling. Ligand binding activates the intrinsic kinase activity, leading to phosphorylation of the receptor. This results in recruitment of Shc and Grb2/SOS/Ras. Ras activates a kinase cascade consisting of Raf/MEK/ERK, which leads to activation of transcription factors such as Elk-1 and the induction of target genes. Also, ligand binding leads to activation of PI3K and ultimately AKT, leading to inhibition of apoptosis.

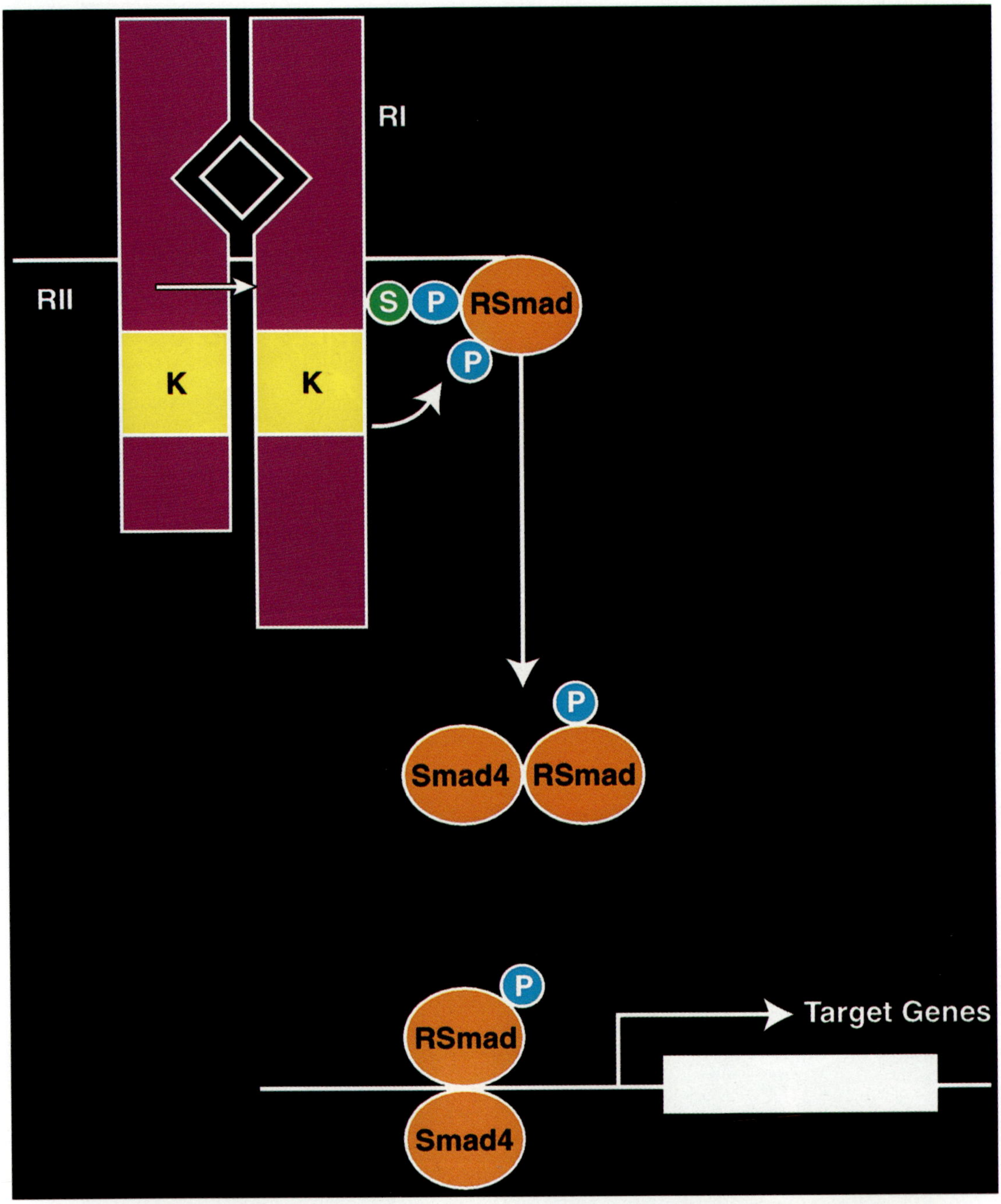

FIG. 12.6. Schematic representation of TGF-β receptor family signaling. TGF-β binds to the type II receptor, a serine/threonine kinase. This causes recruitment of the type I receptor, also a serine/threonine kinase. The type I receptor then phosphorylates and activates the type II receptor. Receptor-associated Smad transcription factors (R-Smads) bind the phosphorylated type II receptors and are themselves phosphorylated. Phosphorylated R-Smads dimerize with Smad4 and translocate to the nucleus, where they activate target genes.

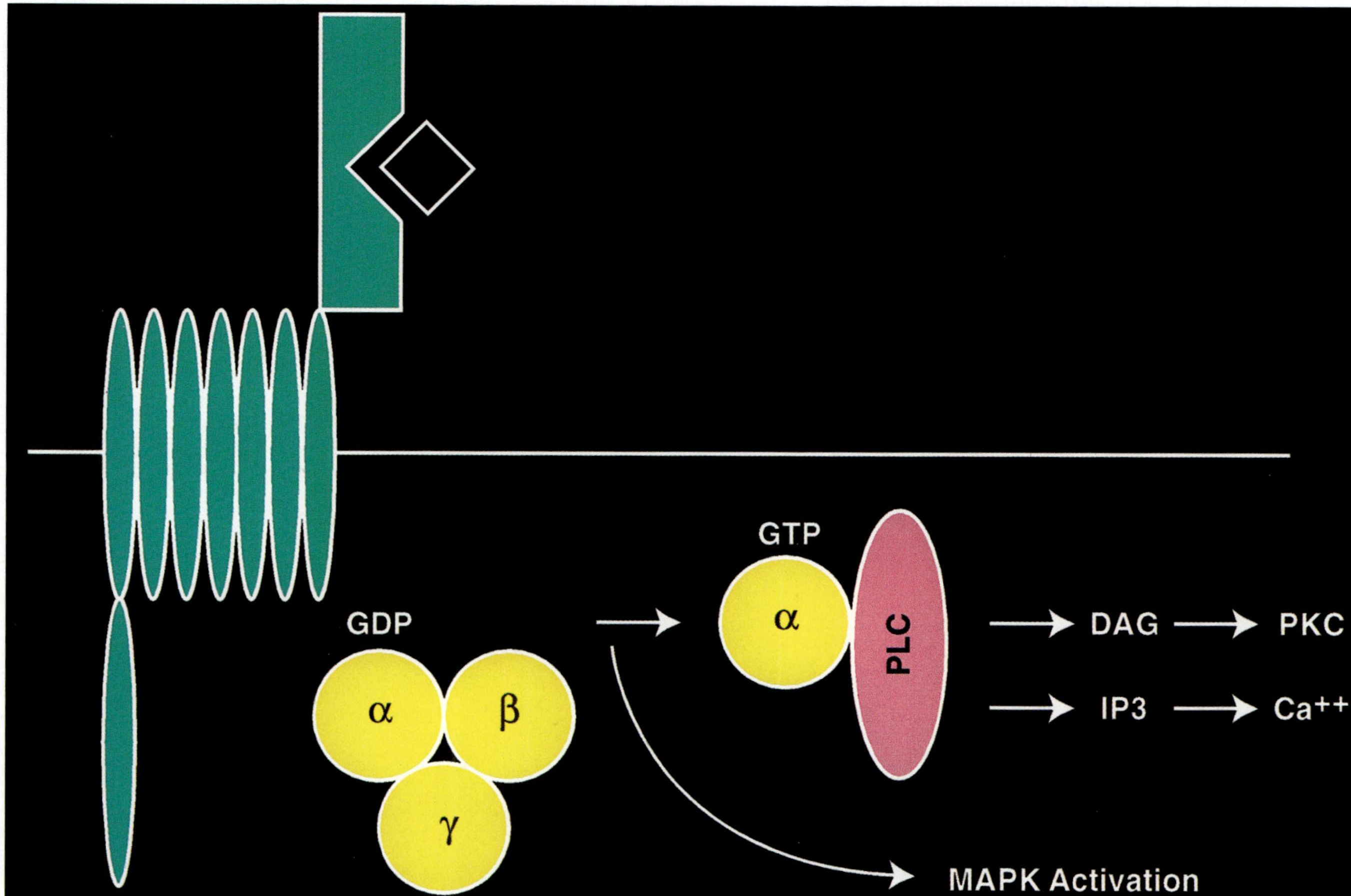

FIG. 12.7. Schematic representation of chemokine receptor activation. Ligand binding results in trimeric G-protein activation and activation of phospholipase-C (PLC). PLC leads to cellular activation by activating protein kinase C (PKC) and by releasing intracellular calcium stores via the second messenger IP3.

55. Moriggl R, Sexl V, Piekorz R, et al. Stat5 activation is uniquely associated with cytokine signaling in peripheral T cells. *Immunity* 1999;11:225.
56. Moriggl R, Topham DJ, Teglund S, et al. Stat5 is required for IL-2–induced cell cycle progression of peripheral T cells. *Immunity* 1999;10:249.
57. Starr R, Hilton DJ. Negative regulation of the JAK/STAT pathway. *Bioessays* 1999;21:47.
58. Shultz LD, Schweitzer PA, Rajan TV, et al. Mutations at the murine motheaten locus are within the hematopoietic cell protein–tyrosine phosphatase (Hcph) gene. *Cell* 1993;73:1445.
59. Bignon JS, Siminovitch KA. Identification of PTP1C mutation as the genetic defect in motheaten and viable motheaten mice: a step toward defining the roles of protein tyrosine phosphatases in the regulation of hemopoietic cell differentiation and function. *Clin Immunol Immunopathol* 1994;73:168.
60. Starr R, Willson TA, Viney EM, et al. A family of cytokine-inducible inhibitors of signalling. *Nature* 1997;387:917.
61. Starr R, Hilton DJ. SOCS: suppressors of cytokine signalling. *Int J Biochem Cell Biol* 1998;30:1081.
62. Endo TA, Masuhara M, Yokouchi M, et al. A new protein containing an SH2 domain that inhibits JAK kinases. *Nature* 1997;387:921.
63. Naka T, Narazaki M, Hirata M, et al. Structure and function of a new STAT-induced STAT inhibitor. *Nature* 1997;387:924.
64. Yasukawa H, Misawa H, Sakamoto H, et al. The JAK-binding protein JAB inhibits Janus tyrosine kinase activity through binding in the activation loop. *EMBO J* 1999;18:1309.
65. Marine JC, Topham DJ, McKay C, et al. SOCS1 deficiency causes a lymphocyte-dependent perinatal lethality. *Cell* 1999;98:609.
66. Marine JC, McKay C, Wang D, et al. SOCS3 is essential in the regulation of fetal liver erythropoiesis. *Cell* 1999;98:617.
67. Alexander WS, Starr R, Fenner JE, et al. SOCS1 is a critical inhibitor of interferon gamma signaling and prevents the potentially fatal neonatal actions of this cytokine. *Cell* 1999;98:597.
68. Chung CD, Liao J, Liu B, et al. Specific inhibition of Stat3 signal transduction by PIAS3. *Science* 1997;278:1803.
69. Dent AL, Shaffer AL, Yu X, et al. Control of inflammation, cytokine expression, and germinal center formation by BCL-6. *Science* 1997;276:589.
70. Ashkenazi A, Dixit VM. Apoptosis control by death and decoy receptors. *Curr Opin Cell Biol* 1999;11:255.
71. Itoh N, Yonehara S, Ishii A, et al. The polypeptide encoded by the cDNA for human cell surface antigen Fas can mediate apoptosis. *Cell* 1991;66:233.
72. Lynch DH, Watson ML, Alderson MR, et al. The mouse Fas-ligand gene is mutated in gld mice and is part of a TNF family gene cluster. *Immunity* 1994;1:131.
73. Watanabe-Fukunaga R, Brannan CI, Copeland NG, et al. Lymphoproliferation disorder in mice explained by defects in Fas antigen that mediates apoptosis. *Nature* 1992;356:314.
74. Fisher GH, Rosenberg FJ, Straus SE, et al. Dominant interfering Fas gene mutations impair apoptosis in a human autoimmune lymphoproliferative syndrome. *Cell* 1995;81:935.
75. Rieux-Laucat F, Le Deist F, Hivroz C, et al. Mutations in Fas associated with human lymphoproliferative syndrome and autoimmunity. *Science* 1995;268:1347.
76. Martin DA, Zheng L, Siegel RM, et al. Defective CD95/APO-1/Fas signal complex formation in the human autoimmune lymphoproliferative syndrome, type Ia. *Proc Natl Acad Sci USA* 1999;96:4552.
77. Rathmell JC, Thompson CB. The central effectors of cell death in the immune system. *Annu Rev Immunol* 1999;17:781.
78. Banner DW, D'Arcy A, Janes W, et al. Crystal structure of the soluble human 55 kd TNF receptor-human TNF beta complex: implications for TNF receptor activation. *Cell* 1993;73:431.
79. Hymowitz SG, Christinger HW, Fuh G, et al. Triggering cell death: the crystal structure of Apo2L/TRAIL in a complex with death receptor 5. *Mol Cell* 1999;4:563.
80. Mongkolsapaya J, Grimes JM, Chen N, et al. Structure of the TRAIL-DR5 complex reveals mechanisms conferring specificity in apoptotic initiation. *Nat Struct Biol* 1999;6:1048.
81. Chan KC, Chun HJ, Zheng L, et al. A domain in tumor necrosis factor receptors that mediates ligand-independent receptor assembly and signaling. *Science* 2000;288:2351.
82. Siegel RM, Frederiksen JK, Zacharias DA, et al. Fas preassociation required for apoptosis signaling and dominant inhibition by pathogenic mutations. *Science* 2000;288:2354.
83. Livnah O, Stura EA, Middleton SA, et al. Crystallographic evidence for preformed dimers of erythropoietin receptor before ligand activation. *Science* 1999;283:987.
84. Remy I, Wilson IA, Michnick SW. Erythropoietin receptor activation by a ligand-induced conformation change. *Science* 1999;283:990.
85. Kischkel FC, Hellbardt S, Behrmann I, et al. Cytotoxicity-dependent APO-1 (Fas/CD95)–associated proteins form a death-inducing signaling complex (DISC) with the receptor. *EMBO J* 1995;14:5579.
86. Huang B, Eberstadt M, Olejniczak ET, et al. NMR structure and mutagenesis of the Fas (APO-1/CD95) death domain. *Nature* 1996;384:638.
87. Eberstadt M, Huang B, Chen Z, et al. NMR structure and mutagenesis of the FADD (Mort1) death-effector domain. *Nature* 1998;392:941.
88. Ashkenazi A, Dixit VM. Death receptors: signaling and modulation. *Science* 1998;281:1305.
89. Nicholson DW, Thornberry NA. Caspases: killer proteases. *Trends Biochem Sci* 1997;22:299.
90. Scaffidi C, Fulda S, Srinivasan A, et al. Two CD95 (APO-1/Fas) signaling pathways. *EMBO J* 1998;17:1675.

91. Hu Y, Benedict MA, Ding L, et al. Role of cytochrome c and dATP/ATP hydrolysis in Apaf-1–mediated caspase-9 activation and apoptosis. *EMBO J* 1999;18:3586.
92. Li H, Zhu H, Xu CJ, et al. Cleavage of BID by caspase-8 mediates the mitochondrial damage in the Fas pathway of apoptosis. *Cell* 1998;94:491.
93. Luo X, Budihardjo I, Zou H, et al. Bid, a Bcl2 interacting protein, mediates cytochrome c release from mitochondria in response to activation of cell surface death receptors. *Cell* 1998;94:481.
94. Strasser A, Harris AW, Huang DC, et al. Bcl-2 and Fas/APO-1 regulate distinct pathways to lymphocyte apoptosis. *EMBO J* 1995;14:6136.
95. Yeh WC, Pompa JL, McCurrach ME, et al. FADD: essential for embryo development and signaling from some, but not all, inducers of apoptosis. *Science* 1998;279:1954.
96. Zhang J, Cado D, Chen A, et al. Fas-mediated apoptosis and activation-induced T-cell proliferation are defective in mice lacking FADD/Mort1. *Nature* 1998;392:296.
97. Irmler M, Thome M, Hahne M, et al. Inhibition of death receptor signals by cellular FLIP. *Nature* 1997;388:190.
98. Rasper DM, Vaillancourt JP, Hadano S, et al. Cell death attenuation by "Usurpin," a mammalian DED-caspase homologue that precludes caspase-8 recruitment and activation by the CD-95 (Fas, APO-1) receptor complex. *Cell Death Differ* 1998;5:271.
99. Goltsev YV, Kovalenko AV, Arnold E, et al. CASH, a novel caspase homologue with death effector domains. *J Biol Chem* 1997;272:19641.
100. Srinivasula SM, Ahmad M, Ottilie S, et al. FLAME-1, a novel FADD-like anti-apoptotic molecule that regulates Fas/TNFR1-induced apoptosis. *J Biol Chem* 1997;272:18542.
101. Van Parijs L, Refaeli Y, Abbas AK, et al. Autoimmunity as a consequence of retrovirus-mediated expression of C-FLIP in lymphocytes. *Immunity* 1999;11:763.
102. Pan G, Ni J, Wei YF, et al. An antagonist decoy receptor and a death domain-containing receptor for TRAIL. *Science* 1997;277:815.
103. Wang J, Zheng L, Lobito A, et al. Inherited human caspase-10 mutations underlie defective lymphocyte and dendritic cell apoptosis in autoimmune lymphoproliferative syndrome type II. *Cell* 1999;98:47.
104. Papoff G, Cascino I, Eramo A, et al. An N-terminal domain shared by Fas/Apo-1 (CD95) soluble variants prevents cell death *in vitro*. *J Immunol* 1996;156:4622.
105. Newton K, Harris AW, Bath ML, et al. A dominant interfering mutant of FADD/MORT1 enhances deletion of autoreactive thymocytes and inhibits proliferation of mature T lymphocytes. *EMBO J* 1998;17:706.
106. Hsu H, Xiong J, Goeddel DV. The TNF receptor 1–associated protein TRADD signals cell death and NF-kappa B activation. *Cell* 1995;81:495.
107. Hsu H, Huang J, Shu HB, et al. TNF-dependent recruitment of the protein kinase RIP to the TNF receptor–1 signaling complex. *Immunity* 1996;4:387.
108. Jiang Y, Woronicz JD, Liu W, et al. Prevention of constitutive TNF receptor 1 signaling by silencer of death domains. *Science* 1999;283:543. [For erratum, see *Science* 1999;283:1852.]
109. Rothe M, Pan MG, Henzel WJ, et al. The TNFR2-TRAF signaling complex contains two novel proteins related to baculoviral inhibitor of apoptosis proteins. *Cell* 1995;83:1243.
110. Rothe M, Sarma V, Dixit VM, et al. TRAF2-mediated activation of NF-kappa B by TNF receptor 2 and CD40. *Science* 1995;269:1424.
111. Park YC, Burkitt V, Villa AR, et al. Structural basis for self-association and receptor recognition of human TRAF2. *Nature* 1999;398:533.
112. Ye H, Park YC, Kreishman M, et al. The structural basis for the recognition of diverse receptor sequences by TRAF2. *Mol Cell* 1999;4:321.
113. Pullen SS, Labadia ME, Ingraham RH, et al. High-affinity interactions of tumor necrosis factor receptor–associated factors (TRAFs) and CD40 require TRAF trimerization and CD40 multimerization. *Biochemistry* 1999;38:10168.
114. Lee HH, Dempsey PW, Parks TP, et al. Specificities of CD40 signaling: involvement of TRAF2 in CD40-induced NF-kappaB activation and intercellular adhesion molecule–1 up-regulation. *Proc Natl Acad Sci USA* 1999;96:1421.
115. Yeh WC, Shahinian A, Speiser D, et al. Early lethality, functional NF-kappaB activation, and increased sensitivity to TNF-induced cell death in TRAF2-deficient mice. *Immunity* 1997;7:715.
116. Heine H, Kirschning CJ, Lien E, et al. Cutting edge: cells that carry A null allele for toll-like receptor 2 are capable of responding to endotoxin. *J Immunol* 1999;162:6971.
117. Beg AA, Baltimore D. An essential role for NF-kappaB in preventing TNF-alpha–induced cell death. *Science* 1996;274:782.
118. Lee SY, Reichlin A, Santana A, et al. TRAF2 is essential for JNK but not NF-kappaB activation and regulates lymphocyte proliferation and survival. *Immunity* 1997;7:703.
119. Baldwin ASJ. The NF-kappa B and I kappa B proteins: new discoveries and insights. *Annu Rev Immunol* 1996;14:649.
120. Baeuerle PA, Baltimore D. I kappa B: a specific inhibitor of the NF-kappa B transcription factor. *Science* 1988;242:540.
121. Karin M. How NF-kappaB is activated: the role of the IkappaB kinase (IKK) complex. *Oncogene* 1999;18:6867.
122. Delhase M, Hayakawa M, Chen Y, et al. 1999. Positive and negative regulation of IkappaB kinase activity through IKKbeta subunit phosphorylation. *Science* 1999;284:309.

123. Li Q, Van Antwerp D, Mercurio F, et al. Severe liver degeneration in mice lacking the IkappaB kinase 2 gene. *Science* 1999;284:321.
124. Tanaka M, Fuentes ME, Yamaguchi K, et al. Embryonic lethality, liver degeneration, and impaired NF-kappa B activation in IKK-beta–deficient mice. *Immunity* 1999;10:421.
125. Li ZW, Chu W, Hu Y, et al. The IKKbeta subunit of IkappaB kinase (IKK) is essential for nuclear factor kappaB activation and prevention of apoptosis. *J Exp Med* 1999;189:1839.
126. Hu Y, Baud V, Delhase M, et al. Abnormal morphogenesis but intact IKK activation in mice lacking the IKKalpha subunit of IkappaB kinase. *Science* 1999;284:316.
127. Li Q, Lu Q, Hwang JY, et al. IKK1-deficient mice exhibit abnormal development of skin and skeleton. *Genes Dev* 1999;13:1322.
128. Shinkura R, Kitada K, Matsuda F, et al. Alymphoplasia is caused by point mutation in the mouse gene encoding NF-κB–inducing kinase. *Nat Genet* 1999;1:74–77.
129. Chin AI, Shu J, Shan Shi C, et al. TANK potentiates tumor necrosis factor receptor–associated factor–mediated c-jun N-terminal kinase/stress-activated protein kinase activation through the germinal center kinase pathway. *Mol Cell Biol* 1999;19:6665.
130. Schievella AR, Chen JH, Graham JR, et al. MADD, a novel death domain protein that interacts with the type 1 tumor necrosis factor receptor and activates mitogen-activated protein kinase. *J Biol Chem* 1997;272:12069.
131. Adam D, Adam-Klages S, Kronke M. Identification of p55 tumor necrosis factor receptor–associated proteins that couple to signaling pathways not initiated by the death domain. *J Inflamm* 1995;47:61.
132. Zheng L, Fisher G, Miller RE, et al. Induction of apoptosis in mature T cells by tumour necrosis factor. *Nature* 1995;377:348.
133. Tartaglia LA, Pennica D, Goeddel DV. Ligand passing: the 75-kDa tumor necrosis factor (TNF) receptor recruits TNF for signaling by the 55-kDa TNF receptor. *J Biol Chem* 1993;268:18542.
134. Chan FK, Leonardo MJ. A crucial role for p80 TNF-R2 in amplifying p60 TNF-R1 apoptosis signals in T lymphocytes. *Eur J Immunol* 2000;30:652.
135. Weiss T, Grell M, Hessabi B, et al. Enhancement of TNF receptor p60-mediated cytotoxicity by TNF receptor p80: requirement of the TNF receptor–associated factor–2 binding site. *J Immunol* 1997;158:2398.
136. Bjornberg F, Lantz M, Gullberg U. Metalloproteases and serineproteases are involved in the cleavage of the two tumour necrosis factor (TNF) receptors to soluble forms in the myeloid cell lines U-937 and THP-1. *Scand J Immunol* 1995;42:418.
137. McDermott MF, Aksentijevich I, Galon J, et al. Germline mutations in the extracellular domains of the 55 kDa TNF receptor, TNFR1, define a family of dominantly inherited autoinflammatory syndromes. *Cell* 1999;97:133.
138. Amakawa R, Hakem A, Kundig TM, et al. Impaired negative selection of T cells in Hodgkin's disease antigen CD30-deficient mice. *Cell* 1996;84:551.
139. Banks TA, Rouse BT, Kerley MK, et al. Lymphotoxin-alpha–deficient mice. Effects on secondary lymphoid organ development and humoral immune responsiveness. *J Immunol* 1995;155:1685.
140. Rennert PD, James D, Mackay F, et al. Lymph node genesis is induced by signaling through the lymphotoxin beta receptor. *Immunity* 1998;9:71.
141. O'Neill LA, Greene C. Signal transduction pathways activated by the IL-1 receptor family: ancient signaling machinery in mammals, insects, and plants. *J Leukoc Biol* 1998;63:650.
142. Whitham S, Dinesh-Kumar SP, Choi D, et al. The product of the tobacco mosaic virus resistance gene N: similarity to toll and the interleukin-1 receptor. *Cell* 1994;78:1101. [For erratum, see *Cell* 1995;81:466.]
143. Dinarello CA. Interleukin-1. *Cytokine Growth Factor Rev* 1997;8:253.
144. Auron PE. The interleukin 1 receptor: ligand interactions and signal transduction. *Cytokine Growth Factor Rev* 1998;9:221.
145. Gillespie MT, Horwood NJ. Interleukin-18: perspectives on the newest interleukin. *Cytokine Growth Factor Rev* 1998;9:109.
146. Kopp EB, Medzhitov R. The Toll-receptor family and control of innate immunity. *Curr Opin Immunol* 1999;11:13.
147. Yang RB, Mark MR, Gurney AL, et al. Signaling events induced by lipopolysaccharide-activated toll-like receptor 2. *J Immunol* 1999;163:639.
148. Poltorak A, He X, Smirnova I, et al. Defective LPS signaling in C3H/HeJ and C57BL/10ScCr mice: mutations in Tlr4 gene. *Science* 1998;282:2085.
149. Qureshi ST, Gros P, Malo D. Host resistance to infection: genetic control of lipopolysaccharide responsiveness by TOLL-like receptor genes. *Trends Genet* 1999;15:291.
150. Sims JE, March CJ, Cosman D, et al. cDNA expression cloning of the IL-1 receptor, a member of the immunoglobulin superfamily. *Science* 1988;241:585.
151. McMahan CJ, Slack JL, Mosley B, et al. A novel IL-1 receptor, cloned from B cells by mammalian expression, is expressed in many cell types. *EMBO J* 1991;10:2821.
152. Wesche H, Resch K, Martin MU. Effects of IL-1 receptor accessory protein on IL-1 binding. *FEBS Lett* 1998;429:303.
153. Cullinan EB, Kwee L, Nunes P, et al. IL-1 receptor accessory protein is an essential component of the IL-1 receptor. *J Immunol* 1998;161:5614.
154. Sims JE, Gayle MA, Slack JL, et al. Interleukin 1 signaling occurs exclusively via the type I receptor. *Proc Natl Acad Sci USA* 1993;90:6155.

155. Liu C, Hart RP, Liu XJ, et al. Cloning and characterization of an alternatively processed human type II interleukin-1 receptor mRNA. *J Biol Chem* 1996;271:20965.
156. Cao Z, Henzel WJ, Gao X. IRAK: a kinase associated with the interleukin-1 receptor. *Science* 1996;271:1128.
157. Wesche H, Henzel WJ, Shillinglaw W, et al. MyD88: an adapter that recruits IRAK to the IL-1 receptor complex. *Immunity* 1997;7:837.
158. Cao Z, Xiong J, Takeuchi M, et al. TRAF6 is a signal transducer for interleukin-1. *Nature* 1996;383:443.
159. Kopp E, Medzhitov R, Carothers J, et al. ECSIT is an evolutionarily conserved intermediate in the Toll/IL-1 signal transduction pathway. *Genes Dev* 1999;13:2059.
160. Singh R, Wang B, Shirvaikar A, et al. The IL-1 receptor and Rho directly associate to drive cell activation in inflammation. *J Clin Invest* 1999;103:1561.
161. Sizemore N, Leung S, Stark GR. Activation of phosphatidylinositol 3-kinase in response to interleukin-1 leads to phosphorylation and activation of the NF-kappaB p65/RelA subunit. *Mol Cell Biol* 1999;19:4798.
162. Adachi O, Kawai T, Takeda K, et al. Targeted disruption of the MyD88 gene results in loss of IL-1– and IL-18–mediated function. *Immunity* 1998;9:143.
163. Lomaga MA, Yeh WC, Sarosi I, et al. TRAF6 deficiency results in osteopetrosis and defective interleukin-1, CD40, and LPS signaling. *Genes Dev* 1999;13:1015.
164. Kanakaraj P, Ngo K, Wu Y, et al. Defective interleukin (IL)-18–mediated natural killer and T helper cell type 1 responses in IL-1 receptor–associated kinase (IRAK)–deficient mice. *J Exp Med* 1999;189:1129.
165. Thomas JA, Allen JL, Tsen M, et al. Impaired cytokine signaling in mice lacking the IL-1 receptor–associated kinase. *J Immunol* 1999;163:978.
166. Medzhitov R, Preston-Hurlburt P, Kopp E, et al. MyD88 is an adaptor protein in the hToll/IL-1 receptor family signaling pathways. *Mol Cell* 1998;2:253.
167. Glaccum MB, Stocking KL, Charrier K, et al. Phenotypic and functional characterization of mice that lack the type I receptor for IL-1. *J Immunol* 1997;159:3364.
168. Ullrich A, Schlessinger J. Signal transduction by receptors with tyrosine kinase activity. *Cell* 1990;61:203.
169. Schlessinger J, Ullrich A. Growth factor signaling by receptor tyrosine kinases. *Neuron* 1992;9:383.
170. Rosnet O, Birnbaum D. Hematopoietic receptors of class III receptor–type tyrosine kinases. *Crit Rev Oncog* 1993;4:595.
171. Sherr CJ. The fms oncogene. *Biochim Biophys Acta* 1988;948:225.
172. Besmer P, Murphy JE, George PC, et al. A new acute transforming feline retrovirus and relationship of its oncogene v-kit with the protein kinase gene family. *Nature* 1986;320:415.
173. Qiu FH, Ray P, Brown K, et al. Primary structure of c-kit: relationship with the CSF-1/PDGF receptor kinase family—oncogenic activation of v-kit involves deletion of extracellular domain and C terminus. *EMBO J* 1988; 7:1003.
174. Weiss A, Schlessinger J. Switching signals on or off by receptor dimerization. *Cell* 1998;94:277.
175. Shoelson SE. SH2 and PTB domain interactions in tyrosine kinase signal transduction. *Curr Opin Chem Biol* 1997;1:227.
176. Buscher D, Hipskind RA, Krautwald S, et al. Ras-dependent and -independent pathways target the mitogen-activated protein kinase network in macrophages. *Mol Cell Biol* 1995;15:466.
177. Tsai M, Chen RH, Tam SY, et al. Activation of MAP kinases, pp90rsk and pp70-S6 kinases in mouse mast cells by signaling through the c-kit receptor tyrosine kinase or Fc epsilon RI: rapamycin inhibits activation of pp70-S6 kinase and proliferation in mouse mast cells. *Eur J Immunol* 1993;23:3286.
178. O'Farrell AM, Ichihara M, Mui AL, et al. Signaling pathways activated in a unique mast cell line where interleukin-3 supports survival and stem cell factor is required for a proliferative response. *Blood*1996;87:3655.
179. Campbell SL, Khosravi-Far R, Rossman KL, et al. Increasing complexity of Ras signaling. *Oncogene* 1998;17: 1395.
180. van der Geer P, Hunter T. Mutation of Tyr697, a GRB2-binding site, and Tyr721, a PI 3-kinase binding site, abrogates signal transduction by the murine CSF-1 receptor expressed in Rat-2 fibroblasts. *EMBO J* 1993;12: 5161.
181. Schlessinger J. How receptor tyrosine kinases activate Ras. *Trends Biochem Sci* 1993;18:273.
182. Downward J. Control of ras activation. *Cancer Surv* 1996;27:87.
183. Dhanasekaran N, Premkumar Reddy E. Signaling by dual specificity kinases. *Oncogene* 1998;17:1447.
184. Cobb MH. MAP kinase pathways. *Prog Biophys Mol Biol* 1999;71:479.
185. Shi ZQ, Lu W, Feng GS. The Shp-2 tyrosine phosphatase has opposite effects in mediating the activation of extracellular signal-regulated and c-Jun NH2-terminal mitogen-activated protein kinases. *J Biol Chem* 1998;273: 4904.
186. Gu H, Pratt JC, Burakoff SJ, et al. Cloning of p97/Gab2, the major SHP2-binding protein in hematopoietic cells, reveals a novel pathway for cytokine-induced gene activation. *Mol Cell* 1998;2:729.
187. Chen HE, Chang S, Trub T, et al. Regulation of colony-stimulating factor 1 receptor signaling by the SH2 domain-containing tyrosine phosphatase SHPTP1. *Mol Cell Biol* 1996;16:3685.
188. Krautwald S, Buscher D, Kummer V, et al. Involvement of the protein tyrosine phosphatase SHP-1 in Ras-mediated activation of the mitogen-activated protein kinase pathway. *Mol Cell Biol* 1996;16:5955.
189. Treisman R. Regulation of transcription by MAP kinase cascades. *Curr Opin Cell Biol* 1996;8:205.
190. Porter AC, Vaillancourt RR. Tyrosine kinase receptor–activated signal transduction pathways which lead to oncogenesis. *Oncogene* 1998;17:1343.

191. Reedijk M, Liu X, van der Geer P, et al. Tyr721 regulates specific binding of the CSF-1 receptor kinase insert to PI 3′-kinase SH2 domains: a model for SH2-mediated receptor-target interactions. *EMBO J* 1992;11:1365.
192. Toker A, Cantley LC. Signalling through the lipid products of phosphoinositide-3-OH kinase. *Nature* 1997;387:673.
193. Datta SR, Brunet A, Greenberg ME. Cellular survival: a play in three Akts. *Genes Dev* 1999;13:2905.
194. Alessi DR, Kozlowski MT, Weng QP, et al. 3-Phosphoinositide–dependent protein kinase 1 (PDK1) phosphorylates and activates the p70 S6 kinase *in vivo* and *in vitro*. *Curr Biol* 1998;8:69.
195. Datta SR, Dudek H, Tao X, et al. Akt phosphorylation of BAD couples survival signals to the cell—intrinsic death machinery. *Cell* 1997;91:231.
196. del Peso L, Gonzalez-Garcia M, Page C, et al. Interleukin-3–induced phosphorylation of BAD through the protein kinase Akt. *Science* 1997;278:687.
197. Brunet A, Bonni A, Zigmond MJ, et al. Akt promotes cell survival by phosphorylating and inhibiting a Forkhead transcription factor. *Cell* 1999;96:857.
198. Kops GJ, de Ruiter ND, De Vries-Smits AM, et al. Direct control of the Forkhead transcription factor AFX by protein kinase B. *Nature* 1999;398:630.
199. Tang ED, Nunez G, Barr FG, et al. Negative regulation of the forkhead transcription factor FKHR by Akt. *J Biol Chem* 1999;274:16741.
200. Rena G, Guo S, Cichy SC, et al. Phosphorylation of the transcription factor forkhead family member FKHR by protein kinase B. *J Biol Chem* 1999;274:17179.
201. Biggs WHR, Meisenhelder J, Hunter T, et al. Protein kinase B/Akt-mediated phosphorylation promotes nuclear exclusion of the winged helix transcription factor FKHR1. *Proc Natl Acad Sci USA* 1999;96:7421.
202. Zha J, Harada H, Yang E, et al. Serine phosphorylation of death agonist BAD in response to survival factor results in binding to 14-3-3 not BCL-X(L). *Cell* 1996;87:619.
203. Cardone MH, Roy N, Stennicke HR, et al. Regulation of cell death protease caspase-9 by phosphorylation. *Science* 1998;282:1318.
204. Ozes ON, Mayo LD, Gustin JA, et al. NF-kappaB activation by tumour necrosis factor requires the Akt serine-threonine kinase. *Nature* 1999;401:82.
205. Romashkova JA, Makarov SS. NF-kappaB is a target of AKT in anti-apoptotic PDGF signalling. *Nature* 1999;401:86.
206. Cantley LC, Neel BG. New insights into tumor suppression: PTEN suppresses tumor formation by restraining the phosphoinositide 3-kinase/AKT pathway. *Proc Natl Acad Sci USA* 1999;96:4240.
207. Damen JE, Liu L, Rosten P, et al. The 145-kDa protein induced to associate with Shc by multiple cytokines is an inositol tetraphosphate and phosphatidylinositol 3,4,5-triphosphate 5-phosphatase. *Proc Natl Acad Sci USA* 1996;93:1689.
208. Lioubin MN, Algate PA, Tsai S, et al. p150Ship, a signal transduction molecule with inositol polyphosphate-5-phosphatase activity. *Genes Dev* 1996;10:1084.
209. Biscardi JS, Tice DA, Parsons SJ. c-Src, receptor tyrosine kinases, and human cancer. *Adv Cancer Res* 1999;76:61.
210. Romero F, Fischer S. Structure and function of vav. *Cell Signal* 1996;8:545.
211. Lupher MLJ, Andoniou CE, Bonita C, et al. The c-Cbl oncoprotein. *Int J Biochem Cell Biol* 1998;30:439.
212. Vignais ML, Sadowski HB, Watling D, et al. Platelet-derived growth factor induces phosphorylation of multiple JAK family kinases and STAT proteins. *Mol Cell Biol* 1996;16:1759.
213. Deberry C, Mou S, Linnekin D. Stat1 associates with c-kit and is activated in response to stem cell factor. *Biochem J* 1997;327:73.
214. Megeney LA, Perry RL, LeCouter JE, et al. bFGF and LIF signaling activates STAT3 in proliferating myoblasts. *Dev Genet* 1996;19:139.
215. Johnson MR, Valentine C, Basilico C, et al. FGF signaling activates STAT1 and p21 and inhibits the estrogen response and proliferation of MCF-7 cells. *Oncogene* 1998;16:2647.
216. Sahni M, Ambrosetti DC, Mansukhani A, et al. FGF signaling inhibits chondrocyte proliferation and regulates bone development through the STAT-1 pathway. *Genes Dev* 1999;13:1361.
217. Massague J. TGF-beta signal transduction. *Annu Rev Biochem* 1998;67:753.
218. Heldin CH, Miyazono K, ten Dijke P. TGF-beta signalling from cell membrane to nucleus through SMAD proteins. *Nature* 1997;390:465.
219. Piek E, Heldin CH, Ten Dijke P. Specificity, diversity, and regulation in TGF-beta superfamily signaling. *FASEB J* 1999;13:2105.
220. Letterio JJ, Roberts AB. Regulation of immune responses by TGF-beta. *Annu Rev Immunol* 1998;16:137.
221. Wrana JL. Regulation of Smad activity. *Cell* 2000;100:189.
222. Raftery LA, Sutherland DJ. TGF-beta family signal transduction in Drosophila development: from Mad to Smads. *Dev Biol* 1999;210:251.
223. Kawabata M, Inoue H, Hanyu A, et al. Smad proteins exist as monomers *in vivo* and undergo homo- and hetero-oligomerization upon activation by serine/threonine kinase receptors. *EMBO J* 1998;17:4056.
224. Imamura T, Takase M, Nishihara A, et al. Smad6 inhibits signalling by the TGF-beta superfamily. *Nature* 1997;389:622.
225. Nakao A, Afrakhte M, Moren A, et al. Identification of Smad7, a TGFbeta-inducible antagonist of TGF-beta signalling. *Nature* 1997;389:631.

226. Weinstein M, Yang X, Deng C. Functions of mammalian Smad genes as revealed by targeted gene disruption in mice. *Cytokine Growth Factor Rev* 2000;11:49.
227. Zhu Y, Richardson JA, Parada LF, et al. Smad3 mutant mice develop metastatic colorectal cancer. *Cell* 1998; 94:703.
228. Yang X, Letterio JJ, Lechleider RJ, et al. Targeted disruption of SMAD3 results in impaired mucosal immunity and diminished T cell responsiveness to TGF-beta. *EMBO J* 1999;18:1280.
229. Ashcroft GS, Yang X, Glick AB, et al. Mice lacking Smad3 show accelerated wound healing and an impaired local inflammatory response. *Nat Cell Biol* 1999;1:260.
230. Galvin KM, Donovan MJ, Lynch CA, et al. A role for smad6 in development and homeostasis of the cardiovascular system. *Nat Genet* 2000;24:171.
231. Zhou S, Zawel L, Lengauer C, et al. Characterization of human FAST-1, a TGF beta and activin signal transducer. *Mol Cell* 1998;2:121.
232. Labbe E, Silvestri C, Hoodless PA, et al. Smad2 and Smad3 positively and negatively regulate TGF beta–dependent transcription through the forkhead DNA-binding protein FAST2. *Mol Cell* 1998;2:109.
233. Liu F, Pouponnot C, Massague J. Dual role of the Smad4/DPC4 tumor suppressor in TGFbeta-inducible transcriptional complexes. *Genes Dev* 1997;11:3157.
234. Luo K, Stroschein SL, Wang W, et al. The Ski oncoprotein interacts with the Smad proteins to repress TGFbeta signaling. *Genes Dev* 1999;13:2196.
235. Stroschein SL, Wang W, Zhou S, et al. Negative feedback regulation of TGF-beta signaling by the SnoN oncoprotein. *Science* 1999;286:771.
236. Yamaguchi K, Shirakabe K, Shibuya H, et al. Identification of a member of the MAPKKK family as a potential mediator of TGF-beta signal transduction. *Science* 1995;270:2008.
237. Shibuya H, Yamaguchi K, Shirakabe K, et al. TAB1: an activator of the TAK1 MAPKKK in TGF-beta signal transduction. *Science* 1996;272:1179.
238. Moriguchi T, Kuroyanagi N, Yamaguchi K, et al. A novel kinase cascade mediated by mitogen-activated protein kinase kinase 6 and MKK3. *J Biol Chem* 1996;271:13675.
239. Wang W, Zhou G, Hu MCT, et al. Activation of the hematopoietic progenitor kinase–1 (HPK1)–dependent, stress-activated c-Jun N-terminal kinase (JNK) pathway by transforming growth factor beta (TGF-beta–activated kinase (TAK1), a kinase mediator of TGF beta signal transduction. *J Biol Chem* 1997;272:22771.
240. Sakurai H, Miyoshi H, Toriumi W, et al. Functional interactions of transforming growth factor beta-activated kinase 1 with IkappaB kinases to stimulate NF-kappaB activation. *J Biol Chem* 1999;274:10641.
241. Berger EA, Murphy PM, Farber JM. Chemokine receptors as HIV-1 coreceptors: roles in viral entry, tropism, and disease. *Annu Rev Immunol* 1999;17:657.
242. Murphy PM. Neutrophil receptors for interleukin-8 and related CXC chemokines. *Semin Hematol* 1997;34:311.
243. Cyster JM. Chemokines and cell migration in secondary lymphoid organs. *Science* 1999;286:2098.

13

Cytokine-Induced Neuropsychiatric Toxicity

Darin M. Lerner, Alan Stoudemire, and *Donald L. Rosenstein

*Weill Medical College, Cornell University, Westchester Division, White Plains, New York; and *Psychiatry Consultation-Liaison Service, National Institute of Mental Health, Bethesda, Maryland*

The cytokines interleukin-2 (IL-2) and interferon-a (IFN-α) are potent biological agents used to treat malignancy, infectious diseases, and neurodegenerative disorders. While these medications show substantial therapeutic promise, the neuropsychiatric toxicity associated with these agents is frequently treatment limiting. The pathophysiology of this toxicity is not well delineated, and CNS adverse effects are often misdiagnosed. This report reviews the preclinical and clinical literature describing the morbidity associated with these agents and suggests appropriate clinical management strategies and future directions for research.

Immunomodulating therapies employing cytokines such as IL-2 and IFN-α are rapidly becoming part of the standard medical armamentarium. The neuropsychiatric toxicity associated with these agents is poorly understood and poses substantial management problems for clinicians. In this paper, we review the literature on the etiology, clinical presentation, and management of the neurotoxicity induced by IL-2 and IFN-α. The correct diagnosis and treatment of these adverse events are essential, given the treatment-limiting morbidity that can occur with these cytokines. Moreover, there is a need both to identify individuals at high risk for developing cytokine-induced CNS toxicity and to develop prophylactic strategies for this common adverse event.

Cytokines—soluble mediators secreted by immune tissues—are promising medications for a wide variety of malignancies, infectious diseases, and neurodegenerative diseases. Cytokines have been used successfully to treat malignancies such as renal cell cancer, malignant melanoma, and leukemias, presumably by promoting an immune response against cancer cells or by altering biochemical pathways in the cell. Similarly, cytokines may disrupt biochemical pathways essential for viral replication in infectious diseases such as human immunodeficiency virus (HIV) and hepatitis C virus (HCV) infection. The process of neural degeneration observed in multiple sclerosis and amyotrophic lateral sclerosis (ALS) may also be susceptible to cytokine therapy as these may be immunologically mediated disorders. Analogous to the treatment-limiting systemic toxicity associated with conventional chemotherapy, the adverse effects of cytokine biotherapy frequently present substantial clinical management problems.

INTERLEUKIN-2

Interleukin-2 (IL-2) is a 15- to 16-kDa protein produced mainly by peripheral $CD4^+$ helper T-cells in response to stimulation by antigens and mitogens. Through a cascade effect, IL-2 activates resting T-cells to initiate DNA synthesis and cell division resulting in the proliferation and clonal expansion of T-cells. The magnitude and duration of this response is determined by the interaction between IL-2 and its high-affinity receptor [found on T-cells, B-cells, natural killer cells (NK), monocytes, macrophages, and neutrophils]. IL-2 regulates its own expression as well as that of other cytokines, notably interleukin-1 (IL-1), tumor necrosis factor (TNF), and interferon-γ (IFN-γ) (1).

Clinical trials of recombinant IL-2 have targeted malignancies with low response rates to traditional chemotherapy, such as metastatic malignant melanoma and renal cell cancer (2). These malignancies are responsive to IL-2, with tumor suppression rates of up to 60% for melanoma and 40% for renal cell cancer (1). No direct cytotoxic effect on tumor cells by IL-2 itself has been detected; rather, IL-2 is thought to mediate tumor regression by stimulating the proliferation and activation of cytotoxic cells such as NK cells, and tumor specific T-cells. Additionally, IL-2 may act indirectly by stimulating other cytokines and hormones (1).

IL-2 is administered either systemically (intravenously as bolus or continuous infusion or subcutaneously) or locally to specific tumor sites. It has been used as monotherapy, as part of adoptive immunotherapy, and in gene therapy protocols. Treatment protocols typically vary in duration from 3 days to 2 weeks. The cumulative systemic exposure is a critical factor in determining toxicity, with longer exposure conferring greater risk. However, both therapeutic efficacy and toxicity appear to be dose related.

Neuropathophysiological Mechanisms

While the underlying mechanisms of IL-2–induced CNS toxicity are not known, several potential explanations have emerged from animal and human studies. Increased water content in the gray and white matter has been observed by magnetic resonance imaging (MRI) in IL-2–treated patients (3). It has been suggested that IL-2 can impair the functioning of the blood–brain barrier and lead to a capillary leakage syndrome (1). Capillary leakage is a prominent aspect of IL-2 toxicity in other organ systems. Water retention may also be increased via a CNS-mediated increase in ADH synthesis (1). Whether IL-2 is able to readily cross the blood–brain and blood–CSF barriers and thereby mediate direct effects on brain functioning is unknown. While IL-2–induced brain edema is associated with significant neurotoxicity in the presence of brain metastases, it is uncertain whether it is etiologically important in those patients without metastases. At least one study revealed no correlation between the severity of CNS symptoms and vasogenic edema (3). However, other authors (1) suggest that the capillary leakage syndrome is likely to be associated with CNS toxicity through the increased access to the brain of neuroactive substances.

Preclinical studies by Hanisch (1) have localized endogenous IL-2 and IL-2–related molecules to the frontal cortex, septum, striatum, hippocampal formation, hypothalamus, locus ceruleus, cerebellum, pituitary, and fiber tracts of the corpus callosum. In addition, IL-2 can affect gene expression, neuronal activity, and release of neurotransmitters in brain regions subserving sleep and arousal, memory and cognition, locomotion, and neuroendocrine function. IL-2 is a potent and specific regulator of neurotransmitter release in the frontal cortex, hippocampus, striatum, and the hypothalamus. In laboratory animals and *in vitro,* neurotransmission by acetylcholine, dopamine, and norepinephrine can be modulated by IL-2 in a dose-dependent, biphasic manner. Furthermore, there is strong evidence of IL-2 interference with neural activity in the hippocampus, suggesting that it may modulate memory formation (1).

IL-2 modulates the release of several hypothalamic and pituitary peptides and, for most pituitary hormones, is even more potent in regulating secretion than hypothalamic releasing and inhibiting factors (1). IL-2 induces release of corticotropin-releasing factor (CRF), arginine vasopressin (AVP), and somatostatin from the hypothalamus; and adrenocorticotrophic hormone (ACTH), thyroid-stimulating hormone (TSH), and prolactin-releasing hormone (PRH) from the pituitary (1). In cancer patients experiencing their second exposure to IL-2 treatment, peak serum ACTH levels were four times higher than in patients with Cushing's disease (4). An increase in the release of the opioid β-endorphin was similarly observed (4). IL-2 inhibits growth hormone releasing factor (GRF) as well as luteinizing hormone releasing hormone (LHRH) release from the hypothalamus and follicle stimulating hormone (FSH), luteinizing hormone (LH), and growth hormone (GH) release from the pituitary (1). In cholinergic neurons, IL-2 stimulates nitric oxide (NO) production and thereby CRF release (1). Hence, dysregulation of the hypothalamic pituitary adrenal (HPA) axis may play a crucial role in IL-2–induced neurotoxicity.

Forms of Toxicity

High-dose intravenous IL-2 is associated with substantial systemic toxicity involving multiple organ systems (2,5,6). Many patients complain of a flu-like syndrome characterized by decreased energy, fatigue, anorexia, and malaise. Hypotension, arrhythmia, angina, and myocardial infarction have been reported, (5,6). The hemodynamic pattern observed is quite similar to that seen in septic shock. Hypotension is typically corrected with intravenous fluid administration and, when indicated, vasopressors. High-dose intravenous IL-2–associated arrhythmias include sinus bradycardia, atrial fibrillation, and ventricular tachycardia; supraventricular tachycardias are the most common and are responsive to conventional treatments. In early trials (5), ischemia or myocardial injury occurred in 2% to 10% of patients during the first days of treatment with intravenous IL-2. Some patients with evidence of myocardial infarction had normal coronary arteries, suggesting a direct cardiotoxic effect (5). Anemia and thrombocytopenia were common side effects, with other hematological abnormalities occurring more rarely. With high-dose intravenous IL-2 therapy, up to 88% of patients have required RBC transfusions (5). Moderate to severe thrombocytopenia that resolves upon IL-2 discontinuation was observed in up to 63% of patients (5). Infectious complications may include staphylococcal sepsis, due to neutrophil dysfunction, typically occurring in prolonged courses of therapy (5). While IL-2 does not cause neutropenia, it may lead to decreased neutrophil chemotaxis and, thus, an increased susceptibility to bacterial infections (2). Cholecystitis, hyperbilirubinemia, and hepatomegaly may occur but return to normal after IL-2 discontinuation (5). Acute renal failure due to high-dose intravenous IL-2 therapy usually shows rapid resolution following cessation of IL-2 (2,5). Hypophosphatemia without phosphaturia has been described (5). Diarrhea, nausea, and vomiting occur in most high-dose IL-2 recipients and quickly resolve (5). Pulmonary complications due to the capillary leak syndrome are seen at high doses (5). Dose-dependent dermatological complications, including erythema and pruritus, have been observed, and life-threatening bullous eruptions and exfoliative dermatitis have been reported (5). The morbidity and mortality associated with high-dose systemic administration of high-dose IL-2 have improved dramatically over the last decade with more experience accumulated and a better understanding of the dose-related toxicities.

Compared to intravenous IL-2 therapy, lower dose subcutaneous administration of IL-2 is associated with fewer overall adverse effects, is not associated with a capillary leakage syndrome, and may be administered on an outpatient basis (7).

Neuropsychiatric Toxicity

Neuropsychiatric symptoms observed in patients receiving IL-2 therapy include behavioral changes, agitation, cognitive impairment, disorientation, delusions, and hallucinations. The first report of clinically significant neuropsychiatric toxicity associated with systemic IL-2 administration appeared in 1987. Denicoff et al. (8) conducted a prospective evaluation of 44 cancer patients treated with IL-2 alone or IL-2 administered with adoptive immunotherapy (lymphokine-activated killer cells). Twenty-two of the 44 patients demonstrated severe cognitive changes as measured by the Mini-Mental State Exam, the Digit-Symbol Test, and the Trail-Making Test. All 22 patients met DSM-III criteria for delirium. Significant behavioral changes were noted in 15 patients, with symptoms ranging from brief agitation requiring minimal supervision to severe agitation and combativeness, lasting several days and requiring the use of neuroleptics and physical restraints. Seven patients developed frank delusions during treatment. Neuropsychiatric symptoms typically appeared at the end of each IL-2 treatment phase and were dose-related. Seventeen of 24 (71%) patients who received IL-2 at 100,000 U/kg showed moderate to severe neuropsychiatric changes, whereas only six of 19 (32%) patients who received a lower dose did. No specific psychiatric risk factors were identified by any of the measurement instruments or self-reports used in this study. Weight gain (representing vascular leakage and fluid accumulation) was not correlated with the development of a neuropsychiatric syndrome.

While the neuropsychiatric toxicity associated with IL-2 is best characterized as a delirium, several longer lasting neuroendocrine (e.g., thyroiditis) and memory disturbances (including permanent neurological damage) have been described in humans and animals (1). Karp (9) reported eight patients who developed new focal neurological abnormalities while receiving IL-2 therapy for cancer or HIV infection. In these patients, initial delirium evolved into ataxia, hemiparesis, seizures, cortical blindness, and coma. MRI studies revealed multiple white and gray matter lesions, particularly in the occipital poles, the centrum semiovale, and cerebellum, which resolved with clinical improvement. Pace (10) reported overall diffuse frontal EEG slowing in 20 patients treated with IL-2 and also described increased P300 latency in cognitive evoked potentials.

Consistent with the modulatory effect of IL-2 on the HPA axis, we have observed IL-2–induced mood changes such as depression and hypomania in some cancer patients, although there have been no clinical studies published to date describing these adverse effects. While the depressive and hypomanic symptoms of many patients will decrease or remit following discontinuation IL-2 therapy, other patients have persistent depressive symptoms requiring antidepressant treatment. In our experience, none of the patients with hypomanic symptoms have required mood-stabilizing therapy.

Hypothyroidism is a frequent complication of IL-2 administration (1,5) and may be associated with psychiatric symptoms. Some patients develop a marked decline in T3 or T4 levels, while others have clinical signs of hypothyroidism, including goiter (5). Abnormal thyroid indices usually develop 2 weeks after starting treatment and resolve several weeks after the discontinuation of IL-2 therapy. Thyroxin replacement may be required in advanced cases. An autoimmune mechanism is suspected but has not been conclusively demonstrated (5).

Direct intraventricular IL-2 for leptomeningeal metastases resulted in subcortical brain damage in one patient. This patient had no subsequent evidence of malignancy after treatment but developed a delayed CNS syndrome thought to be secondary to IL-2 (1).

Clinical Management

Clinician and patient education are key to early diagnosis and treatment. Patients and staff should be informed about potential psychiatric adverse effects such as conceptual disorganization, disorientation, feelings of fear or mistrust, and perceptual distortions or hallucinations. Patients should be reassured that these symptoms almost always resolve completely after treatment and encouraged to communicate symptoms at their first appearance. Even with awareness of these effects, prodromal symptoms of CNS toxicity are frequently missed or misattributed to the effects of the underlying disease, poor psychological adjustment, or a preexisting psychiatric disorder (11).

The treatment approach to managing IL-2 neurotoxicity is similar to that for any delirium. With the emergence of neuropsychiatric symptoms, other medical causes of mental status change such as electrolyte or endocrine abnormalities, and infectious processes should be excluded. It may be necessary to hold or reduce the IL-2 dose in order to minimize toxicity. As with other nonsedative/hypnotic withdrawal deliria, neuroleptics are the first-line medications for patients experiencing severe agitation or psychosis. Haloperidol (Haldol), the most commonly used neuroleptic for delirium, can be instituted at a low dose (0.5 mg po or IV) and increased as necessary to manage symptoms. The use of better tolerated atypical neuroleptics such as risperidone, olanzapine, and quetiapine may be considered, whereas drugs with more anticholinergic properties, such as low-potency neuroleptics, might exacerbate a medication-induced delirium. Risperidone has been effective in the treatment of delirium secondary to other medical conditions (12), and olanzapine has efficacy comparable to that of haloperidol for treatment of delirium in medical patients (13). Efficacy has yet to be reported for quetiapine. Sleep disturbance is a frequent complication of IL-2 treatment and is often treated with benzodiazepines. However, benzodiazepines may exacerbate the delirium. We recommend avoiding benzodiazepines, anticholinergics, and antihistamines. As with antidepressant treatment in other medically ill patients, selective serotonin reuptake inhibitors (SSRIs) should be considered the first-line treatment of patients with IL-2–associated depression.

INTERFERON-α

Interferon-α (IFN-α) is a 19-kDa protein, shown to be an effective therapy for condyloma acuminatum, chronic myelogenous leukemia, hairy cell leukemia, Kaposi's sarcoma, and hepatitis C virus (HCV) infection. It is also being investigated as a treatment for malignant melanoma and other tumors (14). The formulation, dose, and frequency of administration of IFN-α varies depending on the medical condition for which it is used. The typical approach for HCV infection is to administer 3 to 6 million international units (MIU) of IFN-α subcutaneously three to six times per week.

Neuropathophysiological Mechanisms

While it is known that IFN-α can disrupt the vascular endothelium in tumors, no evidence yet indicates that it can disrupt the blood–brain barrier (11). Several lines of evidence (15) suggest that IFN-α may mediate neurotoxicity via neuroendocrine, neurotransmitter, cytokine, and free radical pathways.

IFN-α shows concentration-dependent biphasic activation or inhibition of the HPA axis. Antigenic and amino acid structural similarities (sharing of a 24–amino acid sequence at the NH_2-terminal) among IFN-α, ACTH, and γ-endorphin suggest possible receptor interactions (16). IFN-α binds to brain opiate receptors, and its CNS activity may be reversed by opioid antagonists such as naltrexone (17). Dysregulation of the HPA axis [via increased corticotropin releasing hormone (CRH) secretion] and the hypothalamic–pituitary–thyroid axis have been implicated in the pathophysiology of some subtypes of major depression and may be involved in cytokine-induced depression (11). Although not well characterized, IFN-α may dysregulate the frontal-subcortical dopamine system through an opiate-associated mechanism (17). Moreover, the clinical syndrome observed in IFN-α neurotoxicity (psychomotor slowing, cognitive dysfunction, and dysphoria) resembles the symptomatology of diseases associated with dopamine depletion. Therefore, IFN-α–induced CNS pathology could be related to the neurocognitive and executive deficits seen in Parkinson's disease. Alterations of noradrenergic receptor and serum tryptophan levels have been observed in both IFN-α therapy and in the AIDS dementia syndrome (17). Serotonin depletion may be responsible for the dementia and depression seen in both syndromes (17).

Other cytokine systems, second messengers, and nitric oxide may also mediate the neurotoxicity seen with IFN-α (15). IL-1, TNF-α, and IL-2 can be directly or indirectly induced by IFN-α in the brain. These cytokines have been implicated in disturbances of memory mechanisms in the hippocampus and neuroendocrine activity in hypothalamus; other evidence an association with neurodegeneration and neuron apoptosis (11,15). As discussed previously, nitric oxide may mediate some aspects of cytokine neurotoxicity (15) as well as some aspects of alcohol intoxication and withdrawal (18).

Forms of Toxicity

Renault et al. (19) described the adverse consequences of IFN-α administration in HCV patients and divided these effects into early and late categories. Early effects include a flu-like syndrome, beginning as soon as 2 to 4 hours following the first IFN-α injection, characterized by mild fever, chills, headache, arthralgias, and myalgias. These adverse effects usually attenuate with repeated dosing and are rarely treatment limiting except at extremely high doses (e.g., >20 MIU three times per week).

Other symptoms appear insidiously after 2 to 6 weeks of therapy. A catabolic state with loss of up to 10% of body weight, hair loss, and decreased libido may be observed. Higher doses may lead to nausea, vomiting, hypotension, tachycardia, and rashes (19).

Hematologic abnormalities resulting from bone marrow suppression are common with sustained IFN-α therapy (20,21). Leukopenia is observed in 69%, thrombocytopenia in 42%, and anemia in 60% of patients. Cytopenias are usually mild, self-limited, and well-tolerated provided that patients have no preexisting blood cell disorders (20). Hypotension, hypertension, and uncomplicated tachycardia occur in 5% to 15% of IFN-α recipients in a dose-dependent manner (20,21).

During prolonged IFN-α courses, autoantibody titers may rise (20). Most frequently, the thyroiditis associated with hypo- or hyperthyroidism is associated with autoantibodies. Hypothyroidism occurs with two to three times the frequency of hyperthyroidism. Clinical symptoms may occur 2 months after the beginning of IFN-α therapy but most frequently become apparent after 4 months. The median occurrence of hyperthyroidism is at 2 to 4 months of treatment; the median occurrence of hypothyroidism is at 6 to 12 months of treatment (20). Most patients respond well to thyroid replacement therapy, with long-term substitutive treatment needed only in those patients with severe and sustained hypothyroidism after IFN-α discontinuation (20).

In a multicenter, randomized clinical trial of IFN-α (3, 5, or 10 MIU three times per week) in HCV infection (22), 29% of patients required dose modification due to adverse effects, most of which occurred in the first 12 weeks of treatment. Ten percent discontinued treatment secondary to adverse effects. Six percent of all patients developed an elevated TSH following treatment, which may have etiologic significance for IFN-α–associated mood disturbance.

Neuropsychiatric Toxicity

CNS adverse effects of IFN-α include irritability, depression, personality changes, impaired concentration, fatigue, insomnia, and delirium. While some reports have questioned the frequency and clinical significance of IFN-α–induced neuropsychiatric symptoms (23,24), the bulk of published evidence demonstrates that the CNS adverse effects of IFN-α are substantial and potentially treatment limiting. Ten of 58 patients with chronic HCV infection treated with recombinant human IFN-α at the NIH Clinical Center (19) developed psychiatric syndromes believed to be secondary to IFN-α treatment. These symptoms increased in incidence with extended treatment. Irritability and anxiety superimposed on fatigue frequently occurred after the second or third month of treatment and presented as problems in the workplace, problems with relationships, or domestic discord. Patients may describe overreactions to minor frustrations, such as uncontrollable tearfulness out of proportion to the circumstance (19).

There are several case reports of manic episodes occurring in middle-aged patients who had no psychiatric histories and who had been receiving IFN-α therapy for several years (25–27). A previously healthy 40-year-old patient had IFN-α–induced manic and depressive episodes that persisted for 3 years after the discontinuation of IFN-α and required maintenance treatment with mood-stabilizing and antidepressant medication (26). In two patients who developed depression while receiving IFN-α, the abrupt discontinuation of IFN-α resulted in the development of manic symptoms. These symptoms were particularly marked in a patient who had been treated with paroxetine for depression for nearly 1 year (27).

The diagnosis of depression in patients treated with IFN-α presents problems similar to depressive syndromes associated with other medical illnesses. In addition to the symptoms of sadness, anhedonia, guilt, and poor self-esteem, patients often experience fatigue, sleep disturbance, decreased appetite, weight loss, decreased libido, slowed thinking, and poor memory. These symptoms may reflect manifestations of hepatitis, direct physiological effects of IFN-α, or a secondary depression. In our experience, depression associated with IFN-α is more severe and occurs with greater frequency than what is typically experienced by medically ill patients with similar degrees of functional impairment.

Neuropsychological and personality profiles in patients with leukemia or ALS treated with IFN-α (28,29) indicate delayed recall of verbal material, impaired speed and efficiency of cognitive processing, deficits in executive function, and personality and mood disturbances. Patients treated with IFN-α demonstrate electroencephalographic changes consisting of frontal slowing (with return to baseline following discontinuation) and shortened latencies for visual evoked potentials and brainstem auditory evoked potentials (30).

Few predictors for psychiatric adverse effects due to IFN-α therapy exist. Capuron and Ravaud (31) suggested that the magnitude of scores on a depression rating scale administered before initiation of IFN-α therapy predicted the intensity of depression in patients after 4 weeks IFN-α. However, previous reports do not concur with this finding, and an assessment period of longer than 4 weeks is necessary to adequately establish whether depressive symptoms occur in these patients (32). Pariante et al (33) suggested that patients with preexisting mood and anxiety disorders are no more likely to discontinue IFN-α therapy than patients without a history of psychiatric disorder. The NIH (19) study found that irritability and mood disturbances occurred with the highest incidence in patients who had relatively minor hepatitis, who received the highest dose (10 MIU) of IFN-α, and who lost weight during treatment. Delirium tended to occur in patients with severe hepatitis, previous brain dysfunction, or drug and alcohol abuse. One interesting caveat in this regard is that patients with a prior history of alcohol or substance abuse may develop an intense craving for alcohol and drugs, as well as symptoms of insomnia and anxiety late in the course of IFN-α therapy (18).

The neuropsychiatric toxicity associated with IFN-α therapy appears to be a function of dose, duration, and route of administration. In patients with chronic myelogenous leukemia (28), duration of treatment accounted for 55% of the variance in mood measures and neuropsychological test scores.

Clinical Management

As with IL-2 therapy, it is important to inform the patient and the family about the possible adverse effects of IFN-α, and to enlist their aid in early detection and management. It should be emphasized that, while IFN-α frequently causes psychiatric symptoms, they are usually of mild to moderate severity and resolve following treatment. Irritability and depression are the most common mood problems caused by IFN-α and often occur insidiously. In the case of HCV infection, the onset of these mood symptoms often occurs just as the patient's hepatitis is beginning to respond to therapy. Consequently, the clinician should inquire about subtle changes in mood, behavior, and cognition that may be overlooked in the context of overall medical improvement. When the irritability is moderate to severe and impacts on social functioning or is associated with poor impulse control, the IFN-α dose should be reduced if possible. Such reduction frequently leads to symptom alleviation within 48 to 72 hours. Careful monitoring is required as the irritability or agitation can persist.

Depression should be treated aggressively when it occurs. With severe depression, it is essential to reduce or stop the IFN-α. In this clinical situation, reassurance and watchful waiting, while important, are not sufficient. Janssen (34) reported two attempted suicides and one completed suicide in patients who became depressed during or shortly after the initiation of IFN-α therapy for chronic viral hepatitis. While antidepressants are commonly used for IFN-α–induced depression, there is little existing efficacy data. Case reports indicate success using fluoxetine and nortriptyline in IFN-α–treated patients with hepatitis C. SSRIs may be beneficial in the IFN-α–treated oncology population (17). In our experience, patients receiving IFN-α are somewhat less likely to respond to antidepressants than patients with primary depression. Nonetheless, first-line treatment is with an SSRI because these agents are safe and well-tolerated by medical patients. One recent double-blind, placebo-controlled study in 38 patients receiving high-dose IFN-α for malignant melanoma suggested that prophylactic use of the antidepressant paroxetine (Paxil) is effective in preventing IFN-α–induced depression. Confirmation of this finding would have significant implications for the preventive management of neuropsychiatric toxicity in vulnerable medical populations (35).

Hospitalization and reducing or stopping the IFN-α dose is mandatory for treatment of delirium. Neuroleptics should be used to treat the associated symptoms of agitation and attentional disturbances (36). Consistent with laboratory findings, an open-label pilot study (reviewed in 17) showed that the opiate antagonist naltrexone alleviated neurotoxic symptoms. Although one group reported using naltrexone most frequently for IFN-α–induced cognitive impairment, there was no documented improvement in any particular symptoms in the open-label study. Additionally, opiate-antagonist use was problematic in patients requiring pain control with opioid agents (17).

Occasionally, IFN-α must be discontinued because of irritability. For irritability, anecdotal reports indicate that methylphenidate is effective in reducing the number and severity of episodes (36). However, the stimulant properties of methylphenidate could lead instead to increased irritability, as is sometimes observed when treating major depressive disorder. Other agents that may be useful in treating irritability include SSRIs and the atypical neuroleptic risperidone (Risperdal). Risperidone has been used to treat pathologic irritability in a range of psychiatric disorders, including those occurring in hospitalized medical patients (37).

CONCLUSION

Cytokine therapy has become increasingly important in the treatment of a wide range of medical diseases. While such immunotherapy offers great therapeutic potential, its CNS toxicity frequently limits treatment. Improved awareness of the clinical presentation of IL-2 and IFN-α neurotoxicity can lead to appropriate diagnosis of these effects. The pathophysiology of cytokine-induced neuropsychiatric toxicity remains poorly understood, and there is a clinical need to identify those individuals most at risk for cytokine-induced CNS toxicity. Without reliable predictors of susceptibility to CNS toxicity to guide individual care, the high incidence of psychiatric morbidity associated with IL-2 and IFN-α treatment calls for controlled trials of psychotropic premedication in patients receiving cytokine therapy. Consultation psychiatrists play a large role in the care of patients receiving cytokines and should be involved early in management of neuropsychiatric complications.

REFERENCES

1. Hanisch U-K, Quirion R. Interleukin-2 as a neuroregulatory cytokine. *Brain Res Rev* 1996;21:246–284.
2. Rosenberg SA, Yang JC, Topalian SL, et al. Treatment of 283 consecutive patients with metastatic melanoma or renal cell cancer using high-dose bolus interleukin 2. *JAMA* 1994;71:907–913.
3. Saris SCPN, Rosenberg SA. The effect of intravenous interleukin-2 on brain water content. *J Neurosurg* 1989; 71:169–174.
4. Denicoff KD, Durkin TM, Lotze MT, et al. The neuroendocrine effects of interleukin-2 treatment. *J Clin Endocrinol Metab* 1989;69:402–410.
5. Vial T, Descotes J. Clinical toxicity of interleukin-2. *Drug Saf* 1992;7:417–433.
6. Kammula US, White DE, Rosenberg SA. Trends in the safety of high-dose bolus interleukin-2 administration in patients with metastatic cancer. *Cancer* 1998;83:797–805.
7. Palmer PA, Atzpodien J, Philip T, et al. A comparison of two modes of administration of recombinant interleukin-2: continuous intravenous infusion alone versus subcutaneous administration plus interferon-alpha in patients with advanced renal cell carcinoma. *Cancer Biother* 1993;8:123–135.
8. Denicoff KD, Rubinow DR, Papa MZ, et al. The neuropsychiatric effects of treatment with interleukin-2 and lymphokine-activated killer cells. *Ann Intern Med* 1987;107:293–300.
9. Karp BI, Yang YC, Khorsand M, et al. Multiple cerebral lesions complicating therapy with interleukin-2. *Neurology* 1996;47:417–424.

10. Pace A, Pietrangeli A, Bove L, et al. Neurotoxicity of antitumoral IL-2 therapy: evoked cognitive potentials and brain mapping. *Ital J Neurol Sci* 1994;15:341–346.
11. Meyers CA, Valentine AD. Neurological and psychiatric adverse effects of immunological therapy. *CNS Drugs* 1995;3:56–68.
12. Siphahimalani A, Masand PS. Use of risperidone in delirium. *Ann Clin Psychiatry* 1997;9:105–106.
13. Sipahimalani A, Masard PS. Olanzapine in the treatment of delirium. *Psychosomatics* 1998;39:422–430.
14. Triozzi PL, Kinney P, Rinehart JJ. Central nervous system toxicity of biological response modifiers. *Ann NY Acad Sci* 1990;594:347–354.
15. Licinio J, Kling MA, Hauser P. Cytokines and brain function: relevance to interferon-alpha–induced mood and cognitive changes. *Semin Oncol* 1998;25:30–38.
16. Blalock JE, Smith EM. Human leukocyte interferon: structural and biological relatedness to adrenocorticotrophic hormone and endorphins. *Proc Natl Acad Sci USA* 1980;77:5972–5974.
17. Valentine AD, Meyers CA, Kling MA, et al. Mood and cognitive side effects of interferon-α therapy. *Semin Oncol* 1998;25(suppl 1):39–47.
18. Adams ML, Cicero TJ. Alcohol intoxication and withdrawal: the role of nitric oxide. *Alcohol* 1998;16:153–158.
19. Renault PF, Hoofnagle JH, Park Y, et al. Psychiatric complications of long-term interferon-alpha therapy. *Arch Intern Med* 1987;147:1577–1580.
20. Vial T, Descotes J. Clinical toxicity of the interferons. *Drug Saf* 1994;10:115–150.
21. Pardo M, Marriott E, Moliner MC, et al. Risks and benefits of interferon-alpha in the treatment of hepatitis. *Drug Saf* 1995;13:304–316.
22. Lindsay KL, Davis GL, Schiff ER, et al. Response to higher doses of interferon-alpha$_{2b}$ in patients with chronic hepatitis C: a randomized multicenter trial. *Hepatology* 1996;24:1034–1040.
23. Caraceni A, Gangeri L, Martini C, et al. Neurotoxicity of interferon-α in melanoma therapy results from a randomized controlled trial. *Cancer* 1998;83:482–489.
24. Okanoue T, Sakamoto S, Itoh Y, et al. Side effects of high-dose interferon therapy for chronic hepatitis C. *J Hepatol* 1996;25:283–291.
25. Strite D, Valentine AD, Meyers CA. Manic episodes in two patients treated with interferon-alpha. *J Neuropsychiatry Clin Neurosci* 1997;9:273–276.
26. Monji A, Yoshida I, Tashiro K, et al. A case of persistent manic depressive illness induced by interferon-alpha in the treatment of chronic hepatitis C. *Psychosomatics* 1998;39:562–564.
27. Carpiniello B, Orru MG, Baita A, et al. Mania induced by withdrawal of treatment with interferon-alpha. *Arch Gen Psychiatry* 1998;55:88–89.
28. Pavol MA, Meyers CA, Rexer JL, et al. Pattern of neurobehavioral deficits associated with interferon-alpha therapy for leukemia. *Neurology* 1995;45:947–950.
29. Poutianien E, Hokkanen MLN, Farkkila M. Reversible cognitive decline during high-alpha interferon treatment. *Pharmacol Biochem Behav* 1994;47:901–904.
30. Forman AD. Neurologic complications of cytokine therapy. *Oncology* 1994;8:105–110.
31. Capuron L, Ravaud A. Prediction of the depressive effects of interferon-alpha by the patient's initial affective state. *N Engl J Med* 1999;340:1370–1370.
32. Rosenstein DL, Lerner D, Cai J. More on the depressive effects of interferon-alpha. *N Engl J Med* 1999;341: 849–850.
33. Pariante CM, Orru MG, Baita A, et al. Treatment with interferon-α in patients with chronic hepatitis and mood or anxiety disorders. *Lancet* 1999;354:131–132.
34. Janssen HLA, Brouwer JT, van der Mast RC, et al. Suicide associated with alpha-interferon therapy for chronic viral hepatitis. *J Hepatol* 1994;21:241–243.
35. Musselman DL, Lawson DH, Gummick JF, et al. Paroxetine for the prevention of depression induced by high dose interferon alpha. *N Engl J Med* 2001;344:961–966.
36. Renault PF, Hoofnagle JH. Side effects of alpha interferon. *Semin Liver Dis* 1989;9:273–277.
37. Lerner DM, Schuetz L, Holland S, et al. Low-dose risperidone for the irritable medically ill patient. *Psychosomatics* 2000;41:69–71.

Subject Index

Page numbers ending in *f* refer to figures. Page numbers ending in *t* refer to tables.